AIDS Treatment News
Issues 1 through 75

Issues 1 through 75
April 1986 through March 1989

AIDS
TREATMENT
NEWS

JOHN S. JAMES

CELESTIAL ARTS
Berkeley, California

The publisher assumes no liability for any injuries sustained in conjunction with use of any therapy, substance, protocol, or treatment described in this book. Individuals are cautioned that this material appears for informational use only, and the publisher advises that individuals seek professional medical counsel regarding any therapy described in this book.

CELESTIAL ARTS Publishing
Post Office Box 7327
Berkeley, California 94707

The author gratefully acknowledges that some of this material appeared, in somewhat different form, in *DAIR UPDATE* (published by the Documentation of AIDS Issues and Research Foundation, Inc.), in the *San Francisco Sentinel,* and in *Coming Up!/Bay Times.*

Cover design by Nancy Austin
Text design by Nancy Austin
Index by Ira Kleinberg
Editorial Consultation by Denny Smith
Composition by HMS Typography, Inc.
Production by Mary Ann Anderson

Library of Congress Cataloging-in-Publication Data

James, John S., 1941-
    AIDS treatment news : 1 through 75 / John S. James.
      p. cm.
    Includes bibliographies and index.
    ISBN 0-89087-553-7
    1. AIDS (Disease)—Treatment. 2. AIDS (Disease)— Alternative treatment. I. Title.
    RC607.A26J35 1989
    616.97 '9206—dc20   89-7399
                                                                CIP

First Printing, 1989

0 9 8 7 6 5 4 3 2 1

Manufactured in the United States of America

Contents

Statement of Purpose

AIDS Treatment News reports on experimental and complementary treatments, especially those available now. It collects information from medical journals, and from interviews with scientists, physicians, and other health practitioners, and from persons with AIDS or ARC.

Long-term survivors have usually tried many different treatments and found combinations that work for them. *AIDS Treatment News* does not recommend particular therapies, but seeks to increase the options available.

We also examine the ethical and public-policy issues around AIDS treatment research.

Annotated Contents

HIV CLINICAL CARE PROGRAM OPENED BY COLUMBIA UNIVERSITY STUDENT HEALTH SERVICES/278

NATIONWIDE AIDS DEMONSTRATIONS, APRIL 29-MAY 7/279

IMMUNOTOXIN TREATMENT FOR AIDS?/279

The Theory/280 * Proposed Treatment: An Immunotoxin/282

NEW MAI (MYCOBACTERIUM AVIUM INTRACELLULARE) TREATMENTS/282

Preface

HISTORY

AIDS Treatment News began in May 1986 as a biweekly column in the *San Francisco Sentinel*, a gay newspaper. The column appeared there for over two years; starting January 1989 it moved to a monthly San Francisco newspaper, *Bay Times/Coming Up!*. (The newsletter remains biweekly of course.)

This writer was first involved with AIDS in 1985, and went "shopping" for an organization which could use research and writing skills. Mobilization Against AIDS suggested the Documentation of AIDS Issues and Research Foundation (DAIR) in San Francisco. DAIR most wanted articles on experimental treatments, and suggested about a dozen for us to research. The first article that came together successfully happened to be about AL 721, and it was published in DAIR's newsletter in April 1986; the same article is also issue number 1 of *AIDS Treatment News*. (DAIR still publishes its newsletter, *DAIR Update*, and it also maintains an AIDS archive open to the public. For more information, call DAIR; see Appendix B for their phone number.)

Several months later there was so much demand for back issues that we started the newsletter. The first issue was in January 1987, but we republished the earlier columns as back issues.

This writer had no medical training, but had worked several years doing statistical computer programming for medical research projects, and also had some journalistic experience. (He is known in the computer field for a series of articles on then-little-known computer language called Forth, and also for developing a computer-communication program called The Conference Tree.)

How was *AIDS Treatment News* financed? In 1986, there was no prospect of funding for this work, because of our lack of credentials, and because of the disinterest and hostility toward treatments in the AIDS service community. "Beautiful death" ideas were strong in San Francisco, and treatment information was regarded as quackery, false hope which interfered with the process of accepting death. We realized that the newsletter would have to be self-financed, so we set a regular price in the low-to-middle range of professional newsletters, and a much lower PWA price; the latter was computed to cover the incremental cost of sending each issue (including labor), allowing circulation to expand indefinitely even at the low rate. Meanwhile the professional-rate subscriptions pay for research and overhead. We spent $10,000 starting *AIDS Treatment News*, not counting donation of our own time, but it could have been done for much less; for example, we were so concerned to get the material out that we did not send bills for eighteen months, but kept sending issues whether subscribers paid or not. Exposure in the *Sentinel* was crucial, however, as *AIDS Treatment News* has seldom advertised; it is hard to establish its credibility except by word of mouth, and the issues themselves are the most effective advertisements.

AIDS Treatment News is organized as a sole proprietorship—which any business is if it does not file papers to become something else. Recently we considered incorporating as a nonprofit, but the disadvantages outweighed the benefits. As a nonprofit we would in fact have become an organization specializing in raising money from corporations and foundations. Funding organizations have handled AIDS poorly, first ignoring it entirely and now flocking from theme to theme as each new idea gets its moment in the sun. We have succeeded in large part because we have answered only to our subscribers, avoiding the pressures which have shaped almost everything else in AIDS.

OPERATION TODAY

At this time the paid circulation is over 5,000. About two-thirds have paid the PWA rate, but we do not have exact figures, because for additional confidentiality protection we put no indication into our database of what rate subscribers chose. This policy causes bills to always have both the PWA and professional-rate options, no matter what the subscriber paid before. Of course we never give out the list, but we took this precaution so that in case a copy were stolen, it would have no information about the health status of subscribers.

Who works at *AIDS Treatment News*? Four people (including the publisher) work full time, and two work part time. Besides the publisher, the regular-hours staff consists of:

- Denny Smith—treatment information;
- Thom Fontaine—subscription services;
- Tim Wilson—office operations and marketing; and
- Debra Kelly—administrative support and special projects.
- Philippe Roques—computer operations and German/French translations.

Where do we get our information? Some people think that *AIDS Treatment News* must have inside connections, but in fact we have surprisingly little access to non-public information. We are press, and officials seldom tell us anything they are not telling the rest of the press.

Instead, we spend much time on the phone, and we usually first hear of a new treatment during a conversation about something else. Then we use online research databases for background information, so that we can interview experts intelligently; without access to computerized databases this newletter would have been impossible. Then we talk with physicians, patients, scientists, or anyone else with first-hand experience with the treatment, and write the article based on these conversations.

How do we decide what to publish? There is no simple answer. We try to avoid imposing medical ideas or biases of our own. Instead we look at the quality and credibility of information available. What has been published about a proposed treatment, and by whom? What are the reputations of the people behind it? What are their vested interests? What human experience is available? Has data been collected and assembled properly, and fully reported? Is there any independent confirmation? And if the information is correct, would it be useful to our readers?

THE FUTURE

We feel that it is our duty to continue to provide the kind of reporting our readers have come to expect.

Our main focus is treatment information. But we believe that community organizing and public-policy awareness are also essential for saving lives. For the treatments now available cannot guarantee survival, even for those who can pay for anything. Individual action alone is not enough; only community action can assure that research and access are not obstructed by red tape, mindless rules, and indifference.

AIDS Treatment News has focused on covering the most promising treatments rather than debunking others. There are several reasons for this practice:

- Readers want to hear about what is promising, not what isn't.

- For every treatment we do cover, there are ten others we would cover if only we had time. It takes as long to investigate a bad treatment as a good one, so we choose to focus on the latter.

- A debunking publication must spend considerable effort on legal preparation or defense. We could do so, but we would have to become a different kind of organization.

- We want to keep information channels open; therefore, we want people to be able to approach us without fear of being trashed, no matter how unconventional their ideas may be.

- We want to avoid the easy mistake of rejecting unfamiliar ideas prematurely.

On the other hand, times have changed. Two years ago so little was happening in AIDS treatment development that anything that moved was welcome. Now much is happening, so there is more concern that shallow but heavily promoted ideas can divert community attention and waste energy which is critically needed to address the real treatment issues.

On these and other matters, we want to hear from our readers. While we cannot answer all our mail, we always read it and consider it with respect.

Editor's Note

When John S. James published the first 50 issues of *AIDS Treatment News* in one bound volume, the demand for these back issues was immediate, indicating a heretofore-unmet need for public access to information about AIDS treatments, research, alternative approaches, and truthful reporting about the controversies and facts surrounding these issues.

This book, comprised of the first 75 issues, was conceived shortly after the appearance of the volume of 50 back issues. The author and the publisher felt that the information here needed to be widely accessible—at a substantially-reduced cost—and thus this collection of 75 issues was born in paperback book form.

The grassroots AIDS movement of patients and activists has been one of the remarkable achievements to emerge from the troubled times of the epidemic. These newsletters reflect both the dedication and heroism of the many men and women who have devoted time and energy in the ongoing search for answers to the serious challenges posed by AIDS.

ACCURACY OF INFORMATION

These newsletters are filled with referrals to names, addresses, phone numbers, and costs. In each instance, every effort was made to assure that the referral is up-to-date (as of July 1989). In nearly all cases, the referral address or phone number is listed in Appendix B at the back of the book, with a parenthetical notation in the text telling the reader to "see Appendix B." This has been done so that, in future printings of this book, we will be able to update regularly these names and addresses, without disturbing the presentation of the standard text itself.

But of course, addresses, contact persons, and so on change—often frequently in a rapidly-advancing field such as AIDS research. And so, even with our updatings, a name, number or address may no longer be viable. If you do have trouble reaching a referral, please contact *AIDS Treatment News* for help (see Appendix B for phone number).

In a very few instances, referrals have been deleted because of absolute certainty that the referral is no longer available or useful. Even in such cases, we have noted that we have done so, in the interests of presenting the most complete edition of these issues as possible, as well as in the interest of preserving the historical usefulness of this document.

HISTORICAL DOCUMENTATION

Readers should be aware that the editors regard these collected newsletters as not only a profound resource for patient information and advocacy, but also as an historical document, chronicling the immense issue of AIDS treatment research. For this reason we have preserved the newsletters nearly intact, including information that is updated pages later. Please understand that as you use this book, it is best to consult the index, referring to the latest entries as possible. Earlier entries provide necessary background for understanding the complexities of the issues, substances, and research.

For this reason—that we believe these newsletters constitute a remarkable chronicle of the history of AIDS treatment, AIDS activism, and the response of the community to the epidemic—much outdated material remains in this volume. Again, this is because these early newsletters represent more than an information resource; they represent a historical document of our times.

A NOTE ON EGG-LECITHIN-LIPIDS AND "AL 721"

Additionally, readers should note that "AL 721" is now a registered product name for the egg-lecithin-lipid substance manufactured by Ethigen Corporation. In these newsletters, the term "AL 721" refers generically to the entire spectrum of egg-lecithin-lipids as they were originally referred by the general community, not specifically to the product of Ethigen Corporation. We retain the "AL 721" terminology here for its fidelity to the historic development of alternative AIDS therapies. In later issues (beginning with issue number 70), the term "egg lecithin lipids" is used, reserving the term "AL 721" for the Ethigen product only. See page 427 for further clarification of this point.

HOW TO USE THIS BOOK

This book has been thoroughly indexed by Ira Kleinberg. Readers interested in specific treatments should first consult the index and consider their needs in doing so—do you wish to read the entire background and development of a treatment or therapy? Or are you most interested in the latest reports? Bearing these questions in mind will help you decide whether to read all entries for a treatment, or only the most recent.

FUTURE EDITIONS

The publisher plans to update this volume as necessary in subsequent printings and to collect future issues into a similar volume, should the need remain to do so. It is our plain hope that, shortly, such information will become completely obsolete and of no use whatsoever to anyone—because a good, effective therapy or cure has been found. Until that time, this book offers some practical guidance, information, and a call to activism.

—Paul Reed
August 1989
San Francisco

Introduction

by John S. James

OVERVIEW: AIDS Treatment Research and Public Policy—Yesterday and Today

A look through these 75 issues published during the last three years, from April 1986 to March 1989, shows that surprisingly few of the treatments covered have proven either effective or ineffective for treating AIDS during this time. The promising but unproven drugs of three years ago are still promising but unproven today. The research to test them just was not done. This slow pace of *practical treatment* research and development, and the lack of access by patients and physicians to treatments known to be valuable and sometimes lifesaving, reflects major public-policy failures in medical research—failures highlighted by the AIDS epidemic.

Only in the last year have these policy failures been addressed and acknowledged within the mainstream leadership of U.S. science, medicine, and government. And practices still in place guarantee years of delay before promising treatments visible today get to pharmacy shelves.

With the exception of AZT—a valuable drug but one with many drawbacks—the U.S. system was profoundly hostile to practical research on treatment options available now. And since U.S. institutions control most of the money, public and private, spent anywhere in the world on AIDS, they set many of the policies, rules, and standards of credibility which research anywhere must live with.

Many people today express surprise that two years after AZT, no comparable drug is available (and none is near approval). *AIDS Treatment News* is not surprised. For three years we have shown that research was being conducted in such a way that no successful outcome was possible. The problem was not that drugs failed, but that they were not tested. Very few potential treatments even reached the point of failure. The research which was done addressed questions with little relevance to stopping the epidemic—no matter how the answers came out.

Many observers have looked at the great successes in basic research on AIDS, such as investigations into the genetics of HIV, and concluded that "AIDS research" is therefore going well. But most of this high-tech basic science, which has indeed achieved impressive successes and may eventually lead to a cure, could not possibly produce practical treatments for many years—too late for those now ill.

The real logjam is in human testing of dozens of promising agents already in existence, many with extensive track records of safe human use, to learn whether and how they should be used—and in making available drugs already known to be helpful, including improved treatments for opportunistic infections. For many of the potential treatments discussed in *AIDS Treatment News*—treatments well supported by credible, published evidence—nothing whatever was done and we are no closer to answers today than we were last year or two years ago.

What went wrong?

Officially sanctioned drug development responded to commercial and institutional interests, not scientific, medical, or humanitarian concerns. It allowed professional, corporate regulatory, and political self-interest to eclipse the interests of patients. Until recently it closed itself off to input from persons with AIDS, and usually even from their physicians. This is why an "alternative" AIDS treatment movement developed in the first place.

And the alternative-treatment movement has done well. It does not, of course, have a cure for AIDS. No treatment yet known works for everybody; instead, people keep trying one relatively safe treatment possibility after another, abandoning those that fail for them and accumulating those that seem to work for them. AIDS is a complex disease, very different in different people; until we have a "magic bullet," or major advances in diagnosis, informed trial and error may remain the best way to select treatments for each individual.

In this desperate situation where there are no perfect answers, the alternative-treatment movement assembled a credible, useful menu of choices for people to try—in addition to, not in place of, AZT or other treatments which their physicians may prescribe.

What should be done now? We believe that *treatment advocacy* may be the most cost-effective way to save lives. Private AIDS organizations, as well as official bodies such as Congressional staffs, must build independent in-house expertise through long-term, committed work, day in and day out.

Other public issues—such as economic, environmental, legal, or foreign-policy concerns—have independent centers of expertise which can ask tough questions and insist that their issues be addressed. In AIDS treatment research, however, official statements from experts dependent on Federal grants were until recently simply swallowed whole. Legislators, reporters, AIDS activists, and others may have been suspicious, but without independent expertise they had no basis for sustained skeptical questioning.

AIDS treatment research and access issues were for years filled with horror stories which could never stand the light of day. Today some of these problems are being acknowledged and corrected. Many others remain.

BEGINNINGS OF REFORM

In the last year we have seen major improvements. Policy makers and researchers on one hand, and people with AIDS and their physicians on the other, are talking with each other. Impressive centers of expertise are developing in the AIDS advocacy movement. Problems are being acknowledged. Yet even in 1989 we are still following paths which guarantee thousands of unnecessary deaths.

One example will illustrate. Today the enlightened idea is to provide early, compassionate access to experimental treatments while clinical trials continue. This is a big improvement. Last year it was fashionable to deny patients access to experimental treatments, in the name of "science" (but only in the case of AIDS—cancer patients have long had such access, without having "science" invoked against them).

The new compassion is about drugs *all but known* to work, but not yet "proved" effective. This proof consists of prolonged, expensive, and therefore profitable scientific rituals—procedures never designed for an AIDS-type emergency, but which do work well for building entrenched constituencies of powerful vested interests. Years-long delays and tens of thousands of deaths have been accepted with little question in order to reprove what is already known. "Compassionate" treatment access while these rituals grind on will save some of these lives, but will never reach many others who need it.

No one disputes the legitimate need to learn more about any drug, to test long-term side effects before a new drug is widely distributed. But these concerns must be addressed directly, not held hostage to unrelated and ill-considered "efficacy" trials, designed to fit the requirements of academics and regulators, not to save the lives of patients.

Research rituals will continue until the national will to save lives becomes stronger than the inertia of business as usual. Only then will standards of knowledge appropriate to the emergency be accepted, and research directed accordingly toward practical questions, strategies, and goals.

We hope this book will contribute to public understanding of how opportunities have been lost in AIDS treatment development, and how past and present problems can be corrected. A humane, informed, and articulate public and professional consensus can save lives.

FROM THE PREFACE TO THE 1988 EDITION
OF COLLECTED BACK ISSUES

Readers may be bewildered by the mass of the information assembled here—especially since this volume collects dozens of newsletters, each intended to be read separately, and presents them chronologically, not reorganized by subject matter. Which information is most important today?

The author is neither a physician nor a scientist—so we try to avoid imposing our own ideas about which treatments are best. Instead we try to report community consensus among those informed about each particular treatment.

And besides treatments, we also report on public-policy issues. Here we have had to formulate our own views. For even the most grievous public-policy concerns on AIDS treatment and research often had no public opinion at all, let alone a consensus. The reason is that almost nobody had examined them or come to terms with them in any way, let alone formed an opinion or expressed one.

For both treatment and public-policy information, we recommend the latest issues as the most important.

These years of *AIDS Treatment News* include "sleepers" which have slipped by public awareness. Some of these articles originally appeared not as a newsletter, but in a free newspaper which seldom came to professional attention; we retrieved old word-processor files for this reprinting. Journalists, policy makers, and medical researchers, as well as persons with AIDS and their physicians, will find information here which they do not have, but should.

HOW TO USE THIS BOOK

AIDS Treatment News reprints 75 newsletters reporting from the front lines of the war against AIDS over a three-year period. Because AIDS information is changing so rapidly today—and also because this writer is not a physician—we emphasize that this book must *not* be taken as medical advice.

Instead, it provides a unique reference and background on many practical treatments which are likely to be in use for years to come—for AIDS and/or to treat other diseases or conditions.

It also provides an unvarnished history of public-policy failure in AIDS treatment research and development. This history, much of it not readily available elsewhere, gives a living context to the reform efforts now being discussed.

Potential activists and historians alike will find unique source material on the birth of the AIDS treatment movement—its three-year evolution from virtual nonexistence and being instantly dismissed, to involving tens of thousands of people and affecting the national agenda of the debates on drug-development and health-policy reform.

If you read this book straight through like a novel, you will encounter the oldest and least current material first. It is better to start with the index to find a particular treatment, person, organization, locality, or other entity of interest. Or start by browsing in the annotated table of contents, index, or the newsletters themselves. When you find anything of interest, the index can help you trace themes and stories backwards and forwards over the three-year period covered by this volume.

AIDS Treatment News is still being published as a biweekly newsletter. To receive the current issue free, together with information on how to subscribe, send a self-addressed stamped envelope to: *AIDS Treatment News*, P.O. Box 411256, San Francisco, CA 94141; or phone, 415-255-0588.

—John S. James
August 1989
San Francisco

Issue Number 1
April 11, 1986

AL 721: EXPERIMENTAL AIDS TREATMENT

Update 1989: We have left these articles unchanged, to preserve the historical context. Naturally, much treatment information has changed since they were published.

AL 721 is an unusual lipid mixture which acts differently from other drugs being tested against AIDS. It removes cholesterol from the outer membranes of cells and perhaps of viruses, increasing the fluidity of the membranes and apparently making it harder for viruses to attach to receptor sites, part of the process by which they infect the cell. Unlike most of the other drugs being tested, AL 721 appears to be entirely safe.

In human trials on elderly subjects, AL 721 restored immune functioning (lymphocyte proliferative capacity) which had been lost due to the normal aging process (Shinitzky and colleagues, cited by Sarin and colleagues, 1985). In recent laboratory tests at the U.S. National Cancer Institute and elsewhere, AL 721 greatly reduced infection of human cells by the AIDS virus (Sarin and colleagues, 1985). Apparently it can cross the blood-brain barrier: "Mixture 721 ('active lipid') was previously shown to be of practical use for membrane fluidization of brain tissue both in vitro and in vivo" (Lyte and Shinitzky, 1985).

However, AL 721 has not yet been given to persons with AIDS or any related condition, to our knowledge. Due to the history of disappointing drugs which looked good in the laboratory, we should avoid raising hopes prematurely, before a treatment has passed the key test of improving the condition of patients.

Background

AL 721 was developed several years ago at the Weizmann Institute of Science in Rehovot, Israel, by Meir Shinitzky and others. It is composed of three lipids, mixed in a ratio which has much more effect on cell membranes than other ratios tested. "AL" stands for "active lipid"; "721" is the ratio, 7:2:1, of the ingredients. Lyte and Shinitzky, 1985, tested the effects of different ratios on human lymphocyte and erythrocyte cells in the laboratory.

The three lipids are: (1) various neutral lipids, prepared by a published procedure, 70%; (2) phosphatidylcholine (purified lecithin), 20%; and (3) phosphatidylethanolamine, 10%. All three components were extracted from egg yolks. They were thoroughly mixed, using ultrasound. The procedure for making AL 721 has been published (Lyte and Shinitzky, 1985). AL 721 can be given either orally or by injection; in at least one animal study, injection was difficult but more effective (Heron and colleagues, 1982).

Researchers suspect that the "aqueous dispersion of this mixture consists of chylomicron-like assemblies where the neutral lipids provide the hydrophobic core on the surface of which phospholipids are spread as a monolayer" (Lyte and Shinitzky, 1985). Lecithin is the active ingredient, and the other components cause it to be applied effectively.

Clinical studies in France are testing AL 721 against cystic fibrosis in children (*Research* newsletter of the Weizmann Institute of Science, Rehovot, Israel, cited in UPI news story September 2, 1985). Laboratory and animal studies have suggested that AL 721 might also be useful against certain other viruses such as herpes (see AP News stories November 13 and 14, 1985), and other conditions including opiate and alcohol addiction (Heron and colleagues, 1982), and faulty neurotransmitter activity in the aging brain (*Research* newsletter). These different possibilities rest on the same mechanism: removing cholesterol, which normally increases with age, to restore fluidity (mobility of proteins) to the membranes. Researchers hope that this "membrane engineering" could eventually provide a whole new method of treatment for many conditions.

Safety

AL 721 appears to be safe. All three ingredients are contained in food. AL 721 has even been proposed as a dietary supplement for the elderly (*Research* newsletter).

In the trials on normal elderly patients mentioned above, each person took 10 to 15 grams of AL 721 orally per day for six weeks, with no adverse effects (Shinitzky, references above).

One possible concern for some patients is the hypothesis that decreasing, not increasing, membrane fluidity may be useful in treating some cancers. "Rigidification of membrane lipids may be of great potential for exposure of tumor-associated antigens, which may render tumor cells with specific immunogenicity. This approach can elicit antitumor immune reactivity both in vivo and in vitro" (Shinitzky, 1984, vol. 1 page 38).

Could Diet Help?

Could special diets provide some of the effect of AL 721?

Shinitzky discusses treatment possibilities in the "Towards Membrane Engineering" section of *Physiology of Membrane Fluidity,* Volume 1. "The obvious candidate for membrane fluidization both in vitro and in vivo is lecithin from natural sources (e.g. egg yolk)." But the efficacy depends on how the lecithin is presented to the membranes. The AL 721 mixture forms physical structures which transport the lecithin to the membranes effectively.

Heron and colleagues (1982) found that lecithin alone had some effect in increasing fluidity in mouse brain membranes, though much less than AL 721. Crude egg lecithin had a slightly greater effect than pure egg lecithin—possibly because the impurities included the other ingredients—although this difference was not statistically significant. (All three ingredients of AL 721 are contained in egg yolk.)

The same paper also mentioned a report published over fifty years ago that lecithin relieved morphine withdrawal symptoms in mice (Wen-Chao Ma, 1931)—an effect which would be expected from increased membrane fluidity.

Discussion in the same paper also suggests the possibility that AL 721 may do much better what lecithin has done all along. "Diets with a high lecithin content have been frequently recommended for a variety of disorders on the basis that they replenish choline" (Zeisel et al., 1980). However (data presented in the article) indicate that the previously proposed rationale for lecithin treatment covers only a minor aspect of this approach, and that treatment of deteriorated functions with AL could be much more effective in alleviating symptoms associated with lipid imbalances and in restoring the normal membrane lipid fluidity."

Other mysteries remain. In all the membrane fluidity work we have seen, the lecithin used was extracted from eggs; how would lecithin from other sources compare? We have not seen any study on whether egg yolk in diet could affect membrane fluidity. Also, we don't know of any work on how AL 721 passes through the digestive system; it would probably be digested into its components, suggesting that the special mixing of the ingredients might not be necessary.

In short, it might or might not be possible to produce some of the effect of AL 721 by diet, if AL 721 itself is not available. No one knows at this time.

Clinical Testing and Availability

As of mid January 1986, clinical tests of AL 721 against AIDS are being planned, but have not received final approvals. The first human trials will use only a handful of patients. We have heard that the earliest possible date that results of very limited clinical tests could be available is late spring.

Clinical trials are also being planned or carried out in Europe. We don't know if these are against AIDS.

AL 721 is licensed to Praxis Pharmaceuticals in Beverly Hills, California, and is manufactured by its subsidiary, Matrix Research Laboratories in New York. According to a report in a business publication dated September, 1985, Praxis believed that it would be at least four years before the FDA allows any commercial sale (Scrip, 1985). Naturally we expect that it would not take so long if AL 721 does show usefulness against AIDS.

We should continue to watch AL 721, along with the other proposed new treatments for AIDS. It is important that testing and availability not be blocked by bureaucratic inertia and red tape, especially when, as in this case, safety concerns are minimal. Drugs must be proven effective as well as safe before being released for general use; but here it seems that no one outside of a single company is in a position to take initiative to bring about formal testing, or even to find out whether timely and adequate studies are planned. Research and treatment for life-threatening illnesses must not be held up to suit the schedule of a handful of researchers or companies. Physicians must be able to participate in studies which place the welfare of their patients first.

For More Information

Shinitzky's 2-volume *Physiology of Membrane Fluidity* (reference below) gives extensive background information on the science behind AL 721. However, neither volume mentions AIDS.

The only published information we could find concerning AL 721 and AIDS is the letter to the *New England Journal of Medicine* by Sarin, Gallo and others (see below); wire-service reports which interviewed some of its authors (AP and UPI, November 13 and 14); a UPI report September 2 on the Weizmann Institute's newsletter *Research;* and a business report on Praxis Pharmaceuticals (*Scrip,* reference below).

The most recent scientific background on AL 721 is the article by Lyte and Shinitzky, 1985.

Acknowledgements

The author wishes to thank Dennis McShane, M.D., for reading and commenting on a draft of this article. All statements are of course the author's responsibility.

REFERENCES

Associated Press (Boston), "AIDS," November 13 and 14, 1985.

Heron, D., M. Shinitzky, and D. Samuel, "Alleviation of Drug Withdrawal Symptoms by Treatment with a Potent Mixture of Natural Lipids," *European Journal of Pharmacology* 83 (1982), pp. 253–61.

Lyte, M. and M. Shinitzky, "A Special Lipid Mixture for Membrane Fluidization," *Biochimica et Biophysica Acta* 812 (1985), pp. 133–8.

Ma, Wen-Chao, "A Cytopathological Study of Acute and Chronic Morphinism in the Albino Rat," *Chinese Journal of Physiology* 5 (1931), pp. 251–74.

Sarin, P.S., R.C. Gallo, D.I. Scheer, F. Crews, and A.S. Lippa, "Effects of a Novel Compound (AL 721) on HTLV-III Infectivity *In Vitro*," *New England Journal of Medicine* 313 (November 14, 1985), pp. 1289–90.

Scrip (ISSN 0143-7690), "Praxis' Offering Yields $3.7 M," *Scrip* 1032 (September 9, 1985), p. 8.

Shinitzky, M. (ed.), *Physiology of Membrane Fluidity,* Vols. 1 and 2, (Boca Raton, Florida: CRC Press, 1984).

Shinitzky, M., D. Samuel, L. Antonian, and A.S. Lippa, "AL 721, A Novel Membrane Fluidizer," *Drug Development Research* (in press).

United Press International (Boston), (November 14, 1985), "AIDS Drug."

United Press International. (London), (September 2, 1985), "Eggs."

Issue Number 2
April 25, 1986

AIDS/ARC TREATMENT: A ROLE FOR LECITHIN?

Two separate bodies of medical research suggest that lecithin may be helpful in the treatment of AIDS or ARC.

The first information comes from the development of AL 721, now being tested as an experimental treatment against AIDS in drug trials. AL 721 has been shown to reduce AIDS virus infection of human T-cells in the laboratory (Sarin *et al.*, *New England Journal of Medicine*, November 14, 1985). It works by changing the cell membrane so that the virus cannot attach itself to receptor sites, and therefore cannot infect the cell.

The active ingredient of AL 721 is lecithin; the rest of the mixture apparently makes the delivery of the lecithin more effective. Much evidence suggests that ordinary lecithin can produce the same "membrane fluidization" effect, which is believed to be the basis of the antiviral action of AL 721, though probably to a lesser degree.

Unfortunately, AL 721 is tied up in the corporate and regulatory red tape of new-drug approval. Doctors and patients cannot get it, and they may not be able to get it for years. Lecithin could be tried now, at least as a stopgap until AL 721 becomes available.

Meanwhile, different research teams have found purified lecithin useful in the treatment of viral hepatitis. A computer literature search turned up four clinical papers; three of them are not readily accessible, and therefore easily overlooked. All four papers reported controlled studies which found strong evidence of effectiveness, and definitely recommended the treatment. Since the antiviral effect of AL 721 is not believed to be specific to AIDS, the hepatitis results may demonstrate a practical clinical use of the same effect shown to prevent AIDS infection of cells in the laboratory.

No published work so far has discussed lecithin and AIDS. A Medline computer search found over 3800 papers concerning AIDS, and over 4100 concerning phosphatidylcholines (lecithin and related substances), but only a single item which discussed both—the AL 721 letter cited above.

While the information collected here cannot prove whether or not lecithin could be useful in the treatment of AIDS or ARC, it certainly suggests that lecithin be tried—especially since it is safe, inexpensive, and readily available.

AL 721 Background

AL 721 is an experimental AIDS treatment derived from lecithin. It was developed from several years' research on "membrane fluidity" by dozens of scientists, work spearheaded by Meir Shinitzky, an immunologist doing cancer research at the Weizmann Institute of Science in Israel. AL 721 is known to be safe for human use, and is known to reduce AIDS infection in laboratory cultures, as mentioned above. Unfortunately, clinical tests have barely begun and no results are yet available, so we have no direct evidence one way or the other on whether AL 721 will prove useful in the treatment of AIDS or ARC.

AL 721 is a mixture of three lipids (fats), in a 7:2:1 ratio; hence the name (the "AL" stands for "active lipid"). The three ingredients are phosphatidylcholine (purified lecithin—called "PC" in this article—which makes up 20 percent of AL 721), phosphatidylethanolamine (PE—10 percent—a related substance also contained in commercial lecithin preparations), and neutral lipids which apparently serve as a carrier to present the active ingredients to the cell membrane more effectively. The particular 7:2:1 ratio proved to be the most effective proportion.

All of the ingredients of AL 721 are extracted from ordinary egg yolks.

AL 721 increases the "fluidity" of cell membranes—the degree to which proteins can move around. It does this by removing cholesterol and increasing the ratio of phospholipids (lecithin and related compounds) to cholesterol in the membrane. Increasing the fluidity apparently makes it harder for viruses to attach to receptor sites, which are proteins in the membrane. Unless it can attach to a receptor site, the virus cannot enter and infect the cell.

Incidentally, membrane fluidity decreases with age; and AL 721 has been found to restore certain functions lost with aging. Since increased fluidity should make it harder for the AIDS virus to infect the cell, this theory would predict that susceptibility to AIDS might increase with age.

AL 721 does cross the blood-brain barrier.

AL 721 and Lecithin

A number of published articles outline the science behind AL 721. These papers contain fragmentary but extensive indications that lecithin has the same membrane fluidization effect as AL 721, although to a smaller degree.

No one has collected and organized this evidence; the scientists working with AL 721 have, not surprisingly, sought to highlight how that preparation is special. Instead of marshaling the information here, which would turn this short section into a separate paper, we refer the reader to papers by Shinitzky, Lyte, Heron, and the co-authors who appear with them in the References section, below. Also see *Physiology of Membrane Fluidity,* edited by Shinitzky, for a thorough presentation of the scientific background behind the membrane fluidity theory and the development of AL 721.

The prospectus of Praxis Pharmaceuticals, Inc., of Beverly Hills, California (the licensee and commercial developer of AL 721), provides other information about this preparation and its relationship to lecithin. In human trials, AL 721 has been shown to restore immune function (lymphocyte proliferative capacity) lost due to the aging process; the restored immune functions were comparable to those of young adults. Animal studies have shown that AL 721 may also be useful for treating alcohol and morphine withdrawal, and to prevent relapses in the treatment of dependency on these drugs. Both these effects are believed due to membrane fluidization. AL 721 also shows promise for treating cystic fibrosis in children, but through a different mode of action.

The prospectus also suggests AL 721 as "a more efficient source of lecithin" for treating bipolar affective disorder, compared to soybean-derived lecithin, which earlier studies had shown might be effective for this condition.

And aside from these therapeutic uses, "AL is a relatively pure form of lecithin derived from egg yolk and may be used as a nutritional supplement."

Previous Lecithin Therapy

We have examined dozens of abstracts from nearly 200 studies of lecithin administration or therapy published in medical journals during the last ten years. Most of these studies were based on very different theories of lecithin's mode of action. They used the substance either to increase the amount of choline in the brain, or to reduce fat deposits in blood vessels. For a review of these studies, see Wood and Allison, 1982.

Conspicuously absent from almost all work so far have been studies of lecithin to help the body fight viral diseases. Until the AL 721 study published last November (cited above), there was little or no reason to look for an antiviral effect.

Lecithin and Viral Hepatitis

Our literature search found four papers on use of lecithin or related substances to treat hepatitis.

Jenkins and others, 1982, reported a double-blind trial on 30 patients with non-A non-B hepatitis. This study compared 15 patients given three grams per day of polyunsaturated phosphatidylcholine ("Essential Phospholipid", Nattermann & Cie, Germany) for one year with those given a placebo; all patients simultaneously received other hepatitis therapy. The study concluded that the phosphatidylcholine definitely helped in the treatment of this condition. In addition, two of the controls but none of the treatment group suffered relapses during the study.

This paper did not consider the possibility of an antiviral effect, but suggested prevention of autoimmune damage as a possible mode of action. It did mention the membrane fluidity work, but no antiviral effects of increased membrane fluidity were expected at that time.

Atoba et al., 1985, in a study in Nigeria, used matched treatment and control groups, each with 30 patients with acute hepatitis B. The treatment group used 1.8 grams of "essential phospholipid choline", and the control group used vitamin-B complex. The treatment group showed faster improvement on almost all measurements. For example, the initial bilirubin and transaminases were comparable for both groups, but after four weeks, 77 percent of the treatment but only 37 percent of the control patients showed normal serum transaminase levels. After six weeks, 93 percent of the treated patients but only 53 percent of the controls had normal levels of both bilirubin and transaminase.

This study was not double blind, as the patients had to buy their own drugs. Cost was a problem, and may have contributed to the decision to use the smaller dose; Jenkins and others, who used three grams, mentioned that they had done a pilot study in which 1.8 grams had proved effective.

(Incidentally, it is difficult to find the Atoba paper, as it was published in an Indian journal received by only four medical libraries in the United States. Copies can be obtained through a commercial research service.)

Kosina *et al.*, 1981, found improvements in clinical signs, laboratory tests, and number of relapses in 80 patients with hepatitis A or B, compared to controls. This study used "essential cholinephospholipids (Essentiale forte)"; we don't know the dose. The paper is in Czech and we have read only an English abstract; we would appreciate any help with translation.

We have read only the English summary of Visco, 1985. This Italian study reported successful treatment of viral hepatitis with phosphatidylcholine, in a controlled trial.

How is the potential usefulness of lecithin against viral hepatitis relevant to AIDS? The membrane fluidity theory is not specific to the AIDS virus—the theory just happened to be tried first against it in the laboratory. It is quite possible that membrane fluidization is the mechanism of action of lecithin in these hepatitis trials. If so, it would show that oral lecithin can produce in the body an effect already found to prevent infection by the AIDS virus in the laboratory—an effect clinically useful against another virus disease.

Even if the effect of lecithin against hepatitis is not due to any antiviral action but rather to the prevention of autoimmune damage, as some of the authors of the papers suggested, there might still be a use against AIDS. A number of researchers suspect that AIDS has an autoimmune component.

Dosage and Side Effects

As lecithin has yet to be studied as a treatment for AIDS or ARC, we can only review dosage levels used to treat other conditions. Fortunately, the doses used in the hepatitis studies turn out to be within the range which has long been recommended by the manufacturers of the lecithin granules which have been sold in health-food stores for years.

Jenkins *et al.*, 1982, used three grams of phosphatidylcholine per day. Most commercial lecithin granules contain about 22 percent PC, so three grams is equivalent in PC content to about 14 grams of the granules. This amount happens to be about the same as the two-tablespoon maximum daily dose traditionally recommended by commercial vendors of lecithin granules.

Some studies have used higher doses, as much as 100 grams per day of commercial lecithin. These high doses produced unwanted side effects, such as nausea, diarrhea, depression, and loss of appetite, but apparently no lasting ill effects. Therapists giving high doses of lecithin should monitor the patients, particularly for depression (Wood and Allison, 1982).

Most patients could tolerate up to 25 grams of commercial lecithin per day without side effects. Also, most patients could tolerate up to 40 grams of purified (85 percent) PC, meaning that several times as much PC can be administered in the purified form.

On the other hand, a very small dose would probably be ineffective, because many foods already supply lecithin; adding only a little more would not change much. The amount of lecithin supplied by food varies with diet, but is in the range of one to five grams per day (Wood and Allison, 1982).

Ultimately the only way to determine a dose might be by trial. If T-cell counts are being monitored, they might be the first place to look for an effect, since membrane fluidization (with AL 721) was found to prevent the infection of human T-cells in the laboratory. For those who don't wait for a scientific trial, which might or might not take place, the obvious approaches would be to try the maximum dose recommended for the product (equivalent to the dose used in the Jenkins hepatitis study), or to try larger doses to see what seemed to work.

Lecithin is classified as GRAS (generally recognized as safe). In the Medline database since 1980, out of over 4000 references concerning phosphatidylcholines, only five concerned adverse effects. Still, we should note possible problems. Long-term feeding of large doses to pregnant animals has interfered with the development of the fetus (Bell and Lundberg, 1985). And one study of commercial lecithin preparations found that all of the ones tested were contaminated with potentially dangerous methylamines, probably from spoilage (Zeisel *et al.*, 1983). It would seem reasonable to store lecithin properly, refrigerated in small bottles, to keep it away from moisture, light, and air, and to discard any with a rancid taste or smell.

An alternative source of lecithin is egg yolk. Egg yolk contains all the ingredients of AL 721. It also contains much cholesterol, which might counteract the effect of AL 721; we don't know whether or not this would be a practical problem, and would appreciate advice from nutritionists.

There are slight chemical differences between the PC in egg yolk, and the PC in soy lecithin (the kind sold in health-food stores). We don't know whether or not this difference has any practical effect. The scientific work which developed AL 721 used egg lecithin, while most other studies of lecithin therapy used the soybean variety.

Summary

The published information collected here suggests that lecithin might be useful in the treatment of AIDS or ARC. This possibility seems to have been overlooked; a computer literature search turned up no papers which discussed it.

We hope that researchers will examine this information, and run clinical tests if justified. There is little danger of harm, and some chance of benefit.

REFERENCES

Atoba, M.A., E.A. Ayoola, O.Ogunseyinde, "Effect of Essential Phospholipid Choline on the Course of Acute Hepatitis-B Infection," *Tropical Gastroenterology* 6(2) (April–June, 1985), pp. 96–9.

Bell, J.M. and P.K. Lundberg, "Effects of Commercial Soy Lecithin Preparation of Development of Sensorimotor Behavior and Brain Biochemistry in the Rat," *Developmental Psychobiology* 18(1) (1985), pp. 59–66.

Heron, D., M. Shinitzky, and D. Samuel, "Alleviation of Drug Withdrawal Symptoms by Treatment with a Potent Mixture of Natural Lipids," *European Journal of Pharmacology* 83 (1982), pp. 252–61.

Jenkins, P.J., B.P. Portmann, A.L.W.F. Eddleston, and R. Williams, "Use of Polyunsaturated Phosphatidyl Choline in HBsAg Negative Chronic Active Hepatitis: Results of Prospective Double-blind Controlled Trial," *Liver* 2 (1982), pp. 77-81.

Kosina, F., K. Budka, Z. Kolouch, D. Lazarova, and D. Truksova, "Essential Cholinephospholipids in the Treatment of Virus Hepatitis," (English translation of title), *Casopis Lekaru Ceskych* 120(31-32) (August 13, 1981), pp. 957-60.

Lyte, M. and M. Shinitzky, "A Special Lipid Mixture for Membrane Fluidization," *Biochimica Et Biophysica Acta* 812 (1985), pp. 133-8.

Praxis Pharmaceuticals, Inc., "Prospectus," (January 17, 1985).

Sarin, P.S., R.C. Gallo, D.I. Scheer, F. Crews, and A.S. Lippa, "Effects of a Novel Compound (AL 721) on HTLV-III Infectivity *In Vitro*," *New England Journal of Medicine* 313(20) (November 14, 1985), pp. 1289-90.

Shinitzky, M. (ed.), *Physiology of Membrane Fluidity*, Vols. 1 and 2, (Boca Raton, Florida: CRC Press, 1984).

Shinitzky M., D. Samuel, L. Antonian, and A.S. Lippa, "AL 721, A Novel Membrane Fluidizer," *Drug Development Research* (in press).

Visco, G., "Polyunsaturated Phosphatidylcholine in Association with Vitamin B Complex in the Treatment of Acute Viral Hepatitis B. Results of a Randomized Double-blind Study," (English translation of title), *Clinica Terapeutica* 114(3) (August 15, 1985), pp. 183-8.

Wire-service reports on Al 721: UPI, (September 2, 1985 and November 14, 1985); AP, (November 13, 1985 and November 14, 1985).

Wood, J.L. and R.G. Allison, "Effects of Consumption of Choline and Lecithin on Neurological and Cardiovascular Systems," *Federation Proceedings* 41 (1982), pp. 3015-21.

Zeisel, S.H., J.S. Wishnok, and J.K. Blusztajn, "Formation of Methylamines from Ingested Choline and Lecithin," *Journal of Pharmacology and Experimental Therapeutics* 225(2) (1983), pp. 320-4.

Issue Number 3
May 9, 1986

WHAT'S WRONG WITH AIDS TREATMENT RESEARCH?

Any review of AIDS research must distinguish between the basic science studying the biology of the disease, and the applied work to develop practical treatments and make them available to patients.

The basic research has performed very well, compared to the time required to understand diseases in the past. This scientific success, however, does not reflect competent Federal management or public policy. Instead, the scientific achievements have stemmed from the great progress in biology in the last two decades—and from the dedication and sacrifices of individual scientists who for years managed to carry on their work without proper support.

While public policy for basic research has been merely poor, that for treatment development has been abysmal, amounting to a system of human sacrifice which could hardly be worse even if deliberately designed to have people die. Community organizations must develop independent expertise on treatments, which they have not done so far. To rely solely on official institutions for our information is a form of group suicide.

Here are some examples. The first one concerns the most promising treatment now under development:

(1) Azidothymidine (AZT). The general public, and even most AIDS organizations and activists, do not yet realize that we already have an effective, inexpensive, and probably safe treatment for AIDS.

The scientific and newspaper reports on AZT have been buried in an avalanche of other AIDS stories. The press, evidently advised not to raise "false hopes," has reported the news but not highlighted its importance. As a result, doctors do not need to deal with the anger of persons who know they are being left to die unnecessarily. And public officials do not need to deal with political demands for a change.

In the only published clinical study of AZT (*Lancet,* March 15, 1986), 19 subjects with AIDS or ARC gained an average of five pounds each during a six to eight week course of treatment. Fifteen of the 19 showed increases in the number of helper T-cells. Other improvements included two cases of nailbed fungus infections which cleared up with no anti-fungal treatment, six patients who developed normal skin-test reactions when they had none before, and six who had an end to night sweats or a greatly improved sense of well-being. At the highest doses tested, AIDS virus disappeared from the blood. Only KS did not improve, perhaps because the treatment was not continued long enough, or because specific treatment for KS may be needed in addition. Side effects were minor.

Eleven of these 19 patients had AIDS—six with pneumocystis, four with KS, and one with both. One of the most important results of this study is that it showed that the immune system can re-build itself if the virus is stopped, contrary to what many doctors had believed. It is not necessary to write off persons who have already developed AIDS.

AZT does cross the blood-brain barrier.

The drug is not a cure. It will probably have to be taken indefinitely, and we don't yet have proof of long-term safety or effectiveness. The study did report on the condition of the patients later, four to eight months after entry to the study; except for one who was taken off the study due to advancing KS and who later died, they were generally in good shape, although two cases of pneumocystis, and some other opportunistic infections, developed several months after the patients had been taken off AZT.

So what's happening now? The study ended with the conclusion that long-term, controlled studies would be needed. Yet during the several months which have elapsed since the benefits of AZT were known, very little clinical work has been done. Large-scale studies are at least two more months away. If all goes well, your doctor might be able to get AZT in about two years.

Of course there are risks in using a drug before the effects of long-term use are known. There are also long-term risks from untreated AIDS.

We should point out that ten thousand people are expected to die of AIDS in the next year. And with deaths doubling every year, a little math shows that a two-year delay between when a treatment is known to work and when it becomes available means that three quarters of the deaths which ever occur from the epidemic will have been preventable.

Incidentally, a biochemist can easily make AZT. The only reason it's not already available through a grey market is that people don't yet understand its importance.

(2)   AL 721. AZT represents a shining public-policy success compared to what has happened with AL 721.

AL 721 has been around for years and is known to be safe for humans. And at least since November 1985, it has been known to prevent the AIDS virus from infecting human T-cells in the laboratory. But it still hasn't been tested on any person with AIDS or ARC, to our knowledge; there are rumors that secret tests, with only a handful of patients, may have started in April 1986.

AL 721 is composed entirely of substances found in ordinary egg yolk. As such, it could legally have been sold as a food supplement—not as an AIDS medicine, but in fact made available to patients immediately.

Instead, its licensee, Praxis Pharmaceuticals of Beverly Hills, California, treated AL 721 as a high-tech AIDS drug, using it last year to raise 3.7 million dollars in the stock market. The company itself predicted that it would be at least four years before the FDA approved any commercial sale.

Thus one of the most promising treatment leads available was lost to years of red tape. It's hard to get investors to put millions into a food supplement.

Praxis has cloaked its AL 721 work in secrecy. We don't know how well they're handling it, but what is known isn't encouraging. Meanwhile, the licensing forms a legal barrier which prevents anyone else from touching AL 721.

Would a promising treatment be handled this way in any other deadly epidemic?

(3) A little arithmetic shows that an AIDS cure will be much more profitable in a few years than it would be now. In fact, today it would cause a big loss to the company which developed it. There is no commercial incentive to develop an AIDS cure too early.

Today it costs at least 50 million dollars to get a new drug through all the testing required for Federal approval. Divide 50 million by the ten thousand people in the U.S. who now have AIDS, and you can see that a company would have to make five thousand dollars clear profit on each person just to pay off its development expenses—not including interest, insurance, and costs of operation.

But in a few years, the picture will change dramatically. With cases doubling every year, we will have a ten-fold increase within four years. That's ten times the potential profit.

Of course it would look bad for a company to hold up an AIDS treatment just to make money. Here the Federal bureaucracy provides a service to industry, withholding new-drug approval and forcing the private company to take the profitable path.

Of course the government shouldn't look bad, either. So under the spotlight of publicity it makes the right decisions. For example, the FDA approved testing of HPA-23, no longer one of the most promising treatments but the one Rock Hudson went to Paris to receive, in an unheard-of five days.

(4) Doctors genuinely care what happens to their patients. But doctors don't rock the boat. Very few will speak out or otherwise step out of the context which the larger system has given to them.

Doctors seldom initiate treatment trials. Even at the leading AIDS hospitals, doctors run trials when drug companies bring them something to test, not before. This fact is important because, as we have seen, drug companies have very different incentives than doctors in this matter.

It's also important because it virtually guarantees that a treatment which cannot be patented or licensed exclusively to some company—such as preventing ARC from developing into AIDS by eliminating suspected cofactors—will not be tested seriously.

(5) What can be done? Plenty.

The most important thing we can do is to build awareness—within AIDS organizations, within the high-risk communities, and among the general public—of what is going on and where the problems are. So far, community-based AIDS organizations have been uninvolved in treatment issues, and have seldom followed what is going on. No wonder the gay community and the general public don't know, either.

With independent information and analysis, we can bring specific pressure to bear to get experimental treatments handled properly. So far, there has been little pressure because we have relied on experts to interpret for us what is going on. They tell us what will not rock the boat. The companies who want their profits, the bureaucrats who want their turf, and the doctors who want to avoid making waves have all been at the table. The persons with AIDS who want their lives must be there, too.

Organizations with treatment expertise can find out exactly where the delays are. They can analyze the current plans to centralize Federal AIDS research. They can identify and publicize important leads which have been dropped. They can expose gross mis-allocation of funds, such as attempts to inject homophobia, racism, or other political hobby horses into AIDS research policy. When black markets develop, they can receive samples and have them tested by reputable laboratories, to protect people against fraudulent or inferior products. We have not had this kind of advocacy so far, and we have suffered for it.

We must of course talk with everyone, cooperate with everyone, be willing to work together. But no longer can we rely entirely on government-sponsored organizations or on the medical-industrial complex for our understanding of what is happening with treatment research and development. The people there may have their hearts in the right place, but they must follow the dictates of a system which fails to follow up opportunities, does not make saving lives a high priority, and is not always directed in good faith.

Issue Number 4
May 23, 1986

PROBLEM WITH AZT?

Our last column summarized the only published report so far of clinical tests with the experimental drug azidothymidine. This early trial brought clear benefits and few side effects to the 19 patients in the study group.

Later we heard anecdotal reports that several patients in later trials in two cities (not including San Francisco) developed pancytopenia, a serious bone-marrow disease. We called Burroughs-Wellcome Corporation, which is developing AZT; they told us that there have been some changes in hematological measurements in both phase 1 and phase 2 tests, but that sometimes these changes occur in persons with AIDS without any therapy, so more study is necessary before we can draw conclusions.

We will have to wait for more information. Meanwhile, here are some points to consider about all clinical tests on experimental drugs, not only AZT.

First, this writer and many others have been urging faster action on the development of new treatments. Often there is a trade-off between speed and risk; for example, researchers could reduce the risks of side effects by scheduling months or years of animal tests before any human trials begin. But persons with AIDS should have the right to make their own decisions about accepting the risks of trying new treatments, instead of being given a flat "No". And everyone benefits when treatment research moves quickly ahead. For these reasons, we should not criticize but commend researchers and physicians who make decisions which are right at the time, even if wrong in hindsight—which balance the risks of doing something against the risks of doing nothing. They are taking a personal risk when they could so easily cover themselves by refusing to do clinical trials until exhaustive preliminaries had been completed.

Also, we should make sure that no treatment gets lost unnecessarily, even effects occur. For example, AZT worked very well in at least one clinical trial (p in *Lancet*, March 15, 1986). Problems discovered in other trials may be m For example, side effects could be dose-related; the published results of this possibility, as the higher doses tested sometimes produced a B-c though never a serious one. Perhaps it will prove possible to predict who will react adversely to a drug, or to monitor blood tests in order to catch problems in time. Side effects can even result from impurities in experimental drugs, which are not regularly manufactured but often made up in a new batch for each study, by scientists who have probably never prepared that substance in pharmaceutical purity before. And even if it's not possible to avoid a danger, the benefit of the treatment may outweigh it.

Unfortunately, research institutions which conduct a test which fails due to side effects may never find it in their interest to publish or announce the results, due to fear of legal liability or other reasons. If they don't publish, other clinicians who have heard of the problems but don't have the details won't dare to try the drug again, and a useful treatment which might be safe if used differently will be lost. Sometimes we may have to insist that when persons have risked their lives in drug trials, the public has at least a moral right to have the results published so that they can help other scientists and doctors to save lives in the future.

FDA MAY TRY TO RESTRICT VITAMINS—AGAIN

Ten years ago the U.S. Food and Drug Administration tried to regulate vitamins as drugs if they contained more than one and a half times the recommended daily allowance. All but the smallest doses of vitamin C, for example, could have been banned from over-the-counter sale.

That proposal touched off one of the most massive public outcries in history. Not only did the FDA have to kill its plan, but an act of Congress prohibited the agency from regulating food substances like drugs in the future, unless it could prove that they were dangerous.

Earlier this month the FDA, working with the American Dietetic Association and with support from the American Dairy Board, set into motion a sophisticated plan which could lead to new restrictions on food supplements. While not directed against treatments for AIDS, resulting new rules might affect or even ban a number of "alternative" therapies.

So far, all that's happened is that the FDA has warned that Americans might be poisoning themselves, and asked physicians to voluntarily report any suspected adverse effects of vitamin overdose, on the same form already used to report side effects of drugs. No one has objected to collecting such information, which could be used legitimately to warn vitamin users and doctors about any dangers. The health-food industry has been complacent, apparently expecting the data to vindicate its claim that vitamins and other food supplements are safe.

The problem is that asking all the doctors in the country to report suspected bad effects of supplements, and only the bad effects, will produce such masses of data and more than enough horror stories to fill any number of Congressional hearings. No one else could do so, even if the vitamins were innocent. The FDA will collect the stories and use them at the times and places of its own choosing. And patient confidentiality will probably prevent independent

Then Congress will have the choice to let babies be poisoned, etc., or to do something. And if Congress does act, it will most likely grant broad regulatory authority, instead of narrow powers which would have to be re-legislated every year as situations changed. In this way the FDA will satisfy that driving hunger which is the ultimate motivation of any active bureaucracy—the relentless quest for more power.

What can we do? It's hard to protest, because so far there's nothing to protest against. If horror stories do get used, it will be hard to protest without appearing heartless. The plan is a masterpiece of strategy for taking away peoples' power over their own lives, and putting that power into the hands of a medical establishment which is not only expensive, but usually unwilling to run the legal risks of trying alternative treatments at any price.

One thing we can do is to make sure that people know what's going on. And we can raise the question of whether we are a nation of people who make their own decisions, using warnings and advice from the experts, or whether a committee of experts should decide what's best for you, and use police powers to enforce your compliance.

Issue Number 5
June 6, 1986

DANGER IN HYDROCORTISONE

Update 1988: We have not heard any news about hydrocortisone in some time. But the current consensus seems to be that small amounts used externally in ointments can be okay, when recommended by a physician.

Scientists are using hydrocortisone to stimulate the growth of the AIDS virus in the laboratory. They have published a warning that the drug may be harmful to HTLV-III positive persons. But the warning has failed to reach physicians, their patients, and support organizations.

Hydrocortisone, a steroid used to reduce inflammation, is sold over-the-counter in skin ointments. Doctors can prescribe larger doses, which can be given by injection. People should be on guard about prescribed use of hydrocortisone.

The warning appears in the paper, "Hydrocortisone and some other hormones enhance the expression of HTLV-III", by Markham, Salahuddin, Veren, Orndorff, and Gallo, published in the *International Journal of Cancer,* January 15, 1986. The researchers needed to grow the virus in order to develop a more effective test for it. Hydrocortisone significantly increased the ability of the virus to infect human blood cells. Some other steroids also helped the AIDS virus (but to a smaller extent), and others had no effect.

The paper cites earlier studies in which similar steroids caused an increase in opportunistic infections and cancer.

There may be times when hydrocortisone can be justified even for persons exposed to the virus. Physicians must decide case by case. But it's important that the risk be known and that people think at least twice before using the drug at this time.

HELP FROM GAMMA GLOBULIN

A new paper from the Albert Einstein College of Medicine reports important benefits from gamma globulin treatment of children with AIDS. An earlier study by the same group had already found the treatment clearly valuable for adults with pneumocystis.

Gamma globulin, a normal component of human blood, contains antibodies produced by the immune system. Doctors have routinely used it for years as a temporary boost for persons with certain immune-system deficiency (other than AIDS), or to prevent a contagious disease from developing after a normal person has been exposed to it. In the work reported here, gamma globulin was used to prevent or treat secondary infections, not the underlying AIDS itself.

During the three years of the latest study, most of the children in the control group deteriorated or died, while there were no deaths in the gamma-globulin treatment group. Since the study, however, eight of the fourteen children who received the treatment have died. We don't know whether or not the gamma globulin had been discontinued.

Helper T-cell counts improved in 42 percent of the treatment group, compared to seven percent of the controls. There were far fewer cases of fever and of serious blood infections in the treatment group.

A new study will test hyperimmune globulin, which contains AIDS antibodies and might be more effective.

For more information, see the paper by Rubinstein and Calvelli in the May/June 1986 issue of *Pediatric Infectious Diseases.*

The earlier study (Silverman and Rubinstein, "Serum lactate dehydrogenase levels in adults and children with acquired immune deficiency syndrome (AIDS) and AIDS-related complex: possible indicator of B cell lymphoproliferation and disease activity; Effect of intravenous gammaglobulin on enzyme levels", in *The American Journal of Medicine, May 1985)* reported on the treatment of adults as well as children. One major finding was that gamma globulin was more effective than conventional treatments (trimethoprim/sulfamethoxazole and pentamidine) for pneumocystis. Of the adults with pneumocystis, all five in the control group died. Two of the four who received gamma globulin died after several months; we don't know if the treatment had been continued. The other two were in stable condition with no evidence of pneumonia a year later, when the paper was written.

This work is important because gamma globulin is safe, very well known, and routinely available to doctors. In fact, the issue of the journal where this article appeared carried an advertisement filling three full pages for the same preparation used in the study. The ad listed "immunodeficiency" (but not AIDS) as the primary indication for its use. Gamma globulin would seem to be an obvious choice to try against AIDS—even before a leading authority on the disease (Dr. Arye Rubinstein) documented its use against pneumocystis a year ago. It could be used now and would almost certainly save lives, in the treatment of pneumocystis at least.

Yet practically nothing has been done A computer search of over 4000 papers on AIDS turned up only nine which involved gamma globulin; of these nine, three were from the Albert Einstein group mentioned above, and three others only measured gamma globulin but did not administer it to patients. We know of only one report of failure to obtain benefit, and that study involved just two patients.

Researchers may have overlooked this treatment because there were theoretical reasons to doubt its effectiveness. For instance, persons with AIDS already have very high levels of gamma globulin in their blood, even without any treatment. Perhaps the gamma globulin which is already there lacks some of the necessary antibodies. In any case, we hope that the new report from the Albert Einstein College of Medicine will bring this promising therapy the attention which it deserves.

Issue Number 6
June 20, 1986

INTESTINAL PARASITES AND AIDS

Several years before the AIDS epidemic, many gay men became infected by intestinal parasites which previously had occurred mostly in the tropics. These diseases—mainly amebiasis and giardiasis—started to spread through sexual transmission, to infect as many as 60 percent of gay men. Once infected, persons can carry the parasites for years unless they are treated. Many gay men show only slight symptoms or none at all, yet they may have a loss of energy, and can spread the infection to others.

Now scientists are studying the relationship of intestinal parasites to AIDS. Many of them suspect that the AIDS virus usually cannot cause the disease by itself, but that other factors usually help it to infect. These "cofactors" do not cause AIDS, but may make it more likely that exposure to the virus will develop into the disease. Some experts believe that the continuing epidemic of parasites among gay men has been a cofactor for AIDS and a major contributor to its spread.

This theory has important practical value, because it suggests ways to reduce the risk of AIDS, both in those not yet exposed and in those have a positive antibody test and may already have the virus. Doctors and scientists still differ in their interpretation of the available information about parasites and AIDS, but there is little argument about what people need to do to protect themselves. Gay men should get tested regularly for parasites, have them eradicated if they are found, and take steps to avoid transmission.

But since scientists don't know for sure that parasites contribute to AIDS, national public policy has largely ignored this approach, as it has ignored so many promising leads toward AIDS prevention and treatment. Individuals must take the initiative and learn on their own how to get the best possible protection for themselves and others. Fortunately, the San Francisco Health Department does have an active program for parasite eradication; and many private physicians here have experience in handling this problem. Still, each individual must make the decision to take advantage of the services which are available.

Evidence That Parasites May Help Cause AIDS

The scientific case against parasites is complex, and scattered in many different publications. Here we will outline some of it, and the possible mechanisms involved; then we will suggest other sources for detailed information.

- Laboratory studies have shown that the AIDS virus is much more infective against helper T-cells which are "activated"—meaning that they are doing their job in fighting disease. Ordinary minor diseases and infections increase activation of the T-cells for a few days or so, but the parasites (like other chronic infections) can cause a permanent increase.

- Parasites also can suppress other components of the immune system, perhaps as part of the mechanism by which they protect themselves against it.

- Suppressed immunity can open the door to the AIDS virus. For example, in one incident in Scotland, 300 hemophiliacs were given a blood product later found to contain the AIDS virus. Only about half of them became antibody positive. Scientists then studied frozen blood samples taken before these people were exposed, and found that the main difference between the groups was that those who became positive had had a suppressed immune system to start with. In those with good immunity, the virus did not get far enough to cause the antibodies to be produced.

- Parasites may damage the intestinal wall, which may make it easier for the AIDS virus to get into the bloodstream. Also, intestinal damage allows undigested proteins in food to get into the blood, causing further activation of the T-cells because they try to fight this protein.

- Parasites and intestinal damage cause malabsorption and resulting malnutrition, further weakening the body and the immune system.

- All the populations which have developed AIDS have had cofactors, either parasites or other conditions which could have the same effect on the immune system. For example, central Africa, Haiti, and Belle Glade, Florida, where AIDS is epidemic through heterosexual transmission, all have warm climates and poor sanitation, conditions which lead to prevalence of parasitic diseases; and those with the parasites are much more likely to test positive for the AIDS virus than those without. Hemophiliacs and transfusion recipients seldom have parasites, but they regularly receive foreign substances in the blood, which may cause similar immunological effects. The same applies to intravenous drug users.

- One group which should have the highest risk for AIDS in fact has practically none. Of about two hundred "needlestick" cases—medical or laboratory workers who cut themselves with contaminated needles or other instruments, thereby introducing the AIDS virus directly into their bloodstream—almost nobody has developed even a positive antibody response, let alone ARC or AIDS. It is possible that lack of parasites or other cofactors contributed to the very low rate of infection.

Diagnosis and Treatment Issues

Symptoms of parasites can include loose stools, flatulence (gas), or diarrhea (usually mild), and especially malaise—feeling ill, depressed, or tired. Often these problems come and go, so people don't recognize them as symptoms. They think they are tired because they work hard, or because that's just the way they are. In one study, for example, about half the gay men in San Francisco who had amebiasis did not recognize any symptoms at all.

Diagnosis is by examination of stool samples. Unfortunately, the parasites are easy to miss in the lab. Taking three stool samples gives about an 80 percent chance of finding them if they are there.

The available treatments have drawbacks. Flagyl, the oldest antibiotic for treating amebiasis and giardiasis, causes unpleasant side effects, and very large doses have caused cancer in laboratory animals. But flagyl is very effective, and it kills a wide variety of disease-causing organisms. It is often used for infections acquired in the tropics, and it has a long history of being used safely.

The sexually transmitted amebiasis is less virulent than the strains found in the tropics, so physicians can usually use milder drugs, such as humatin (also called paromomycin). Humatin does not leave the digestive system, so it does not have side effects elsewhere in the body. It is about 95 percent effective for amebiasis. One disadvantage of humatin is the expense; it costs about sixty dollars for the treatment. All of these drugs can cause serious side effects in rare cases, so they must be used carefully by doctors. It is best to consult a physician who has experience in treating these parasites; you could get referrals through the San Francisco Health Department, or through various organizations concerned with AIDS or other sexually transmitted diseases.

Persons who live or work in San Francisco can use the screening program run by the San Francisco Health Department. There is a small clinic fee which can be waived if you do not have the money. If you test positive, you can be treated by your own physician, or at a Health Department clinic. This program is strictly confidential to protect your privacy. For more information about San Francisco's program of screening for parasites, call the San Francisco City Clinic (see Appendix B).

Other Treatment and Prevention Issues

• Any kind of drug may be more dangerous to persons with ARC or AIDS. Only an experienced physician can recommend the treatment appropriate for each individual.

• It's very important that sexual partners be diagnosed for parasites and treated together, to prevent re-infection.

• The safe-sex guidelines for preventing AIDS will not always stop transmission of parasites. In addition to safe sex, persons must also avoid transmission of feces, for example through toys or by careless handling of condoms after use. Tiny amounts of feces, too small to see or smell, can contaminate hands, other parts of the body, or other objects, and later get into the mouth during eating, smoking, or other activities, causing an infection.

• Some intestinal protozoa (single-celled animals) are called "non-pathogenic", meaning that they do not cause obvious disease. They might be cofactors for AIDS; no one knows at this time. Also, they may be "markers" for the more serious organisms that were missed in the test. Physicians differ on whether treatment should be given if only non-pathogens are found.

• Some people use Chinese medicine or other herbs as an alternative to antibiotics like flagyl or humatin. These may be effective in some cases, but you should be tested afterwards to see if the treatment worked.

Summary

Most people exposed to the AIDS virus do not get AIDS. That's why it is so important to look for "cofactors," to find out what factors can reduce or increase the risk of AIDS in those who are exposed to it. By eliminating suspected cofactors, we can help to protect ourselves against AIDS.

At this time there is no conclusive proof that parasites are a cofactor, but there is considerable evidence. In any case, the parasites are a serious health problem which is epidemic in our community. All gay men should get tested periodically, have these diseases eradicated if they are found, and take care to avoid transmission. This is one measure that all of us (and especially those with a positive antibody test) can take to protect ourselves and others against AIDS.

REFERENCES

Archer, Douglas L. and Walter H. Glinsmann, "Enteric Infection and Other Cofactors in AIDS," *Immunology Today* (October 1985).

Pearce, Richard B., "Intestinal Protozoal Infections and AIDS," *The Lancet* (July 2, 1983).

————, "Parasites and AIDS: Evidence of a Link," *DAIR Update,* Number 1, published by the Documentation of AIDS Issues and Research Foundation.

Zagury, D., *et al.,* "Long-term Cultures of HTLV-III-infected T-cells: A Model of Cytopathology of T-cell Depletion in AIDS," *Science* (February 21, 1986).

Issue Number 7
July 4, 1986

ISOPRINOSINE BY MAIL

Update 1989: The Hauptmann Institute is no longer in business.

Many persons with AIDS or ARC have had to travel abroad for treatments which are probably helpful but have not been approved for marketing in this country. The most common of such treatments are ribavirin and isoprinosine, which have been approved in dozens of countries and are often sold over the counter in pharmacies. At this time, Americans are usually allowed to bring in about one month's personal supply of these pharmaceuticals from Mexico. (To find out more about doing so, call Project Inform; see Appendix B for address and phone number.)

The problem, of course, is the expense and stress of repeated trips to Mexico, especially the continued uncertainty about what will happen at the border. Also, many people who need these medicines are too ill to travel, and it is illegal for anyone else to bring in a supply for them. That's why we were interested to learn that at least one company sells unapproved drugs to Americans by mail from abroad, has been doing so for at least two years, and currently does sell isoprinosine.

Apparently the key legal fact which makes this business possible is that the sellers are foreign nationals operating outside of the U.S., and therefore they are not subject to the jurisdiction of U.S. laws. U.S. Customs cannot afford to unwrap every package which comes in, so they use spot checks instead. Some of the shipments are seized and destroyed, resulting in loss of what the buyer paid; but the seller has had some time to develop expertise in how to ship packages so that most of them get through. Customs has more important priorities, such as narcotics, which come under entirely different laws; stopping small amounts of medicines ordered for personal use to save someone's life is a lower priority for them.

Conceivably the buyer could be charged with "conspiracy" with the foreign suppliers to cause international shipment of the unapproved pharmaceuticals—but we have never heard of such a case and consider it very unlikely, providing that the quantities involved are intended only for personal use. Prosecuting a person with AIDS or ARC for this reason would make the government look bad. And the prosecutor would have to prove that you had placed the order—hard to do if reasonable precautions were taken such as paying anonymously by money order, and refusing to discuss the matter with any official or investigator, in the unlikely event that anyone inquired. Usually, if a shipment does get seized, Customs will merely write to the addressee, giving him or her the choice of forfeiting the material, or appearing in court to contest the seizure. People usually have it forfeited if this occurs.

So far, this writer knows of only one company which sells isoprinosine by mail to U.S. customers: (Reference to the Hauptmann Institute deleted by editor; this Institute is no longer operating.) Unfortunately, the price is $148 for a bottle of 100 500-mg tablets. This is over ten times the current price in Mexico ($2.47 for a box of 20). Incidentally, The Hauptmann Institute also sells other unapproved drugs, unrelated to AIDS, which are not overpriced; they cost about the same as if purchased in Mexico. (Editor's note: references to the Hauptmann Institute and this discussion of prices are reprinted here for historical purposes; the Institute is not in operation.) At this price, few will want to buy by mail—especially since The Hauptmann Institute does not sell ribavirin also, so those who want to use both will still have to make the trips abroad. But what's important is that such a business can operate, as this one has done for some time. If it becomes well known that companies can sell by mail into the U.S., and that there is demand, then others will follow. Many people would pay a reasonable markup to avoid repeated trips abroad; so a small business might even fill orders through retail purchases off pharmacy shelves, avoiding the need to finance and maintain an inventory.

Anyone considering using unapproved drugs should note several points:

(1) Get the advice of your physician. But if you ask, "Should I use (an unapproved drug)", the physician almost has to say no. Instead, if you say that you plan to do it, then an informed and sympathetic physician can discuss the pros and cons, offer advice on how to do so safely, or why you should not do it at all.

(2) Watch out for fraudulent operations, such as counterfeit pills or companies which just take the money. We can expect to see profiteering and other rip-offs, and it will be hard to stop them by legal action. But we do have control in that most of the sales will depend on repeat customers—who are organized and talking to each other. We may need to find labs to analyze samples and make sure the products are legitimate. Any company in business for the long haul will have lots of incentive to build and preserve its reputation, its most valuable asset.

(3) To help guard against counterfeits, and also to prevent chemical deterioration, customers should expect medicines sealed in their original containers by the manufacturer. In one case we heard about, isoprinosine tablets became discolored after being removed from their individual sealed wrappers and exposed to air for two months.

(4) Ultimately we should insist that beneficial or necessary drugs be available legally in an emergency. The problem isn't anything wrong with these medicines, but that all new prescription drugs must go through a separate U.S. approval process which takes years and costs tens of millions of dollars. This procedure might make sense for pharmaceuticals intended for mass marketing, when alternatives are available; but in an emergency, people should have more freedom to make an informed choice and weigh risks and benefits for themselves.

In current practice, decision making first reflects the interests of the most powerful—major corporations and Federal regulatory bureaucracies. Only after their demands have been met are the needs of patients considered. It is unconscionable to continue locking medical decisions into this straitjacket of institutional convenience.

COMPASSION IN RESEARCH?

Last week, at the international AIDS conference in Paris, an associate professor at the Harvard Medical School presented results of a study of ribavirin. This study gave it to 15 persons with AIDS or ARC, and reported good results and no toxicity from the drug after eight weeks. But when the treatment was stopped, the virus returned.

This is the same ribavirin which people have been taking for months on their own, if they can keep making trips to Mexico to bring back the permitted one-month personal supply (to find out more about doing so, contact Project Inform; see Appendix B for address and phone number). (If someone is too ill to travel, it is illegal for anyone else to bring in their supply for them.) It is the same ribavirin which has been approved as an antiviral in dozens of countries around the world.

Then why, in the middle of an epidemic, isn't it allowed here? The main reason seems to be that if the government made an exception to the lengthy approval process, due to the AIDS emergency, then other companies would complain that their products didn't get an exception, too.

If it has taken until now for officially-sanctioned researchers to publish a trial with fifteen patients, imagine how long it takes for the complete approval process—even for a medicine already known to be beneficial.

Another problem is that the manufacturer, which has a legal monopoly on ribavirin, recently imposed a major price increase even though the drug was already expensive and a serious financial burden to its users. Insurance will not pay for ribavirin because it is not officially approved.

Federal new-drug approvals, intended to protect the public from unsafe or ineffective drugs, have in fact become chips in a corporate bartering process. They impact stock prices, determine the fate of investments, and set the ground rules for an institutional game of inside tracks and old-boy networks. The patients are not represented.

Why are you and your doctor not allowed to consider ribavirin, which is quite safe, well known, well tested, and in use in dozens of other countries? Not for your good, but rather because the manufacturer has not yet earned the right to market it in the U.S. Therefore no one can sell or provide it here, aside from limited and restricted experimental trials, even when persons with AIDS or ARC could clearly benefit by having the option.

Why are you and your doctor not allowed to weigh the risks and benefits of azidothymidine, which is more dangerous than ribavirin but also more effective? Why not AL 721, almost certainly completely safe, although we do not know how effective because trials were delayed for months and began just recently, on only eleven patients, and in secrecy? Why are persons with AIDS or ARC told to wait a year or more, for definitive results on treatments already known with fair-to-high confidence to offer important benefit?

A special legal status called "compassionate use" approval is supposed to provide an emergency exception to such roadblocks. But a drug company must apply for compassionate use, and the U.S. Food and Drug Administration must grant approval. The process includes lots of red tape, and considerable expense to the company. We are hearing that there is less interest in compassionate use for AIDS or ARC than for other diseases which affect far fewer people. Once again we see that the institutions of this country are refusing to respond to AIDS as an emergency.

Repeated appeals to change these hideous policies have had little success. Perhaps we need to let more people know exactly what is happening, how business decisions and government regulations are delaying the most promising research, and prohibiting doctors from using what is here now to save lives. Perhaps we will need lawsuits by the friends and families of those denied access to the best treatments available. Certainly we need to develop our own understanding of the situation, and our own channels for getting things done.

Issue Number 8
July 18, 1986

AIDS, AL 721, AND LECITHIN

Update 1989: Today there is little interest in lecithin as an antiviral, although it has not been definitely ruled out.

This writer's research into the experimental AIDS treatment AL 721, and the scientific background behind it, turned up unexpected information that ordinary lecithin, widely available in health-food stores, probably has the same kind of effect as AL 721, and may help to strengthen the body's defenses against certain virus infections, including AIDS.

Six weeks ago I sent this information to more than a hundred AIDS experts. Of over ten who responded, almost all were encouraging; no one found any reason that it couldn't work. But unfortunately, it is unlikely that anyone will test this possibility scientifically, due to bureaucratic and commercial constraints. So rather than see it dropped, I decided to present the information to everyone, hoping that alternative healers and AIDS/ARC support groups can see if it works, and report to each other by word of mouth, as a kind of direct democracy in medical research. This article is the first published report of the possible usefulness of lecithin—still an unproven possibility, since no one has yet tried it for AIDS or ARC.

Briefly, scientific studies suggest that lecithin and some related substances change the membranes of cells in ways that make it harder for viruses to get in. The treatment does not kill the virus, but helps prevent new cells from being infected. And animal experiments with one form of lecithin have shown that it does cross the blood-brain barrier and affect brain cells in a way likely to be protective; we don't have more direct evidence on its usefulness in the brain, because no studies have been done.

Three completely separate bodies of information support the theory that lecithin might be helpful in treating certain viral diseases. First, laboratory tests of AL 721, which is a form of lecithin, have shown that it inhibits AIDS virus infection of human cells. Second, there have been four published clinical studies which used the main ingredient of lecithin to treat viral hepatitis in humans; all of these were controlled studies, and all reported clearly successful results. Third, there are fragmentary anecdotal reports of lecithin being useful in treating viral conditions such as herpes.

Here we will only summarize the information. For a technical paper with the literature references, see *AIDS Treatment News,* Issue Number 2.

AL 721 and Lecithin

The general public first heard of AL 721 from news reports of a letter published in the *New England Journal of Medicine,* November 14, 1985. Several scientists, including some of the leaders in AIDS research, reported finding that AL 721 reduced infection of human blood cells by the AIDS virus, apparently by interfering with the process by which the virus first binds to the cell.

AL 721, developed as a "membrane fluidizer" by the Weizmann Institute of Science in Israel, had been used experimentally for several years. It had been used in humans at least once, to reverse certain immune deficiencies resulting from the normal aging process.

AL 721 is a mixture of three ingredients, all of them extracted from egg yolks. The two active ingredients—phosphatidylcholine (PC) and phosphatidylethanolamine (PE)—are also the active ingredients of lecithin. Under the electron microscope, AL 721 dispersed in water forms little balls with the PC and PE on the surface. The third ingredient apparently forms a framework which presents the PC and PE to cell membranes more effectively.

Scientists believe that AL 721 works by increasing the ratio PC and PE to cholesterol in the membranes of cells and/or viruses. Reducing the cholesterol increases the "fluidity" of the membrane, making it harder for viruses to attach to receptor sites, which are protein molecules in the membrane which the virus must use to enter the cell.

Does ordinary lecithin do what AL 721 does? This question is controversial. AL 721 was developed to have the best ratio of its three ingredients, for membrane fluidization in the test tube. But when used orally, the usual route, digestion breaks AL 721 into its components. Since the special structure has been destroyed, and the special ratio has been changed because all three ingredients are also found in many ordinary foods, there may be less difference between AL 721 and lecithin in the body than in the test tube.

Another question is whether soybean lecithin, the kind easily available in health-food stores, is as effective as the egg lecithin used to make AL 721. There is a small chemical difference; no one knows whether it has any practical consequence. Most medical research on lecithin has used the soybean variety, but the AL 721 work used egg lecithin instead.

The big advantage of lecithin, of course, it that you can get it. It is virtually impossible to get AL 721, in any country at any price, and it may be impossible for years.

Lecithin and Hepatitis

All four published attempts to treat viral hepatitis with purified phosphatidylcholine (the main ingredient of lecithin) were successful. But these studies are not well known in this country, because the papers are hard to get. One is in Italian, and one in Czech; of the two in English, one, which reports research in Nigeria, was published in an

Indian medical journal received by only four libraries in the United States. The remaining paper, published in England, is readily available but four years old.

The English study (Jenkins *et al., Liver,* 1982) was a double-blind trial with 30 patients with chronic active hepatitis; it measured effectiveness by examining liver biopsies. Fifteen patients were given three grams of PC per day, and the other fifteen received a placebo, for one year; all received standard hepatitis treatments in addition. After the year, biopsies showed that the treatment group clearly did better. In addition, none of the treated patients but two of the controls suffered relapses during the study.

The Nigerian study (Atoba *et al., Tropical Gastroenterology,* 1985) used smaller doses, 1.8 grams or less for six weeks, probably because the cost of the drug was a serious burden to the patients, who had to buy their own. The treated patients showed faster improvement in almost all measures than the controls. After six weeks, blood tests were normal in 93 percent of the treatment group, but only 53 percent of the controls. (All of the 60 patients had hepatitis B.)

We have obtained the Czech and Italian papers, which were published in 1981 and 1985 respectively, but have only been able to read their English abstracts. Both were controlled studies giving PC to substantial numbers of persons with viral hepatitis, and both reported that the treatment was successful.

How does this evidence that lecithin helps against viral hepatitis relate to AIDS? It relates because the membrane fluidization theory of the action of lecithin is not specific to the AIDS virus. The hepatitis work shows that the antiviral effect predicted by the membrane fluidization theory, and demonstrated against the AIDS virus in laboratory cultures by the AL 721 work cited above, can in fact be used clinically against a viral disease.

Anecdotal Information

The following reports are not persuasive like the scientific studies above. We present them not as evidence, but as leads which could be followed up.

One health-food store in Texas ran a customer survey and asked those who bought lecithin what they were using it for. Two women answered that they had each discovered by accident that it made their herpes sores go away.

The other report comes from this writer's personal experience. For several years I had a repeating virus-like condition which caused sweating and extreme fatigue, with sleeping up to 14 hours a day. It kept getting worse until it was seldom possible to get through a day at work without naps. Attempts to get a medical diagnosis were unsuccessful. Vitamin C, garlic, and echinacea did little good if any.

After learning about some of the work cited above, I started using four tablespoons of lecithin and three eggs per day. Within two weeks there was a dramatic improvement, and for several months since I have been almost entirely free of the problem, for the first time in years.

Lecithin Safety and Cautions

Lecithin is found in many foods, and is used as an additive in processed foods. The U.S. Food and Drug Administration lists it as "generally recognized as safe." Still, some cautions should be noted.

The quality control for commercial lecithin is very poor, and often the substance is rancid when sold to customers. Rancid foods contain potentially dangerous chemicals and should be avoided. One way to reduce the risk is to become familiar with the various smells of different batches of lecithin, and throw away any which has gone bad. Lecithin should be stored under refrigeration, and away from light and air. Some high-priced commercial preparations are supposed to resist spoilage; we don't know how good these are.

Too much lecithin can produce unpleasant side effects, such as nausea, diarrhea, loss of appetite, and mental depression. One medical paper warned doctors to be particularly careful of depression if they give large doses.

Pregnant women should use special care. Animal studies have shown that large amounts of lecithin can harm the fetus.

Could there be any special dangers for persons with AIDS or ARC? There is no information either way about this risk. It would seem prudent to be careful about loss of appetite, one of the side effects mentioned above, because of the importance of maintaining good nutrition.

Fortunately, the doses of PC used in the hepatitis studies are consistent with the standard doses commonly recommended for commercial lecithin. The largest dose cited above, 3 grams of PC per day, is equivalent to about 14 grams of lecithin granules, which contain about 22 percent PC. Fourteen grams happens to be about equal to two tablespoons of the granules, which many of the commercially available packages recommend as the maximum daily amount.

Lecithin is commonly divided into two portions given about 12 hours apart. Those who have never tried it before may want to start with small amounts.

Medical studies have given up to 100 grams of commercial lecithin per day, and found that most patients can tolerate up to about 25 grams without side effects. Much larger amounts of PC can be given if purified preparations are used; but pure PC is expensive and not readily available.

On the low-dose end, the average diet already supplies about one to five grams of lecithin per day. Therefore very small amounts, such as the half-gram or so pills often sold in health-food stores, would probably have little effect.

The Bottom Line

None of this information proves that lecithin will be useful for treating AIDS or ARC. But it certainly suggests that the possibility should be investigated. Unfortunately, researchers have virtually ignored this area; of the nearly 4000 articles on AIDS and over 4000 on PC found by a recent computer search of the medical literature for the last eight years, only a single one concerned both: the AL 721 letter cited above.

Until scientists get the political, administrative, and financial support to do this job, we will have to do it ourselves.

Probably the best forum for researching this and other possible treatments is the AIDS/ARC support groups. Individuals can get advice from others before beginning any therapy; and reports of results can spread easily within the groups by word of mouth.

Scientific studies are more precise, but group experience should be able to determine whether or not there are any major benefits, which is what we need to know.

We do not recommend specific treatments, which must be determined separately for each person. But we do hope that this article will stimulate discussion both in the support groups, and in the medical and scientific communities.

Issue Number 9
August 1, 1986

THE PARIS PAPERS

The massive printed program of the International Conference on AIDS (in Paris, June 23–25, 1986) contains over 700 abstracts of papers and oral presentations given at the conference. Doctors and scientists from around the world rushed to get their reports ready for the meeting, making the resulting collection an encyclopedia of what's going on in almost every medical and scientific aspect of AIDS, except for alternative natural therapies. (For information on an upcoming San Francisco conference on alternative treatments, see below.)

No breakthrough came out of the Paris conference, or at least none recognized as such. We shouldn't expect breakthroughs, because it would be very wrong to conceal important news in order to make a splash at the next meeting. Instead, this conference reported the routine advances which offer major leads for new research. And it portrayed a developing world-wide catastrophe which cries out for appropriate institutional and social response.

There is no way to summarize the abstracts of the conference in this column; the material is so vast that just reading all the titles takes over an hour. Instead, we will mention a few of the highlights selected by several AIDS experts who attended the Paris conference, and who reported on it at a 90-minute session at the "AIDS/ARC: Update '86" conference at the University of California in San Francisco last week. We cannot do justice to this session, and suggest that you get a tape of it if you want to find out more about the results presented in Paris; a phone number for ordering the tape is given below. Meanwhile, here are a few of the important points discussed; comments by this writer are in parentheses.

(1) One panelist reported that there is less emphasis on immune boosters and more on viral inhibition instead. (However, other experts are moving toward drug combinations of antivirals plus immune boosters. Others are emphasizing the importance of infection through direct contact of cells in the blood, which suggests that killing

34

virus particles in the bloodstream may do only part of the job, while drugs like AZT which work inside the cell might be more effective.)

(2)   The question of whether intestinal parasites such as amebas are cofactors which help the AIDS virus establish itself and cause the disease is still up in the air. The tests to find out for sure would be very complicated, and no one seems to be doing that work now.

(Here we see another major failure of public policy in handling the AIDS epidemic. Since much evidence suggests that parasites and other cofactors play an important role, this question should clearly be followed up. Since we aren't going to get a conclusive answer, we should probably assume that the answer is yes, because this way the cost of being wrong will be so much less. Unfortunately, individuals as well as public agencies find it hard to commit themselves unless they have definite answers.)

(3)   In San Francisco, safe-sex education has been notably successful and has dramatically reduced new infections. (Unfortunately, the rate of new cases and deaths here will continue to rise for a time, because these cases represent infections acquired months or years ago, before the widespread change to safe sex.) But in most parts of the world, basic AIDS information has not penetrated. Education could stop the spread of AIDS everywhere, but in most places it isn't being used.

(The Federal government has refused to fund the kind of education which has proved effective in San Francisco. Gay organizations alone don't have nearly enough money to cover the whole country in time. State and local governments seldom fund work outside their borders, and foundations and mainstream churches have largely stood aside.)

(4)   Central Africa is particularly critical. Millions of people may be infected already, by heterosexual contact and by sharing of needles used for medicines. These countries don't have enough resources for effective prevention programs.

An undercurrent at the Paris conference was that the Africans there were not being cooperative. The reality is more complicated. The African scientists had to speak in terms acceptable to their governments, which are afraid that an AIDS panic will damage their shaky economies. Damage has already happened; ships have stopped coming to ports after widespread publicity to unconfirmed reports of AIDS among prostitutes there.

African countries also resent the treatment they often receive from foreign scientists. Research teams come in, take the data out, and then don't share their findings with the country's government or scientists. The excuse is that they cannot release the information before its publication in a technical journal. (This problem is also delaying AIDS research and treatment development in the U.S. Many journals demand that authors keep their results secret until the publication date, usually many months after the scientists submitted the paper. During this time, other researchers who could benefit from the information don't know about it.)

(5)   In the U.S., AIDS is spreading much faster now among IV drug users than among gay men. New studies reported at Paris show that almost all the IV users now know that they can get AIDS from sharing needles. Many have stopped sharing, but most continue to do so because clean needles are not available.

(The obvious solution of making clean needles available, for example by allowing sale without a prescription in drug stores, as needles used to be sold, usually gets blocked by political forces. The best available alternative may be teaching effective sterilization of "works", or use of veterinary needles, which are not controlled. Ultimately, we must inform the public that dirty needles are bringing AIDS into the heterosexual population, where it may become epidemic though sexual contact once a critical mass is reached. Opinions will differ on particular public-health measures, but each should be considered on its merits; political posturing at the expense of AIDS control now threatens not just gays, but everybody.)

The panel of speakers covered many more areas, such as AIDS in women, neurological complications, and the difficulties of vaccine development. A second panel of persons with AIDS or ARC then commented on the reports. You can order a tape of this meeting for $8 (plus $1 shipping) from InfoMedix (see Appendix B for phone numbers). Ask for tape number S226-III, "Report from the Paris Meeting", at the AIDS/ARC: Update '86 conference at the University of California in San Francisco.

NATURAL THERAPIES CONFERENCE IN SAN FRANCISCO

On August 23 and 24, the "Talks on Natural Therapies for Chronic Viral Diseases" meeting will take place at the Cathedral Hill Hotel in San Francisco. Costs vary but are about $125 for the two-day conference; persons with AIDS or ARC can attend at the student rate of $85.

Speakers include: Ranjit K. Chandra, M.D., from Newfoundland, a world-recognized expert on nutrition and the immune system; Laurence E. Badgley, M.D.; Keith D. Barton, M.D.; Robert Cathcart, M.D.; Scott Gregory, C.A., M.S., O.M.D.; Louise Hay; Stephen A. Levine, Ph.D.; Robert McFarland; Louie Nassaney; Jason Serinus; Ann Wigmore, D.D., N.D.; and many other experts on nutrition and immunity. This conference is sponsored by The Human Energy Church and *The Journal of Holistic Health and Medicine*.

Issue Number 10
August 15, 1986

AIDS/ARC AND BHT

Update 1989: Since this article was written, there has been little use of BHT as an AIDS treatment—and no major studies. Some side effects have been reported.

BHT, a chemical used commercially as a food preservative, has also shown antiviral effects in scientific tests. Though no medical uses have been officially approved, many people have used it for controlling herpes, and a few for AIDS or ARC. BHT does cross the blood-brain barrier.

Unlike many other experimental AIDS treatments, BHT is readily available in many health-food stores and by mail order. And expense isn't a problem because BHT costs so little that twenty dollars can buy a three-year supply.

This paper will outline the arguments for and against the antiviral use of BHT, list some precautions, and tell readers how to find out more about it.

The Scientific Case for BHT

Scientists first became interested in BHT as an antiviral by accident, when their virus cultures failed to grow in media containing the substance. More research showed that only lipid-coated viruses were affected. (The AIDS virus, and also the opportunistic infection cytomegalovirus (CMV), are lipid coated.) The team that discovered this effect of BHT, at Pennsylvania State University, published the first paper on it (Snipes *et al.*, 1975).

BHT has been found to inhibit or inactivate every lipid-coated virus against which it was tried, including herpes (Freeman *et al.*, 1985; Keith *et al.*, 1982; Richards *et al.*, 1985), cytomegalovirus (CMV) (Kim *et al.*, 1978), Newcastle disease virus in poultry (Brugh, 1977; Winston, 1980) and other viruses. In the laboratory, it worked especially well against CMV. It does not affect other kinds of viruses that are not lipid coated, such as polio.

No one knows for sure how BHT has this effect. One theory is that it removes the lipid coat, allowing antibodies to attack the core of the virus. Another theory is that it removes a particular protein from the coating of the virus, preventing the virus from attaching itself to a healthy cell. This mode of action may be unique among antivirals.

Since BHT has worked with all lipid-coated viruses tested, and AIDS is lipid coated, it would be worthwhile to try the same laboratory test with the AIDS virus. At least one scientist wants to perform this work, but it has been difficult to get the needed funding, fifteen thousand dollars. (One organization may want to fund this work, but it can only award grants to non-profit institutions like universities, not to individuals or corporations; and no one has yet been found who knows this scene and can make the necessary arrangements. Anyone who could help in getting this research going should contact Stephen Fowkes at the MegaHealth Society (see Appendix B).

What about human or animal tests of BHT with the AIDS virus? No one has done such a study, and as far as we know, there is no official interest in doing one. But a handful of published reports describe tests of BHT with other lipid-coated viruses *in vivo* (in animals or humans, not in a laboratory dish): two in chickens, one in mice, one in guinea pigs, one in rabbits, and one in humans. All were successful, to varying degrees.

The studies using chickens (cited above) tried to determine whether feed additives were responsible for agricultural vaccination failures. An incidental finding in the studies showed that BHT protected chickens against Newcastle disease, caused by a lipid-coated virus.

In mice, BHT reduced the healing time for herpes lesions when applied topically to the sores (Keith *et al.*, 1982). In guinea pigs, topical BHT shortened the time of the original herpes infection, but not of recurrences (Richards *et al.*, 1985. This study is difficult to interpret, since most of the placebo animals died during the initial infection; anyone interested in this report should read the entire paper, not just the abstract.) In rabbits, BHT in their diet reduced the severity and death rate from herpes eye infections (Coohill *et al.*, 1983).

We can find only one published scientific study of BHT used as an antiviral in humans. In this double-blind test, published in 1985, BHT or placebo was applied topically to herpes sores, but late in their development, after the patients had arrived at the clinic. BHT caused a small but definite improvement. Researchers speculated that BHT might possibly be effective even when the virus travels directly from cell to cell (Freeman *et al.*, 1985).

The Case Against BHT

People who use BHT as an antiviral (or who take it to slow the aging process and extend lifespan, an effect found in some animal studies), take about a thousand times as much as most people obtain in the average American diet. The biggest concern about BHT, whether used as a medicine or a food preservative, is that it has promoted cancer in some animal experiments.

Due to the widespread use of BHT in food, many studies have fed large amounts of it to animals to investigate cancer and other risks. The results are complex and contradictory, with experts disagreeing on its safety as a food additive.

What seems to emerge from the recent studies is that BHT does not cause cancer by itself. But in some cases, it can increase the occurrence of tumors in animals exposed to known carcinogens (Ito *et al.*, 1985; Tsuda *et al.*, 1984). In other cases, however, BHT prevents cancer, and actually protects the animals from it. (Incidentally, these studies shown that BHA, another food additive, is more dangerous than BHT, and can cause cancer by itself. Some vitamin companies sell BHA; we suggest that people avoid it.) The bottom line is that nobody really knows what the cancer risk is—if any—from BHT. The possibility cannot be ignored; anyone who uses BHT should consider it.

Another concern is the danger of overdose. BHT cannot be used like vitamin C, which has a huge safety factor. Some people use as much as two grams a day of BHT; animal studies suggest that ten times that amount would be close to a fatal dose.

Last year, two published reports attacked the popular use of BHT for herpes or for life extension. "The Saga of BHT and BHA in Life Extension Myths" (Llaurado, 1985) played down the concern about cancer, but cited a 1957 study by the same author in which he had fed one gram per day of BHT to rabbits through a stomach tube. Not surprisingly, the rabbits died. The author concludes by urging the FDA to ban BHT except for its use as a preservative.

The other report was a letter from two physicians at the University of California, Los Angeles (Shlian and Goldstone, 1986). They cite the cancer danger and the rabbit study, and also report a case of severe stomach problems in a person who ate four grams of BHT on an empty stomach. The patient required hospitalization, but recovered after several days. (We point out that most BHT users recommend that no one should take more than two grams per day, perhaps no more than one; that they should start with small doses and work up, and—probably—not take BHT on an empty stomach.)

BHT and Herpes

Most of the current popular interest in antiviral uses of BHT stemmed from two books by Durk Pearson and Sandy Shaw: *Life Extension: A Practical Scientific Approach,* and *The Life Extension Companion.* Pearson and Shaw began using two grams of BHT per day in 1968, for life extension; in 1974 they reported that a doctor had tried it for 150 patients who had herpes. Almost all of them achieved remission.

Another of the best-informed groups on the antiviral use of BHT is the Mega-Health Society (see Appendix B).Steven Fowkes at MegaHealth has been talking with users and collecting their reports for six years. He also co-authored a book, *Wipe Out Herpes With BHT,* with John Mann, published by the MegaHealth Society and available from them or at some health-food stores. Fowkes is now trying to bring BHT to public attention as a possible treatment for AIDS.

Fowkes has spoken with or corresponded with hundreds of people using BHT for herpes; we asked him about the overall success rate. He said that most of those who call him are the ones for whom it has failed to work. Usually they have taken less than one gram per day of BHT orally, and when they raise the dose, and take the BHT with some vegetable oil or lecithin to help it dissolve, it often works. About a third of those who call are not able to get good results with anything he suggests.

On the other hand, the vast majority of those who write report good results; usually they are writing to offer thanks. Some also report temporary skin reactions; almost always these are people on low-fat diets. Half of those who write say that their skin has improved since they started taking BHT.

BHT can be taken in capsules, or the crystals can be dissolved in vegetable oil. Taking it in oil may be more effective, but most people use the capsules because they don't like working with powders. The capsules should probably be taken with fatty foods, since BHT dissolves in fat, but not in water. Both forms are available in some health-food stores, or from health-products companies such as Vitamin Research Products in Mountain View, California or Twin Laboratories in Ronkonkoma, New York.

BHT and AIDS

Fowkes has barely begun to talk with people who are using BHT for AIDS or ARC. He has been trying to bring the matter to public attention, but it hasn't been easy.

Last August, he wrote a four-page letter on the use of BHT as a possible AIDS treatment to several dozen public officials and scientists. The only response was a single polite thank-you from one scientist. Clearly we cannot wait for any authorities to begin testing BHT. As we have seen repeatedly, after the lip service is done, saving lives is not a priority of U.S. public policy on AIDS—if it is even a goal.

One company, Key Pharmaceuticals in Miami, has a patent on antiviral use of BHT, so it does have an interest in research. This company helped finance the double-blind herpes study mentioned above, and it may receive approval to market a BHT ointment for the treatment of herpes. We have also heard rumors of good preliminary results of human tests of BHT against CMV, an opportunistic infection which, like AIDS, is caused by a lipid-coated virus.

In San Francisco, we spoke with Jim Gulli, who has used BHT for ARC for almost a year. Before using BHT, he had serious health problems; since then he has been in good health. His helper T-cell count was 200 to 300 for two years, but since using BHT it has gone up with every test, and was over 800 when last tested four months ago. Suppressor cells went from 1000 to 1500. His swollen lymph nodes remain swollen, but the night sweats are gone. He had had unusual, sharp headaches for a year; these cleared up within a month of starting BHT, and are gone completely.

Gulli takes one gram of BHT, dissolved in linseed and sesame oils, once daily. Since it takes about a day of occasional shaking to dissolve the crystals, he prepares a month's supply at a time, adding about 35 grams of BHT to 70 tablespoons of the oils; one tablespoon from each of the two oils then provides a total of one gram. He experienced side effects at first—some light-headedness, and loss of appetite for two to three weeks—but no problems after that.

Some Precautions

Here are some warnings which we have heard from people who are using BHT. This list is not complete, and some of the items could be wrong. Do not rely on this article for medical advice; we are reporting these precautions for information only.

• Before deciding to use BHT, consider the risks. BHT should not be used casually.

- BHT should be avoided by anyone with hepatitis or other liver problems.

- Beware of overdose, especially if you measure the crystals yourself. Note that doses should be proportional to body weight. The two people we spoke with who use BHT for AIDS/ARC are taking no more than one gram per day.

- BHT is fat soluble, so thin people may need less. Also, persons on low-fat diets may be more susceptible to side effects.

- BHT can interfere with blood clotting, so it might be a special risk for persons with ITP, hemophilia, or other clotting problems.

- Persons with AIDS, especially KS, can react to medicines in unexpected ways. Since no published studies exists on AIDS and BHT, no one knows whether there are any untoward side effects specific to persons with AIDS. Anyone with personal information on BHT and AIDS is encouraged to contact one of the people listed at the end of this article who will distribute this information to others.

- When BHT is being used, it is a good idea to take vitamin C also.

- Doses of BHT should start small and gradually increase. It is probably not harmful to stop abruptly, however, because BHT stays in the body for several weeks.

- A few people are chemically sensitive to BHT. One study (Fisherman and Cohen, 1973) gave test doses to persons who already had allergy or asthma problems, to see if BHT in food was the cause. In those who reacted to BHT, a 250 mg dose (half that amount for severe asthmatics) caused a flare-up of the problem; some of the asthmatics needed medical treatment to stop the attack. The reactions always showed up within 75 minutes. While such reactions were rare, they do reinforce the advice that small doses be used at first.

- In research studies, BHT has changed the sensitivity of animals to radiation damage. When it is first used, sensitivity is increased; later, sensitivity is decreased. Anyone receiving radiation treatments should be sure to tell their doctor if they are using BHT.

- Maintain a balanced diet. One study gave toxic doses of BHT to rats, and found these doses caused more damage to animals that were on a protein-deficient diet.

- Alcohol should be avoided for at least several hours after taking BHT. Alcohol may have a stronger effect than usual, so be especially careful about driving.

- Some people at least should avoid taking BHT on an empty stomach.

- There may be special risks to using BHT during pregnancy.

- BHT can interact with other drugs. It can either increase or decrease their effects. Some drug interactions may be unknown, but a pharmacist may be able to help.

- Always let your doctor know what you are doing. With BHT, as with any experimental or alternative treatment, you should research and understand the treatment yourself. Share what you have learned with your doctor. Most of them will be more sympathetic if they know that you have done your homework.

- If you use BHT, it may be a good idea to invest twenty dollars in a kilogram of the crystals—a three-year supply—to guard against the possibility that sales might be banned down the road.

Summary

Published scientific evidence strongly suggests that BHT might help in treating AIDS or ARC, as well as certain opportunistic infections, especially CMV, and that the risks can be kept small. It has been proved effective on every other lipid-coated virus on which it has been tried, and has worked as an antiviral in animals and in laboratory tests. The only human antiviral test, topical use for herpes, was also successful.

But we don't know with certainty whether BHT will help for AIDS or ARC, because no one has done the research, either in the laboratory or with patients. An unknown number of people are using BHT for AIDS or ARC on their own, but there is no way to contact them, and many don't want to talk publicly. For CMV, often a major problem with AIDS/ARC, there is more evidence that BHT may be effective, as it has been tested against the virus in the laboratory and worked well; however, there are currently no published human studies.

This writer talked personally with two people now using BHT for ARC. One seemed definitely to have benefitted; the other is enthusiastic but is taking it on faith, and has no clear evidence of whether or not it helped.

No one expects BHT to be a cure. But if it can help in the management of AIDS and/or CMV, it would have value now until better treatments become available.

We urgently need scientific studies which could obtain definite answers on BHT's effectiveness. This research could be done quickly and inexpensively, since BHT is readily available in high purity for human use, and much of the preliminary work such as animal safety studies has already been done. Meanwhile, we should support those who are using BHT on their own, and collect and publish anecdotal information when possible.

For More Information

For background information on BHT as an antiviral or for life extension, contact Steven Fowkes at the MegaHealth Society (see Appendix B). The MegaHealth Society serves as a clearinghouse for BHT information. It also publishes a quarterly newsletter, which will include new developments in the use of BHT for herpes and for AIDS.

REFERENCES

Brugh, M., "Butylated Hydroxytoluene Protects Chickens Exposed to Newcastle Disease Virus," *Science* 197 (1977), pp. 1291–92.

Coohill, T.P., B.R. Ferrell, D. Carson, and L.P. Elliott, "Orally Administered Butylated Hydroxytoluene Inhibits Herpes Simplex Virus (type I) Infection in Rabbits," Paper presented at the Eighty-third Annual Meeting of the American Society for Microbiology, New Orleans, LA (abstract number S41) (March 6–11, 1983).

Denz, F.A. and J.G. Llaurado, "Some Effects of Phenolic Anti-oxidants on Sodium and Potassium Balance in the Rabbit," *British Journal of Experimental Pathology* 38(5) (1957) pp. 515–52.

Fisherman, E.W. and G. Cohen, "Chemical Intolerance to Butylated-hydroxyanisole (BHA) and Butylated-hydroxytoluene (BHT) and Vascular Response as an Indicator and Monitor of Drug Intolerance," *Ann Allergy* 31(3) (March 1973), pp. 126–33.

Franklyn, R.A., "Butylated Hydroxytoluene in Sarcoma-prone Dogs," *The Lancet* (June 12, 1976), p. 1296.

Freeman, D.J., G. Wenerstrom, and S.L. Spruance, "Treatment of Recurrent Herpes Simplex Labialis with Topical Butylated Hydroxytoluene," *Clinical Pharmacology and Therepeutics* 38 (1985), pp. 56–9.

Ito, N., S. Fukushima, and H. Tsuda, "Carcinogenicity and Modification of the Carcinogenic Response by BHA, BHT, and Other Antioxidants," *Critical Reviews In Toxicology* 165(2) (1985), pp. 109–50.

Keith, A.D., D. Arruda, W. Snipes, and P. Frost, "The Antiviral Effectiveness of Butylated Hydroxytoluene on Herpes Cutaneous Infections in Hairless Mice," *Proceedings of the Society for Experimental Biology and Medicine* 170 (1982), pp. 237–44.

Kim, K.S., H.M. Moon, V. Sapienza, R.I. Carp, and R. Pullarkat, "Inactivation of Cytomegalovirus and Semliki Forest Virus by Butylated Hydroxytoluene," *The Journal of Infectious Diseases* 138(1) (July 1978), pp. 91–4.

Llaurado, J.G., "The Saga of BHT and BHA in Life Extension Myths," *Journal of the American College of Nutrition* 4 (1985), pp. 481–4.

Mann, J.A. and S.W. Fowkes, *Wipe Out Herpes With BHT* (Manhattan Beach, CA: MegaHealth Society, 1983).

Pearson, D. and S. Shaw, "The Herpes Epidemic: A Possible Solution," In *The Life Extension Companion* (New York: Warner Books, 1984).

Richards, J.T., M.E. Katz, and E.R. Kern, "Topical Butylated Hydroxytoluene Treatment of Genital Herpes Simplex Virus Infections of Guinea Pigs," *Antiviral Research* 5 (1985), pp. 281–90.

Shlian, D.M. and J. Goldstone, "Toxicity of Butylated Hydroxytoluene," *New England Journal of Medicine* (March 6, 1986), pp. 648–9.

Snipes, W., S. Person, A. Keith, and J. Cupp, "Butylated Hydroxytoluene Inactivates Lipid-coated Viruses," *Science* 188 (April 4, 1975), pp. 64–6.

Tsuda, H., S. Fukushima, K. Imaida, T. Sakata, and N. Ito, "Modification of Carcinogenesis by Antioxidants and Other Compounds," *Acta Pharmacol Toxicol* 55 (Supplement 2) (1984), pp. 125–43.

Winston, V.D., J.B. Bolen, and R.A. Consigli, "Effect of Butylated Hydroxytoluene on Newcastle Disease Virus," *American Journal of Veterinary Research* 41(3) (1980), pp. 391–4.

Witschi, H.P., "Enhancement of Lung Tumor Formation in Mice," *Carcinogenesis* 8 (1985), pp. 147–58.

Issue Number 11
August 29, 1986

AL 721 UPDATE AND RECIPE

Recently we received a 50-page document used in gaining British government approval for clinical tests of the experimental AIDS treatment, AL 721, in England. The anonymous person who sent this document included a simple kitchen recipe, allegedly suggested by persons running the trials, for a stopgap substitute to use until the real AL 721 becomes available. Here are some highlights of the document—and the recipe.

Background on AL 721

AL 721, a form of lecithin derived from egg yolk, has greatly reduced infection of human cells by the AIDS virus in the laboratory. It acts on the membranes of viruses and/or cells, preventing the virus from attaching itself to a receptor site and thereby entering the cell.

In human trials (not with AIDS), AL 721 restored immune functions which had declined with age in the elderly. This result suggests that AL 721 may serve as an immune enhancer, as well as an antiviral.

The researchers who have worked with AL 721 believe it is completely safe. Human and animal tests have shown no problems. And besides, AL 721 consists only of ingredients normally found in food, so it could legally be sold as a nutritional supplement without medical claims. Unfortunately, the license holder decided to gain the necessary government approvals to market AL 721 as a drug, a lengthy process which has already delayed its legal availability by almost a year since its potential usefulness for AIDS was known, and which may cause even longer delays in the future.

It is easy to make AL 721 in a laboratory. The document we obtained describes the procedure, apparently to fulfill British government requirements for licensing for human testing. This process involves using potentially hazardous chemicals such as acetone, and could not be done safely by untrained persons.

For more background on AL 721, see two previous articles by this author: "AIDS, AL 721, Lecithin" in the San Francisco *Sentinel* (July 18, 1986); and "AL 721: Experimental AIDS Treatment" in *DAIR Update, #2*, (April 1986), published by the Documentation of AIDS Issues and Research Foundation. These articles pointed out that the scientific background of AL 721 suggests that ordinary lecithin and egg yolks probably have some of the same pharmaceutical effect. The new information we report here confirms and extends this theory.

The Document

"AL 721: Particulars of Medicinal Product and Clinical Trial", dated December 1985, provides information required under the British "Medicines Act of 1968". It tells what the product is, how to make it, how it works, and what has been learned from human and animal studies. Much of the information is extremely detailed, and much has already been published. Here are some highlights.

• Besides possible antiviral use, AL 721 is also being studied for relieving alcohol and opiate withdrawal symptoms. However, only animal studies have been published to date.

• The proposed AIDS study involved only 11 patients, all with persistent generalized lymphadenopathy but without AIDS/ARC symptoms. The study restricted itself to these patients for several technical reasons. First, those persons at the earlier stage of the disease may have more of the virus than those with more serious symptoms, making it easier to test whether or not the drug works. Their condition was more stable, so there would be less confusion between effects of the drug and changes in their condition which would have happened anyway. And in principle, antivirals are more likely to be effective early in the infection. However, nothing in the document suggests that AL 721 could not work later; in fact, we have received two anecdotal reports of its effectiveness with AIDS (described below).

• The study design called for giving 10 grams per day of AL 721 to the 11 patients for one month. If benefits were found, it would be given for another month. There was no control group or placebo; the study design was to reject the drug if nobody benefitted, and otherwise study it further.

• The study planned to use "virological, immunological, and clinical criteria" to measure effectiveness. Specifically, it would use reverse transcriptase assay as a measure of viral activity, T-cell counts and skin hypersensitivity as immunological tests, and also clinical condition as another measure of effectiveness.

• Unfortunately, we don't know the results of this study. The document we have was used to obtain approval for human testing, prior to the study itself.

An AL 721 Substitute

The person who provided the above report also gave us a simple recipe for a substitute to use for now until physicians and patients can get AL 721. We believe this recipe is credible. It is consistent with everything else we know; and it came from a person who also provided the above document, which is not generally available. In addition, it accompanies a written formula for how to make AL 721.

The recipe is simply to mix a heaping tablespoon of good-quality lecithin from a health food store, with one raw egg yolk from which all the white has been removed. (One way to remove the white is to carefully pass the yolk from hand to hand, discarding the white, until the yolk is almost dry. A paper towel may help.) This mixture can be stirred into a glass of water or fruit juice, and taken once or twice a day on an empty stomach. For it to be effective, other fats should not be eaten for at least two hours. We should warn readers that some physicians regard raw foods as unsafe for persons with AIDS, because they may contain bacteria.

Two Testimonials

While the above study only involved persons with lymphadenopathy, we heard of someone with KS who used AL 721 in a drug trial and was convinced that it saved his life. We have not spoken directly with this person, but heard about the case from Tom Jefferson of Project Inform in San Francisco.

The other testimonial comes from the cover letter which accompanies a formula for how to make AL 721:

> I am a PWA. I was desperately ill all of January. By February I was totally disabled and moribund. . . .
>
> I have been on the medication for two months. My T4 helper cells have doubled. I feel good. I have gained ten pounds. My friends who are taking it have shown similar good results. . .
>
> If you take the medication morning and evening you can expect a noticeable improvement in your condition within three weeks. The count of T4 helpers will rise slowly over many months.

The formula for making AL 721 which accompanies this letter is identical to that submitted to the British government to gain approval for human testing. Therefore we are convinced that it is authentic.

While we cannot confirm these anonymous testimonials, we decided it was better to publish them than not to. They gave almost all of the information available on human use of AL 721 for AIDS or any related condition.

Conclusion

AL 721 is a serious treatment possibility for AIDS or ARC. It should have been available long ago, especially since the risks are insignificant. Not only is it not sold, but we have no idea when physicians or their patients will be able to get it.

Fortunately, AL 721 is easy to manufacture. We will need medical, legal, political, and other community involvement in order to research and then find ways around the obstacles to its availability.

Issue Number 12
August 29, 1986

AIDS TREATMENT PRACTITIONERS PRESENT NATURAL THERAPIES

Twenty-five leading physicians, scientists, healers, and care-givers discussed their experience with AIDS last weekend in San Francisco. Several hundred people attended the conference, "Talks on Natural Therapies for Chronic Viral Diseases," sponsored by The Human Energy Church and the *Journal of Holistic Health*.

Some of the highlights:

• Robert McFarland, who had most AIDS symptoms and was bedridden for two years, prepared himself to die in 1982. But instead he began treating himself nutritionally, and has been active and doing well since 1984. McFarland sought out an alternative healer, and read constantly on AIDS treatments, turning his bedroom into a library. Some of the treatments which he described as most important are:

Garlic. He chops it up and eats it all the time, often eight to ten cloves per day. Once, for pneumonia, he boiled a garlic preparation and inhaled the vapors for several days, and also used very large amounts of vitamin C, until the pneumonia was gone. He also uses garlic and ginger tea.

Vitamin C. He usually takes 20 grams per day, using it every two to three hours, and always takes calcium, magnesium, and potassium with it. He now uses the pill form instead of powders, because pills are convenient to carry around during the day. Some of his many friends call him "The vitamin C and garlic man."

Taheebo (pau d'arco). He now takes one or two cups of the tea per day, but used to take four or five.

BHT. He used it for shingles, and reported "fantastic" relief. Although he had a very severe case, the pain went away in several days.

Macrobiotics.   McFarland is a vegetarian, and he combined macrobiotics with other health diets.

Acupuncture.   Sessions gave him more energy, at first just for a day or two, but eventually they seemed to bring lasting improvement.

Other.   The regimens included dozens of other vitamins and herbs, including vitamin A, all of the B vitamins, vitamins D and E, PABA, biotin, pantothenic acid, folic acid, choline, inositol, lecithin, zinc, chromium, selenium, amino acids, glandular extracts, RNA, DNA, evening primrose, shiitake, comfrey, echinacea, Chinese herbs, acidophilus milk, juice fasts for arthritis problems, and GH3. For detailed information, readers can order cassette tapes of McFarland's two talks (see "For More Information," below). Both talks were on Saturday, August 23.

McFarland emphasized that persons with AIDS must take responsibility for their own health, and he was distressed that many of his friends who died would not listen and consider his experiences. Part of the problem, he said, is that you are dealing with both a man and a little boy; the man doesn't want anybody to know he is sick, and the boy wants to roll up in a blanket and let mom handle it. McFarland criticized teaching people to prepare for death.

He emphasized that you do not have to die with AIDS. But you have to work on it yourself. You can't expect the doctors to do it for you, he stated, and there are no magic bullets.

We can only mention a few of the others. Tapes of all talks are available.

 • Keith D. Barton, M.D., a physician who practices in Berkeley, has developed an AIDS treatment protocol based on the work of Russell Jaffe. For a list of five categories of lifestyle, diet, and treatment recommendations, see his article in the San Francisco *Sentinel* (January 31, 1986). Dr. Barton distributed this article at the conference.

 • Robert Cathcart, M.D., a physician well known for his use of vitamin C and ascorbate, provided some of the practical and theoretical background of his work. He explained the rationale of bowel-tolerance doses, and why smaller amounts, such as four grams per day, may not be effective. He outlined how to use the large doses properly. Of particular importance was his use of ascorbate to block allergic reactions to drugs used to treat pneumocystis. This possibility deserves wide attention and prompt investigation, because drug reaction is a major problem in pneumocystis treatment. Dr. Cathcart has never had a patient die purely of pneumocystis if they were a good vitamin C taker.

 • Stephen Levine, Ph.D., a research biochemist who has done original and highly-regarded work on allergies, discussed a wide range of subjects, including free radicals, oxygen, and the use of germanium compounds.

 • Robert A. daPrato, M.D., has developed a theory of AIDS based on stress and relative excess of adrenal gland cortical output.

 • Ranjit K. Chandra, M.D., Professor of Pediatric Research, Medicine, and Biochemistry at Memorial University of Newfoundland, and nominated for a Nobel prize in medicine in 1985, presented detailed evidence of the influence of malnutrition on disease. He said that while some infections, like smallpox or yellow fever, attack anyone regardless of nutrition, others, including pneumocystis and herpes, are known to occur more in persons who are malnourished. Dr. Chandra discussed the role of nutrition in production of thymic factor and mature helper T-cells, and mentioned 15 essential trace elements and four toxic elements. Besides his public talks, Dr. Chandra also gave a three-hour intensive for practitioners, also available on tape.

• Jason Serinus, author of *Psychoimmunity and the Healing Process*, sees AIDS as a disease of the heart chakra, which corresponds to the thymus gland. He sees the visualization process in the work of people like Louise Hay as the key to healing this disease. The tape of his sessions includes healing tones.

• Louise Hay, well known for her AIDS services, described her work on self esteem. Serinus particularly recommends that people get the tape of her session, even if they have her other tapes, because here she answered many practical questions from practitioners who work with people with AIDS.

• Patrick Donovan, N.D., and two other naturopathic physicians from John Bastyr College of Naturopathic Medicine in Seattle, Washington, presented an AIDS treatment protocol, including lifestyle modification and nutrition, based on a study of over 200 medical, biochemical, and pharmacological articles. This work won one of the two awards for research papers given by the conference organizers. Naturopaths are not allowed to practice in California, but physicians can get the treatment protocol through Dr. Donovan.

• Michael L Culbert, D.Sc., won the other award for his paper on a multifunctional approach to AIDS/ARC. Dr. Culbert is also the author of *AIDS: Terror, Truth, Triumph*, available from American Biologics in Chula Vista, California.

• Laurence E. Badgley, M.D., a physician practicing in San Bruno, California and the principal organizer of the conference, also presented a preliminary report of his own study (with mycologist Henry Mee, Ph.D.), on the use of the "Somacin" formula, composed of extracts of several edible Chinese mushrooms. A three-week course of treatment clearly helped at least four out of six patients with ARC or AIDS, and no toxic effects were found.

(We should point out that this study, apparently done with no outside funding, is exactly what is needed to screen new ideas and select treatment options reasonably likely to work. Even a study with only six patients can move a treatment out of the realm of rumor, hearsay, and commercial claims and counterclaims. The Federal research establishment has refused to study most of the promising treatments, making the contribution of individual physicians and other practitioners especially critical.)

There were many other talks which this writer could not attend because two sessions ran simultaneously. Tapes of all the talks are available.

For More Information

To order audio tapes of the "Talks on Natural Therapies for Chronic Viral Diseases", get an order blank from the Conference Recording Service (see Appendix B for address and phone number). You can reach many of the speakers through telephone information. For others, contact Laurence Badgley, M.D., at the Human Energy Press (see Appendix B).

Issue Number 13
September 12, 1986

AIDS CONSPIRACY JUST A THEORY?

We keep hearing more today about AIDS conspiracy theories. While this writer finds problems with most of the germ warfare scenarios, the other kind of allegation—severe and perhaps deliberate mismanagement of the public-health response to the epidemic—is hard to refute.

The evidence supports an urgent call for action by physicians, scientists, AIDS organizations, church and civic groups, and others. For the real value of a conspiracy theory is to wake us up to today's holocaust and to augment ongoing efforts to save lives.

This article looks briefly at the germ warfare theories, and then examines in depth the unconscionable neglect and mismanagement of AIDS treatment research. Related topics, such as the swine flu theory, official neglect or mismanagement of prevention, education and patient support efforts, or the drastic cutbacks in Federal support for public health, are beyond our scope here.

Germ Warfare Theories

These theories view AIDS as a weapon, developed by someone's germ warfare experiments and released accidentally or deliberately. Proponents have done an excellent job of collecting background information on germ warfare and how it may relate to AIDS. Rather than reviewing this information in detail, we will tell you where to obtain it for yourself. (For background on AIDS and germ warfare theory, contact the Information Network Against War and Fascism; see Appendix B; audio tapes and books are available on AIDS and germ warfare.)

There are problems with the germ warfare theory. Almost all the evidence supporting it concerns only the possibility that germ warfare may have happened, not whether it actually did. The key technical issue is whether anyone knew enough to have created the AIDS virus.

The hardest task in generating a new human disease would be to get it spread as an epidemic. It would be easier to concoct a disease for delivery to the battlefield, to kill people there and then die out. It would be even easier to start an epidemic with an existing disease, which can already spread from one individual to another—the hardest thing for a disease to do. But creating the AIDS virus and making sure it worked would have taken many human experiments which would have killed the people involved. Every test would have taken months or years because of the long incubation period. Bureaucrats would be afraid to approve a project that would kill human subjects. It's hard to believe that an effort of this scale could have been accomplished by a small group without management authorization.

The other problem with the germ warfare theory is that it doesn't lead us to any productive action now. Even if true, it would be almost impossible to prove. Even if proved, we could only punish the guilty, not save lives.

The germ warfare theory, then, distracts from a better use of our energies. There is another possible conspiracy which, if proved, could wake people up from a terrible silence and neglect which now prevails.

Mismanagement or Sabotage of Treatment Research

This writer's previous articles have documented an appalling consistency of neglected treatment opportunities, leads not followed up, and lack of priority on saving lives. We don't have the smoking gun—proof of public policy made for the deliberate purpose of letting people die. But there is no excuse for continuing to leave treatment research to "the experts," without independent monitoring and overview. The experts are focused on their own specialties and constrained in many ways by those who control their funding, who have agendas of their own.

When we look at some specifics to follow, keep in mind these general patterns, which prevail almost without exception:

• The only AIDS treatment research seriously pursued by established institutions concerns options which will not be widely available to physicians for a long time, at least a year and probably several years.

(Many developments in conventional treatments for opportunistic infections do become available sooner, but these do not address the underlying condition of AIDS, and do little to change the ultimate outcome.)

• Even the superstars of AIDS research (let alone the unknowns) must continually plead for money to keep their work alive. They are kept on short leashes. They therefore do not criticize what is going on, but stick to their own specialties; they act only under guidelines with prior institutional approval.

Suppliers who sell drugs or equipment to doctors know that in any field there are only a handful of leaders, and thousands more who follow the prevailing conventional wisdom. These followers do not evaluate new treatments on their merits.

And in today's science and medicine, the leaders are those able to bring big money into their institutions. They remain leaders only so long as they remain acceptable to the political forces which control that money.

• AIDS organizations have done excellent work in prevention, education, and support. But they have neglected to monitor what is going on in treatment research.

In leaving the research to the experts, they have contented themselves with the image of brilliant scientists working day and night to find a cure.

The result? No one is watching. There is unbelievable mismanagement which could never have been so bad under an informed public.

The Squandered Treatments

Here are some of the ignored opportunities and mismanaged treatments that have been described in depth in earlier installments of this column:

* BHT has proved effective against every lipid-coated virus tested, both *in vitro* (in a laboratory dish) and *in vivo* (in animals or humans). The AIDS virus is lipid coated, but no one has tested BHT with AIDS *in vitro* or *in vivo,* and we know of no institutional plans or effort to do any such test.

We aren't claiming that BHT necessarily works for treating AIDS or ARC. But when so much evidence suggests that it might, why is there no institutional interest in finding out? This case is one of many which shows that U.S. public policy treats the AIDS epidemic as less than an emergency.

* AL 721 shows considerable promise as both an antiviral and immune enhancer; its action is different from other drugs and thus doesn't completely fit the above categories. Since AL 721 is composed entirely of ingredients found in food, and appears to be completely safe, it should have been tested immediately. But AL 721 has been withheld from physicians pending proof of effectiveness. It took most of a year just to start the first preliminary test on a handful of subjects, and it may take years more before physicians are allowed to use their professional judgement on trying AL 721 for their patients.

* AZT may be the best AIDS treatment to date, although it may have serious side effects. We hereby publish—apparently for the first time anywhere—the fact that AZT has a hidden history, blacked out of all current scientific and popular articles about it. Eight years ago several published papers described its antiviral effects, and named the same mode of antiviral action being discussed today. Today's work represents little scientific advance over eight years ago; it only adds the performance of obvious tests with the AIDS virus and with AIDS/ARC patients.

The public believes that Burroughs-Wellcome developed AZT; instead what the company did was to keep everyone else away by buying up the worldwide patent rights, and the world supply of the key ingredient used in its manufacture. (The company deserves credit, however, for bringing the compound to public attention; otherwise, it might have been lost.) The serious ethical concerns with the conduct of the current clinical trials on AZT have been documented elsewhere. (On the ethical issues underlying the current AZT trials, see the article in *Discover* magazine, August 1986. On the favored treatment of the late Roy Cohn, who apparently used political influence to get AZT when it was denied to others, see several syndicated Jack Anderson columns in July and August, 1986.)

* Intravenous gamma globulin has shown good results in treating pneumocystis and other opportunistic infections—despite the paradox that the patients already had gamma globulin levels which were too high. Gamma globulin infusion should be

considered for toxoplasmosis, a brain infection which is becoming more prevalent and is hard to treat with drugs now employed. Doctors can use gamma globulin routinely—its intended use is for immune deficiencies other than AIDS—but only a handful of AIDS or ARC patients have received it. Apparently, no one has promoted it to doctors; the manufacturer is prohibited from doing so because its use for AIDS/ARC is not officially approved. Obtaining such approval would take much time and money.

• Natural therapies—ranging from well-known ones like vitamin C and garlic to newer botanicals like shiitake and chlorella—clearly deserve attention. But they have been almost completely ignored by institutional AIDS research.

By contrast, some natural remedies for other conditions—such as the herb feverfew for preventing some migraine headaches—have been rigorously tested in patients by simple double-blind trials, and are now known to work. It would be ethically and scientifically justified to test natural remedies in random double-blind trials, with patients who also received all standard medical treatments recommended by their physicians.

We can get solid answers about natural remedies, but to get them fast requires financial and policy support for doctors and scientists who can do the work. In the U.S., such support has been virtually nonexistent. (The study of feverfew and headaches was done in England.)

Rumors of Worse

We have heard credible, but unconfirmed reports of worse mismanagement. We are publishing these reports so that others who have additional information can help us confirm or disprove them.

• Several years ago, a government committee of scientists reviewing research grants may have been ordered to not fund any AIDS research, as Congress was under pressure from a fundamentalist campaign. The scientists reportedly complied. Anyone with specific information, especially the names and dates that would identify specific files for a Freedom of Information Act lawsuit, should contact this writer. It is important to put the facts on the record to wake people up to the more subtle forms of sabotage probably happening now.

• In 1985, a disastrous study of the drug suramin is generally agreed to have killed several people. Now this study is being used to impede further research by denying AIDS/ARC patients and their physicians access to other experimental treatments.

Yet, a number of persons close to the suramin trials believe that the deaths and other damage stemmed from dosage and other errors in how these tests were conducted—errors that were preventable based on previously available information. (The doses and other procedures were set centrally, not by the individual doctors or hospitals which ran the trials.)

We need more information. The big concern is to prevent this unfortunate event from causing thousands of additional deaths by impeding AIDS treatment research now and in the future.

• We are investigating reports of antivirals virtually unknown in this country. U.S. doctors were reportedly denied permission to test one of them, although other treatments like HPA-23, with less medical merit but widely publicized (due to Rock Hudson's involvement), were quickly approved.

Summary

The mismanagement of AIDS treatment research is far worse than the public—or even AIDS experts—realize. The incidents we have cited appear to be only the tip of an iceberg.

We must have independent analyses of treatment research and related policy issues and decisions. The official experts are too close to their own specialties and overly dependent on the continued good graces of funding sources to do this job for us.

AIDS activists and organizations who have avoided treatment research because they don't have a scientific background, should realize that they don't need to be experts because the most important need is for organizing. Physicians and scientists already have pieces of the information, and they need someone they can talk to who can put the pieces together and let people know what is going on. Non-scientists can fairly easily grasp treatment-research issues; these don't require an extensive background in biology or medicine.

For several months this writer has published reports of potentially life-saving treatments that have been ignored or grossly mismanaged; no one has yet found any errors in this reporting. What is most unbelievable is that no one else has been bringing out this information. With thousands dead, millions of people affected, and thousands of doctors, scientists and journalists involved, there has been a conspiracy of silence around the central issues of AIDS treatment research.

The consistent, severe mismanagement of this research will stop when doctors, scientists, journalists, and organizers stop passing the buck to other experts, and begin to inform one another and the public.

Issue Number 14
September 26, 1986

DNCB AIDS/ARC TREATMENT

Update 1989: Years later there is still interest in DNCB, still a scientific case for it, still a number of users—and still no study. Instructions for use have changed, however; and today there are many other treatment options available.

There's more to DNCB than meets the eye. This writer had ignored the story, because it appeared confusing and not very important. But patients using DNCB persuaded me to take a closer look—and a very different picture emerged.

Researchers have not completed rigorous clinical studies of DNCB, so we don't have definitive scientific proof of its effectiveness. But the evidence we do have clearly places DNCB among the most hopeful treatment possibilities currently available. And the ongoing work with DNCB is providing new insights into AIDS, and into the differing treatment needs of different classes of patients.

DNCB is other stories, too. The lack of institutional DNCB research has led to a network of "guerrilla clinics", now in 14 U.S. cities and growing almost daily. These groups are supplying each other with batches of DNCB lotion and instructions for use, on the condition that the lotion never be sold but always given away free.

The dangers may be small, but doctors are concerned at the lack of scientific testing and of medical supervision. And yet, for most people, the guerrilla clinics will remain the only alternative—until institutional science and medicine gives this treatment the attention it deserves. (At this time we know of physicians using DNCB in only five cities: San Francisco, Berkeley, Los Angeles, San Diego, and New York.)

A Brief History

DNCB (dinitrochlorobenzene) is a chemical that affects the body much like poison oak. It penetrates the skin and binds onto protein there, rendering these proteins much more likely to stimulate an immune reaction. In a person who has normal immunity,

55

DNCB causes a rash like poison oak. The pure chemical is so strong that it must be diluted almost a thousand times before use.

Immunologists have used DNCB extensively in their research. Several years ago, Dr. L. Bruce Mills—then a Stanford research dermatologist studying the biochemistry of certain enzymes—observed that DNCB successfully treated a kind of severe warts, in children, that could not be effectively treated conventionally. Not only did the treated warts disappear, but all the other warts on the body, too. It turned out that the DNCB stimulated the development of T-cells, correcting the immune defect which had allowed the warts to develop. The DNCB treatment—for certain kinds of warts—has become generally recognized as effective.

Next, Dr. Mills, now a physician in private practice in San Francisco, tried DNCB for treatment of KS lesions in persons with AIDS. Not surprisingly, it turned out that KS was more difficult to treat than the warts. But there were dramatic improvements in many cases, and not only for KS. Recently, Dr. Mills has distinguished four groups of AIDS/ARC patients. Different treatments are appropriate to the different groups.

The Autoimmune Theory of AIDS/ARC

Before describing the four groups of patients, it is important to outline a new theory of AIDS now being developed by a number of researchers, including Dr. Mills.

In the conventional theory, the AIDS virus (formerly called HTLV-III, or LAV, now named Human Immunodeficiency Virus, or HIV) infects the T-cells, especially the T4, or helper T-cells, that control the immune system. The helper T-cells normally recognize foreign proteins, and instruct the B cells (a different part of the immune system) to produce specific antibodies which attack the invading organisms.

In AIDS, the virus kills most of the helper T-cells, so the immune system cannot identify the disease-causing organism. The B cells do generate lots of antibodies, but they are the wrong ones. Therefore, the body cannot resist certain opportunistic infections and cancers which, normally, it could easily control.

New T-cells are being produced all the time, at least until the person is gravely ill. But, according to the conventional theory of AIDS, the virus keeps killing them.

The autoimmune theory accepts all of the conventional view outlined above. But it also says that a different mechanism can keep killing the T-cells, even if the virus is no longer a problem in some patients.

This theory states that the high level of wrong antibodies produced by the B cells can begin attacking normal body cells, especially the T-cells themselves. The result is a vicious circle—with the T-cells unable to control the B cells, and the B cells producing antibodies which in turn kill T-cells. Many separate observations support the autoimmune theory: for example, the recent discovery of a new kind of anti-platelet antibody that is specific to AIDS/ARC patients.

The Four Groups of Patients

Dr. Mills' patients not only receive DNCB; they also receive extensive monthly laboratory blood tests, whenever financially possible. The resulting data has led Dr. Mills to the following classification of patients:

The first question asked when he groups AIDS/ARC patients is whether the level of gamma globulin (immune globulins) is extremely high, close to 3000 or worse. If so, there is a problem from too much antibodies. Dr. Mills calls these patients Group III (discussed below).

Group I patients get the most dramatic benefit from DNCB. Their immune globulin level is not too high, and these patients respond well to DNCB in three to six months—in laboratory tests and by clinical improvement. These patients may not need any other treatment than DNCB.

Note that it does take time to get results, however. That is because DNCB works by stimulating the growth of new T-cells, and it takes time for these cells to be produced and to mature.

Group II patients also have a reasonable immune globulin level, but they do not respond well to DNCB in three to six months. Dr. Mills believes these patients may also need an antiviral.

Group III, mentioned above, has the problem of too much antibodies. For these patients, many of the other lab results are unreliable. Dr. Mills hopes that about a year of treatment with DNCB can reduce the immune globulin level.

Group IV is end-stage AIDS. DNCB may raise the T-cell counts a little, but it is too late to save the person's life. Note that Mills' classification is different from the normal distinction of ARC vs. AIDS, and that many patients with pneumocystis or KS (for whom most doctors have all but given up) would not be in group IV, but in one of the other three groups.

How Is DNCB Used?

Usually, a small amount of DNCB (2/15 of one percent) is dissolved in Vaseline Intensive-Care lotion. Sometimes other solutions are used. Once a week, the doctor paints a small patch on the arm, covers it with gauze, and tells the patient to remove the gauze and wash off the DNCB lotion in a certain number of hours. The DNCB should cause a rash to appear on the skin. Patients with a suppressed immune system will not react at first, but everyone tested so far has eventually achieved a reaction.

In KS conditions, the DNCB is painted directly on the KS lesions, but usually only after a skin reaction has already been achieved on the arm.

Dr. Mills also has patients take about a dozen blood tests. These include T-cell subsets, immune globulins, lymphocytes, and platelets. Also included are blood lipids, liver function, and other tests to warn of any dangerous side effects of the DNCB; so far, none has been found. In addition, he runs standard tests for rheumatoid arthritis, lupus, and syphilis, even though the patients do not have these conditions, because positive results may indicate a malfunctioning immune system.

A Case History

We spoke with one patient—not referred to us by Dr. Mills—who is considered a star patient, because there are no complicating factors in his case. He started treatment early, while severely immune suppressed but not otherwise ill. He took no other treatments and had no opportunistic infections or other illnesses during the treatment. He received extensive lab work on several occasions, so there is much data available to study. And he continued the DNCB treatments without interruption in the ten months he has been Dr. Mills' patient.

When he began treatment, his helper/suppressor ratio was .22, and absolute helpers 118. At that time, he read an article that claimed that it was impossible to reconstitute the immune system if the helper number was less than about 245.

For the first five months, the number went up, but just a little: 118, 265, 295, 365. At that time he was discouraged and had no further tests done for four months, but he continued the DNCB. When retested, in June 1986, the helpers were 529, (within the normal range of 447 to 1284). This month (September) they rose to 707. Total T-cells went from 686 at the beginning, to 2259. The helper/suppressor ratio had climbed from .22 to .63—not yet normal, but a major improvement.

Meanwhile, all the other lab tests moved in the right direction (or stayed normal). Immune globulins decreased from 2600 to 1830 (normal range is 540 to 1480). Lymphocytes increased from 1400 to 2700 (normal is 800 to 3200). Hemoglobin improved from 12.7 to 15.3 (normal is 13.9-18). The lupus and rheumatoid arthritis tests went from positive to normal; the "syphilis" antibodies dropped.

The patient told us that Dr. Mills believes that it may eventually be possible to stop using the DNCB, but he isn't sure yet.

Despite these results, the patient is unsure how many others will have the persistence to follow the treatment consistently, even though the results are slight for the first several months. When he started DNCB, he was feeling well; he had only a positive antibody test. Fortunately, he then took the T-cell subset lab test, which showed that though he was feeling well, he was living on borrowed time; it is surprising that he had not already developed pneumocystis or other problems. He began the DNCB treatment immediately and stayed with it.

Since this patient was well throughout, there was no opportunity to observe clinical improvement. Many others have shown major clinical improvement, including a resolution of nailbed fungal infections, KS lesions (even severe ones) that have almost disappeared, and generally feeling better and having more energy.

What's Needed Now?

The above case history, and the 26 others summarized by Dr. Mills in his letter published in the June 1986 *Journal of the American Academy of Dermatology,* are not scientifically conclusive. The reason is that patients in a private practice are self selecting. Those who don't think the treatment is working usually leave, so that only the good results tend to be reported. We need well-designed, controlled clinical studies to prove the effectiveness of DNCB, and to provide further information on exactly how to use it most effectively.

We have heard reports that such studies are now beginning in New York and Los Angeles, but have not been able to investigate these reports by press time.

In San Francisco, Dr. William L. Epstein, Chairman Emeritus of the Department of Dermatology at U.C. Medical Center, wants to perform a study of DNCB (and also urushiol, the active ingredient of poison oak) for AIDS as well as other immune diseases. Dr. Epstein is President of the American Academy of Dermatology and the world's foremost expert on contact skin sensitization (such as caused by poison oak or DNCB). But, so far, the study has not been approved. The rumor we have heard—not from

Dr. Mills, nor from Dr. Epstein, who was not contacted for this story—is that the study was first denied funding, and then also denied permission to use patients; and that the reason the study was prohibited was rooted in the politics of personal and professional rivalries, including the fact that cancer specialists—not immunologists—have held political control of AIDS research.

Any physicians interested in studying or using DNCB for AIDS or ARC should note that, as far as we know, there have never been harmful effects from such use, except that with occasional patients the expected skin reaction can be severe. Dr. Mills does not know of any kind of AIDS/ARC patients who should *not* get DNCB, although clearly it will help some groups of patients more than others. DNCB is already used in medical practice, and a pharmacy can mix it for use. The cost is negligible. Application requires only a cotton swab, once a week, plus ordering standard laboratory tests. In short, there are no technical obstacles to wider use of DNCB, nor to conducting the kinds of studies needed to get definitive answers on its value for AIDS or ARC.

For More Information

Published information can be found in the June 1986 *Journal of the American Academy of Dermatology,* pages 1089-1090. Also, see Michael Helquist's articles in *Coming Up!* (October 1985), and in *The Advocate* (November 12, 1985, April 4, 1986, and November 25, 1986), and Pat Christen's article in the *Bay Area Reporter* (June 19, 1986). Ann Guidici Fettner has a short article in the *New York Native* (June 23, 1986). Also see "Autoimmune Drug Discovery Published", in *Update,* June 11, 1986.

Most physicians are not set up to handle large numbers of calls, and they can seldom return calls except from their patients or from other physicians.

The best person to call for information about DNCB and the guerrilla clinics is Jim Henry (see Appendix B for phone number). He can tell you whom to contact near your area about using DNCB.

Another information source is Project Inform (see Appendix B).

Issue Number 15
October 10, 1986

WHAT'S HAPPENING WITH AZT?

Four months ago when this column first reported on AZT, the problem was digging out the information. Now the problem is digging out from under the avalanche of press coverage released by a public-relations juggernaut that may be unprecedented in medical history. The current campaign for AZT involves a major drug company, several agencies and branches of the Federal government, and a number of major medical centers—all working in a concerted push planned months ago, even before the test results were in.

The dilemma around AZT is that the best information now existing is the results of the recent study in which 145 persons with AIDS took AZT (and 137 others received the placebo, or dummy pill, in the "double blind" trial). Yet physicians, reporters, or independent scientists cannot see these results; they only hear those conclusions which the institutions pushing AZT choose to release. The first scientific report may be weeks or months away (we have heard that the writing has just started). So for now, persons with AIDS and their physicians may have to make decisions based on what amounts to little more than press releases, plus a 15-page protocol giving treatment information for physicians.

Why not simply trust the experts who have the information, and the recommendations and policies they publish? Because no one familiar with how AIDS has been handled could reasonably trust the authorities with his or her life. Remember that the last officially announced miracle was suramin, which was a disaster in the trials.

The past behavior of the "AZT juggernaut" also does not inspire confidence:

• The government-corporate-university combine behind AZT blacked out all reference to previous antiviral work with the compound, effectively concealing this information from the scientific community. Several papers mentioning antiviral laboratory tests of AZT were published eight years ago, but researchers are unlikely to find them without references.

60

The references are available from this writer who, incidentally, sat on this information for several months to avoid any risk of damaging the AZT campaign by embarrassing it before it had acquired economic and political momentum.

• The conduct of the double-blind trials did not show compassion for the patients. We are particularly appalled by the admitted fact that much of the reason for denying AZT to practically everybody with AIDS was to force several hundred subjects into double-blind trials (which the experimenters believed no one would have entered if they had other access to the drug). We also question whether double-blind trials were necessary at all in this case, since it was clear, even before the trials began, that AZT was helpful; see the study in *The Lancet* (March 15, 1986), as well as anecdotal press reports. (We believe that double-blind experiments are both scientifically and ethically appropriate only when the experimenters really don't know which of two options is better.) For an in-depth report on the ethical issues of the AZT trials, see the article by Denise Grady in *Discover* magazine (August 1986).

• It may be coincidental, but informal information channels on AZT seem to be drying up at this time. Also perhaps coincidentally, a lot of competing information is being kept out of the news.

(This problem goes far beyond AZT. Scientists who want to publish their results or want to be funded in the future, or drug companies who want Federal approval for their products, are both highly vulnerable and therefore easily pressured. Medical journals want results kept secret until they get around to publishing them, so that, at publication, it will make news. Government officials don't want political pressure, or anguished calls from the public that complicate their lives. Scientists and corporations—both competitive—don't want their rivals to overshadow them in public attention. For all these reasons, insiders enter into a virtual conspiracy to keep the public in the dark about important news; they justify their actions as avoiding "false hopes" until they have done "more research", which may take years.

This writer, too, has withheld important treatment news, when the scientists feared that if it leaked out in the press, major medical journals would refuse to publish it, regardless of merit. Then their results would be effectively lost, not taken seriously by the medical establishment, and therefore not used for treating AIDS at this time.

This system of concealment prevents patients and their physicians from knowing about promising treatment possibilities, many of which would certainly be tried if the available information were considered and the patient's interest were put first.)

What Is Known About AZT?

AZT does look like the best treatment news in a long time. We know that it can help some people, though it is not a cure. And we know that its use involves serious risks, though we don't know how serious.

AZT is a simple chemical compound; it closely resembles another chemical which is a normal component of DNA, the substance which carries the genetic code of living things. AZT enters the cell (including brain cells, since it crosses the blood-brain barrier), and interferes with a key step in the reproduction of a certain kind of virus, (the retrovirus), of which the AIDS virus is one example. A retrovirus, unlike almost all other life forms including other viruses, does not contain any DNA. Instead, its genetic information is in RNA, and this information must be transcribed into DNA by an unusual process inside the cell. AZT interferes with this process, apparently by providing false building blocks which get incorporated into the DNA being created by the virus.

AZT slows or stops the reproduction of the virus, but does not kill it. So AZT is not a cure for AIDS, but must be taken indefinitely until something better is found.

Fortunately, however, the fact that AZT only inhibits the virus does not mean that it only keeps AIDS from getting worse. Most people who used AZT had significant or major improvement—including weight gain, clearing up or prevention of opportunistic infections, improvement in T-cell counts, and generally feeling better. In the latest trial, 17 patients in the placebo group died but only one in the AZT group died.

How bad are the side effects? We have heard contradictory reports. The main problem seems to be anemia and bone-marrow damage, which can be severe in some cases. At press time, this writer has not found out how well physicians have learned to control these problems—by using smaller doses, doing blood tests for early warning, or in other ways. A spokesperson at the official AZT hotline justified the strict controls being placed on the use of AZT by calling it a "highly toxic experimental drug."

There is also concern that AZT might cause long-range problems which have not yet manifested, especially since it might affect human DNA. Apparently this worst-case scenario is just a theoretical concern at this time; and as long as AZT is used only by those who are already seriously ill and would probably die without it, this possibility doesn't seem like a big worry. But any future move to use AZT as a preventive measure for the millions of people who have been exposed to AIDS but are still well, must be scrutinized very carefully.

Researchers are trying new compounds which might be similar to AZT, but are less toxic. However, these new chemicals have had little or no human testing yet.

How To Get AZT

(Editor's Note: AZT is now available as a prescription drug; the following information is retained as part of the historical record.)

Here is what we have heard:

• At this time only persons who have had pneumocystis will be allowed to receive AZT. The drug will be provided without charge, under a special plan for greatly expanding the ongoing clinical trials. It is believed that about six thousand people with AIDS will be eligible to get AZT under this rule.

• The patient must not currently be getting any other drug for an AIDS-related condition, or cancer chemotherapy, or any drug which could harm the kidney or bone marrow. He or she must have healthy kidneys, liver, and bone marrow. There may be some requirements for red and white blood cell counts.

• Children under 12, pregnant or nursing women, or women taking birth-control pills will be excluded at this time.

• Any medical doctor can prescribe AZT. However, the doctor must first submit special forms, including proof that the patient has had pneumocystis. Then the

AZT will be shipped to a nearby pharmacy. To start this process, the doctor can ask for a packet of forms from the hotline.

• We have heard conflicting reports about when AZT will be made available to persons with opportunistic infections other than pneumocystis. One leading researcher was quoted as saying that would happen when greater supplies were available. But the AZT hotline denied that supply was an issue, and said that AZT was being made available to persons with pneumocystis now because patients had shown statistically significant greater survival time, and that it could be made available to persons with other opportunistic infections when other studies had been completed.

Discussion

• The exclusion of persons with KS, but not pneumocystis, may not be as arbitrary as it sounds. In the earliest AZT trial (the study in *The Lancet* cited earlier), most patients with KS got worse or did not improve. But this study involved only a handful of patients, so there should be more testing.

• We need detailed reports of the new study just completed, but not yet published. With 145 persons on AZT, and 137 on the placebo, information must have come to light on opportunistic infections other than pneumocystis, and perhaps on KS also.

• We have seen repeatedly that treatment research will seldom move unless there is political pressure. In the near future we will urgently need to make sure that AZT is made available to others who should have it, especially those with serious ARC such as toxoplasmosis, meningitis, or infection of the brain by the AIDS virus. Often no conventional treatment has worked for these people. There is no excuse to wait for a new study, which could take months just to set up, when all available evidence supports the use of AZT.

• We are hearing recent reports that the AIDS virus does not kill nerve cells when it infects the brain, so the damage might be reversible if the virus could be stopped. Since AZT is known to halt reproduction of the virus, to bring major clinical improvement to some people, and to cross the blood-brain barrier, why not let persons try it now when there are neurological complications and no other treatment is effective, instead of handing these people a death sentence?

If the decision makers need more evidence, they can have a researcher spend a few days comparing the records of the 145 AIDS patients who received AZT with those of the other 137 who got the placebo. Although all these subjects were chosen for the trial because they had had pneumocystis, some of them must surely have developed neurological problems also—in the placebo group at least.

• The case of the AZT trials shows once again that the division between AIDS and ARC is arbitrary and not medically justified. It serves mainly as a bureaucratic excuse to deny people the help they need.

• The availability of AZT, the first AIDS treatment considered effective by conventional medicine, must not be allowed to hamper the development of other experimental or alternative treatments. Remember that the development of antibiotics did not stop with penicillin—and AZT is far less effective than penicillin was.

• The use and control of AZT will raise privacy issues, especially for the large number of doctors and patients who have not officially been reporting AIDS. Fortunately, the names of patients receiving AZT will not go to Washington; only code numbers will be used. The local pharmacies will know the patients' names, however.

• A number of practical questions still need answers. How long should one continue taking AZT if it doesn't seem to be helping? Are there any problems with stopping its use? Users will still need to wake up in the middle of every night to take a pill, in order to maintain blood levels of the drug; is this requirement really worth it for patients who should get good rest and reduce stress levels? Will doses, etc., be set and changed entirely for the patient's benefit, or also for purposes of collecting clean data? Some of these questions may be answered in the treatment protocol for doctors, available through the hotline.

A Personal Note

After following AZT for several months, what would this writer do? Would I use AZT?

If I needed it, yes. If I had pneumocystis, probably yes, but it would depend on my condition, history, etc. The difference in death rates in the double-blind trial, the published results of the earlier trial, and the anecdotal results which have leaked out of these studies, are all impressive.

But whether or not I qualified for or used AZT, I would also look closely at other experimental treatments: DNCB, AL 721, ribavirin and isoprinosine, naltrexone (see future article), and BHT, more or less in that order. Information on DNCB, in particular, indicates that this treatment might be especially valuable to those least helped by an antiviral such as AZT; see our article on DNCB, in Issue Number 14 (September 26, 1986).

I would also look closely at diet, vitamins, and herbs; at physical exercise; at avoiding drugs, intestinal parasites, and other illnesses; and at attitudinal and spiritual healing, through affirmations, visualization, or whatever worked best for me. I would attend AIDS/ARC support groups.

At this time, AZT shows more proven benefit than any other single treatment—partly, at least, because it has been tested more. But we do know for sure that it is not a cure. It has not made anything else obsolete, nor has it overcome the need for individuals to learn about treatments and take responsibility for putting together a total program that works for them.

Toward that end, this column will continue to point out the treatment options which appear most promising—whether they are experimental, alternative, or conventional—and to report on the scientific background behind them, and on the experiences of their users.

Issue Number 16
October 24, 1986

NALTREXONE FOR AIDS/ARC

DISCLAIMER: This article is based primarily on interviews with Bernard Bihari, M.D., of the Downstate Medical Center in Brooklyn, New York. However, some information came from other sources, and Dr. Bihari did not see the draft before it went to press. Any errors are the sole responsibility of this writer (—John S. James).

Naltrexone is an experimental treatment which physicians can use now. It is inexpensive, and a gentle treatment which mobilizes the person's own healing power. It has no known side effects or dangers. About 20 physicians and several hundred persons with AIDS or ARC—most of them in the New York City area—are now using naltrexone.

How effective is it? We cannot report about results, because a technical paper is being prepared for a medical journal, and if the results get out in the press, the journal will not publish it. All we can say is that those using this treatment believe it clearly holds promise—even though it is also clear that naltrexone alone does not help everyone.

As a treatment for AIDS/ARC, naltrexone is new. Although clinical trials started 14 months ago, we do not know any physician on the West Coast who is now using it. Until the results of trials are published, patients and physicians will have to hear about naltrexone by word of mouth, or through articles like this one, and then take the initiative to find out more.

The bottom line is that your physician can talk to the head researcher running clinical trials on naltrexone, at the phone number given, and/or to a physician using the drug in private practice for AIDS and ARC, to find out what he or she needs to know about whether this treatment would be appropriate for you, and how to use it properly. Anyone with AIDS or ARC should consider this option. The most important point of this article is that these doctors are happy to talk with other physicians.

Naltrexone's Standard Medical Use

Naltrexone has been approved by the FDA for about two years, for use as a "narcotic antagonist," to keep heroin or other opiate addicts off the drugs. Naltrexone works by blocking the "opiate receptors"—sites on the cell membranes where opiates have their effect. If a person on naltrexone later takes heroin or another opiate, it will have no effect. But the person must be completely off narcotics before starting naltrexone, or it will cause an immediate, extreme withdrawal reaction.

Naltrexone itself is not a narcotic, and not at all addicting. It is taken by mouth, not injected, in doses of 50 mg per day for preventing addiction. It has also been tried in very large doses, 200 to 300 mg per day, for treating obesity. At these doses, there are toxic side effects.

Naltrexone for AIDS or ARC

For treating AIDS or ARC, naltrexone must be used in very small doses—only about one-twentieth of the dose used by ex-addicts. Too large a dose would be ineffective, and might even have the opposite of the intended effect. Because the only tablets available in pharmacies contain the large dose for ex-addicts, the pharmacy must dissolve one pill (more than a two-week supply) and give the patient instructions for measuring out an exact amount of the liquid.

No side effects have ever been found at the small doses used for treating AIDS or ARC.

Also, because of the small dose, the daily cost of the medicine alone is only about fifteen cents. Of course the actual cost will be more, because of the special preparation which the pharmacy must do.

Naltrexone is an immune enhancer. It may need to be combined with an antiviral or with other treatments, for some patients. One doctor at least is now testing naltrexone on patients who, on their own, are simultaneously taking ribavirin. (U.S. doctors cannot prescribe ribavirin, although it has been approved for medical use in over 30 countries, and is showing increasingly good results when used for AIDS or ARC.)

We caution the reader not to dismiss naltrexone as only a minor treatment, because of the small dose. Many of the patients using it have AIDS or severe ARC.

How Does It Work?

The theory behind the low-dose naltrexone treatment for persons with AIDS or ARC is very complex. But this theory has a special importance, because it may also explain the physiological mechanism by which physical exercise, and even positive mental attitudes, can help in healing AIDS.

We can only outline some of the elements of this theory, based on results of immunology research over the last several years. Dr. Bihari and his colleagues used these results to develop the low-dose naltrexone treatment, which might be valuable for other diseases, including cancer and autoimmune diseases, as well as for AIDS. They started a three-month double-blind trial for AIDS and ARC in mid 1985. After the three months, they started treating all the patients with naltrexone. The original patients have now been using it for up to 14 months; others joined the study later.

The theory of naltrexone is based on endorphins. Endorphins, produced by the pituitary gland, could be described as the body's natural opiates. The endorphin system—the endorphins themselves, and the opiate receptor sites in cells, which is where they act—help the body respond to stress. Endorphins are responsible for the "runner's high," the good feeling people get after exercise.

In the last several years, immunologists have also discovered that endorphins are a major link in communication between the brain and the immune system. Every cell in the immune system—T-cells, B-cells, platelets, etc.—has opiate receptors, that respond to endorphins.

Unlike most other immune modulators, which only affect one or two parts of the immune system, endorphins seem to be a natural up-regulator of the whole system, and probably a normal means by which the system heals itself. For unknown reasons, AIDS seems to interfere with this process of healing, perhaps by causing a very high level of alpha interferon (see below).

Naltrexone temporarily blocks the opiate receptors which are part of the endorphin system. But at the same time, it increases the amount of endorphins, and also the number and sensitivity of receptors. Both these effects increase the overall activity of the endorphin system.

The blocking effect of the low naltrexone dose wears off within several hours, but the up-regulation of the endorphin system works even during the blocking period, and then lasts throughout the day. The naltrexone must be taken at night as the pituitary produces most endorphins in the early morning.

The key test of whether naltrexone is working is not T-cell counts, but rather a reduction in the abnormally high level of alpha interferon found in persons with AIDS. Unfortunately, the alpha interferon test is only available to researchers, not to physicians in private practice. But since low-dose naltrexone is not harmful in any case, physicians can use it even though they cannot do the key test of how well it is working. (At this summer's Paris AIDS conference, Dr. Bihari reported that a majority of patients treated with naltrexone showed a drop in alpha interferon levels.)

Miscellaneous

• Physical exercise can increase the level of endorphins. Dr. Bihari suggests that aerobic exercises (not bodybuilding exercises) would be most effective.

• Endorphins may be part of the physical basis of the healing effect of positive thoughts and images, healthy attitudes, and good morale. There is no scientific proof at this time.

• No one has found any problem combining naltrexone with antivirals or with other immune modulators. However, naltrexone must not be combined with any narcotic painkiller, including codeine, percodan, morphine, or demerol. The painkillers would prevent the therapeutic effect of naltrexone. However, the combination is not dangerous, and patients who must go on narcotics should continue taking the naltrexone.

• Patients should continue using naltrexone as long as there is any immune deficiency. It is a long-term treatment. Some patients will see results soon, others will take longer to obtain an effect, and some will not be helped at all (at least not by naltrexone alone).

• It is perfectly legal for physicians in private practice to prescribe naltrexone for AIDS or ARC, even though the drug was approved for other purposes. The physician must find a pharmacy willing to prepare it. Physicians in New York have not found it hard to have pharmacies dissolve the naltrexone tablets, once they explain how to do it. At least four pharmacies in New York are now preparing naltrexone this way; we don't know of any on the West Coast. (Most San Francisco pharmacies do not usually stock naltrexone, although they can order it.) *(Update 1989: Most San Francisco pharmacies now carry naltrexone and are experienced in its routine preparation for this purpose.)*

Information for Physicians

Physicians may call Bernard Bihari, M.D. at the Downstate Medical Center, Brooklyn, New York (see Appendix B). He developed the low-dose naltrexone therapy, and is running the clinical trials.

Very little published information is available at this time. All we know about is the abstract of Dr. Bihari's Paris poster session, and a three-page writeup about the ongoing trials in *Experimental Drugs for AIDS and ARC: A Directory of Clinical Trials* (September 1986 draft, published by the American Foundation for AIDS Research).

The author thanks Martin Delaney and David Winterhalter, of Project Inform, for calling my attention to the naltrexone research, and for putting me in touch with Dr. Bihari.

Issue Number 17
November 7, 1986

LICORICE, GLYCYRRHIZIN, AND AIDS/ARC

Update 1989: There has never been much public interest in glycyrrhizin as an antiviral. There is still some scientific interest.

In the last few weeks, Japanese researchers have found that a component of ordinary licorice can stop the growth of the AIDS virus in test tube cultures of human lymphocytes.

Many substances can stop the AIDS virus in the laboratory. But this discovery, by a joint project of researchers at Fukushima Medical College and Yamaguchi University Medical School, is particularly important for the following reasons:

* The licorice ingredient, glycyrrhizin, is already clinically used in Japan as an antiviral, especially for treatment of hepatitis B. Good results have been reported.

* Side effects are mild to moderate.

* Concentrations of 50 mg per (ml?) almost completely protected human blood cells from the AIDS virus. We don't know the concentrations reached during normal medical use of glycyrrhizin, but the usual daily doses are 40 to 200 mg, and much larger doses have been used.

* While many Japanese physicians use an intravenous glycyrrhizin preparation apparently not available in the U.S., others have given it orally. Researchers believe that oral administration can provide comparable doses (Fujiwara *et al.*, 1983). Apparently, physicians use the intravenous preparation because it avoids other possibly unwanted ingredients in licorice; includes other substances to minimize the side effects of pure glycyrrhizin or of licorice; and helps standardize the treatment by avoiding variability in absorption from the digestive systems of different individuals.

* Licorice root, commonly available in health food stores and in licorice candy, can deliver medically effective doses of glycyrrhizin. These sources may provide a

workable alternative, should red tape impede clinical AIDS/ARC tests of glycyrrhizin or U.S. availability of the Japanese pharmaceutical preparation.

The Japanese team announced its results on September 22, 1986, and apparently reported them at a meeting of the Japanese Society of Virologists on October 14. We have not yet seen any report of that meeting, only a story in the *Japan Times Weekly* (October 11, 1986), based on a telephone interview with Masahiko Ito, a professor at Fukushima Medical College.

The team has not yet tested glycyrrhizin on persons with AIDS or ARC.

The U.S. press has not picked up this story, and few physicians have heard of glycyrrhizin or licorice as a potential AIDS/ARC treatment. As far as we know, this San Francsico *Sentinel* article is the first mention of it in any U.S. publication.

Licorice and Glycyrrhizin

The most interesting ingredient in licorice is the chemical glycyrrhizin (a word derived from the biological name of the licorice plant, glycyrrhiza glabra). Glycyrrhizin, fifty times sweeter than sugar, is responsible for the sweet taste of the infusions, tinctures or other preparations made from the licorice root. (The Chinese name for licorice is "gan cao", meaning "sweet weed".)

Licorice also contains a number of other medically relevant components, such as glycyrrhizic acid and glycyrrhetinic acid. In one study, the latter showed a "remarkable" effect on the Epstein-Barr virus, although glycyrrhizin itself had none (Okamoto *et al.*, 1983). Most of the Japanese studies used purified glycyrrhizin instead of licorice for experiments and for medical treatment. (We don't know if pure glycyrrhizin is available in the U.S. Licorice root, and various extracts from it, are available in health food stores or from herbalists.)

Medical Experiments and Uses

A recent Japanese study found that glycyrrhizin enhanced interferon gamma production by human blood cells treated with hepatitis B antigen or another immune stimulus (Shinada *et al.*, 1985). Glycyrrhizin alone did not cause the cells to produce interferon. But pre-treatment with glycyrrhizin enabled the cells to produce more interferon gamma (by a factor of as much as eight) when they were challenged with an immune stimulus (such as hepatitis B antigen). Collaboration between T-cells and macrophages was needed to obtain the greatest effect.

Interferon gamma is one of the experimental AIDS/ARC treatments now being tried. According to one recent report (AmFAR, September 1986), these trials have not produced much clinical improvement. However, injecting interferon gamma may not have the same effect as the use of glycyrrhizin to assist the body in producing more of its own interferon as necessary.

Glycyrrhizin has shown antiviral activity in the laboratory (Pompei *et al.*, 1979) and has been widely used in Japan to treat chronic active hepatitis B (Shinada *et al.*, 1986).

The eminent herbalist, Subhuti Dharmananda, discussed licorice in a paper on immunodeficiency syndromes (Dharmananda, 1986). He reported that it has demonstrated both immune enhancing and immune suppressive effects. Licorice has been used for treating gastric ulcer and arthritis; traditional uses in Chinese medicine have included treatment of laryngitis. But licorice is almost always used in combination with other herbs in Chinese medicine.

To learn more about the traditional uses of the herb, we consulted with Quan Yin Acupuncture and Herb Center of San Francisco. They also recommended an herbalist, Brian K. Weissbuch of KW Botanicals, in Fairfax, California. Both explained that while licorice is widely used in Chinese herbal formulas, it generally constitutes only a small part of the preparation (usually less than four percent). Our discussion with Mr. Weissbuch largely concerned precautions and reasons for avoiding indiscriminate use.

Cautions and Adverse Effects

A New Zealand study examined black licorice candy use among 603 high school students (Simpson and Currie, 1982). While these researchers did not search for nor find ill effects among the students, their paper provides a convenient summary of common adverse effects of licorice reported up to that time.

The most common problems were high blood pressure, edema (swelling, often of the ankles, wrists, or face), and muscle pain, weakness, or paralysis. Most of these people had eaten several hundred grams or more of licorice per week, often for months or years. The effects ceased when they stopped using licorice. Licorice acts as a natural cortisone, and may cause sodium and water retention and potassium depletion. Doctors have occasionally found severe or life-threatening reactions requiring medical treatment.

The authors of the New Zealand study warn that persons with heart disease, high blood pressure (or a family history of high blood pressure), or who eat a lot of salt or take certain diuretics, should be especially careful of licorice.

Later studies have shown much greater risks to persons who are taking insulin, or who have alcoholic cirrhosis. Even small amounts of licorice can cause severe reactions.

The authors of the New Zealand study suggested that, for healthy people, eating more than about 200 grams per week (about one ounce a day) of black licorice candy sticks might cause adverse health effects. Some kinds of licorice are believed to have a stronger effect than the sticks. About five percent of the high school students studied ate more than the amount believed potentially harmful.

Miscellaneous

• One problem with licorice candy is that it is difficult to determine how much licorice is being consumed. And the candy has other ingredients, including oil from anise seeds, which may cause untoward side effects in some people. It also has sugar, molasses, or other sweeteners, and salt. Licorice candies and liquors have caused a number of cases of medical problems, as stated earlier. It may be safer to use the root, which can be found in herb or health food stores and prepared according to a practitioner's instructions, or according to directions in herb books.

• What dose ought to be used? One book (John Lust, *The Herb Book*) suggests one teaspoon of the root, prepared as an infusion, with one cup of water, and used slowly throughout the day. One should check with a physician, practitioner, or at least a good herb book before using licorice. It is clearly advisable to tell one's physician what one is doing, even though few physicians are familiar with medical uses or dangers of licorice, and no one knows how it might affect persons with AIDS or ARC.

- One particular caution: water retention can cause a sudden weight gain of several pounds. This dangerous side effect which can be caused by too much licorice or glycyr-rhizin should not be taken as a sign that the treatment is working.

- For those who want to gather licorice in the wild, Weissbuch cautioned that many people confuse the licorice plant with wild fennel, an entirely different plant.

To summarize, glycyrrhizin or licorice might help in treating AIDS or ARC, although no one has tested it with patients at this time. If one does try it, the advice we have been hearing is to use caution, especially in long-term use, to avoid taking too much, and to be aware of one's particular health problems that may rule out the use of licorice, and of symptoms that might be caused by its use.

This column will publish more information about glycyrrhizin or licorice as treatments for AIDS or ARC, as it becomes available.

REFERENCES

AmFAR (American Foundation for AIDS Research), *Experimental Drugs for AIDS and ARC: A Directory of Clinical Trials,* (New York: The American Foundation for AIDS Research, September 15, 1986).

Dharmananda, Subhuti, "A New Herbal Combination for the Treatment of Immunodeficiency Syndromes," Institute for Traditional Medicine and Preventive Health Care, 2442 S.E. Sherman, Portland, OR 97214 (1986).

Fujiwara, Y., R. Kikkawa, K. Nakata, E. Kitamura, T. Takama, and Y. Shigeta, "Hypokalemia and Sodium Retention in Patients with Diabetes and Chronic Hepatitis Receiving Insulin and Glycyrrhizin," *Endocrinol Japon* 20 (1983), pp. 243–9.

Japan Times Weekly, "Component Halts AIDS Virus Growth," (October 11, 1986).

Okamoto, H., D. Yoshida, and S. Mizusaki, "Inhibition of 12-O-tetradecanoylphorbol-13-acetate-induced Induction in Epstein-Barr Virus Early Antigen in Raji Cells," *Cancer Letter* 19(1) (May 1983), pp. 47–53.

Pompei, R., O. Flore, M.A. Marccialis, A. Pani, and B. Loddo, "Glycyrrhizic Acid Inhibits Virus Growth and Inactivates Virus Particles," *Nature* 281 (1979), pp. 689–90.

Shinada, M., M. Azuma, H. Kawai, K. Sazaki, I. Yoshida, T. Yoshida, T. Suzutani, and T. Sakuma, "Enhancement of Interferon Gamma Production in Glycyrrhizin-treated Human Peripheral Lymphocytes in Response to Concanavalin A and to Surface Antigen of Hepatitis B Virus," *Proceedings of the Society for Experimental Biology and Medicine* 181 (1986), pp. 205–10.

Simpson, F.O., and I. J. Currie, "Licorice Consumption Among High School Students," *New Zealand Medical Journal* 95 (January 27, 1982), pp. 31–3.

Issue Number 18
November 21, 1986

COULD YOU GET AZT?

Update 1989: *Naturally much has changed on AZT since November 1986. These early articles are mainly of historical interest.*

The third human drug trial of AZT is beginning now. About half of people with AIDS will be allowed to use AZT in this trial. The rules about who can and cannot get AZT can seem bizarre; and physicians are not allowed to override them even when urgently necessary for the best interest of the patient. We here reprint the entire patient selection criteria, normally sent only to physicians, so that you can tell in advance whether you or a friend probably would or would not be allowed to use AZT at this time. And we spotlight some urgent ethical issues of this trial, and what the community can do to promote more rational and humane treatment development in the future.

Note:

• This article looks at who has the option to use AZT, not whether it is wise to do so. Surprisingly few patients have chosen to sign up so far.

This author's bias is to favor AZT, but with strong reservations. It clearly has saved lives; the latest statistics (November 12) are three deaths in the AZT group, in the double-blind study just completed, compared to 30 with the placebo. AZT can cause serious side effects; about 25 percent of the patients who have received it so far have needed at least one blood transfusion, often many transfusions. Doctors and scientists are seriously concerned that there may be unknown long-term dangers, but no one has yet used AZT long enough to know whether there will be such problems or not. The drug is not a cure, but a treatment that needs to be continued indefinitely, until something better is available. We will know more about AZT when detailed results of the recently completed study are released.

• Anyone considering AZT should know about alternative AIDS treatments—none of them yet recognized by U.S. medicine. Ribavirin is the closest to being recognized. Other articles by this author have documented five treatment possibilities with strong scientific indications that they might be helpful, but with little medical attention or testing so far: these are DNCB, AL 721, BHT, naltrexone, and glycyrrhizin. I reviewed these treatments because they have been largely unknown or ignored, and urgently deserve more attention.

In addition, persons with AIDS and ARC have tried many treatments including herbs, other Chinese medical approaches, vitamins, nutrition, exercise, and healthy emotions and attitudes. Typically, those who have survived in reasonably good health for three years or longer after an AIDS diagnosis have tried many different approaches and put together their own individual programs out of the ones that worked for them. You can learn more about these alternatives through organizations such as the San Francisco AIDS Alternative Healing Project (an organization that refers people with AIDS or ARC to holistic practitioners or to relevant books and articles; see Appendix B). A new book, *Psychoimmunity and the Healing Process* (edited by Jason Serinus, published by Celestial Arts) discusses many of these options.

• The rules on who can get AZT apply only to the current study. There will be other studies, with different rules. And when AZT is licensed, physicians will be able to prescribe it whenever it is in their patients' best interest.

We have heard reports that better forms of AZT, equally effective but much less toxic, have been developed but not yet tested on humans; the decision may be to rush these through testing instead of making AZT itself generally available. If these reports are true, the bad side of the good news is that licensing could be delayed.

• The current study will not use a placebo; everyone will get AZT. Some future studies probably will use a placebo, usually for patients less severely ill, probably to see whether the benefits of AZT as an AIDS preventive outweigh its side effects and dangers.

• Although the current study provides the AZT without charge, patients will still be billed for visits, for required lab tests, and for any treatments required for side effects caused by the AZT. Insurance companies might not pay these costs, because the treatment is considered experimental.

At a public forum on AZT, sponsored by Mobilization Against AIDS in San Francisco, Paul Volberding, M.D., chief of the AIDS Activities Division at San Francisco General Hospital and one of the foremost experts on AZT and on the treatment of AIDS, said that MediCal would pay for these costs for persons with AIDS (ARC is a separate problem). He thought that other states would pay through comparable programs (all these programs are tied to Federal standards). He thought it was likely that private insurance companies would be willing to pay, when they realized that the alternative would be to pay much greater costs due to the progression of AIDS.

When AZT is licensed, it will be available through physicians without arbitrary restrictions, but it will no longer be free. Probably it will be very expensive.

Who Can Get AZT Now?

Physicians who want to use AZT must obtain a packet of instructions and paperwork; they can get this information by calling the AZT hotline. Anyone can call for AZT information, but the packet sent to non-physicians contains little detailed information.

Here are the patient selection rules, sent to physicians:

3.0   Patient Selection

3.1   Inclusion Criteria

3.12   AIDS patients who have recovered from one or more episodes of histologically confirmed pneumocystis carinii pneumonia without AIDS-defining conditions(s) (see MMWR May 23, 1986) presently requiring systemic chemotherapy.

3.13   All patients must have a Karnofsky performance status >= 60 at entry (see appendix I).

3.14   Laboratory parameters—All patients will have the following present at entry:

     a.   Total granulocyte count >= 1000/cubic millimeter

     b.   Hemoglobin >= 9.0 gm/dl

     c.   Platelet count >= 50,000

     d.   SGOT <= 3 times upper limit of normal value e. Serum creatinine <= 1.5 mg/dl. (or upper unit of normal)

     f.   Positive antibody for HTLV-III/LAV confirmed by any federally licensed ELISA test kit.

3.2   Exclusion Criteria

3.21   Patients younger than 12 years of age.

3.22   Pregnant women, nursing mothers or women of childbearing potential not employing barrier contraception or abstinence.

3.23   Patients receiving any potentially myelosuppressive drug (such as trimethoprim-sulfamethoxazole (Septra—ed), pyrimethamine-sulfa or DHPG), nephrotoxic agent (such as amphotericin B or aminoglycosides), or cytotoxic or other experimental chemotherapy for any reason.

There is no section 3.11.

Comments on Patient Selection

• Persons with ARC are excluded, even though they were included as part of the last study. This decision might be due to limited supplies of the drug; we have heard conflicting reports on whether or not there are supply problems.

It is possible that persons with ARC benefitted less from AZT than persons with AIDS, in the last trial. We don't know because very little of the results have yet been released. We have heard that while AZT greatly reduced the death rate compared to the placebo, it had only a small effect on the number of opportunistic infections, and was not very good either at getting rid of the virus or at restoring the immune system.

- Persons with KS but not pneumocystis are excluded. Again we don't know why, although in the very earliest test, with 19 patients, AZT seemed less helpful for the 5 patients with KS.

A new study now being planned will test AZT on some persons with KS. The plans call for using low and high dose groups, and a placebo.

- The blood counts are apparently required because a prominent side effect, in some patients, is a reduction in these counts, probably due to bone-marrow damage.

But even with rational medical justification, these rules still presents ethical problems. They demand a blanket exclusion which ignores everything about the individual case, shutting the patient and physician out of any role in the decision.

Children and the Disabled

The innocuous-sounding "Karnofsky performance status" rule (in the inclusion criteria) excludes anyone ill enough to be disabled. The Karnofsky scale rates how sick a person is; it goes from 100 (no evidence of disease) to zero (dead). The level 60, required to get AZT in this trial, is "requires occasional assistance but is able to care for most of his needs." Anyone more seriously ill cannot get AZT at this time.

It is hard to find any medical grounds for this exclusion. AZT has shown good results in people who have been seriously ill. These are the people who have the most need for the drug and the most reason to risk its dangers.

Volberding thought that one reason for excluding the seriously ill might have been fear of biasing the study. If people took AZT and died anyway, the licensing authority might think that AZT had killed them.

(We would suggest separate categories in the study to avoid that problem, essentially giving AZT on a compassionate basis to those will now be excluded because they are too ill. But it looks like the real bottom line is cost, as the manufacturer would be paying to provide the drug without getting back the data it wanted to support licensing. Regulations do not allow patients themselves to reimburse this cost.)

The automatic exclusion of children also makes no sense from the viewpoint of patients' welfare. It may stem from scientific and administrative convenience. AIDS is different in infants, so their results might need to be analyzed separately. And including children would force dosage to be calculated by body weight, whereas the current study gives the same dose to everyone, allowing all the pills to be the same.

Whatever the reasons for these exclusions, an all-too-obvious political reality makes it easier to get away with them. The disabled are too ill to organize much protest in their behalf. And of children with AIDS, 80 percent are black or Hispanic, often of impoverished parents who acquired AIDS from needles. These parents are unlikely to generate effective protest or political pressure for their children.

Humane Treatment and Medical Ethics

The handling of AZT shows how patients are treated when the medical-regulatory system completely controls the only recognized promising treatment for a deadly disease.

- Life and death decisions are simply announced with no input whatever from most of the persons affected, or their physicians.

- Secret plans go through secret regulatory review, then get approved as a unit. Therefore short of an act of Congress, it is seldom possible to negotiate any change after the plans become public. Too many different organizations would have to sign off on the change.

- The decisions of who does or does not get experimental drugs are not made primarily for the patients' benefit, but for the convenience of those most influential in the conduct of the trials. Corporate profit comes first, since without the money incentive the tests would never happen at all. Then come the needs for institutional and administrative convenience, clean data, and elegant science (whether necessary or not for the emergency at hand). All these take priority over getting the medicine to persons who need it.

- During the placebo trials recently completed, a serious, repeated argument for denying AZT to ten thousand people with AIDS was to force a few hundred into the placebo study as their only chance to get the drug (*Discover* magazine, August 1986, p. 78). Experimenters feared that they wouldn't have subjects if people could get AZT any other way.

- Congress appropriated 47 million dollars to make AZT available to people with AIDS. But only about half of them will be able to get it. Did Congress intend that children under 12, and anyone ill enough to be disabled, would be automatically excluded from receiving AZT?

- Where did the money go? Burroughs-Wellcome says that AZT is very expensive to produce. Maybe so—but without a public accounting, we cannot know.

The "cost" of a project like this, carried out within the ongoing operations of a large organization, can easily depend more on accounting decisions than anything else. For example, capital expenses such as plant construction may serve both this and other projects; how do they get allocated? Chemical companies often do batch runs which in a few days may produce a year's supply of a substance—leaving the equipment free for other uses the rest of the time.

- The real information usually gets withheld from the public, which instead gets whatever PR insiders choose to put out. For example, people are deciding whether or not to sign up for AZT, and at this time they cannot now get the results of the study just completed. These results should be released immediately, not wait for publication delays so that some medical journal can enhance its reputation.

What Can We Do?

- Organizations can influence treatment policy, and they need our support.

For one example, take Mobilization Against AIDS (MAA), which organized the recent public forum with Volberding. According to Paul Boneberg of MAA, in July 1985 they were the only organization to call for a massive increase of Federal AIDS research funding to 500 million dollars in fiscal year 1987 (beginning October 1986). MAA successfully converted the other AIDS organizations, and then many members of Congress, to support massive increases.

The House Budget Committee scheduled hearings in five cities, and AIDS was not on the agenda. In four of those cities, the local AIDS organizations did not know that the hearings were coming. MAA got them to organize an AIDS presence at the hearings, and call for the 500 million.

In January of this year professional lobbyists were saying that massive increases for AIDS research were impossible because of the budget crisis, and that it would be a miracle to avoid cuts. Friends in Congress thought it was irresponsible to demand the impossible from them. But Congressional committees discussed amounts from 500 million down. And the final result was over 400 million dollars appropriated for the current fiscal year, up from about 220 million the year before.

This victory represents the work of many people and organizations. The unique contribution of MAA was to put the massive increases on the agenda.

You can help in future projects by contacting Mobilization Against AIDS (see Appendix B) and offering your support.

• The best way you can contribute is to get involved in the organization or project of your choice, enough to learn what is going on. Financial support is urgently needed; and since AIDS organizations are typically very efficient in their use of funds, your contribution can go a long way.

• The recent report of the National Academy of Sciences, entitled "Confronting AIDS," is a milestone in the development of a serious national commitment against AIDS. We can all work to make sure that its recommendations are followed. (A copy of the report can be ordered from the National Academy of Sciences; see Appendix B.)

• Today we are seeing the beginnings of a sensible attitude toward AIDS in the national mainstream—reflected, for example, in the Surgeon General's report, the recent CBS documentary, and the National Academy of Sciences report mentioned above. Still needed, though, is a humane and rational approach to treatment development. Persons with AIDS or ARC, and their physicians, need much more influence in the conduct of human trials, so that the interest of the patient will be represented.

• Perhaps we could form alliances with those concerned with other diseases, such as Alzheimer's, on treatment issues. Alzheimer's disease is as severe as AIDS, and affects millions of people. Recently a major breakthrough discovered an effective treatment (not a cure), but red tape threatens to delay it for years. The discoverers are still trying to get a patent on pharmaceutical use of the chemical—which has been known for decades—so that some drug company will get interested and then begin the long process of obtaining Federal approval. Nothing can justify so cruel and unworkable an approach to providing treatment for a fatal disease.

We also need a national commitment to test the simple AIDS treatment possibilities like DNCB and BHT—relatively safe, well known in human use, inexpensive, easy to use, readily available or easy to manufacture, unproven because they have not been well tested, but overwhelmingly supported by all available information as likely to be helpful, although not a magic cure.

As AIDS becomes a mainstream issue, the gay community will have a crucial role in pointing out what is actually going on, and making sure that the newly-minted institutional commitment gets translated into effective action.

Issue Number 19
December 5, 1986

SHIITAKE, LENTINAN, AND AIDS/ARC

Update 1989: A study of lentinan as an AIDS treatment, which should have started no later than 1984, started instead in 1989. This small trial in San Francisco, funded by a Japanese company, does not reflect any U.S. commitment to control the epidemic, but rather Japan's commitment to become the world leader in biotechnology.

Shiitake is a kind of edible mushroom traditionally cultivated in Japan, and now used as a delicacy in cooking throughout the world. Lentinan, a substance found in shiitake, has important effects on the immune system, and is now widely used in Japan for treating cancer. Recently there has been increasing interest in medicinal use of shiitake or the lentinan derived from shiitake, as well as other medicinal mushrooms that contain different active ingredients, as possible treatments for AIDS or ARC.

Published medical studies, mostly from Japan, strongly suggest that lentinan may be valuable. But U.S. physicians cannot obtain the medicine, because of bureaucratic and commercial barriers—a situation unlikely to change soon since apparently no formal research is being conducted on AIDS and lentinan in the U.S., in Japan, or anywhere else.

Meanwhile, the mushrooms are available in grocery stores, and health-food stores sell shiitake extracts. Researchers believe that lentinan could be effective orally if used properly. However, much of the commercial-product literature does not reflect information obtained from the scientific studies and medical trials. Anyone using lentinan should know what has been learned about how it should or should not be used.

This article will discuss the Japanese use of lentinan with cancer and with a single case of ARC, and mention some of the many immune effects of this substance. Then we will look at the shiitake preparations available now in the United States, and what should be known about using them.

In this article we can only touch on the very large subject of immune potentiators and antivirals from medicinal fungi.

Lentinan and Cancer

Japanese physicians have used highly purified lentinan as an immunotherapy in clinical trials with hundreds of patients with gastric and other cancers. Study after study found that lentinan combined with chemotherapy worked better than chemotherapy alone. For a review of the immune effects of lentinan, and its use in cancer treatment, see Aoki, 1984 (reference below). Tadao Aoki is the world's leading authority on the medical use of lentinan. Dr. Aoki has repeatedly urged that lentinan be tested for ARC or AIDS.

Early animal studies of lentinan found no anticancer effect; later, scientists realized that the cause of this failure was that too large a dose had been used. With a correct dose, lentinan caused complete regression of certain cancers in mice (see Aoki, 1984). The doses which failed were ten to 80 times too large, suggesting that the effective range may not be too critical.

Lentinan has many immune effects. Researchers are now most interested in its enhancement of "natural killer" (NK) cells, which, like T-cells, are a subgroup of white blood cells. Lentinan can also increase gamma interferon production.

One study found that lentinan alone was not very effective in treating human cancer. For better results, doctors combine it with chemotherapy. The lentinan should be started first (Aoki, 1984).

In both humans and animals, lentinan did not work if there was a protein deficiency (Akimoto, 1986).

Physicians have found that to get the greatest effect, they should avoid giving lentinan every day. Aoki, 1984, suggested a dose of 1 mg twice a week. More recently, this dose has been given every other day.

Doctors usually administer lentinan by injection, either intravenous or intramuscular. It can also be taken orally, but about five times the dose is required.

We can find just one published case of lentinan used to treat KS. The patient, an 84 year old man who also had lung cancer, did not have AIDS. The KS lesions quickly improved, and disappeared in a couple months (Aoki et al., 1981).

Lentinan and AIDS

There is only one published case where doctors used lentinan for treating AIDS or ARC. But this case is crucial, because a person with ARC became antibody negative and remained that way even without the drug. She also improved clinically and is in good health today, two years later.

The published report of this case appeared two years ago in The Lancet (Aoki et al., Lancet). The researchers also released a more detailed report (Aoki et al., Proceedings). This writer learned of the current status through private communication.

The patient, apparently exposed to AIDS by a transfusion, had grown progressively weaker, and repeatedly tested positive for AIDS antibodies. The T4 count was under 300, and other blood tests also suggested ARC.

One mg per day of lentinan was given daily for five months; at that time the doctors did not know that giving it less often would be more effective. The patient's condition improved, and the blood counts went in the right direction. The T4 count reached about 500, although the T4/T8 ratio declined because the T8 count increased faster.

After four months, the AIDS antibody test became negative and remained that way. Two years later, the patient is healthy. We do not know recent blood counts.

Political Problems

Obviously this case should be followed up, especially since lentinan has no serious side effects. But two years after publication in one of the most widely circulated medical journals, we know of no other person with AIDS, ARC, or a positive test who has received lentinan, anywhere in the world. U.S. physicians cannot obtain the drug; Japanese physicians can use it, but they have few AIDS/ARC patients.

At this time, the Bristol-Meyers corporation has an option to buy U.S. license rights to lentinan. We have heard that they have applied to the U.S. Food and Drug Administration for an IND—permission to test an experimental drug—but have not yet received it. We do not know whether Bristol-Meyers is interested in AIDS; the obvious commercial use for lentinan would be for treating cancer. Even if they are interested in trying it as an AIDS treatment, it could take years before it even gets tested on a handful of patients.

The U.S. National Institutes of Health could obtain lentinan and test it, but so far has shown little interest. A colleague of Dr. Aoki sent a thousand doses to Dr. Anthony Fauci, director of the National Institute for Allergy and Infectious Diseases, but received no reply. Perhaps the package got lost in the mail.

The U.S. National Cancer Institute has added lentinan to a list of over 80 drugs which people have suggested as possible treatments for AIDS. Its AIDS Drug Selection Committee plans to consider whether or not to follow up.

What's Available Now?

It may be possible to get lentinan treatment abroad.

We have heard conflicting reports about whether persons known to have AIDS, ARC, or a positive antibody test can enter Japan for medical treatment, or for any other reason. The Japanese consulate was non-committal, which suggests that there may be a problem, and that we might not find out until someone tries to go.

It may also be possible for clinics in Mexico or other countries to buy lentinan from Japan.

Another approach is to develop this treatment from available materials, outside of the official research system. The shiitake mushrooms, which contain lentinan, and various extracts sold in health-food stores, are readily available.

Researchers believe that lentinan can be effective when taken orally, if five times the injected dose is used. In November 1986, Dr. Aoki visited the U.S. National Institutes of Health and reported on the treatment of 59 patients for an immune deficiency called low natural killer cell condition; they received intravenous lentinan in the hospital, then took maintenance doses orally as outpatients. The natural killer cell activity improved greatly, an effect likely to be important for treating KS and other cancer.

What we don't know is how much lentinan is in the mushrooms or the commercial preparations. We don't yet know of any company which has tested its material and calibrated its pills or powder so that users know what they are getting. The chemical test is not available commercially, but could be done in a university lab.

It is important that the products be tested, because too much lentinan can be not only ineffective, but harmful, because it can have the opposite of the intended effect. In one of the cancer studies, overdoses ten times too high markedly depressed the immune response (Aoki, 1984). But side effects of proper doses, which can include skin rashes and a feeling of heaviness in the chest, are rare and not serious when they do occur (Aoki, 1984). They clear up when the lentinan is stopped.

Lentinan is "heat stable" (Aoki, 1984), which probably means it survives normal cooking. One paper reported 30 cases of skin rashes and itching, seen by dermatologists over nine years, caused by eating shiitake as an ingredient of oriental cooking (Nakamura and Kobayashi, 1985). The dermatologists believe that these effects were caused by lentinan, suggesting that it may be possible to get an effective dose through normal use of shiitake as food. Shiitake has long been a folk medicine for cancer in Japan and other Asian countries; and until U.S. physicians can get lentinan, traditional ways of using the mushroom may be the best available.

Much of the commercial health-product literature for shiitake preparations fails to inspire confidence. One flyer claims that its shiitake tablet "may be effective" for "allergy, hypertension, liver trouble, tumor, kidney trouble, post-operative discomfort, lymphnode, infectious hepatitis (B) (sic), collagen disease, rheumatism, gout, diabetes mellitus, gonorrhea, AIDS, common cold or flu, loss of energy". Another suggests what might be called the Godzilla theory of medicine:

"It is believed that the mycelium in the earth had the strength to push its way through a thick layer of concrete. Obviously, if this tremendous power could be utilized for the good of the human body, amazing results could be expected."

People facing death deserve better. We can let the public and professionals know the importance of this potential AIDS/ARC treatment, and the fact that it has been neglected for two years for no medical or scientific reason. A medicine known to be safe, easy to use, and outstandingly effective in the single case tried, at least deserves a second look. If more people were close enough to AIDS treatment research to know what is going on, they would insist that some way be found through the red tape and commercial obstacles which now block testing of some of the most promising treatment leads.

REFERENCES

Akimoto, M., T. Nishihira, and M. Kasai, "Modulation of the Anti-Tumor Effects of BRM Under Various Nutritional or Endocrine Conditions," *Gan To Kagaku Ryoho* 13(4/part 2) (April 1986), pp. 1270–6 (English summary).

Aoki, T., "Lentinan," IN Fenishel, R.L., and M.A. Chirgis, editors, *Immune Modulation Agents and Their Mechanisms* (New York and Basel: Marcel Dekker, Inc., 1984), pp. 63–77.

Aoki T., H. Miyakoshi, Y. Horikawa, and Y. Usuda, "Staphage Lysate and Lentinan as Immunomodulators and/or Immunopotentiators in Clinical and Experimental Systems," IN Hersh, E.M., M.A. Chirgis, and M. Mastrangelo, editors, *Augmenting Agents In Cancer Therapy* (New York: Raven Press, 1981), pp. 101–12.

Aoki, T., H. Miyakoshi, Y. Usuda, J.C. Chermann, F. Barre-Sinoussi, R.C. Ting, and R.C. Gallo, "Antibodies to HTLV I and III In Sera From Two Japanese Patients, One With Possible Pre-AIDS," *The Lancet* (October 20, 1984), pp. 936–7.

Aoki, T., H. Miyakoshi, Y. Usuda, R.C. Ting, and R.C. Gallo, "Lentinan Treatment of Japanese Cases Infected With Human T-Lymphotropic Retroviruses HTLV-I and -III)," *Proceedings of the Sixth*

Symposium on Rationale of Biological Response Modifiers In Cancer Treatment (August 31–September 1, 1984), Hakone, Japan.

Nakamura, T., and A. Kobayashi, "Toxicoderma caused by the edible mushroom shiitake *(lentinus edodes)*," *Hautarzt* (October 1985), pp. 591–3 (English summary).

Wakui, A. *et al.*, "Randomized Study of Lentinan on Patients with Advanced Gastric and Colorectal Cancer," *Gan To Kagaku Ryoho* (April 1986), (English summary).

Issue Number 20
December 19, 1986

SUPPRESSOR CELLS
AND ALTERNATIVE AIDS/ARC TREATMENTS

Last week, researchers at the University of California San Francisco (UCSF) published two landmark scientific papers on AIDS; summaries appeared in last week's San Francisco *Sentinel*. One of the papers (Walter *et al.*, 1986) reports a finding likely to be one of the most important of the year. This article examines the impact on this finding on two alternative treatments—DNCB, and lentinan.

The UCSF paper did not mention these treatments; and we did not discuss this article with the scientists. Statements made here are solely the responsibility of this writer.

The UCSF researchers decided to study why only some people infected with the AIDS virus become ill, while many others remain healthy. They unexpectedly found that the suppressor T-cells of the healthy individuals prevented the virus from growing. In several different laboratory tests, the virus could grow in helper T-cells from those persons, but only if the suppressor cells were removed.

This finding surprised the scientists, since normally suppressor T-cells have an opposite function. Instead of attacking invading organisms, they turn off the immune response initiated by the helper T-cells, restoring the normal balance after the immune reaction has done its job. But now we know that these same suppressor cells also stop the growth of the AIDS virus directly (although they do not kill it). The scientists suspect that they stop the virus by secreting some chemical, currently unknown.

Jay Levy, M.D., head of the research team at what is widely considered one of the three leading centers for basic AIDS research in the world, described the new finding as "the first indication that individuals have in themselves a means of controlling the virus."

Implication for Alternative Treatments

Mainstream science and medicine, on one hand, and "alternative" AIDS treatments on the other, have unfortunately kept apart, forming two different worlds which seldom talk seriously with each other. The UCSF paper does not discuss alternative treatments; it may have been necessary to omit them in order to keep credibility or even to be published in the mainstream world. The UCSF paper could only suggest the potential treatment of growing a patient's suppressor cells outside the body and then putting them back in—an idea likely to take years before it is ready for widespread use.

But meanwhile, the UCSF findings explain better than ever before how certain alternative treatments are working. They highlight the urgent need for research institutions to take these treatments seriously, and test and develop them quickly.

DNCB and Lentinan

For in-depth information about these alternative treatments, see earlier articles in this series: "DNCB AIDS/ARC Treatment," (Issue Number 14) and "Shiitake, Lentinan, and AIDS/ARC," (Issue Number 19). Here the important fact is that both treatments greatly increase T-cell counts.

The T-cell subset blood tests report T-4 (helper-inducer) and T-8 (suppressor-cytotoxic) counts. A low helper/suppressor ratio can be used as an early warning of trouble, but today researchers are learning that this ratio can be misleading, especially in monitoring the effectiveness of a treatment. The actual cell counts are more important than the ratio.

With DNCB treatment, what commonly happens is that both cell counts go up, but at first the suppressors increase faster. The ratio looks like it is getting worse; but later the helpers go up, and the ratio moves toward normal.

The new UCSF finding makes possible a good guess at what is happening. The treatment itself causes all T-cells to increase. But at first the helper T-cells increase only slowly, because the AIDS virus, which infects only these helper cells, keeps killing them—either directly, or by provoking the body's own immune system against them. The suppressor cells keep increasing, however, until there are enough of them to stop the virus. Then the helper cells can increase, and the ratio improves.

Another alternative treatment, the drug lentinan, derived from the shiitake mushroom and now well accepted by physicians in Japan to increase T-cells for cancer treatment, showed this effect to a spectacular degree in the only case where lentinan has ever been tested for AIDS or ARC. Before treatment, the helper/suppressor ratio had decreased to .92, and the helper T-cell count was 172. During several months of lentinan treatment, the ratio continued downward to .37; but meanwhile the helpers had risen to 597. During treatment, the patient went from positive to negative on the AIDS antibody test (from just above to just below the line in the test being used). Two years later she is in good health—and does not need to continue using lentinan. (The absolute test values, and current condition of the patient, were not published but obtained by this writer through private communication.) A reasonable guess at what happened here is that the lentinan treatment pushed this patient over the line from someone on the way to developing ARC and/or AIDS to someone whose suppressor cells could stop the virus.

Suppressor Cell Levels in AIDS/ARC

If suppressor cells can stop virus growth, why do some people with AIDS or ARC have a high T-8 (suppressor-cytotoxic) count?

An earlier UCSF study carefully analyzed T-cell subsets in healthy volunteers and persons with AIDS (Stites *et al.*, 1986). Most of the T-8 cells are the cytotoxic kind, not suppressors; and the study found that the cytotoxic cells appeared to be responsible for most of the T-8 increase in AIDS. In other words, the high T-8 count may not be due to large numbers of suppressor cells.

If correct, this hypothesis would be good news, because it leaves open the possibility that there is nothing wrong with the suppressor cells in persons with AIDS or ARC. All that is needed to stop the virus may be to increase their numbers—which DNCB, and lentinan also, can do.

The new UCSF finding does not completely answer the question why some persons infected with the virus get AIDS or ARC while others do not. But a reasonable guess is that, although the suppressor cells can control the virus, the body lacks a systematic way of mobilizing this defense. Indeed the feedback mechanism may work in the wrong direction with a virus like AIDS, which attacks the helper T-cells. Since suppressor cells normally respond to helper cells, killing the helper cells may also reduce the number of suppressors, reducing the ability to stop the virus.

If this hypothesis is correct, the human defenses against AIDS may be balanced on a knife edge. Often the suppressor cells can keep the virus in check. But if for any reason the virus gets a start, it could indirectly reduce the number of suppressors and allow the virus to multiply further.

The obvious therapy would be to use a treatment to mobilize the suppressor-cell defense.

A handful of physicians have used DNCB for treating AIDS and ARC, for as long as two years. While they have had very good results both in blood counts and clinically, it is also clear that DNCB alone is not enough for everybody. Some patients may also need an antiviral. And some have very high levels of immune globulins, and it is not known whether these will eventually return to normal. Other treatments may be needed in combination with DNCB.

AIDS Research Politics

At this time several leading AIDS researchers want to do a clinical study of DNCB. They have not been able to get funding.

Lentinan, the other T-cell growth treatment, is not available in the U.S. One company has an option to license it here, but has not said whether it is interested in AIDS or ARC. Others are kept away by the license restrictions. The U.S. National Cancer Institute has put lentinan into a suggested-treatment file for eventual consideration by a committee.

It is all too clear that AIDS treatment research will not be handled properly until there is a political demand every step of the way. To build an effective demand, AIDS organizations and others must pay attention to treatment research issues; virtually none have yet done so. The experts can do the job, but we must reduce the political and institutional obstacles in their path.

Alternative Information Now

For DNCB information you can call Jim Henry (see Appendix B). Lentinan is found in the shiitake mushrooms, and Japanese scientists have learned that the drug can be used orally. The problem is that we don't know how much is in the mushrooms, and too much can have the opposite of the intended effect and be worse than useless. We do know that lentinan should not be used every day; every other day, or every fourth day, have worked better.

Traditionally, shiitake has been a folk remedy in Japan, part of the Oriental tradition of medicinal foods. Traditional cooking recipes may give the best available information about how much of the mushroom to use, and how to prepare it. We asked Misha Cohen at Quan Yin Acupuncture and Herb Center in San Francisco to recommend a cookbook; she suggested *Aveline Kushi's Complete Guide to Macrobiotic Cooking,* by Aveline Kushi, published by Warner Books. You could also contact the Gay Macrobiotic Network in San Francisco (see Appendix B).

REFERENCES

Stites, D.P., C.H. Casavant, T.M. McHugh, A.R. Moss, S.L. Beal, J.L. Ziegler, A.M. Saunders, and N.L. Warner, "Flow Cytometric Analysis of Lymphocyte Phenotypes in AIDS Using Monoclonal Antibodies and Simultaneous Dual Immunofluorescence," *Clinical Immunology and Immunopathology* 38 (1986), pp. 161-77.

Walter, C.M., D.J. Moody, D.P. Stites, and J.A. Levy, "CD8+ Lymphocytes Can Control HIV Infection in Vitro by Suppressing Virus Replication," *Science* (December 19, 1986).

Issue Number 21
January 2, 1987

AL 721, AND THE DEADLY SILENCE

Update 1989: Michael May, who was interviewed here, died of AIDS-related cryptosporidiosis in the summer of 1988.

The statement below was written by a friend of mine who was near death from AIDS in early 1986, but now is healthy. His experience adds urgency to the increasing weight of scientific evidence suggesting that AL 721 can be a major help to some people with AIDS or ARC. (This treatment, extracted entirely from egg yolks, could legally qualify as a food; it has no known side effects or dangers. It is easy to make and inexpensive.)

Why can't you get AL 721? Why has Federal research funding effectively black-listed safe, promising treatments available now, such as AL 721, DNCB, and lentinan? I don't know.

Why haven't physicians and their professional organizations informed themselves about treatments like AL 721, and insisted on rational public policies for research and availability? Here the answer seems clear.

In the past, most physicians have not considered it part of their job to learn about, let alone use or advocate, unapproved or experimental treatments. But today we have an emergency where the Federal government has abdicated its responsibility to research the most promising treatments available now. Treatment research has been driven almost entirely by commercial motives which, due to the costs and complexity of getting any new drug approved in the United States, necessarily favor high-tech, novel, patentable treatment options—the very ones unlikely to be available for years.

Since malpractice insurance seldom covers use of unapproved treatments, physicians naturally are reluctant to recommend or use them. But the bigger problem, and our focus here, is that physicians and medical organizations have refused to even look at those treatments they have refused to use. Apparently the medical profession has avoided this conflict between the welfare of their patients and their own need for insurance protection. It is easier to insist, even against the evidence, that there are no workable treatments available, that everyone with AIDS will die. This view gets them off the hook, but becomes a self-fulfilling prophecy.

Parents of a child with AIDS obtained AL 721 from an Israeli physician. But the child's U.S. physician, an AIDS specialist, said that he would withdraw from the case if the child used AL 721, since he knew nothing about the treatment. The parents gave the medicine away.

AIDS organizations, too, have shirked their duty to study treatment issues and then advocate in the interests of persons with AIDS. For example, although the San Francisco area has 50 AIDS organizations, only two, to my knowledge, have taken any steps whatever to inform themselves or anyone else about AL 721, and very few have worked to change public policy to make this and other treatments more available.

Again it's not hard to see why. To involve themselves in public policy issues concerning non-approved treatments, after physicians had refused to do so, would embarrass the medical profession, from which funding agencies take their cue. An atmosphere has developed where it is safe to hold the hands of the dying, but risky for organizations to even study the treatments available now which all available evidence suggests are likely to save lives.

Consider another possible treatment: BHT (see Issue Number 10) In every laboratory and animal test, it has inhibited every lipid-coated virus against which it was tested, including herpes, CMV, and many other viruses; in the laboratory it was especially effective against CMV, an opportunistic infection which causes many deaths of persons with AIDS. Agricultural scientists studied BHT after its use as a feed preservative caused vaccination failures, apparently by blocking the action of live-virus vaccines; the scientists found that BHT in the diet protected animals against major diseases caused by lipid-coated viruses.

The AIDS virus is lipid coated, and therefore probably vulnerable to BHT. BHT crosses the blood-brain barrier. It's use in humans (as a food preservative) is well known, and the risks are small. It is inexpensive and readily available in high-quality form prepared for human use. Obviously this highly promising treatment deserves scientific testing for AIDS or ARC, but nothing whatever has been done. Both the medical profession and the AIDS organizations have maintained an eerie, near-total silence about this failure to follow up on one of the most promising treatment possibilities we have.

Journalists are eager to report on AIDS treatment neglect and mismanagement. But most news organizations forbid their employees to cover medical-treatment stories until after they are published in medical journals.

And so some of the best treatment research leads have fallen between the cracks.

Why wait for history to record that many deaths were unnecessary, that another holocaust happened because so many were silent?

We can make a change. All that's needed is to get people involved in treatment research issues, closely enough so that they can make independent judgments and decisions. The facts are so compelling that if only people knew what was happening, improvement would be inevitable.

The following statement is by a person with AIDS who has used AL 721 for most of a year. While we know that testimonials do not prove a medicine effective, we published this one for several reasons. First, years of the most reputable laboratory study have strongly suggested that AL 721 might work for treating AIDS or ARC, especially for persons who do not have KS or other cancers; early results of clinical trials are highly encouraging. Second, so little human testing has been done that every case adds significantly to our knowledge. And third, we don't present this case as proof, but as an urgent attempt to bring the treatment to wider medical and public attention. U.S. physicians and their patients should be allowed to use it now, especially since it is entirely safe, instead of being told to wait months or years for more studies. The biggest obstacle to availability is that worldwide licensing restrictions have kept everyone away from AL 721 except for one small company, which has not chosen to market it in any country at this time.

"My Illness"

"I noticed a difficulty with my health during the summer of 1985. I had a painful separation from a job. My energy dropped. I attributed it to mental depression.

"During the fall I suffered with strange illnesses: an ear infection that wouldn't respond to antibiotics; athlete's foot; frequent colds. In January of 1986 I had the worst 'flu' of my life, and it wouldn't go away. Toward the end of the month I developed a tightness in my chest and a bad cough. Then I went to the doctor. The ELISA test, T-lymphocyte subsets, and a viral culture confirmed what I did not want to hear. AIDS.

"I was given Bactrim for the pneumocystis, and the cough abated. But my strength was gone. I could no longer work. During February and March, I developed painful sores. A fungus spread to my legs and arms. My skin was scaly, with red blotches. I had fits of perspiration at night; I had fevers. I couldn't eat; I became thin. Worst of all was the generalized feeling through my body that I was dying. Indeed, I was dying."

"My Treatment With Active Lipids (AL 721)"

"At this time a good friend of mine—an Israeli citizen—was doing some investigation on my behalf. She discovered a treatment developed at the Weizmann Institute of Science in Rehovot, Israel. By express mail she sent me a most remarkable document—a letter full of promise. As I read it, my condition had deteriorated to the point where I had hardly the strength to breathe. I knew my death was imminent.

"So I took a leap of faith—I had nothing to lose anyway. After writing goodbye letters to my friends and loved ones, I was taken, in a wheelchair, to the El Al plane, along with my mother and my closest friend. I don't know how I endured that long flight. My Israeli friend met the plane, and took us to our hotel.

"The next day I began treatment with AL 721, a potent form of lecithin which makes your cell membranes resistant to viral attacks. It is derived from egg yolks. AL 721 looks and tastes like butter; you spread it on your bread and eat it morning and evening. My Israeli doctor said to me, 'The Americans don't like our treatment. It's too simple for them.'

"During the first week of treatment there was no change in my condition. The three of us were planning how to deal with a corpse so far from home. But after two weeks of treatment, lo and behold! I did feel stronger. My diarrhea seemed less severe. I began to eat. During the first month I gained some weight.

"I consumed these Active Lipids through April, May, and part of June. When I came back to the U.S.A. I walked off the plane—no more wheelchair. I continued my treatment by taking a heaping tablespoon of granulated lecithin mixed with a raw egg yolk daily. During June my T-4 count continued to rise, even without the Active Lipids. My sores and skin rashes disappeared.

"By the end of August, however, the T-4 numbers were heading down again. Since AL 721 is not available in the U.S.A., I once again flew to Israel. Another month of treatment lifted my T-4 number significantly."

"Post AIDS"

"In February and March my moribund condition had forced me to let go of my plans, my hopes, my loves, my career, my possessions, and life itself. The pain was unspeakable. When it came over me that some unfathomable hand of fate had determined that I would not die, but live, I became semi-hysterical. I remained that way through most of the summer. Why should I have been allowed to receive this miraculous treatment when it had been denied to so many others?

"As I write this, I have no more physical symptoms. The infections have gone; the night sweats have stopped; I have no more fevers. I am able to eat again, and my weight is close to normal. The last symptoms to disappear were the red blotches and scaling on my face. In October these, too, went away.

"I am trying to make sense of all this. I tell my story in hopes that it may help someone. I remain easily excitable. When you have been to Auschwitz and survived, I think you never get over it."

Issue Number 22
January 16, 1987

RIBAVIRIN. PEPTIDE T.

Update 1989: Small, scattered tests of peptide T are still beginning, two and a half years later.

Update 1987: PEPTIDE T. A report on the four near-terminal AIDS patients treated in Sweden with peptide T appears as a letter in The Lancet *(January 17, 1987), page 159. This half-page letter mentioned that there was no clinical deterioration or weight loss during the test. Central nervous system measurements (by magnetic resonance imaging) improved substantially. One case of psoriasis improved and was in complete remission four weeks after the peptide T treatment was ended. Lymphocytes increased, in one case sixfold. There was little or no problem with side effects.*

This letter also specifies the doses used and frequency of administration.

Meanwhile, we are hearing by word of mouth that top researchers are especially interested in peptide T and the approach it represents.

RIBAVIRIN NEWS AND CONFUSION

Last week the manufacturer of ribavirin released key results from a double-blind study of that drug's effectiveness in preventing persons with lymphadenopathy syndrome from progressing to AIDS. Although questions remain, the results are good.

Unfortunately much confusion grew from the ribavirin announcement. The extensive media reports have not told what is going on.

The announcement, by ICN Pharmaceuticals of Costa Mesa, California, at a Washington, D.C. press conference, essentially consisted of six numbers. Of 56 patients who received a placebo, ten developed AIDS in the 24-week trial. Of 55 who received 600 mg per day of ribavirin, six developed AIDS. Of 52 who received 800 mg, none developed AIDS.

These results raised two questions. First, few physicians believe that the difference between 600 and 800 mg could be as significant as these results suggest; therefore we should not assume that 800 mg dose was completely effective, because it is more likely that the fact nobody at all progressed to AIDS was partly due to lucky chance. Also, the total number who developed AIDS in the first two groups was much higher than would be expected, and no one knows why.

While the scientists' work continues, people must make life and death decisions. There is little doubt that these results taken as a whole add powerful support to the already powerful case that ribavirin can be an important treatment for some patients. Still, you have to get it in Mexico, and physicians are reluctant to advise you to do so.

Behind the Scenes

Here is some background information we have not seen reported:

Last-minute change.   The January 9 (1987) press conference had been planned to announce not only the results above, but also Federal approval of an extended IND (investigational new drug) application. ICN already has an IND for ribavirin, which gave it permission to use the drug in the trials mentioned above. The new IND would have allowed much larger trials, probably with thousands of patients, under a detailed protocol somewhat like the one used for AZT. In fact, the FDA agreed to handle ribavirin like AZT, in order to treat the two manufacturers equally.

But unexpected events days before the press conference prevented final completion and approval of the plan. ICN and the FDA quickly agreed, one day before the press conference, that the company would go ahead with the announcement but release only the principal result at this time.

Unfortunately, the ensuing confusion in the first day's media reports made everyone look bad. ICN appeared to be raising false hopes in order to promote itself, by getting front-page publicity for partial results which left important questions unanswered. And the widely circulated report in early editions of the January 10 *New York Times* implied that both ICN and the FDA were passing the buck; it quoted ICN as saying it had no plans to make ribavirin available until the FDA approved, and quoted the FDA as saying that ICN had not submitted a formal request for approval. Technically both statements are true, but a well-placed source reports that the agency and the company are in fact working well together, that together they have produced a plan for large-scale distribution which came within a hair's breadth of release on January 9, and that the plan is now under review and likely to be released, possibly in as little as two weeks.

The ARC study.   The results given January 9 concerned only persons with lymphadenopathy. A separate part of the same study tested whether ribavirin could prevent development of AIDS in persons more seriously ill with ARC. These results are expected shortly—along with the release of the plan mentioned above. We have heard that 24 of the ARC patients developed AIDS, but we don't know the breakdown of the 24 into the three treatment groups (placebo, 600 mg, and 800 mg).

Dosage. Some people believe that 1000 or even 1200 mg would be better than 800, for those persons who can tolerate that much. Apparently almost everyone can tolerate 800; we heard that no one had to be taken off the ICN study due to side effects, and no one needed a transfusion.

Ethical Issues

The gay community and others involved with AIDS must address and clarify certain ethical issues concerning experimental treatments.

False hope or false hopelessness?   Is it raising false hope to spread good news about promising but as yet unproven treatments? Or is it false hopelessness to teach people to ignore new developments and prepare for death?

The conventional approach is to leave treatments to the experts until they are proven safe and effective and released for marketing. But we should remember that final proof and approval take years even after a drug has proven itself well enough to get many scientists, physicians, and investors behind it.

The other way is to run with every reasonable treatment lead until we know whether or not it works. The risks are often very small, and in any event they must be balanced against the risks of doing nothing. AIDS has killed perhaps a thousand times more people as all the experimental treatments put together. And any published results help doctors and scientists develop better treatments in the future. Why give up on all new treatments just because several have been disappointing?

Publicity and secrecy.   Researchers have been criticized when they report results to the press and public, rather than through medical journals or meetings. But it takes months to get published in a medical journal, and during this time most journals insist that the results be kept secret from the press and public, and therefore also from most scientists and physicians. This secrecy enables journals to make a splash in the news when their issues come out, but it has seriously slowed AIDS and other research. This research depends on public interaction among scientists who may be in different lines of work and unable to communicate privately since they do not personally know about many others who are doing work relevant to them.

In recent years the public has shown an unprecedented interest in and demand for detailed medical knowledge. Books like the *Physician's Desk Reference* have become bestsellers. This trend is part of the growing movement for persons to take more responsibility for their health, instead of leaving it to the experts.

Persons with AIDS and ARC and their physicians must make treatment decisions, including decisions about unapproved treatment options. It is wrong to withhold the information they need.

Availability.   Ribavirin has been sold for human use for 12 years. It is now approved in about 40 countries, including many in Western Europe and elsewhere which have sophisticated drug-testing requirements. For over two years, growing evidence has suggested that this broad-spectrum antiviral might be useful for AIDS.

Now ribavirin has shown good results in a major double-blind placebo trial. Still, U.S. physicians cannot prescribe it, and patients must get it in Mexico. This is inexcusable.

The U.S. drug-approval system reflects the interests and needs of giant pharmaceutical companies far more than the interests and needs of persons with AIDS. Government drug approvals have in fact become corporate assets, like patents, licenses, stocks, and other forms of wealth. This web of vested interests, not concern for patients' welfare, has controlled the regulatory response to the AIDS emergency. Corporations which played by the rules, and earned their drug marketing approvals at the cost of tens of millions of dollars each, would object to the government now giving quick and free summary approvals to their rivals. Consider, for example, the current Federal decision to treat ribavirin and AZT equally, although one has been in routine human use for 12 years while the other is brand new and known to have serious risks. Corporate interests, not patients' interests, came first.

This system will continue to deny medically sound treatments to persons who are seriously ill until medical associations, patients' organizations, and other public-interest groups start advocating far more forcefully for patients' rights to treatment, telling Congress, the media, and others that the current system which purports to protect the welfare of patients is in fact undermining it.

We can start by remembering the third of the Four Moral Appeals of the ARC/AIDS Vigil:

"We appeal to the FDA to immediately allow American physicians to prescribe medicines and treatments for ARC and AIDS that are available to their colleagues in other countries."

PEPTIDE T

An experimental substance called "peptide T" may represent a major research breakthrough, and it could be available soon for human use.

Peptides are short chains of amino acids (the building blocks of proteins). Peptide T is a chain of eight amino acids, namely AlaSer-Thr-Thr-Thr-Asn-Tyr-Thr (using conventional three-letter abbreviations). The name came from the fact that four of the eight amino acids happen to be threonine (abbreviated 'Thr', or 'T').

Scientists discovered the above formula by computer matches of protein sequences in the AIDS virus and elsewhere, and then they synthesized peptide T in the laboratory.

Peptide T seems to be the small piece of the AIDS virus which attaches to a receptor site on the surface of the helper T-cell. The virus must attach to this site in order to infect the cell. Apparently peptide T attaches instead, preventing the virus from doing so.

In laboratory tests, extremely small amounts of peptide T reduced infection of human helper T-cells. Slight variations of the peptide could greatly improve or diminish its effectiveness. The best variant inhibited AIDS virus infection at concentrations of about one part in ten million. The researchers see this result as only the beginning of the development of a whole new class of treatments for AIDS and other conditions.

Peptide T has already been given to four terminally ill AIDS patients in Sweden; their condition improved and all are still alive. According to the Public Affairs Branch of the Office of Scientific Information, National Institute of Mental Health (NIMH), the NIMH together with the National Institutes of Health have applied to the U.S. Food and Drug Administration for an IND (approval to use an investigational new drug), and hope to begin human trials very soon. The spokesperson did not know of any funding problems or any other barriers which would prevent the trials from starting as soon as the IND is approved. However, another official at NIMH said that animal toxicity tests would be needed first.

More information about peptide T can be found in the highly technical article published in the *Proceedings of the National Academy of Sciences* (December 1986). A description appeared in *The New York Times* (December 16, 1986), page 18. The results of the test with four patients in Sweden will be published in *The Lancet* (January 17, 1987).

The public, through its AIDS, medical, and other public-service organizations, must continue to watch the development of peptide T, as well as other treatment research. In the past, too many promising AIDS treatment leads have been strangled in red tape or left on the shelf to collect dust instead of being tested promptly. Only continuing public vigilance can make sure it doesn't happen again.

Issue Number 23
January 16, 1987

AEROSOL PENTAMIDINE:
NEW PCP PROPHYLAXIS AND TREATMENT

Update 1989: We believe this is the first article ever published about aerosol pentamidine. The FDA approved this treatment in June, 1989.

AIDS Treatment News has learned of a new treatment which may be a major advance in preventing pneumocystis in persons with AIDS. About 100 patients in New York and 30 in San Francisco are now using this experimental therapy, but so far there has been little publicity and most physicians are unfamiliar with it. Until the current trials are finished, the treatment must be considered unproved; but so far it appears to be close to 100 percent effective in preventing pneumocystis, with few if any side effects.

(Meanwhile, a completely separate study in San Francisco is now enrolling patients for aerosol pentamidine treatment after pneumocystis has already been diagnosed. For more information, see below. It is important to start this treatment early.) The new prevention procedure was developed by Edward Bernard, M.D., and other investigators; he is a researcher in infectious diseases at the Memorial Sloan-Kettering Cancer Center in New York, where the aerosol pentamidine prophylactic treatment has been used for about 11 months. Due to the great demand and a huge waiting list to get into the study, the Sloan-Kettering team has provided information to other physicians who are interested.

In San Francisco, Pacific Presbyterian Medical Center is treating about 30 patients with the aerosol pentamidine prophylaxis. While the treatment is not generally available at this time, physicians can probably find ways to obtain it for their patients when necessary.

Rationale of Aerosol Pentamidine

Pentamidine has been used for over 40 years as an anti-parasite drug. In Africa, it was learned that one treatment every six months could prevent sleeping sickness. Ten million people have used the drug; due to the duration of its effect, it has been called "the chemical vaccine." The reason for the long-lasting protection is that pentamidine stays in the tissues and is eliminated very slowly.

Pentamidine is effective against pneumocystis, but when sufficient amounts are given in the conventional way, by IM or IV injection, it can cause severe side effects. Studies have shown that only a very small portion of the injected drug reaches the lungs. Much more of it goes to the liver, kidney, spleen, and other organs, where it is useless for preventing pneumocystis and may cause toxicity.

To deliver the medicine more selectively to where it is needed, researchers tried administering it by a very fine aerosol spray which could be inhaled deeply into the lungs. They tested the treatment with animals first, because the drug had never before been given in that way, and there is little experience with using aerosols for any infection. Aerosol pentamidine did reach effective levels in the lungs, and very little went to other organs. Even ten times the effective dose showed no evidence of harmful effects in the animals. The half-life of the medicine in the lungs—the time required for half of it to disappear—was 35 days, meaning that one treatment every two weeks could maintain a reasonably constant drug level.

How Is the Preventive Treatment Used?

Every two weeks, patients come to the clinic and inhale the medicine from a machine called a nebulizer, which produces a very fine spray. Sloan-Kettering uses an ultrasonic, hand-held model; it is known in the clinic as "the green machine." For safety, the Sloan-Kettering team provides a separate machine for each patient; it imports them from West Germany for investigational use. Patients administer the medicine at their own pace. The treatment takes 15 to 30 minutes.

For the first month, treatment is used once a week, to build up protection quickly.

How safe and effective is the preventive use of aerosol pentamidine? In the Sloan-Kettering study with about 100 patients so far, a few mild cases of pneumocystis occurred in the early stages of treatment, before the researchers began starting patients on a once a week schedule for the first month to build protective levels quickly. After the change to the new schedule, there have been no cases at all in anyone on the treatment. And as far as we know there have been no side effects.

Of course this treatment has no effect on the underlying AIDS infection or immune deficiency, so for continued protection it must be used indefinitely. Also, the aerosol treatment cannot protect against other opportunistic infections which are not in the lung, a factor which should be considered before other preventive treatments are discontinued.

What Happens Next?

The Sloan-Kettering team wants above all to get this treatment thoroughly tested and approved, so that any physician can prescribe it; they are working with the U.S. Food and Drug Administration toward this end. But usually it is necessary to do a double-blind placebo trial as part of the approval process. The Sloan-Kettering researchers do not want to use a placebo, and have not done so. To get approval without a placebo trial requires a much stronger showing than usual. The researchers are trying to prove that the treatment is at least 95 percent effective in preventing pneumocystis. Getting conclusive proof of safety and effectiveness is especially complicated because many of the patients have other opportunistic infections or KS, and many are also using other treatments such as AZT.

For More Information On Prevention

Because this treatment is experimental, some researchers at least don't think it is quite ready for routine use in physicians' offices, and instead prefer to see it used at a medical center or university hospital, where institutional review boards provide additional protection for patients.

In San Francisco, a number of pulmonary specialists are familiar with the aerosol pentamidine treatment. Other physicians can consult with them about where to obtain it for their patients.

Almost nothing about this treatment has appeared in print, except for two brief references in the abstracts of the Paris AIDS conference last June (poster sessions number 300 and 294). In three months, a medical journal will report on the early animal studies at Sloan-Kettering. The team presented the earliest report of its work at a March, 1986 meeting of the American Society for Microbiology. It issued a press release at the time, but apparently nobody picked it up.

Aerosol Pentamidine To Treat Pneumocystis

A completely separate group of researchers has developed an aerosol pentamidine treatment for use after pneumocystis has already been diagnosed. Two hospitals in San Francisco are now ready to accept patients. As far as we know, the treatment is not yet available outside of San Francisco.

Some of the researchers at Sloan-Kettering doubt that aerosol pentamidine would be effective after pneumocystis has developed; they fear that congestion would prevent the medicine from reaching the parts of the lung where it is most needed. However, a team of researchers at the University of California San Francisco Medical Center carried out numerous animal studies and found that aerosol pentamidine could be highly effective if pneumocystis was present but in its less severe forms. Some of the animal results were published in the January 1987 *Antimicrobial Agents and Chemotherapy.* Although these studies used rats, the results are likely to apply also to humans, because in previous experiments, the effects of new treatments on pneumocystis in the rat have been highly predictive of their effects in humans.

Robert Debs, M.D., the principal investigator in the animal studies, calls pneumocystis the perfect disease to treat by aerosol, because the infection is in the air spaces at the end of the airways, where the medicine goes, and ordinarily it does not occur outside of the lung.

Two hospitals within the University of California San Francisco system have received approval from the FDA and are currently enrolling patients with established pneumocystis pneumonia for treatment with aerosol pentamidine. Treatment will be given once a day for fourteen days; each administration takes about half an hour. There is no control group; everyone enrolled will receive the drug, and the results will be compared with recent studies of IV pentamidine or septra. Physicians may contact either Bruce Montgomery, M.D., at San Francisco General, or Jeffrey Golden, M.D., at Moffitt. If physicians suspect that pneumocystis is present, it is important to enroll the patient early for this treatment.

Acknowledgements

We wish to thank Edward Bernard, M.D., of Memorial Sloan-Kettering Cancer Center in New York, Robert Debs, M.D., of University of California San Francisco Medical Center, Robert Fallat, M.D., of Pacific Presbyterian Medical Center, San Francisco, and two patients who must remain nameless, for their assistance with this article.

Issue Number 24
January 30, 1987

HOW TO MAKE AL 721

Five weeks ago I published a report that Americans could receive treatment in Israel with AL 721, an experimental AIDS/ARC medicine developed in that country at the Weizmann Institute of Science. Since that time the research project which accepted Americans has been shut down, as a result of pressure from within the U.S., so the treatment is no longer available.

What is the politics behind this shutdown of AIDS research and treatment? Not only have individuals lost a treatment option, but also the highly esteemed immunologists working at Weizmann have lost learning opportunities. The political answers are unclear, but the following sketch, which we have not been able to confirm, seems to reflect the understanding of those close to the situation:

• The patent licensee which owns the rights to AL 721 in the U.S. and many other countries is Praxis Pharmaceuticals, Inc., of Beverly Hills, California. Tiny by drug-industry standards, this public company has only six employees, according to its "10-K" disclosure form. This company strongly objected to the use of AL 721 in Israel to treat American patients.

How can a U.S. company shut down some of the AIDS research at the world-famous Weizmann Institute? Why can't the public policy of the United States find a way to make an exception to business as usual during the AIDS emergency?

• Praxis is seeking approval from the FDA to market AL 721 for AIDS and other diseases. But this small company faces an uphill fight because much larger and more influential corporations have their own AIDS treatments on the Federal agenda. Apparently there are important Federal officials who want AL 721 to never be approved, because they are committed to other treatment approaches instead. The owners of Praxis are apparently very concerned that any protest or publicity, such as could be generated by Americans traveling to Israel to receive treatment there when it is unavailable here, could deprive them of the allies they do have in the FDA, and kill the AL 721 treatment regardless of medical or scientific merit.

Praxis has been outspoken in telling Congress about certain problems in the Federal management of AIDS research, and it may have suffered as a result.

* It is believed that there is no chance whatever for FDA approval until well into 1988—over a year from now—even though the medicine is known to be completely safe and there is nothing to lose by trying it.

If the above reports are true, then all the communities concerned with AIDS have a decision to make. Should we put this issue on the public agenda to try to change national policy, to demand that saving lives be given a higher priority, or keep quiet to avoid risking further damage to AIDS treatment research and development?

AL 721 Quick Background

AL 721 was first developed at Weizmann as a medicine for other diseases, long before its possible relevance to AIDS was known. The U.S. patent (number 4,474,773, October 2, 1984) does not mention AIDS. AL 721 may be the first of a new class of medicines using what has been called "membrane engineering"—modifying cell membranes to achieve treatment goals. AL 721, which consists entirely of a mixture of three lipids (fats) found in ordinary food, increases the "micro fluidity" of cell membranes, by increasing the ratio of phospholipids to cholesterol. Increased membrane fluidity makes it harder for viruses to attach to receptor sites and enter the cell.

The meticulously careful and thoroughly documented scientific work which developed the theory behind AL 721 is illustrated by the two-volume book *Physiology of Membrane Fluidity,* edited by Dr. Meir Shinitzky, a cancer researcher at the Weizmann Institute and the principal developer of AL 721, and published by CRC Press, Boca Raton, Florida.

The first reference to AL 721 and AIDS was in a letter to the *New England Journal of Medicine* (November 14, 1985), by several researchers including Robert Gallo, M.D. and Dr. Prem Sarin of the U.S. National Cancer Institute. The letter reported that AL 721 could prevent the infection of human T-cells by the AIDS virus in the laboratory. Theory suggests that in addition to AIDS, AL 721 might also help against other lipid-coated viruses, such as herpes, CMV, and Epstein-Barr. It was found to be effective against herpes in one animal test, reported October 1986 at a symposium in New Orleans.

Since AL 721 had been known to be safe and had previously been tested in humans in Israel, it would seem that the encouraging laboratory results with the AIDS virus would quickly be followed by clinical tests. But in the 14 months since the laboratory report was published, we only know of eight people who have received AL 721 in clinical trials, all mildly ill lymphadenopathy patients at St. Luke's/Roosevelt Hospital Center in New York. The results were encouraging, with large reductions in viral activity (about 80 percent) in five of the seven patients for whom measurements were available. Tests with AIDS patients are now about to begin. (We had heard that this study was full, but now it is rumored that it may be expanded. We don't know whether or not a placebo will be used.) One person who was near death from AIDS a year ago and is now in good health after AL 721 treatment wrote about his experience (*AIDS*

Treatment News, Issue Number 21). The treatment works slowly; it took two weeks to feel any effect, and months before T-cell counts rose significantly. Probably the treatment must be continued indefinitely.

The picture emerging is that AL 721 can be effective as an antiviral for many people, but that therapy might be improved by also using an immune treatment, such as a thymus hormone, after the virus infection had been slowed or inactivated.

AL 721 is not a cure, not a magic bullet, although it probably can save lives and restore many people to health. Since there are no dangers or drawbacks to AL 721, there is no justification for stopping people who want to use it.

AL 721 Formulas

We publish the following to open doors. There are three approaches to making AL 721: a laboratory formula, a substitute which can be made at home, and new methods likely to be available soon.

AL 721 is easy to make in a laboratory, but companies cannot do so openly because they could be sued for patent infringement. Also, no useful instructions for making the substance have previously been published. The U.S. patent, and also a published scientific paper, give two different procedures for making AL 721, but neither of them is useful in practice. So this writer obtained professional assistance in expanding the sketchy instructions disclosed in the patent into the formula given below. The patent applies in many but not all nations, so it would be legal to make AL 721 in some countries, and legal to advertise openly that Americans or others could go there for treatment. No one has yet set up such an operation as of this writing.

The substitute home formula was developed by a chemist in the New York City area in January 1987, and distributed at AIDS support meetings there. It is made by mixing butter or cooking oil with a concentrated lecithin formula widely available in health-food stores and in some drugstores. The proportions of the three ingredients of AL 721—phosphatidyl choline, phosphatidyl ethanolamine, and neutral lipids— are not exact but are well within the range of at least one set of specs for the official product. However, there are slight chemical differences between ingredients derived from eggs (used in AL 721) and those from the other sources used here. There is no known reason why this home substitute could not work like AL 721. Every expert I have spoken to suspects that it probably will work, at least to some extent; but nobody has proven that it will.

The third approach is based on special food products not yet entirely available. Just before press time, this author learned of a suitable egg lecithin now being sold in the U.S. at a reasonable price ("Phosphatidyl choline 60 percent from egg yolk", which also contains about 30 percent phosphatidyl ethanolamine); but unfortunately the chemical company which sells it does not allow any of its products to be used for human consumption.

Neutral lipids would need to be added; butter or cooking oil could be used as in the home formula. But it would be better to obtain neutral lipids from egg yolks as described in a scientific article on AL 721 (Lyte and Shinitzky, "A Special Lipid Mixture for Membrane Fluidization," *Biochimica et Biophysica Acta* 812, (1985), pp. 133-8). When food companies can supply both the egg lecithin and the egg neutral lipids, which would be entirely legal to do and technically easy, then it will be possible to make a product virtually identical to AL 721 in anyone's kitchen.

There are no known problems in combining this food with any other AIDS drug or therapy.

AL 721 should be stored frozen, and moved to the refrigerator a few hours before use. It should not be allowed to stand at room temperature, as the components may separate; for best absorption they should remain well mixed when the product is used. AL 721 should be taken on an empty stomach, preferably in the morning and/or evening, with little or no fats eaten for at least two hours afterwards. Each dose is 10 grams of the lipids.

Patients should discuss any treatments they are using with their physicians. At this time few physicians are familiar with AL 721.

AL 721 Laboratory Formula

Caution: the process below uses highly flammable materials and must be done with proper facilities. This is *not* a home recipe.

We have combined this information from many sources, and have *not tested* the version written here. We publish this information as a starting point for professional development, *not* as a guaranteed method ready for use.

Use of this formula in the U.S., and in some other countries, may infringe patent rights.

1. Dissolve 4 grams of tocopherol acetate (vitamin E) in 40 ml of ethanol, add this to 40 liters of acetone and combine with 20 liters of hen egg yolks. Mix five minutes at room temperature. We believe that dried yolks can be used.

2. To the solid material produced in step 1, add 40 liters of acetone and 800 ml aqueous solution of 0.1 M CaCl2 and 0.1 M MgCl2. Bring to 47 degrees C for one hour, while mixing thoroughly. Filter *while hot*, and discard the solids.

3. Cool to −20 degrees C for at least 16 hours; the AL 721 precipitates. Filter with a metal mesh, discard the liquid. Transfer the product to an evaporation vessel of about 5 liter capacity, and mix with 4 grams of tocopherol acetate dissolved in 40 ml of ethanol. There should be 1.5 to 2 Kg total at this step.

4. Evaporate the solvent in the 5 liter flask by using a water pump for 1 to 2 hours, then an oil pump for 2 to 6 hours. In the final step, put the container in a water bath at 40 to 50 degrees C., to help in evaporating the solvent. Mix the final product well. About 1 to 1.4 Kg of AL 721 should be produced—enough to last one person for at least 50 days.

5. Quality control:

a. The final product should contain about 70 percent neutral lipids (including 2 to 4 percent cholesterol), 20 percent phosphatidyl choline, and about 7 percent phosphatidyl ethanolamine. At room temperature the product will separate into two phases, with the neutral lipids on top. Part of the upper layer can be removed if necessary to adjust the proportions.

b. Acetone in the final product should not be more than 300 ppm.

c. To help avoid bacterial contamination, pasteurized egg yolks are used. Store the product at −20 degrees C.

AL 721 Substitute—(Home Formula)

The following instructions have been distributed at PWA meetings in New York. The text has been slightly changed here. More information is available by calling the phone number below.

PC-55™ is a high-strength lecithin concentrate made by Twin Laboratories, Inc., Ronkonkoma, New York. It contains two of the three ingredients of AL 721; they are in a 5:2 ratio, close to the 2:1 used in AL 721. Neutral lipids can be added to PC-55™ making it a membrane fluidizer comparable to AL 721. This material is a food nutrient, it is not a drug. It is safe.

Combine five tablespoons of PC-55™ and 12 tablespoons of water in a bowl, and whip with an electric mixer or blender. Slowly add 6 tablespoons plus one teaspoon of butter which has been melted (measure the butter before melting). Whip thoroughly three to five minutes. This mixture divided into ten even doses gives slightly over 10 grams of the lipids per dose. Each dose should weigh about 30.4 grams or 1.06 ounces.

The individual doses can be placed into plastic sandwich bags for freezing. If you don't have a scale, you can measure out two tablespoons to each bag, then add a much smaller amount to divide the remainder. One person separates the doses in an ice-cube tray. Move each dose from the freezer to the refrigerator a few hours before use. This preparation spoils very rapidly at room temperature; it must be frozen unless used immediately.

(An earlier version of this formula used cooking oil instead of butter. The proportions are 5 tablespoons PC-55™, 5 tablespoons + 1 teaspoon oil, and 10 Tbsp water.)

The material is best eaten in the morning, spread on fat-free bread or mixed with fruit juice. The user should eat a fat-free breakfast which might consist of fat-free cereals, skim milk, fruits, or vegetables. There are no restrictions on lunch or dinner. An additional dose might be taken before going to bed. Patients treated in Israel are given two doses a day for about four weeks, then single doses for most of one year. Some people with AIDS might experience diarrhea with this membrane fluidizer, especially with the additional dose. Eat brown rice and other solid foods.

You can help others and yourself by keeping a record of your experience—doses, dates, and any resulting effects.

Issue Number 25
February 13, 1987

CHINESE FU ZHENG THERAPY:
THE IMMUNE ENHANCEMENT PROJECT

Fu Zheng is a traditional Chinese herbal therapy now being used by modern Chinese physicians in combination with radiation and chemotherapy for treatment of cancer. Major studies in China have found that this combination can work better than the Western methods alone. Fu Zheng therapy helps to overcome the immune deficiencies caused by the chemotherapy or radiation.

By 1986 the well-known U.S. herbalist Subhuti Dharmananda, Ph.D., had developed a theory of immune enhancement based on principles of traditional Chinese medicine. He brought this work to the attention of herbalists Susan Black and Jay Sordean, C.A., who developed a protocol for a test to see if this approach could be helpful to persons with ARC or AIDS. In 1986 the Immune Enhancement Project, led by Susan Black, a student of Dr. Dharmananda, began the test. The first persons are now completing the six months planned for the trial. The results so far have been very good, better than expected by those who designed and conducted this study.

The Immune Enhancement Project is not the only group using this treatment. But as far as we know it is the only one which is keeping extensive records to support publication of results.

How the Study Was Done

Participants learned about this study through small notices published in the San Francisco *Sentinel*, *Bay Area Reporter*, and *Coming Up!*, or through an article in the *Daily Californian* last summer. Many others found out by word of mouth. Everyone who expressed interest in joining the study received a four-page detailed health questionnaire. The 85 persons who returned the questionnaire were screened, and 35 were invited to participate.

Those selected had to have a positive antibody test or known exposure to the AIDS virus, as well as symptoms consistent with the criteria for ARC/AIDS used by the U.S. Centers for Disease Control. They had to make a six-month commitment to the project, and agree to keep records and be available for periodic checkups. No other Oriental herbs could be used, but Western treatments were okay; for example, three participants began using AZT during the six-month study.

At first, this project planned to work only with persons with ARC. But two people developed pneumocystis while waiting for the study to begin, and they were allowed in. Later, a few other persons with AIDS were also accepted. However, only those who had ARC but not AIDS at entry to the study were included in the statistics. No one progressed from ARC to AIDS after the herbal supplements were started.

The basic protocol called for two herbal combinations, each available as commercial products. One is Astra-8™, a formula designed by Dr. Dharmananda, in accordance with traditional Chinese usage, for strengthening the immune system. The other is Rei-Shi-Gen™, a preparation from the shiitake and ganoderma mushrooms, from Cascade Mushrooms in Portland, Oregon.

Chinese medicine treats each patient uniquely, more so than Western medicine, which often uses a prescribed regimen for a particular disease. The two combinations above were only a starting point; the amounts used could be varied as required, and many other herbs might also be added. So once a month the participants met as a group with the herbalist, to adjust each person's regimen as required; participants could also reach the herbalist between meetings if necessary. These meetings became general support groups, in which people could discuss their experiences with various kinds of treatments.

Because of the frequent need to vary the herbs as each patient's condition changed, the Immune Enhancement Project does not recommend trying fu zheng without a practitioner. However, since usually it is necessary to meet the practitioner only once a month, clients may find it feasible to travel to do so, if they cannot find anyone qualified locally.

Each month participants also filled out a questionnaire consisting of a lengthy check-list of symptoms. They could mark each symptom with one, two, or three checks, or leave it blank. Three checks meant that the condition was a primary problem for them. Two checks meant that it was a problem, but not primary at that time. One check meant that the symptom existed but was not significant.

At the time of this writing, the only results tabulated are the three-check symptoms analyzed for the first three months, for the 20 persons with ARC who had completed three months by the time of the tabulation. (Participants entered the study at different times.) From the dozens of symptoms asked about in the questionnaire, the 19 which caused significant problems are listed in the accompanying table. This table shows the number in the group of 20 patients who listed each symptom as a primary problem on entry into the study, after one month, after two months, and after three months.

Results

The 20 ARC patients showed improvements in almost all of the tabulated symptoms. In reviewing this table, the herbalist commented that fatigue and lymphadenopathy showed perhaps the biggest changes. In addition, diarrhea and night sweats were virtually eliminated as problems. Sinus problems have increased again (not shown on this three-month table); here fu zheng may have had least effect.

One of the goals of the study was to enable patients to reduce antibiotic use, to prevent possible suppression of the immune system. Eleven of the 20 patients were using antibiotics at the start of the study, compared with only one at three months.

Note that the table lists night sweats along with other symptoms such as insomnia, frequent urination, and vivid dreaming. In Chinese medicine, all these conditions are considered signs of "yin deficiency." It turned out that when one of them disappeared, the others did also.

This study could not give regular T-cell subset tests, due to financial constraints. But of the six participants who were tested as a result of their participation in other studies, all showed increases in T-4 counts. Only one of these six appeared to be explainable as a result of treatment received elsewhere. The Immune Enhancement Project hopes to follow up with a funded study which can measure T-cell subsets systematically.

Financial

This study charged participants only for the cost of the herbs, less than $50 a month. A sliding scale reduced this charge below cost in case of need. The herbalist's time was donated. It may not be possible to provide services below cost in the future.

The Institute for Traditional Medicine and Preventive Health Care (Dr. Dharmananda's group) provided a grant of $250 per month, and a private donor occasionally contributed several hundred. The grant that started the project came from the Peoples' Life Fund of the War Tax Resisters League.

The Immune Enhancement Project hopes to obtain funding of about $50,000 for a larger study with 50 people and with extensive blood testing.

For More Information

The best single background paper about the treatment used in this study is "Chinese Herbal Therapies for the Treatment of Immunodeficiency Syndromes," by Subhuti Dharmananda, Ph.D., published by the Institute for Traditional Medicine and Preventive Health Care (see Appendix B). This article is an extensively revised version of Dr. Dharmananda's "A New Herbal Combination for the Treatment of Immunodeficiency Syndromes;" the earlier article was published in the *Pacific Journal of Oriental Medicine* (Spring 1986), pp. 20–30.

Several recent papers on fu zheng have been published in Chinese. Most of these appeared with English abstracts, but we have not been able to obtain the abstracts by press time.

The Immune Enhancement Project will publish the complete results of its study in the *Oriental Healing Arts Journal*. Articles may also appear in other journals.

Fu Zheng Therapy Results: 20 Patients With ARC

SYMPTOM	BEGIN	1 MO	2 MO	3 MO
Fatigue	17	4	5	2
Diarrhea	5	1	1	0
Constipation	2	0	0	1
Weight Loss	1	0	0	0
Nausea	2	0	2	0
Gastrointestinal	1	0	0	1
Hairy Leukoplakia	2	1	0	0
Night Aberrations (sweats, frequent urination, insomnia, vivid dreaming)	9	7	0	1
Lymphadenopathy	20	5	2	3
Sinus Problems	13	3	4	4
Oral Fungus	8	1	1	0
Skin Problems	7	1	1	1
Leg/Knee Weakness	5	0	0	0
Tumors	3	0	1	0
Herpes	5	1	1	0
Neurological Changes	1	0	0	0
Emotional Instability	6	3	3	1
Antibiotic Use	11	0	1	1

This table shows the number of patients, from among the 20 with ARC who had completed the first three months of the study, who listed each symptom as a primary problem on entry to the study, and after one, two, and three months. Reduction in antibiotic use is also shown. No one progressed to AIDS.

Issue Number 26
February 27, 1987

COENZYME Q: NEW KIND OF IMMUNE MODULATOR?

Coenzyme Q, a naturally occurring substance found in many foods and necessary for life in every cell of the body, is sold in pure form in capsules in most health-food stores. No scientific studies have tested it as a treatment for AIDS or ARC. But animal studies have shown that coenzyme Q might be a new kind of immune modulator. It may not increase the total number of T-cells. But correcting a deficiency of coenzyme Q, which may develop especially in illness, can make each cell more effective and may restore the balance between different types of T-cells. Coenzyme Q also has other, better known medical uses, and a history of beneficial synergy when used together with certain other treatments.

No toxicity or harmful side effects have ever been reported; safety has not been an issue. This treatment possibility appears to have no drawbacks or dangers. But since persons with AIDS can respond to treatments in unexpected ways, safety cannot be guaranteed until medical tests have been done. Unfortunately we cannot find any evidence of plans or preparations to test coenzyme Q in the treatment of AIDS or ARC.

What Is Coenzyme Q?

Coenzyme Q, abbreviated "CoQ" (pronounced "co-cue") and also known as ubiquinone, is like a vitamin; many ordinary vitamins in fact work as coenzymes. However, CoQ does not meet the technical definition of the word "vitamin", because the body can produce its own supply in some cases.

Like vitamins, CoQ is essential to life. It plays an essential role in the complex series of biochemical reactions by which cells perform respiration and release energy. A 25 percent deficiency can cause disease, and a 75 percent deficiency can cause death. But if there is already enough CoQ, taking more will not help.

Only one form of coenzyme Q, namely coenzyme Q-10, is used in human metabolism, and by most other vertebrates. Other animals and plants may use other forms,

such as Q-9, Q-8, etc. The numbers refer to the length of a chemical chain which is part of the molecule.

In the body, the highest concentration of CoQ is found in the heart—not surprisingly, since CoQ allows cells to release energy, and cells of the heart must release abundant energy. High concentrations are also found in the liver, and in the cells of the immune system. The heart, and probably also the liver and immune system, are especially vulnerable to CoQ deficiency. The need for CoQ may increase during illness.

The most concentrated "natural" source of CoQ readily available in the American diet is beef heart and other red meat. Spinach, peanuts, and some other foods also contain significant amounts.

For many years CoQ was a laboratory curiosity, after its discovery in 1957, because of the expense of purifying it from sources such as beef hearts. But today Japanese companies have learned to produce large amounts cheaply, using micro-organisms in a fermentation process. Japan is the undisputed leader in the development and use of CoQ, and the only country to produce it in quantity.

Medical Uses

In Japan, over ten million people use CoQ as a prescription medicine, usually for the treatment or prevention of heart disease. Major scientific tests involving a total of thousands of heart patients have found that CoQ helped over 70 percent of them. These people had serious illnesses such as congestive heart failure and angina.

One double-blind heart disease study found "extraordinary clinical improvement" in patients who had been "steadily worsening and expected to die within two years under conventional therapy" (Langsjoen and others, 1985).

In the U.S., CoQ is not approved as a prescription medicine for any purpose—although it is sold over the counter in health-food stores. We interviewed Emile Bliznakov, M.D., a leading CoQ researcher and author of the only popular book on the subject (see reference below). He emphasized that the U.S. Food and Drug Administration is not the problem, and does not oppose efforts to get CoQ approved. Today CoQ is in "phase II" clinical trials, meaning large-scale tests of its effectiveness (not for AIDS or ARC, however). The time required for phase II depends on "money and organization". Since no major pharmaceutical company is pushing for U.S. approval for CoQ, the trials must be done piecemeal, through small-scale tests at universities and research institutes. Fortunately the FDA today will sometimes accept evidence from foreign studies; it used to require these tests to be repeated in the United States.

Since CoQ occurs naturally in foods, U.S. law permits it to be sold over the counter, but only without medical claims. Most doctors don't use unapproved treatments, however, so few of the patients who could benefit from CoQ have heard about it. We have a confusing situation of a completely safe, probably lifesaving medicine which patients can find out about and use on their own, but usually not through their doctors.

CoQ has also shown dramatic results in treating periodontal (gum) diseases. It has been used in cancer treatment, mainly to reduce heart damage caused by the anti-cancer medicine adriamycin. It shows promise for reducing high blood pressure, and for helping some people lose weight. Researchers are testing CoQ as a treatment for several other diseases, including muscular dystrophy and allergies or asthma, but its effectiveness is unknown.

Some people are using CoQ in the hope that it could extend the human lifespan. Obviously no human proof is available, but an animal study found that CoQ extended the lifespan of mice up to 50 percent. The treated animals remained youthful looking during that time. CoQ becomes deficient in aging animals, and supplying it can correct much of the immune deficiency which develops in aging. CoQ is also a strong antioxidant, like vitamin E, and believed to be highly effective in neutralizing free radicals.

Dr. Karl Folkers, one of the world's leading researchers on CoQ, has proposed the term "diseases of bioenergetics" for conditions which result from lack of sufficient energy release in the metabolism of cells.

Immune Effects

Unfortunately most of the research on immune effects of CoQ stopped around 1981. What we do know from the several animal studies which had been done by then suggests that this treatment deserves another look.

A 1981 paper by Dr. Bliznakov (see reference below) reviewed some of these studies, and stated several conclusions:

• A number of different measurements, including resistance to viral and parasitic infections, showed that CoQ was an immune modulator; it was especially effective when given with other drugs.

• Animals could develop deficiencies of CoQ during illness, and/or during aging.

• The effects appeared to be due to increased activity of existing cells, not an increase in the number of cells.

• Dose can be important. No toxic effects have ever been found, even at high doses. But certain other immune modulators can become ineffective or even counterproductive if very large amounts are used, and CoQ might behave similarly.

• Since no harmful side effects were known, CoQ should be tried "for clinical application in disease states in which the immune system is not operating on an optimal level."

Six years later, in January 1987, Dr. Bliznakov published his popular book on CoQ. Millions of people have used CoQ in Japan with no harmful effects. The new book has a chapter on AIDS; it describes animal studies showing that the level of CoQ in the thymus declines with age, and that CoQ given to elderly animals restored immune response associated with the thymus to almost youthful levels.

In our telephone interview, Dr. Bliznakov explained that in animals CoQ has significantly prevented or corrected several different kinds of immune deficiencies—caused by three different immunosuppressive chemicals (adriamycin, cyclophosphamide, and hydrocortisone acetate), by aging, and by a virus. The inference is that it might also help prevent or correct immune deficiencies caused by ARC or AIDS.

In a completely separate study, Dr. Karl Folkers found that CoQ could increase the level of antibodies in the blood of humans (Folkers *et al.*, 1982). This effect might be either helpful or harmful to persons with AIDS. It took a long time—35 to 132 days depending on the patient—for an observable increase to occur.

CoQ has been largely ignored in the United States, and so far this writer has talked to only one person with AIDS who has been using it (we have heard of others). The person I talked to could not comment on effects he experienced, because he was also trying so many other experimental treatments that he could not tell which ones were responsible for which results. It is notable that this person, during the one evening we met, had so much energy that he would have stood out even among those who do not have AIDS and are completely healthy.

This Writer's Experience

As part of the research for this article, I tried CoQ, and have been using it for twelve days as of this writing. Having heard that it could take three weeks or more to notice results, I decided to try a moderately large amount for one month, and then if there were any beneficial effects, find a smaller dose which would maintain them. I tried 60 mg per day of the Twinlab CoQ10™ product, two 10 mg capsules with each meal. The 60 mg dose is twice the maximum recommended on the bottle, but about in the middle of the range of therapeutic doses commonly used in medical studies (30–100 mg per day). The cost, incidentally, was a little over one dollar a day; careful shopping could reduce it greatly.

The main result has been feeling far less fatigue during the daytime, and needing less sleep. I have felt more energy than I've felt for several years, and have been able to do at least an hour's additional productive work each day. Other effects have included being less sensitive to cold and finding that cuts heal faster.

Subjective results can easily reflect a placebo effect. In this case, however, all of these outcomes were unexpected.

I first noticed results after only three hours, and have heard that people trying CoQ as a food supplement often feel effects quickly, within a day or two. However, the medical studies usually find that it takes three weeks or longer to obtain benefits. This discrepancy may reflect the fact that the medical patients were very ill, often with life-threatening conditions. And medical studies usually look for physical, measurable results, rather than subjective reports on how people feel.

The Future

Apparently no one plans to do any scientific test of CoQ for treatment of AIDS or ARC. And even if researchers started now, it would be years before the studies were designed, funded, conducted, analyzed, published, and accepted—in addition to the time required to get government approval. In short, it will take years for U.S. medicine to get CoQ to persons with AIDS or ARC, even if everything goes right and happens as fast as possible.

The lack of testing raises public policy questions about the management of AIDS research. The case for trying this treatment was almost as strong six years ago when AIDS was first recognized as it is today—through information available on the shelves of any large medical library. In these six years nothing has been done concerning CoQ and AIDS. Apparently it wasn't anybody's job to search out promising scientific leads and make sure they were followed up.

Meanwhile, most health-food stores sell CoQ over the counter. Millions of people have used it in Japan as a prescription medicine, without any toxicity or harmful effects. This food supplement is inexpensive and easy to use. Clearly people will try it and see if it works for them, with information spreading by word of mouth, grass-roots organizations, and informal publication. Some physicians are willing to try promising treatments without waiting for official approval, or at least monitor their patients' use of them. Hopefully these physicians will help to collect information systematically and let their patients know of any news which develops.

No one expects CoQ to cure AIDS or ARC. The question is whether it can be helpful as part of an overall treatment program—for some people at least. Until tests are done we cannot be sure. The information available does suggest that CoQ is a plausible treatment possibility which deserves attention.

For More Information

The only popular book is *The Miracle Nutrient Coenzyme Q-10*, by Emile G. Bliznakov, M.D. and Gerald L. Hunt, (published by Bantam Books, January 1987). This book includes over a hundred references to medical and scientific papers. Dr. Bliznakov is one of the leading researchers on CoQ and the immune system and is also president and scientific director of the Lupus Research Institute.

Omni magazine has a one-page article about CoQ (February 1987, page 24).

Hundreds of technical papers have been published. A major recent book is *Coenzyme Q: Biochemistry, Bioenergetics and Clinical Applications of Ubiquinone*, edited by G. Lenaz (John Wiley & Sons, 1985). Four international symposia have been held, in 1976, 1979, 1981, and 1983, and the proceedings have been published.

REFERENCES

Bliznakov, E.G., "Coenzyme Q, the Immune System, and Aging," IN *Biomedical and Clinical Aspects of Coenzyme Q*, Volume 3, (Elsevier/North-Holland Press, 1981), pp. 311-21.

Folkers, K., S. Shizukuishi, K. Takemura, *et al.*, "Increase in Levels of IgG in Serum of Patients Treated with Coenzyme Q-10," IN *Research Communications in Chemical Pathology and Pharmacology* 38 (2) (November, 1982).

Langsjoen, P.H., S. Vadhanavikit, and K. Folkers, "Response of Patients in Classes III and IV of Cardiomyopathy to Therapy in a Blind and Crossover Trial with Coenzyme Q-10," IN *Proceedings of the National Academy of Sciences USA 82* (12) (June, 1985), pp. 4240-4.

Issue Number 27
March 13, 1987

AIDS TREATMENT NEWS FROM PROJECT INFORM

Project Inform, one of very few organizations willing to collect and disseminate information about medical treatments for AIDS and ARC not yet approved by the U.S. Food and Drug Administration, has become a unique resource center. In phone and mail contact with thousands of patients and hundreds of physicians and scientists, this organization may be the first anywhere to spot certain themes or trends concerning what treatments people are using, and which ones seem to be most successful. We interviewed some of the founders and staff of Project Inform, asking them for information which might be useful to our readers.

About the Organization

Project Inform, a community organization based in San Francisco, is sponsored by the non-profit Documentation of AIDS Issues and Research Foundation, Inc. (DAIR). (This writer is a member of the board of directors of DAIR, and has been familiar with Project Inform in that capacity.) Although officially a project of DAIR, Project Inform is in fact autonomous. Existing independently before its affiliation with DAIR, Project Inform sets its own policy, raises its own money, and is the larger and more widely known of the two organizations.

Project Inform first came to public notice by organizing an "underground" medical research study, of the effects of a combined AIDS/ARC treatment consisting of an antiviral and an immune modulator (ribavirin and isoprinosine). Official researchers strongly prefer to study a single drug at a time, and they had not researched the combination therapy despite a growing expert consensus that it was appropriate.

Later, some of the members started BARIG, the Bay Area Ribavirin Interest Group, which organized monthly trips to Mexico to purchase ribavirin at a special group price. BARIG no longer operates because the manufacturer of ribavirin, ICN Pharmaceuticals, no longer makes the group price available.

Last June, Project Inform received a grant from ICN to hire a research professional to analyze the results of its study of ribavirin and other alternative treatments. The first group of questionnaires has been compiled, and the tabulations are being analyzed.

The people of Project Inform include Joe Brewer and Martin Delaney, founders and directors; Tom Jefferson, full-time administrative manager (formerly Acting Director/Special Projects Coordinator of the San Diego AIDS Project); Bill Woods, Ph.D., research director; David Winterhalter, Ph.D., general resource person; and many volunteers. Two physicians and two statisticians serve as consultants. The mailing list includes two hundred physicians.

Project Inform currently provides information on six different treatments: antivirals ribavirin and d-penicillamine; immune modulators naltrexone, isoprinosine and DNCB; and aerosol pentamidine for prevention of pneumocystis. Two other treatments now being considered but not included in the official list at this time are AL 721 (antiviral) and imuthiol (immune modulator).

The organization has an office in San Francisco which answers about 75 phone calls and mails 40 to 50 information packets per day. In other cities—including New York, Chicago, Tulsa, and Long Beach—it is helping local groups develop similar treatment-information resources.

You can reach Project Inform by phone or mail (see Appendix B for their address and phone numbers) to obtain its packet of treatment information. Physicians can request a much more detailed packet—including for example a bibliography of over 500 medical papers on ribavirin going back to 1972. Note that Project Inform can only supply information about the six treatments listed above, or others added later; it is not prepared to answer questions about some of the additional treatments mentioned in this article below.

Physician/Patient and Treatment Themes

We asked Martin Delaney, Tom Jefferson, and Joe Brewer what they were hearing from their communication with thousands of people around the United States and abroad. The following themes emerged.

(Note: Project Inform provides information about experimental treatments, but it does not give medical advice. Only the appropriate medical professionals can evaluate each case and make recommendations for a particular patient.)

• There is a growing consensus that treatment should begin at the earliest reasonable time. By monitoring changes in T-cell subsets and other blood parameters, physicians can spot early signs of trouble. Patients can then make decisions about beginning treatments.

• Patients need a physician who will support and help them pursue a future. The attitude could be something like "let's try to find out how to keep you alive." If a doctor seems to write a patient off as dead, the patient may set out to find another doctor.

• Patients often want to participate with their physicians in evaluating treatment options, and to choose among them. They have a right to know, to follow the research, have an opinion, and get physicians to discuss their choices.

• Many scientific and medical experts believe that multiple treatments for HIV infection will be necessary. Unfortunately, official AIDS research has only recently begun to test a combination antiviral and immune restorative treatment, a strategy long urged by Project Inform and others.

• There is also a growing belief among physician researchers in the need to combine more than one antiviral tactic, not necessarily at the same time. In addition, Project Inform is increasingly hearing from people who are using more than one immune modulator. Fortunately the ones being combined are usually mild, such as naltrexone, isoprinosine, and DNCB, and Project Inform has not heard of any problems due to drug interaction.

• Many patients at risk for pneumocystis will want to consider preventive treatment with pentamidine aerosol. Many patients define being at risk as including those who have serious ARC, and others with very low T-helper cell counts, as well as those who have already had pneumocystis, or who are beginning chemotherapy treatment for KS.

Physicians and patients should be aware of this new aerosol pentamidine preventive treatment, which appears to be close to 100 percent effective in preventing pneumocystis with practically no side effects, and apparently no interactions with other drugs. Project Inform can refer physicians to experts who can answer their questions about how to use this treatment.

A number of persons taking AZT are also using aerosol pentamidine, as the rules of the AZT clinical trial permit its use.

• Project Inform is seeing a growing belief in the use of acyclovir, either in combination with AZT or ribavirin, or alone to prevent or treat certain opportunistic viruses.

• A Congressional committee or other investigative body should devote full attention to what is going on with AL 721. This promising, inexpensive, and completely safe antiviral has suffered from severe and unjustified delays in research and in availability to patients. Baffling delays in approval of ribavirin by the U.S. Food and Drug Administration also need investigation.

• Certain attitudes are helpful or harmful. Avoid the "treatment of the month club"; instead, choose knowledgeably and give a treatment a chance to work (not ignoring side effects, of course). Long-term, consistent use is important. Many treatments take six weeks to three months before they have an effect. Preventive treatments, of course, may never show proof that they have worked.

A central theme of Project Inform is that patients have a right to take an active role. Nobody has the answer on AIDS treatment.

Patients and physicians urgently need better access to information and expert advice—especially for persons who are antibody positive and are considering treatment options now. Project Inform exists because we cannot wait for certainty, but must use the best information available.

Issue Number 28
March 27, 1987

AZT, ALTERNATIVES, AND PUBLIC POLICY

Last week's Federal approval for prescription sale of AZT has raised major concerns of cost and insurance, as well as questions about the objectivity of the regulatory process and the overall direction of U.S. AIDS treatment research.

AZT

Last week the U.S. Food and Drug Administration approved limited sale of the AIDS treatment AZT. Because of confusion about exactly what was approved, we here reproduce a text distributed by a physician to the March 20 meeting of the California AIDS Advisory Committee in Sacramento:

"Indicated for the management of certain adult patients with symptomatic HIV infection (AIDS and advanced ARC) who have a history of cytologically confirmed *pneumocystis carinii* pneumonia or an absolute CD4 (T4 helper/inducer) lymphocyte count of less than 200/mm³ in the peripheral blood before therapy is begun.

"NOTE: This is the official FDA indication for zidovudine (Retrovir), formerly known as azidothymidine (AZT). This information was obtained verbally from the Division of Anti-Infective Drug Products of the FDA."

Note that AZT now has two new names: Retrovir, the proprietary trade name, and zidovudine, apparently a new generic. This writer will continue to use "AZT" as long as it is the one best known to the public. The name is being changed for commercial reasons, despite added confusion for the tens of millions of people who have already heard of AZT.

Two immediate concerns confront persons with AIDS and ARC: the medical merits of AZT, and the serious financial and practical problems likely to develop around it in the coming months.

This writer is not qualified to judge the medical merits, but can only relate impressions from conversations with physicians and other experts. There seems to be a consensus among most physicians familiar with the drug that AZT can benefit many people. Many others cannot use it because of severe side effects, yet some tolerate it with few side effects or none.

AZT works by providing a counterfeit building block used by the virus in assembling DNA, stopping or hindering reproduction of the virus. A number of scientists and physicians fear that AZT could have unknown long-term side effects by interfering with the body's own DNA. No one knows whether this theoretical concern is a real problem. Since the use of AZT started gradually, with a few people initially, any long-term effects will probably show up first in those who have been using the drug the longest, giving some warning to others.

Scientists are developing new drugs which work like AZT but may be less toxic. One example is dideoxycytidine (DDC).

For some people the medical decision to use or not use AZT will be a difficult one. The community could help by insisting on prompt release of detailed scientific results from clinical trials—which didn't happen after last year's major double-blind study of AZT.

Cost

AZT will cost about $750 to $1000 per month. In California, MediCal will pay, because of a law previously passed by the legislature. New York's Medicaid will also pay for AZT; each state will make its own decision. However, Medicare (the Federal program) has announced that it will not pay.

No one knows what private insurance companies will do. The best guess is that most of them will theoretically pay for AZT like any other prescription drug (commonly 80 percent of cost), but that many will work hard to evade the responsibility.

Companies will probably insist on exact compliance with all rules, such as the official FDA indication quoted above. If they can find any flaw in the paperwork, they could send the forms back—after a delay. Meanwhile the patient must front close to a thousand dollars a month; if someone cannot do so and has to go off the drug, the company will not owe for the money not spent. Insurance companies have long known that difficult paperwork, selectively applied, can discourage people and prevent many from ever collecting money due them.

The best defense against such abuses is to support organizations like National Gay Rights Advocates, or Mobilization Against AIDS (both headquartered in San Francisco). NGRA has been highly effective against discriminatory practices in the insurance industry, and MAA has stopped other instances of corporate discrimination against persons with AIDS.

Persons without insurance are already making medical decisions based on ability to pay. The expense of AZT will drain the savings of many individuals, and their families and friends.

Why does AZT cost so much? Prices of proprietary pharmaceuticals have little to do with the cost of manufacture.

Financial analysts expect that the manufacturer of AZT, Burroughs-Wellcome, has priced the drug at three times its usual profit margin and will make $100 million or more profit from AZT alone within the next year, providing no competitor becomes available. The only other AIDS antiviral which has advanced far enough in the regulatory process for possible U.S. approval within a year is ribavirin. Since hundreds of millions of dollars could rest on the FDA decision of whether or not to approve ribavirin, this decision might not be made solely on scientific and medical merit.

Another possible competitor, AL 721, is well over a year away from completing the steps required for FDA approval. AL 721 is entirely safe; in fact it could legally qualify as a food. It appears to be effective for most patients, but we are far from having conclusive proof because so little testing has been done—even though AL 721 has existed for years, and been known to be effective against the AIDS virus since November 1985. The Israeli physician most experienced with AL 721 told this writer that there is no rational reason not to use it now. Yet allowing immediate use would break the rules—and jeopardize hundreds of millions of dollars of AZT profits, as well as disrupting the business and financial planning which relied on the assurance that no AIDS antiviral except AZT or ribavirin could possibly be approved any time in the near future.

(There may be an alternative outcome for AL 721. Most informed persons known to this writer believe that the patent on AL 721 is weak and could not survive a serious test in court. And since AL 721 legally qualifies as food, anyone selling it as a nutritional supplement without medical claims could bypass the FDA entirely. The same name could not be used, but the list of ingredients on the generic products would leave no doubt.)

Another serious concern about Federal drug research and regulation is that U.S. government research agencies have licensing arrangements whereby they will receive royalties from the sale of some AIDS antivirals, but not others. Naturally these agencies are likely to champion the drugs in which they have a financial interest—a serious conflict when the same agencies also control Federal research funds, which could assist in the development of their rivals. And since the FDA must work with the research agencies in deciding whether to grant drug approvals, the objectivity of the Federal regulatory process could also be affected. Any such conflicts of interest would be extremely serious because they could greatly delay the development and availability of AIDS treatments. This writer cannot personally conduct an adequate investigation of this matter, and suggests that others do so.

AIDS organizations have had no knowledge of research and regulatory issues and no influence on them, as they have refused to involve themselves with treatments not already approved by the FDA.

Alternative and Experimental Treatments

This article is the 28th in the author's series on AIDS/ARC treatments. Earlier articles covered such potential medicines as AL 721, DNCB, lentinan, aerosol pentamidine, fu zheng, coenzyme Q, BHT, naltrexone, and ribavirin. How do these compare with AZT?

It seems clear that all of them are much safer than AZT. We know less about effectiveness, often much less, because research hasn't been done. As with AZT, it appears that none of the alternatives is a cure. (Lentinan may have produced a cure in the only case reported; the patient became antibody negative and is healthy three years later. Unfortunately this research, which was published over two years ago, was not followed up. There are now solid rumors of secret corporate research in the United States, and reports of recent clinical trials in Japan. We are seeking more information.)

While none of the above treatments has been proven effective, all are plausible options which might work; most have little risk. Most can be used in combination, so using one does not rule out other treatment options. The problem is that physicians are seldom familiar with unapproved treatments. Physicians get most of their information about new treatments from drug companies, which are forbidden to tell them about new drugs (or new uses for existing drugs) not already approved by the FDA.

A critical issue now is how to advise persons who are antibody positive, but otherwise healthy or not seriously ill. Recent statistics have shown that most of those who are antibody positive will eventually develop AIDS or ARC if left untreated; the risk increases greatly five years after infection. Unfortunately it takes a long time to get good scientific data on preventive treatments, since it is necessary to wait for months or years to see how many of those who are treated become ill. We don't have the time.

There is a rational approach. Almost all treatments for infection work best in the early stages. Therefore, any safe treatments which are plausible to use in the later stages of the disease are likely to be plausible as preventives, also. Why not try harmless treatments like AL 721, lentinan, naltrexone, or imuthiol, where safety is well known, even though we do not have final proof that they work? Even if none works, little harm will have been done; if only one works, that is enough.

The central problem is lack of leadership in getting the safe, plausible treatments available now into widespread, scientifically appropriate use. The commercial forces driving AIDS treatment research favor high-tech, patentable options—the very ones which take longest to develop. Simple, available, off-the-shelf treatments, already well known in human use, could be applied much more quickly; but these kinds of treatments have little commercial potential. And the champions of the commercial treatments are working hard to shut out each other, as well as anything else which threatens their markets. We can expect less tolerance for alternatives now that there is an official treatment for sale.

Almost all AIDS organizations have completely ignored the politically dangerous area of unapproved treatments. As a result, patients have had no representation or advocacy in treatment research decisions. Grassroots movements like the guerrilla clinics have developed without mainstream support.

We are now facing the expected deaths of up to a million or more Americans—even if all further spread of the virus could be stopped today. Many improvements but no miracles are about to come out of the research pipeline. There is no excuse for ignoring safe, available, inexpensive treatments, admittedly unproven but supported by all existing evidence, just because they are unpatentable or otherwise lack the profit potential to drive them through the multi-year, multi-million-dollar Federal drug approval process.

AZT Notes

• Many researchers suspect that low-dose AZT combined with oral acyclovir may be more effective and less toxic than AZT alone—and probably much less expensive. But few physicians will prescribe this treatment, as only laboratory results have been published and there are no clinical studies to show safety and effectiveness. At this time the combination is in "phase I" clinical trial, meaning testing for dosage and safety.

• Anyone investigating either the medical merits of AZT or the pricing issue should know that the history of the drug has been edited in a way favorable to the interests of the manufacturer. Most scientists and others believe that antiviral work on AZT started in 1984. In fact, AZT was repeatedly studied for antiviral effects in the 1970s, and apparently given up as too toxic at the high laboratory concentrations tested. Recent papers on AZT blacked out all reference to the earlier work. This writer discovered the missing science by accident during a computer search. (Researchers can find it through two papers by Krieg, Ostertag and others in *Experimental Cell Research*, Volume 116, 1978.)

Issue Number 29
April 10, 1987

DTC (IMUTHIOL): SCIENCE AND UNDERGROUND

Update 1989: The results of the multicenter trial reported here have not yet been released. Apparently the six-month trial is still not finished, because of recruiting difficulties at certain sites.

Update 1987: At the III International Conference on AIDS in Washington, D.C., researchers reported preliminary results of a double-blind placebo study of 80 ARC patients at five medical centers in France. This new information, the best available at the time, clearly showed significant benefit of DTC and little problem with side effects. These French results are not reflected in the article below, which was written earlier. For details, see "Washington AIDS Conference, Part II," (see Issue Number 35).

DTC, also called imuthiol, an immune modulator developed in France, has shown encouraging results in early tests for treating persons with AIDS and ARC. Placebo-controlled clinical trials are now running at six U.S. medical centers, and all these trials are open to accept new patients at this time. (The six U.S. centers are San Francisco General Hospital, USC, and UCLA in southern California, University of Arizona, Institute for Immunologic Disorders in Houston, and Duke University.)

Meanwhile, a few persons with AIDS or ARC have obtained their own DTC, which is a commonly available chemical costing about $40 a pound—enough for a ten-year supply. Although the highly purified DTC, prepared by the French pharmaceutical company Merieux, Inc., has a near-perfect safety record, there may be other dangers in unsupervised use of the reagent-grade chemical, which was not prepared for human use.

DTC Background

DTC (an abbreviation for diethyldithiocarbamate), has long had various chemical and agricultural uses, and in addition has been used in humans for treating nickel poisoning. It first came to attention as an immune modulator when French scientists, guided by certain chemical properties of DTC, selected it as a candidate for an immune modulator likely to be better than the other ones then available (Renoux and Renoux, 1984).

Yet despite this rational selection process, no one knows for sure how DTC works. It is believed to cause the liver to produce a substance which causes the growth of T-cells. A laboratory study indicated that DTC may also have activity against the AIDS virus, and might be helpful for that reason in the early stages of AIDS (Pompidou, Zagury, Gallo *et al.*, 1985), but we know of no published test of antiviral activity of DTC in humans. One French study treated six persons with ARC with DTC, and found clinical improvement in all of them, laboratory improvement in most measures with none getting worse, and no evidence that the increased T-4 counts encouraged growth of the virus (Lang *et al.*, 1985).

The immune modulating action of DTC may start in the brain, causing it to affect the liver and then the T-cells (Renoux *et al.*, 1984).

Toxicity is low. Animal studies have found that the fatal dose in rodents and dogs is over two hundred times the usual human dose, adjusted for body weight. Long-term toxicity studies have found that rodents, dogs, and monkeys could tolerate up to twenty times the weekly human dose, every day for three months, without side effects (Renoux and Renoux, 1984). Apparently no one develops allergic reactions to DTC, even if they are allergic to other drugs. There are no known problems in combining DTC with any other AIDS/ARC treatments (but see "Interactions" below). Patients must avoid alcohol for at least 24 hours before and after taking the weekly dose, as DTC is similar to disulfiram (Antabuse), a drug used to help alcoholics stay sober by making them sick if they drink.

DTC may possibly be useful in treating autoimmune conditions. French physicians reported one case of successful treatment of lupus, a disease known to be autoimmune (Delepine *et al.*, 1985). It is rumored that a number of other people with lupus have also been treated successfully, but we have not been able to confirm this account.

AIDS/ARC Background

Two studies, one in France and one at the University of Arizona but both unpublished so far, have found preliminary encouraging results.

All this writer knows of the French study at this time is contained in one sentence in the "Clinical Trial Abstract" used at San Francisco General Hospital: "Initial study in AIDS/ARC showed significant improvement in subjects, decrease in LAS and KS was noted in treated patients compared to the control group." An earlier French study of six ARC patients was described above.

A UPI press release of March 18, 1987 quoted the chief of infectious diseases at the University of Arizona Medical Center concerning the study of 26 patients there. DTC was found to prevent the progression of ARC, although it was not a cure. The researcher suspected that combining DTC with AZT could produce dramatic results, although combined trials will not start until Fall. (Some patients now enrolling in the DTC trial at San Francisco, and probably the other five U.S. centers also, will be allowed to use AZT simultaneously if they want to, now that AZT has been approved and is no longer considered "experimental". But we have heard that only those with AIDS will be allowed to use AZT during the DTC trial—not those with ARC, even if they meet the Burroughs-Wellcome requirements for obtaining AZT.)

At San Francisco General, physicians Donald Abrams and Robert Gorter are running the DTC trial. Dr. Gorter explained that they decided to join the Arizona study after learning of the preliminary results in France and in Arizona.

I asked how DTC might compare with DNCB, also an immune modulator possibly relevant to the autoimmune component of AIDS. Dr. Gorter had heard that DNCB would raise the number of T-cells in the blood, but that after eight to 12 weeks the number could drop again. With DTC he expected that the effect would last longer, and with much less of a dip.

The San Francisco study will test DTC for six months; 30 patients will get the treatment, 30 will get placebo. Twenty percent of the patients in each group will be persons with AIDS; the other 80 percent will have ARC. KS is okay if stable, but persons with MAI are excluded from this test. Blood tests must show HIV antibodies, as well as other indications such as a T-helper count under 500. Because of a Federal rule that patients can only use one experimental drug at a time, patients will not be able to simultaneously use other such treatments.

The French manufacturer of DTC, Merieux, Inc., is financing this study. The U.S. government is not contributing. Perhaps because of financial constraints, extensive blood tests are being done only at the beginning and the end of the six-month treatment.

"Underground" DTC

If all goes well, DTC could be approved sometime in 1988. First, the six different centers must finish recruiting patients. Then the course of treatment itself lasts six months. Then the data will be analyzed and submitted to the FDA, which will make its decision. Of course additional delays could occur.

Some people have chosen not to wait and have obtained the chemical DTC. But several problems have slowed the development of a widespread "guerrilla clinic" movement such as the one using DNCB. At this time there is a surge of public interest in DTC, and the problems seem close to being resolved.

DTC is usually taken orally. But the acidity of the stomach would destroy it, so capsules must be "enteric coated", designed to pass through the stomach and dissolve in the intestines. People have made enteric-coated capsules at home, but the process has been somewhat difficult to learn and do. Fortunately the medicine is taken only once a week. It may be necessary to put the DTC into several capsules so that they will be small enough to enter the intestine undigested.

Besides enteric capsules, other methods are being tried:

(1) People have neutralized the acidity of the stomach so the DTC can get through. This method has been reported to work but it is unpleasant and may be dangerous, as normal stomach acidity may prevent the entry of microorganisms which could be particularly dangerous to someone with immune deficiencies.

(2) In recent weeks, several underground researchers have found that DTC can be administered rectally, in suppositories or by enema. Successful absorption has been inferred from the chemical taste and smell often characteristic of DTC after it has entered the bloodstream. This discovery may make "guerilla clinic" use of DTC feasible.

(3)   The drug disulfiram (Antabuse), used to keep alcoholics from drinking, is metabolized in part to DTC inside the body. Theoretically it might be possible to obtain DTC by taking disulfiram—a well-understood prescription drug readily available to physicians. We don't know anyone who has tried doing this yet.

Interactions

Note the warning on alcohol, above.

Underground Notes

• The industrial DTC is only rated to be at least 99 percent pure, and at this time we don't know what the impurities are. It is important to find out if there are any dangerous contaminants, and if so how to get them removed.

• The FDA will probably ban the sale of DTC once its use for AIDS/ARC becomes well known. We have heard that the FDA already banned the sale last month after a press report of the Arizona results, then lifted the ban in 72 hours when it appeared that the news would get little publicity; we could not reach anyone in the FDA to confirm or deny this report. Fortunately DTC is widely used, and quite easy to make in a laboratory; an organized community can easily get around a ban.

• Almost nothing is happening with DTC as an AIDS/ARC treatment in any country except France and the U.S. As far as we know, the pharmaceutical grade is not for sale in any country, although the chemical would remain available abroad even if U.S. sales are banned. Since the cost of the chemical is negligible, DTC could be particularly important for poor countries where the cost of other treatments could be prohibitive.

• In the U.S., the best way to handle DTC would be to change the rules to allow prescription sale of the pharmaceutical product. Recently the FDA proposed such a change. If adapted, the new rules will allow limited sale of drugs for life-threatening conditions, when they are known to be safe and show evidence of being effective, but have not yet achieved final approval. Unfortunately at least one gay political organization has opposed this proposal, apparently fearing that drug companies might abuse it.

• This writer believes that any underground use of DTC should follow the lead of the DNCB "guerrilla clinics" in never charging for the medicine, always giving it free. Free distribution may not change the technical legal status, but politically it makes a guerrilla clinic movement much stronger by removing the issue of profiteering. It also prevents fraudulent sale of counterfeit, inactive substances.

But note that we should not insist that all alternative treatments be free. AL 721, for example, represents a different situation, because it costs over a dollar a day to manufacture, and also because it legally qualifies as a food. It could not be effectively distributed free; but as a nutritional supplement it could be handled by buying clubs or by health-products companies. Many other alternative treatments, such as acupuncture, require professional practitioners. Each situation is different.

For More Information

You may be able to learn more about DTC from Project Inform (see Appendix B).

REFERENCES

Delepine, N., J. Desbois, F. Taillard, C. Allaneau, G. Renoux, "Sodium diethyldithiocarbamate Inducing Long-lasting Remission in Case of Juvenile Systemic Lupus Erythematosus," *The Lancet* (November 30, 1985), p. 1246.

Lang, G., F. Oberling, A. Aleksijevic, A. Falkenrodt, S. Mayer, "Immunomodulation with diethyldithiocarbamate in Patients with AIDS-Related Complex," *The Lancet* (November 9, 1985), p. 1066.

Pompidou, A., D. Zagury, R. Gallo, D. Sun, A. Thornton, P. Sarin, "In-Vitro Inhibition of LAV/HTLV-III Infected Lymphocytes by Dithiocarb and Inosine Pranobex," *The Lancet* (December 21/28, 1985), p. 1423.

Renoux, G., J. Guillaumin, M. Renoux, "Favorable Influences of Imuthiol on Mouse Reproduction and Immune System of Offspring," *American Journal of Reproductive Immunology and Microbiology* (July, 1985), pp. 101–6.

Renoux, G., and M. Renoux, "Diethyldithiocarbamate (DTC); A Biological Augmenting Agent Specific for T Cells," IN R. Fenishel and M. Chirgis, Eds., *Immune Modulation Agents and Their Mechanisms* (New York and Basel: Marcel Dekker, Inc., 1984).

Renoux, G., M. Renoux, K. Biziere, J. Guillaumin, P. Bardos, D. Degenne, "Involvement of Brain Neocortex and Liver in the Regulation of T Cells: The Mode of Action of Sodium Diethyldithiocarbamate (Imuthiol)," *Immunopharmacology* (April 1984), pp. 89–100.

Issue Number 30
April 24, 1987

AL 721 WORKALIKES: WHERE TO GET THEM

AL 721 is an experimental AIDS treatment derived from egg yolks. It is known to be safe and without serious side effects. All available information from laboratory studies, clinical trials, and anecdotal reports suggests that although it is not a cure, it appears to be helpful even at severe stages of HIV infection.

The bad news is that despite promising early results, little testing has been done, and only a handful of people can get the "real", official AL 721. For this potential treatment, like a number of others, has fallen victim to a public-policy nightmare of bureaucratic and commercial red tape. All but lost to institutional medicine, AL 721 has joined an underground, grass-roots circuit of rational AIDS/ARC treatments, well supported by all existing evidence but largely ignored by the official research system for institutional (not scientific or medical) reasons.

During the last year a number of AL 721 substitutes have been tried. But only in the last few weeks have good ones become available.

This article reviews the background of AL 721, tells what you can get now or in the near future, and tells where to find more information.

AL 721 Background

AL 721 consists entirely of substances found in ordinary egg yolk, so it could legally qualify as a food. Eating egg yolk would not have the same effect, however, because the ingredients are not in the right proportion (a 7:2:1 ratio), and also because the high cholesterol in egg yolk would interfere.

AL 721 was developed by cancer researchers at the Department of Membrane Research of the Weizmann Institute of Science in Israel. The three components are: phosphatidylcholine (PC), the main ingredient of ordinary lecithin; phosphatidylethanolamine (PE), usually found with PC in lecithin; and "neutral lipids," ordinary fats like cooking or butter, which serve as a carrier for the PC and PE. Scientists found the 7:2:1 ratio (7 parts neutral lipid, 2 parts PC, 1 part PE) through educated trial and error in laboratory tests; this ratio showed a sharp peak in effectiveness in causing certain changes in cell membranes. The researchers were not looking for an antiviral, but for ways to modify the action of receptor sites on cells for other medical purposes, such as helping alcohol or narcotics addicts overcome their habit by relieving withdrawal symptoms.

AL 721 affects the membranes of cells, and also of "lipid coated" viruses, a class which includes AIDS, herpes, CMV, and Epstein-Barr. The first suggestion of possible use against AIDS appeared in a letter to the *New England Journal of Medicine* (November 1985). Several scientists, including Dr. Robert Gallo of the U.S. National Cancer Institute, reported that AL 721 greatly reduced AIDS virus infection of human cells in the laboratory.

Since AL 721 had already been given to humans and was known to be safe, the obvious next step would have been to try it with AIDS or ARC and see if it helped. But in almost a year and a half since the above article, only eight people have received AL 721 in scientific tests—with good results. About 15 others have received it quietly in Israel, often against the wishes of the U.S. licensee to the patent on AL 721, with good to excellent results. This writer does not know of any other human experience with the official AL 721 as an AIDS/ARC treatment, anywhere in the world.

A number of events in late March and early April of 1987 gave AL 721 much-needed public attention and credibility. A Wall Street civil-disobedience demonstration precipitated major media coverage of AIDS treatment research and availability, letting the public know that the issue exists. In Israel, the researchers who developed AL 721 reported that the seven patients in their initial treatment group, all seriously ill in advanced stages of AIDS, all improved clinically with AL 721 treatment. And the U.S. National Institutes of Health announced that its AIDS Treatment Evaluation Units would evaluate AL 721 in a "Phase I" dosage study. Incidentally, the stock of Praxis Pharmaceuticals, the manufacturer of AL 721, almost doubled in price in the last week of March, apparently reflecting the new credibility of that company's only product.

The "Home Formula"

The failure of official AIDS researchers to follow up on AL 721 and test it seriously, from November 1985 until March 1987 at least, has left a vacuum which home experimenters and a few physicians have filled. A number of AL 721 substitutes have been tried, but none worked well enough to attract much interest until the "home formula" (see below) appeared in January 1987 and quickly superceded all the earlier attempts. April 1987 saw the first of a new generation of egg-lecithin AL 721 substitutes which are probably better than the home formula; but we don't have much experience yet since people have used it for less than two weeks at this writing.

For the benefit of those who don't already have the home formula, we reproduce it here:

"PC-55™ is a high-strength lecithin concentrate made by Twin Laboratories, Inc., of Ronkonkoma, New York, and sold in health-food stores. It contains two of the three ingredients of AL 721; they are in a 5:2 ratio, close to the 2:1 used in AL 721.

Neutral lipids can be added to PC-55™ making it a membrane fluidizer comparable to AL 721. This material is a food nutrient, it is not a drug. It is safe.

"Combine five tablespoons of PC-55™ and 12 tablespoons of water in a bowl, and whip with an electric mixer or blender. Slowly add 6 tablespoons plus one teaspoon of butter (6⅓ tablespoons butter) which has been melted (measure the butter before melting). Whip thoroughly three to five minutes. This mixture divided into 10 even doses gives slightly over 10 grams of the lipids per dose. Each dose should weigh about 30.4 grams or 1.06 ounces.

"The individual doses can be placed into plastic sandwich bags for freezing. If you don't have a scale, you can measure out two tablespoons to each bag, then add a much smaller amount to divide the remainder. One person separates the doses in an ice-cube tray. Move each dose from the freezer to the refrigerator a few hours before use. This preparation spoils very rapidly at room temperature; it must be frozen unless used immediately.

"(An earlier version of this formula used cooking oil instead of butter. The proportions are 5 tablespoons PC-55™, 5 tablespoons + 1 teaspoon oil, and 10 Tbsp water.)

"The material is best eaten in the morning, spread on fat-free bread or mixed with fruit juice. The user should eat a fat-free breakfast which might consist of fat-free cereals, skim milk, fruits, or vegetables. There are no restrictions on lunch or dinner. An additional dose might be taken before going to bed. Patients treated in Israel are given two doses a day for about four weeks, then single doses indefinitely. Some people with AIDS might experience diarrhea with this membrane fluidizer, especially with the additional dose. Eat brown rice and other solid foods.

"You can help others and yourself by keeping a record of your experience—doses, dates, and any resulting effects."

Mr. Steve Gavin developed this home formula in January, 1987 and distributed it at meetings of persons with AIDS. This writer published the formula on January 30, 1987. We don't know how many people have used it by this time, but there must be several hundred. So far we have heard only good results; people have been happy with this preparation.

How does this home formula differ from the "official" AL 721? It differs mainly in its use of soy lecithin instead of egg; the PC and PE from soy have minor chemical differences from the egg varieties. And instead of the "egg oil" neutral lipids used in AL 721, it uses butter, a substitute suggested by experts as the closest generally available. The substitutes were used because egg lecithin and egg oil are difficult to obtain. (Apparently the scientists who developed AL 721 selected the egg substances as the closest to those already found in the human body. No published studies anywhere suggested that the substitutes wouldn't work; but none proved that they would, either.)

Three months later those involved have little doubt that the home formula does work. Mr. Gavin has estimated that it may be half to three quarters as effective as the official AL 721; this estimate may be conservative.

Egg-Lecithin AL 721 Substitutes

At the time of this writing (April 20, 1987), only one AL 721 workalike using egg lecithin is on the market: "Eggsact" from INTREND, a new company in Santa Cruz, California. INTREND was started by three people whom this writer has known socially for several years. Knowing that they were involved in the health-food business, I kept them informed about AL 721 and encouraged them to produce a workalike product. To prevent conflict of interest I avoided any financial involvement with the company (as with all other AIDS treatments and companies), and have no role in this operation besides volunteering information.

"Eggsact" uses egg lecithin for the PC and PE, and butterfat for the neutral lipid carrier. Butterfat had proven successful in the home formula; INTREND chose it because of the difficulty of obtaining egg oil, and also to avoid possible legal problems with the AL 721 patent. The lecithin is not irradiated, and is a high-quality, injectable grade usually used for making pharmaceuticals. Although contamination would be unlikely, the product was tested for salmonella and staphylococcus, with none found; the level of peroxides, a measure of possible rancidity, was undetectable in the chemical tests used. The company will make copies of the test results available on request.

The PE ratio is probably low, below the theoretical 10 percent—as it is in the home formula, and indeed in much of the "official" AL 721. Almost no one has controlled the PE level at this time, and many experts doubt that it is critical.

"Eggsact" is nitrogen packed. It must be kept cold, at freezer temperatures for long-term storage. The company plans to provide foil packaging, but for now it is using canning jars to make the product available immediately. Naturally this material can be sold only as a nutritional supplement, not as a medicine, and the company cannot discuss medical claims or uses.

The cost of using "Eggsact" is $3 to $6 per day—compared to 50 cents to $1 per day for the home formula, or $2 to $4 per day for egg-based workalike soon to be available from the PWA Health Group.

Several other companies are believed to be preparing to market AL 721-like products. At this time the only one we can confirm is Jarrow Formulas. Jarrow plans to sell a product packaged so that it may not need refrigeration until opened. He intends to offer a very low rate to nonprofit groups, in addition to standard commercial distribution through health-food stores, physicians, and other health practitioners, but he cannot sell small quantities directly to individuals.

It is rumored that Praxis Pharmaceuticals is considering marketing AL 721 as a nutritional supplement, as well as pursuing eventual approval as a pharmaceutical. If so, its product could become the gold standard against which the others are judged. It would be the only one able to use the name "AL 721."

PWA Health Group and Healing Alternatives Buyers Club

At least two nonprofit organizations, in New York and San Francisco, will soon distribute an egg-based workalike very close to AL 721. Unlike "Eggsact" their product uses egg oil and controls the PE level. Orders must be placed a month or more in advance, as the manufacturer requires a minimum order of 100 kilograms (about $16,000), and then needs time to prepare it. The minimum individual order is one kilogram, for about $200.

The PWA Health Group started within the PWA Coalition in New York, but then became independent, as the charter of the PWA Coalition does not allow sale of a nutritional supplement. In San Francisco, a number of persons including this writer who have placed orders with the PWA Health Group started the Healing Alternatives Buyers

Club, as a vehicle for distributing the local portion of the original order placed through New York. In the future, the Healing Alternatives Buyers Club will buy directly from manufacturers. And it will actively help facilitate the formation of similar groups elsewhere.

AL 721 Precautions

Though AL 721 has few side effects, some cautions must be considered.

Recently physicians have noticed that some people who had used AL 721 become ill shortly after they discontinued it. In fact, two of the eight lymphadenopathy patients who received the treatment in scientific tests developed AIDS four to six weeks after their AL 721 was discontinued. These cases may be coincidence, and there is no evidence that AL 721 made anyone more ill than they would have been without it; but until more is known, physicians are advising persons not to start AL 721 or workalikes unless they plan to continue. It may be necessary to stop gradually, as with a number of other medicines. (Fortunately the home formula is always available in case supplies of AL 721 or other workalikes are interrupted.)

Too much lecithin can cause nausea, diarrhea, mental depression, and loss of appetite, but is not believed to have lasting ill effects. In some cases nausea or diarrhea attributed to AL 721 turned out to be caused by intestinal parasites such as amebas or giardia instead; these parasites can be eradicated by medical treatment.

Animal studies have shown that large doses of lecithin given during pregnancy can accumulate in the fetus and reach very high levels, causing subtle neurological damage in the offspring. Could proper amounts of AL 721 help to protect unborn children of pregnant women who are HIV positive? Medical experts should examine this possibility.

Issue Number 31
May 8, 1987

AIDS INFORMATION BY COMPUTER

Update 1988:

(1) Many new online sources of AIDS information, including free bulletin boards, are now available. Explore the ones listed here to find recent phone numbers.

(2) The best place to get computer-readable copies of AIDS Treatment News is on AIDS Info BBS (see Appendix B at the back of the book, the sub-listing under "AIDS Treatment News" for the phone number of AIDS Info BBS).

Any personal computer which can connect to the telephone lines can open doors to important AIDS information. This article reviews some of the available resources, and discusses their advantages and disadvantages, their cost, and how to use them.

Computers have several advantages for obtaining and sharing AIDS information:

- Location doesn't matter. The smallest towns have the same access as the largest cities.

- Most computer services are very careful to protect the privacy of their users. Some allow you to be anonymous if you want. Most require a name and address for billing, but these services provide information on dozens of topics, not only AIDS, allowing you to be discreet if necessary. And you can obtain the information from the privacy of your home by telephone.

- Computerized information is available around the clock, and you can study it as long as you like.

By contrast, physicians and other AIDS experts may be hard to reach by phone or in person, and then too busy to spend much time. The computer can help you get the background to make conversations with human experts more productive.

- Computerized information can be updated at any time, so it can be kept current. Providers can avoid the delays of publication, order processing, mailing, and so on.

• Many services allow you to leave questions, comments, or other messages for the public.

Disadvantages

Most of these can be overcome by working through support groups or AIDS organizations.

• Costs vary. If you don't have use of a computer already, buying the equipment will probably cost several hundred dollars or more. Also, some of the most useful information services have one-time sign-up costs, often about $50, to open an account.

Many of the services cost less than $10 an hour during evenings and weekends, more during the workday. Some are much more expensive, others are free. Most of the services which do charge money can be reached by a local phone call from most cities, avoiding long-distance phone charges. The free services do require that you call long distance if necessary to wherever the computer happens to be.

• Computers are still somewhat difficult to learn how to use. Beginners should have a friend help them get started, or take a class through adult education or a computer store, or find a consultant.

• The information available varies greatly in quality.

Overview: Three Kinds of Services

Most "online" services—those that communicate with your home or office computer by telephone—can be divided into three classes: information utilities, computer bulletin boards, and research databases.

Information utilities provide large libraries of special-interest material—from general news to astrology, investment advice, airline fares, shopping, games, and so on. These services usually cost about $8 an hour during the evenings and weekends.

The best-known information utilities are CompuServe, The Source, and Delphi. By far the best for AIDS information is Delphi (see "CAIN," below).

Computer bulletin boards, generally run by individuals as a hobby or public service, are usually free. These systems have been called the first two-way medium of mass communication, as most of the information on them comes from the users themselves. The two systems named below allow anonymous users to access the system and read information.

Research databases are expensive and technical but by far the most powerful online systems. They allow immediate search through references to millions of published medical articles for any subjects or words you request. In a few minutes from your home or office you can do research which would take hours to do at the best medical libraries.

Important research databases for AIDS information include Medline, DIALOG, and BRS Colleague; (see details below).

Specific Services

CAIN   (on Delphi): The Computerized AIDS Information Network (CAIN), funded by the California Department of Health Services, Office of AIDS, will probably be the most valuable general-purpose computerized information resource for most persons and organizations. It has large, diverse collection of good-quality information, costs less than $8 per hour on evenings and weekends, and is one of the easiest computer services to learn how to use.

Information on CAIN includes:

* Selected Associated Press (AP) news stories on AIDS. We checked on April 3, 1987 and found 42 stories, dated March 20 to April 30, covering various aspects of AIDS. These stories often have more information than appears in newspapers, which select and edit the material. (The alternative-treatment stories, incidentally, were generally negative and uninformative—not the fault of CAIN, but a reflection of the fact that most of the press accepts government and other institutional statements as its starting point—at least. And official agencies seldom say that what they have not approved has value.)

* A list of service providers including dental care, insurance and legal resources, antibody test sites, medical and service organizations, projects and foundations, health departments, mental health services, and religious/spiritual organizations.

* Reports from the *PWA Coalition Newsline,* and the California Association of AIDS Agencies.

* Computer bulletin boards on which AIDS organizations and the general public can announce conferences, general news, legislative news, funding available for organizations, help wanted, and so forth.

* Educational references including a list of AIDS books (92 of them), newsletters, brochures, audio-visual material, and professional recommendations and policy statements.

* Research information including reports from the U.S. Centers for Disease Control, selected journal articles, and so on.

* Electronic-mail communication facilities—including international electronic mail, perhaps the only fast, effective, and low-cost means of organizing internationally.

* Names, addresses, and phone numbers of hundreds of AIDS organizations, publications, service providers, and others.

To sign up for CAIN, call them at the number given at the back of this book (see Appendix B). Besides the $7.20 per hour cost for evening or weekend access ($17.40 per hour during prime time), there is a one-time signup fee of $49.95. Those who already have an account on Delphi can find CAIN in the Delphi "library" section. CAIN is available internationally, through computer networks. This newsletter is itself available on CAIN.

Computer Bulletin Boards

These small systems, usually free and set up by individuals, allow users to communicate by leaving messages for each other. Most run 24 hours a day. We don't have a current list of those with AIDS information, but will mention two examples in San Francisco. Both are free and run 24 hours a day, and both allow anonymous reading.

AIDS Information BBS   (see Appendix B for modem phone number) has been run by AIDS organizer Ben Gardiner since July 1985. At any given time it has several dozen messages and short articles, reflecting the interests of its users. A new computer will soon allow a greatly expanded body of information, plus multiple telephone lines.

Newsbase   *(Editor's Note: Newsbase is no longer in service)* specializes in political news and discussion, especially on Latin America. Its AIDS section keeps this writer's treatment articles in computer-readable form. (I use Newsbase as a central library for distributing computer-readable copies to those who want them—such as other online systems, or publications which can receive computerized articles for automatic typesetting. Anyone else can read the articles in Newsbase, too.) On both AIDS Information BBS and Newsbase, the software automatically asks new users for a name and address. But the operators don't mind if you use a pseudonym and dummy address in order to preserve anonymity.

Other computer bulletin boards also have AIDS information. Bulletin boards come and go frequently, and we don't have a current list of these systems. If you know of any AIDS computer information services, leave messages on AIDS Information BBS (phone number listed in Appendix B) so that others can find out about them.

Research Databases

Medline: Run by the U.S. National Library of Medicine, Medline lets you do instant searches of citations to millions of articles in published in medical journals. Medline does not have the full text of these articles, but about 40 percent of the citations do include brief abstracts written by the author. Often the abstract is all you need.

This writer has found Medline immensely useful, but it does have limitations. It usually takes several weeks after libraries have received the medical journals for citations to appear in the computer, so the most current article will not be listed. Also, this writer has found that many AIDS articles, probably hundreds of them, have been indexed erroneously and will not be found by a usual search for AIDS—a serious problem, not generally known, which also affects printed indexes used in all medical libraries. (One example: the only medical-journal publication on DNCB as an AIDS/ARC treatment, reporting the treatment of 6 AIDS patients and 12 with ARC, was cited in Medline but not indexed under AIDS. Researchers will not find this article by a computer search, unless they know about it in advance. The National Library of Medicine corrected this particular error in the original copy of the database, but the correction has not appeared in some of the Medline versions offered by private database companies.)

You can subscribe to Medline directly through the National Library of Medicine, but it's easier to use it through any of various other services, such as DIALOG or BRS Colleague.

DIALOG: This online research service allows uniform, systematic access to Medline and over 200 other databases, including sciences, nursing, public health, pharmaceuticals, general news, and business and corporate information. It provides the most extensive database collection anywhere.

Costs are high, but there is no minimum or sign-up fee; except for manuals, training, and an annual account fee, you pay only for what you use. Experienced searchers learn various tricks to keep costs down, and can often do a search for under $10. New users should take a training class in how to use this system.

For more information, call DIALOG Information Services (see Appendix B).

BRS Colleague: This service, designed for physicians, offers several advantages:

• It includes two databases primarily devoted to AIDS—one from England, and one soon to be available from San Francisco General Hospital—as well as Medline and other medical databases. DIALOG does not have the AIDS databases.

• It provides full text of several dozen important medical journals, as well as a number of medical books. Persons without access to a medical library will find this information particularly useful. And BRS Colleague usually does include the current articles—often hard to find in a library, as others are using them.

• BRS Colleague is less expensive than DIALOG, and easier to learn. No training course is required. For more information, call the BRS marketing department (see Appendix B).

Equipment Notes

You should use a 1200 bps modem (telephone interface). The other common speed, 300, is four times slower—and most databases charge by the hour. Speeds higher than 1200 are available, but not all computer services can use them.

If you don't have any idea what computer to get, three options are a "PC clone" (fully compatible with the IBM PC or XT); or an Apple Macintosh; or a "lap-top" or other portable with a built-in modem.

Obtaining Medical Articles or Research Services

DIALOG does not have the full text of articles, and BRS Colleague provides it for only a few dozen of the thousands of medical journals which exist. What if you need the full article, but do not have access to a medical library?

You can obtain a copy of almost any published article in the world from a research company, such as Information On Demand in McClean, Virginia (see Appendix B for phone number). I have used them for articles so hard to find that no library in California has a copy. They have sources around the world and never fail to find my articles within a week or two—usually for $15 to $20 each.

This company and others can also do the whole research job, for those who would rather pay for the work than get a computer and do it themselves. These research companies are very careful about confidentiality, as their clients insist on it for many reasons. You can use them from anywhere in the U.S. or abroad, since they work by phone and mail so you don't need to visit their offices. They are expert on information sources but not on AIDS; you must be able to tell them specifically what you want them to find out about.

Conclusion

A personal computer can provide fast, private access to extensive AIDS information, from any locality. Most groups or individuals could start by using the Computerized AIDS Information Network, and computer bulletin boards. Those who want in-depth medical research information could subscribe to one of the research databases discussed above. Or they could avoid using a computer, and hire a research company to do the work.

Issue Number 32
May 22, 1987

JAPANESE ANTIVIRAL DISCOVERY

A medical professor has found that a combination of two commonly used intravenous drugs completely stops replication of the AIDS virus in the test tube. The discovery is unknown in the U.S.; this article is the only information so far published in English.

The discoverer believes the combination would probably work as an AIDS treatment, at about a tenth the cost of AZT. Other physicians contacted by the writer urge caution, however, as the drugs would be dangerous for some patients and may not be feasible for long-term use. This treatment has never been tried in people. While physicians could easily administer it today, there are no plans for clinical trials, in Japan or anywhere else.

This writer learned about the discovery from James Palazzolo, a professional Japanese translator with an interest in AIDS. Mr. Palazzolo scans Japanese publications looking for information which may not be available in the U.S. He found this news in the April 12, 1987 *Mainichi Shimbun,* one of Japan's major newspapers; later he interviewed the discoverer by telephone. Here is Mr. Palazzolo's translation of the newspaper article, plus notes of the phone interview.

"Dextran Sulfate and Heparin Discovered to Inhibit HIV"

"Assistant Professor Masahiko Itoh (Microbiology) of the Fukushima Prefectural Medical College has discovered that the combination of dextran sulfate, a drug used in the treatment of arteriosclerosis, and heparin, an anti-coagulant, work synergistically to inhibit the replication of the AIDS virus in the test tube. Professor Itoh added that "these drugs are cheaper and have fewer side effects than AZT, a widely used drug in the U.S. which is effective in prolonging the lives of AIDS patients. Although clinical trials will be necessary, it is hoped that this combination will be effective in prolonging life when used in conjunction with an immune booster.

139

"Assistant Professor Itoh first noticed that the combination of dextran sulfate and heparin worked to prevent the replication of the herpes virus. Cells (M01 T-4) of the same antigenicity as the lymphocytes which HIV infects were infected with HIV and various concentrations of dextran sulfate and heparin were added. The temperature was maintained close to body temperature at 37 degrees and the cells were cultured for 7 to 10 days. Cells cultured with either dextran sulfate or heparin expanded and were destroyed. In contrast to this, viral replication was completely inhibited when a dextran sulfate concentration of 12.5 micrograms per milliliter and a heparin concentration of 15 micrograms per milliliter were added and the cells continued to live. Furthermore, cell toxicity which indicates possible side effects did not appear, even when concentrations up to 4 milligrams per milliliter were added. ·

"Assistant Professor Itoh added that "This drug combination has few side effects compared to AZT which suppresses the production of blood by the bone marrow and I believe this drug combination could cost hundreds of dollars instead of the thousands of dollars required for AZT.""

The newspaper included pictures of the T-cells with and without the treatment.

In Mr. Palazzolo's later phone interview, Assistant Professor Itoh made the following points:

• The heparin stops reverse transcriptase. No one knows what the dextran sulfate does.

• Nothing has been published in English. Nothing has been published in Japanese, except for the above story which was carried on a major news service there. It will be "quite a while" before the technical paper is finished; he doesn't know when.

• Of the two kinds of dextran sulfate—low and high molecular weight—Itoh suspects that both will work. He could not tell the us which kind he used, because that information must appear first in his paper.

• There are no plans for clinical trials in Japan.

Assistant Professor Itoh is willing to answer letters from U.S. physicians considering clinical use here. He does not speak English, but Mr. Palazzolo has offered to translate.

U.S. Reactions

We spoke with two U.S. physicians while researching this article.

James Campbell, M.D., head of the research committee of the Bay Area Physicians for Human Rights, cautioned about practical problems with the dextran-heparin treatment. "It would have to be administered intravenously long term, as the retrovirus can reactivate. And both medications are anticoagulants, which could cause bleeding problems, especially with this group of patients. Certainly it would be worthwhile to investigate further and find the basis of any antiviral effect."

The other physician also expressed concern about the need to continue intravenous use of the drugs.

Scientific Background

Both dextran and heparin are "polysaccharides"—chemicals composed of long chains of various sugar molecules. Scientists are also considering other polysaccharides as possible AIDS treatments, mostly immune modulators; examples are glucan, lentinan (derived from the shiitake mushroom), and possibly other chemicals from different medicinal fungi.

Many different laboratory studies have used both dextran sulfate and heparin together. None of them, so far as we know, looked for an antiviral effect. But the dextran/heparin combination had other results of scientific or clinical relevance. For example, here are the titles of four of over 100 scientific articles published in the last eight years which concern both dextran sulfate and heparin in some way:

• "Thrombin inhibitory activity of heparin cofactor II depends on the molecular weight and sulfate amount of dextran sulfate."

• "Abolition by dextran sulfate of the heparin-accelerated antithrombin III/thrombin reaction."

• "Inhibition by heparin and dextran sulfate of stimulated rat pancreatic adenylate cyclase."

• "Heparin and dextran sulfate antagonize PGL2 inhibition of platelet aggregation."

These articles, and dozens of others about heparin and dextran together, may give scientists a head start in understanding the antiviral effect—and perhaps improving on it.

ACIDOPHILUS: FOR DIARRHEA OR THRUSH?

Acidophilus, used in milk in grocery stores and also sold in concentrated form as a health-food product, consists of billions of live, beneficial bacteria, taken to change the flora of the digestive system and help crowd out harmful organisms. Most physicians do not take acidophilus very seriously, but regard it as a health food and do not mention it to their patients; you will probably not hear about it from your doctor. But some physicians do recommend it for their AIDS patients, and recently we have been hearing of a number of persons who are convinced that it has helped them in controlling diarrhea and/or candida (thrush) in the digestive tract.

We don't know of any scientific studies which would prove or disprove these uses; but acidophilus is readily available, inexpensive, easy to use, and evidently helpful to some. It appears to be entirely harmless, but patients should check with their physicians to make sure there are no reasons to avoid trying it.

The several people we talked to made the following points:

• There are many different kinds of acidophilus, as dozens of different kinds of organisms could be used. Most brands contain only one organism (usually L. Acidophilus), but some formulas contain several different ones.

• Perhaps most important, the people this writer spoke with recommended using a non-dairy acidophilus—since persons with AIDS-related digestive problems may have allergies to dairy products.

• This writer is reluctant to name particular brands. However, we have heard highly favorable comments about 'Jarro-Dophilus,' produced by Jarrow Formulas in Gardena, California. It is unusual in containing five different organisms (L. Rhamnosus, S. Faecium 68, L. Acidophilus ATCC, L. Bifidus, and L. Bulgaricus). This brand is sold in health-food stores, or can be ordered wholesale from Jarrow Formulas (see Appendix B), if not available locally.

• Robert Cathcart, M.D., of Los Altos, California, who is well known for his work with vitamin C in the treatment of AIDS and ARC, uses a different brand of acidophilus (Vital Life), which is sold through physicians and unlikely to be found in stores. Patients often start with three organisms (L. Acidophilus, L. Bifidus, and S. Faecium), then continue with L. Acidophilus only.

Major AIDS Conference

The "III International Conference on AIDS", the major scientific conference of the year, will meet June 1-5 at the Washington Hilton and Towers Hotel in Washington, D.C. *AIDS Treatment News* will be there and will be reporting new information in future issues.

New FDA Treatment Rules

A major rule change may allow persons with AIDS or other serious or life-threatening diseases much more access to experimental new drugs. Contrary to widespread press reports, it is not true that these rules only apply to persons believed to be within six months of death.

Comment: This important advance resulted from public pressure; and without continuing pressure it will mean little or nothing. The rule goes into effect in 30 days—but whether or not patients get appropriate treatment depends on how it is implemented. It is urgent that physicians, medical organizations, and AIDS service organizations inform themselves about these rules and serve as advocates to protect the interests of persons who are ill.

Nationwide "Red Tape" Protests June 1

Demonstrations against unconscionable delays in AIDS research and treatment availability will take place June 1 in Washington D.C. and several other cities—including Chicago, Los Angeles, and San Francisco. Both legal picketing and nonviolent civil disobedience have been planned. Supporters anywhere can wear red tape or a red armband to show solidarity.

Issue Number 33
June 5, 1987

About This Issue: *The articles below were written before the Washington D.C. AIDS confer-* *ence (June 1-5). We delayed the mailing in case new information from the conference made* *changes necessary. We left the articles unchanged, but added the following three notes:*

(1)   On monolaurin, some physicians and others have questioned the rationale of this approach, in view of the lack of *in vivo* tests as an antiviral. No one questioned its safety, or its efficacy against viruses if it can get to them. But theory predicts that monolaurin would be digested and not get into the bloodstream, and because the theory said it could not work, no tests have been done.

On the other hand, the same theory says that AL 721 could not work, yet evidently it does. Also, the only results we have heard of people using monolaurin for an extended time for HIV—the two people mentioned in the article below—have been good. They are even more enthusiastic about monolaurin now than when we wrote the article.

We must weigh the opposite dangers of promoting a treatment which may not work, vs. losing one which may. The effectiveness studies we would like to see have not been done; probably they will not be done for years. This article can only present what we know, and clarify the uncertainties which remain.

(2)   We also want to acknowledge the groups which brought monolaurin to our attention—Oklahoma Project Inform, and Nutrico—both in Tulsa, Oklahoma (see article below). Nutrico is one of the first buyers clubs by and for HIV-positive persons.

Today we are seeing a tremendous growth in such buyers clubs, in cities around the country. Their importance goes well beyond the substantial price discounts they obtain for their members on vitamins and other health products. Buyers clubs serve an important quality control function by representing their members in the marketplace. They help people avoid shoddy products, by learning who can and who can't be trusted, and by having their own laboratory tests done when necessary. They can negotiate prices, and find sources of hard-to-locate specialty products which few of their members could obtain on their own. Many of them will ship their products, so you can use their services from anywhere.

Many buyers clubs also provide product information. Nutrico, for example, sends a 100-page package of information free to its members. (Membership costs $12, but at this time they are sending the package free to anyone who asks for it.) Membership also allows purchase of products at a discount, about 25 percent under retail price.

(3) The other article below, "The Quackhunt of '87", was in large part a reply to a June 1 *Newsweek* article, "Preying On AIDS Victims," which cast aspersions on almost every unapproved treatment. Fortunately, the Washington, D.C. conference showed virtually no trace of the quackhunt psychology—understandable, since the scientists themselves could potentially be vulnerable to such accusations. The press also has trouble with a quackhunt, despite its initial attractiveness, because of the obvious legal difficulties of citing specific examples. The war foreseen in my article may hopefully be one we will not have to fight.

MONOLAURIN

Monolaurin, a fatty-acid derivative found in mother's milk, may contribute to the protection of the infant, before the infant's own immune system has fully developed. Monolaurin is known to be effective against several lipid-coated viruses (a class which includes the AIDS virus), and against certain bacteria as well. The U.S. government has approved monolaurin as a food additive for over 20 years; in 1964 the substance was placed on the list of GRAS substances ("generally recognized as safe"). It is a food which appears to be entirely safe to humans, and it has been extensively studied as a non-toxic food preservative which prevents the growth of bacteria and viruses. Monolaurin is inexpensive and readily available.

Yet until recently, researchers have had little interest in using monolaurin as a treatment for disease. Biochemical theories predict that the digestive system would break down monolaurin into the same end products already provided by ordinary foods, making it ineffective for systemic use as an antiviral. But recent experience suggests that these theories may be wrong.

Monolaurin works against lipid coated (enveloped) viruses much like AL 721—an experimental AIDS treatment developed in Israel, and covered in depth in earlier articles in this series. The same theories which predict that monolaurin could not work as an antiviral after passing through the digestive system also predict that AL 721 would not, for the same reason. But human experience now suggests that AL 721 can be effective orally as an antiviral. At least one of the leading researchers on monolaurin believes that if AL 721 can be an antiviral after passing through the digestive system, then monolaurin probably would too—and the combination may be especially effective.

A group in Tulsa, Oklahoma, called Oklahoma Project Inform, has studied monolaurin, and brought it to this writer's attention. Two people in that group have now used the treatment for almost 60 days, and report that it has been effective in reducing severe swelling of lymph nodes when nothing else had helped. Others have used monolaurin for shorter times, not long enough yet to tell whether it works. But no one so far has been unhappy with this treatment or stopped using it for any reason.

Background

Chemically, monolaurin can be described as a monoglycerol ester of lauric acid, a saturated fatty acid. Some commercially available "monolaurin," however, is only 40 to 60 percent pure and may not be effective; at least 90 percent is required (Kabara, 1984).

All experts seem to agree that monolaurin is entirely safe. Animals have been fed huge amounts, up to 25 percent of their total diet for ten weeks, without any sign of harm (Kabara, 1984). However, no human or animal scientific tests have studied its effectiveness when used orally as an antiviral.

Availability

Cardiovascular Research Ltd. (Arteria, Inc.) in Concord, California, a well-regarded health food company, distributes products containing monolaurin. Most of their business is through physicians, but they also distribute 300 mg capsules of monolaurin in health-food stores, under the "Arteria" or "Ecological Formulas" label. The cost of using 1.8 grams per day is about $30 per month. If local stores don't have the product, it can also be ordered from Cardiovascular Research Ltd. (see Appendix B).

REFERENCES

Flournoy, D.J. and J.J. Kabara, "The Role of Lauricidin as an Antimicrobial Agent," *Drugs of Today* 21(8) (1985), pp. 373-7.

Kabara, J.J., "Lauricidin: The Nonionic Emulsifier with Antimicrobial Properties," IN *Cosmetic and Drug Preservation: Principles and Practice*, Jon J. Kabara, Ed. (New York and Basel: Marcel Dekker, Inc., 1984).

Hierholzer, J.J. and J.J. Kabara, "In Vitro Effects of Monolaurin Compounds on Enveloped RNA and DNA Viruses," *Journal of Food Safety* 4 (1982), pp. 1-12.

Sands, J., D. Auperin, and W. Snipes, "Extreme Sensitivity of Enveloped Viruses, Including Herpes Simplex, to Long-chain Unsaturated Monoglycerides and Alcohols," *Antimicrobial Agents and Chemotherapy* 15(1) (1979), pp. 67-73.

THE QUACKHUNT OF '87:
LEGAL ATTACK ON ALTERNATIVE TREATMENTS?

On May 21, California State Attorney General John Van de Kamp announced the creation of a task force to investigate AIDS consumer fraud and quackery—the first such move in any state. This and other such attention might or might not cause problems for legitimate alternative treatments.

With so much unknown about AIDS, and with existing treatments so unsatisfactory, it will be hard to find consensus on how to distinguish legitimate unproven and unconventional treatment attempts from unconscionable schemes to exploit peoples' desperation. The danger, of course, is that everything not already approved by the U.S. Food and Drug Administration could be automatically classed as fraud or quackery, simply because the distinction of whether or not a treatment is approved provides the only dividing line which is easy for officials to use.

A war against treatment alternatives would greatly reduce the options available to persons with AIDS, ARC, or a positive antibody status. Only AZT has been approved for direct treatment of AIDS and ARC, and no other official approvals are near. Yet most people cannot use AZT, either because they cannot tolerate the side effects, do not benefit from the drug, do not qualify for it under current rules, or cannot pay the extraordinarily high price for it. Without the alternatives, these people are left with nothing at all except management of opportunistic illnesses as they occur.

The new FDA rules to liberalize access to experimental treatments should give some patients new options. But these rules apply—as they must—only to treatments already well advanced in official trials. Only drugs with strong commercial and institutional support get that far. Usually these are high-tech, biotechnology products. Such glamor drugs carry inherent risks because of their novelty, and usually they need years of development and testing before they become ready for widespread use. Meanwhile safe and rational low-tech options such as AL 721 and DNCB suffer official neglect and even active roadblocks. Such promising treatments, barred from official consideration by commercial or political constraints, are the ones which alternative treatments movements are making available. The new FDA rules will do little or nothing to improve access to these drugs.

An official myth holds that government and corporate scientists have pulled out all stops and are leaving no stone unturned in attempts to find a cure. In fact, with the exception of AZT which has serious drawbacks, almost all the research attention has gone into options which could not possibly be widely available for years. Appalling scandals not yet known to the public, such as the mishandling of AL 721, DNCB, and lentinan, will show that the Federal government as well as other U.S. institutions have never made a serious commitment to save the lives of those now ill. Now the grassroots efforts to do what the institutions have repeatedly refused to do may face political and legal attack.

A New AIDS Hysteria?

In the last two months at least a dozen mainstream journalists have called this writer; in the preceding year not a single one had called. Most of the callers were looking for frauds. They were convinced, often without having seen a shred of evidence, that the AIDS world teemed with quacks and frauds. And they were determined to find them.

"I know they're out there," was one typical comment. Another journalist asked for a "small scam"—meaning a handy villain to be pilloried, unconnected with a major institution with the means to fight back. Few of the callers had any interest in the public policy failures which had prevented effective AIDS treatment research and development—and prohibited AIDS service organizations which receive public funding from providing the oversight or advocacy to help correct the situation.

The quackhunt now being prepared provides an easy diversion for the public's heartfelt desire to do something about AIDS. It is politically safe, as liberals can accept it to keep persons with AIDS from getting exploited, and conservatives to keep them from getting treatment. It continues the long-standing approach of writing off persons with AIDS as already all but dead—to be helped through the dying process without a finger lifted in any serious effort to save their lives. It updates this approach for a time when the grassroots treatment movements have grown too large and visible to be ignored any longer.

What Can We Do?

The best way to protect access to alternative treatments is to keep our own house in order.

The AIDS community can extend and develop its own consensus on what is and is not legitimate. We have considerable consensus already:

• We insist on openness and disclosure. Secret treatments are not acceptable. People must know what they are using and why, and be able to seek independent advice. Note that the many quacks who rely on secrecy are automatically excluded from our community.

• Misleading claims are not tolerated. It is not legitimate to promise cures, to make other false or unproved claims, or to pretend to certainty when it doesn't exist.

Anecdotal evidence, however, is legitimate. It is better to present the best information we have, honestly labeled as uncertain, than to give up and do nothing until institutional research finds a definitive answer, several years later.

• We are moving toward a consensus that it is not legitimate for proponents of one treatment to urge users to drop out of others.

Unfortunately the drug companies have set a bad example by insisting that participants in clinical trials drop almost all treatments except theirs. They abuse their subjects, and distort their data by insisting on testing in isolation drugs which everyone agrees will be used in combination.

Besides developing consensus, a second way to guard against quacks and quackhunters alike is to maintain open communication.

San Francisco at least has had many treatment alternatives, but remarkable little AIDS fraud, in the sense of unsupported treatments deceptively promoted to make money. Much more would have been expected in so serious an epidemic. The extensive community networking and legitimate information channels have made it difficult for quacks to operate.

It is particularly important that patients can discuss alternative treatments intelligently with their physicians. Then those considering a questionable treatment can ask their doctor's help in checking it out. But physicians who automatically reject everything not already approved by the FDA cannot help their patients with such decisions and are unlikely to be asked.

A legal crackdown on alternatives would impede the very communication which discourages fraud. Not everyone will just give up and die; many will seek help secretly if they must. The growing quackhunt could ironically increase AIDS fraud by destroying the healthy openness and communication which has kept it in check.

The key to protecting this openness is consensus and a sense of legitimacy among persons with AIDS and ARC. Any political and legal attack must purport to be acting in the interest of the persons who are ill. It cannot succeed against a strong and articulate community consensus.

Issue Number 34
June 19, 1987

THE WASHINGTON AIDS CONFERENCE:
PART I—NEW HOPE ON TREATMENTS

The "III International Conference on AIDS," June 1–5 in Washington, D.C., the major scientific conference of the year, may become a watershed event for AIDS treatments.

As expected, no dramatic breakthroughs were announced. AIDS research proceeds with informal discussions among professionals, seldom by sudden surprises. Few, if any, of the treatments discussed at the Conference were brand new to the scientific community.

But the Conference did mark the growing optimism among scientists and physicians on the possibility of effective treatments. Dr. Samuel Broder of the National Cancer Institute, one of the leading U.S. AIDS researchers, summarized the change of attitude:

"Two years ago you could find 1,000 fine doctors who would say you could never stop the natural progression of this virus. Now you can hardly find anyone." (Quoted in *The Washington Post,* June 6, 1987).

Treatment Listing

Below is an overview of some of the treatment information presented at the Conference. Note the limitations of this listing. We have omitted most of the treatments for opportunistic infections. Even the list of treatments for HIV cannot be complete. No one could attend every session—many were simultaneous—nor absorb everything at the sessions one did attend. Some of the most current information comes from conversations in the aisles, which may not reflect all sides of an issue. This writer has not had time to research the background of all these treatments, or to call the researchers involved. This listing can only be suggestive, not authoritative or comprehensive.

The Conference had over 250 papers presented, plus over 1000 "poster sessions;" 700 others were turned down for lack of time and space. The presentations were recorded, and the public can order audio tapes from the address below. The poster sessions were displayed on long rows of bulletin boards in the exhibit area, each for one day, with the researcher there for part of that time to answer questions. Each paper or poster session had a short abstract, submitted in advance and passed out to all Conference goers in a bound volume of over 1200 abstracts. Unfortunately no additional copies of this *Abstracts Volume* are available; the volume has no copyright notice so presumably anyone could reprint copies. Meanwhile this writer will provide copies of those abstracts which are referenced in this article.

The treatment section below refers to the the abstracts by the same numbering system used in the *Abstracts Volume.* The first letter or letters gives the day of the week: 'M', 'T', 'W', 'TH', or 'F.' For poster sessions, a 'P' follows the day-of-week abbreviation. For example, "M 5.1" (which is a talk on Peptide T) refers to Monday, session number five, talk number one in that session. "MP 24" (a poster session on D-Penicillamine) refers to Monday's poster number 24.

Treatment Summaries

DDC (dideoxycytidine). This antiviral works on the same theory as AZT, providing a false building block for the virus; it may be more effective. For laboratory studies, see THP 8, and TP 1. Human trials are currently being conducted and DDC appears less toxic than AZT; the biggest problem seems to be a skin rash which is temporary and usually not severe. At least 20 people are getting DDC in a scientific trial at this time, but it is too early to tell whether the drug will be clinically useful.

DDC has the same kind of institutional push behind it as AZT did, and it will probably move relatively quickly through testing if it continues to look good.

Underground supplies have developed, but at this time people are waiting until more is known.

AMPLIGEN (mismatched double-stranded RNA). This antiviral and immune modulator is getting considerable interest. A poster session at the Conference (MP 216) reported a test with eleven AIDS and ARC patients. No toxicity was found, and there were many improvements; for example, all patients had been anergic on multiple skin tests before treatment, and all reversed this condition. One AIDS patient, however, developed pneumocystis for a second time and died, after having received the treatment for seven weeks.

A new trial with 200 patients has now begun.

Another poster session (MP 5) presented laboratory results suggesting that Ampligen would work well with AZT, and might allow AZT to be used in a fifth or less of its usual dose to get the same effect as the full dose of AZT without Ampligen.

A report is being published this month in *The Lancet.*

AME (amphotericin methyl esther). AME was easy to miss at the Conference but is generating considerable interest among researchers who know about it.

AME, a water-soluble derivative of the antifungal medicine amphotericin B, has been effective against HIV in several ways in laboratory tests. In humans, AME was tested in the U.S. about 10 years ago as an antifungal; apparently it is much less toxic than amphotericin B. But during the testing some of the doses were too high, and people were hurt seriously enough to sue the manufacturer, which then abandoned the product. The importance of this earlier testing is that dosage and toxicity are now known. We have heard that AME is available today in some countries.

The researchers who presented the poster session (MP 226) are now trying to get clinical trials started for AIDS or ARC. AME might be combined with AZT; the researchers suspect that only a tenth the usual dose of AZT may be required.

AZT (Retrovir). More papers reported research on AZT than on any other treatment—not surprisingly since only AZT is officially approved. Most of the published abstracts do not provide much new information. They confirm the picture we already have—that AZT can help some people, but also that it can have serious side effects.

The most important new development with AZT seems to be the possibility of combining it, usually in low doses, with other drugs, such as DDC or AME.

This writer did not attend the AZT talks or panel, however, and could not obtain the tapes by press time. Those who want more information on AZT could purchase these tapes (see below).

Burroughs-Wellcome also presented a special meeting on AZT for physicians, closed to the press. According to one of the attenders, the data analyzed so far shows a one-year survival rate of 90 percent in the experimental group originally on AZT, much less in the group originally on placebo and switched to AZT later. Other points were that side effects go down in time; and AZT is helping with neurological problems. Burroughs-Wellcome also produced an AZT videotape which it recently mailed to physicians.

Another viewpoint will become available through Project Inform in San Francisco, which has just obtained extensive documentation on the approval of AZT through a Freedom Of Information Act request. This documentation is now being analyzed.

Whatever the medical judgment on AZT, this drug has had an important role in overcoming the fatalism about AIDS treatments, thereby opening the door to serious efforts to save lives instead of just preparing people for death. Many professionals cannot take a treatment seriously unless it is approved; others cannot unless it makes money. AZT has made these people aware that treatment for AIDS is possible. AZT may save more lives by this political effect—opening the door to other research—than by its direct medical use.

Alpha Interferon.   A number of papers reported studies of this treatment, often in combination with AZT. No clear picture emerged from the published abstracts.

Peptide T.   This possible treatment, which has had a very limited clinical trial, has become the focus of a major scientific controversy.

Peptide T (TH 1.3, M 5.1—also see *Sentinel,* January 16, 1987) mimics a part of the AIDS virus which, some scientists believe, makes the initial attachment to the receptor site on the T-helper cell. Some studies have found that peptide T prevents infection of these cells, in the laboratory and in humans. However, most researchers have been unable to reproduce the laboratory results—only one other team has recently done so—and the human trial, in Sweden, involved only four patients. Recently the FDA approved further clinical trials in the U.S.

At this time the scientists are divided on peptide T, and most appear skeptical. But even if this particular drug doesn't work, the line of research which produced it may have great value. Already one team which failed to get results with peptide T produced another peptide which inhibited the AIDS virus in the laboratory without harming cells (WP 6).

Ribavirin. The bitter disputes around this drug became more bitter during the week of the Conference, with the FDA and others accusing the manufacturer, ICN Pharmaceuticals of Costa Mesa, California, of unethical conduct. Meanwhile, ICN sued a securities company in a separate dispute.

These conflicts aside, what do we know about whether the drug works?

The major clinical study of ribavirin and HIV gave 800 mg daily, 600 mg, and placebo, to two separate groups of patients; one group had lymphadenopathy syndrome (LAS), and the other was more seriously ill with ARC. On January 9 of this year, ICN released results of the LAS patients, reporting that none using the 800 mg dose progressed to AIDS, while 10 in the placebo group did (see *Sentinel*, January 16).

But later it became known that a number of patients had been accepted by the study even though they were too ill to qualify under the study's rules. And the great majority of these more seriously ill patients ended up in the placebo group. Many of them progressed to AIDS, distorting the study's results. There is a bitter dispute over whether the ribavirin data showed any effectiveness after this error had been adjusted for (see T 8.5).

Meanwhile, results of the ARC patients were presented last week at the Conference (T 8.6). Ribavirin in the doses tested showed no effectiveness. In fact, more people died in the treatment groups than with the placebo, apparently by random chance.

At the same time, however, some small clinical studies continued to show effectiveness (TP 226, WP 224). And many persons continue to be convinced that ribavirin is saving their lives.

The study which failed to show effectiveness of ribavirin used doses only up to 800 mg per day. The ribavirin underground has long said that this dose is marginal or ineffective; but ICN chose to bend over backwards for safety when designing the study.

Some of the leading researchers want to test ribavirin in higher doses. But meanwhile it is clear that this drug came out of the Conference with considerably less credibility than it had going in.

Other Treatments

Scientists also reported about the following treatments and potential treatments, among others, at the Conference. For space reasons we must cover these in future issues.

- Aerosol pentamidine (TP 217)
- AL 721 (M 5.6, TP 223)
- Avarol and avarone (MP 1)
- Bestatin (WP 229)
- Castanospermine (T 4.3)
- Diethylcarbamazine (MP 3)

- D-Penicillamine (MP 24, TP 220)

- DTC (Imuthiol, diethydithiocarbamate) (MP 227)

- Foscarnet (TH 8.1, THP 13, THP 237, THP 238)

- Glycosylation inhibitors (TP 23)

- Granulocyte-Macrophage Colony Stimulating Factor (MP 222)

- HPA-23 (WP 216, WP 218)

- Imreg-1 (MP 218, THP 241)

- Isoprinosine (MP 132)

- Milk from hyperimmune cows (THP 148)

- Naltrexone (WP 227, THP 124)

- Phosphorothioate analogs (T 4.4)

- Rifabutin (ansamycin) (THP 228, THP 233)

- Tumor Necrosis Factor (T 4.5)

- Vaccines (many papers)

We may also comment on several treatment approaches notably absent from the Conference, although they should have been there. Examples are DNCB, herbal and Oriental therapies, and nutrition.

For More Information

Most of the 250 presentations were taped. Anyone can order the audiotapes from InfoMedix (see Appendix B). Ask for program number T205. Most tapes cost $7.50 for one session, which often includes several related talks. There are no tapes for the poster sessions. The complete set of tapes can be ordered for about $400, or you can get a catalog of the tapes to order individually. (For example, tape number T205-T8, "Clinical Trials—AZT and Ribavirin," includes six talks, T 8.1 through T 8.6, and costs $7.50.)

Issue Number 35
July 3, 1987

THE WASHINGTON D.C. AIDS CONFERENCE: PART II

Part I of this article (see Issue Number 34) cited the new optimism among scientists and physicians about the possibility of developing treatments for AIDS and ARC. The leading experts are now moving from seeing AIDS as a certain death sentence, to considering the possibility that it may become like diabetes—usually controllable with continuing treatments, although still without a cure in sight.

The treatments which eventually will make HIV controllable probably exist now. But only the Federal government has the resources to move quickly and get testing underway for a wide range of plausible treatment options. Unfortunately, except for a handful of commercially attractive possibilities (mainly AZT), U.S. public policy has simply not included a serious effort to save lives through treatment development. So today dozens of treatments which could have been tested long ago are seeping out through the cracks of the system, often supported by tiny groups of researchers without the resources to make headway against a government and commercial structure so complicated, expensive, and ingrown that it systematically shuts out all but the best financed and best connected.

Our last article mentioned the treatments most discussed at the Conference: AZT, DDC, Ampligen, peptide T, Ribavirin, alpha interferon, and AME. Here we mention some of others, in alphabetical order. We have not obtained the tapes of the meetings or been able to review all the printed information; this listing is not comprehensive.

For more information on any of the treatments listed here, see below.

Aerosol (nebulized) pentamidine. A University of California, San Francisco study presented results of inhaled pentamidine as exclusive treatment for early stage pneumocystis (nebulized pentamidine is also used to prevent pneumocystis). The treatment was successful in six of the nine patients. Of the other three, one died after five days of treatment; the other two were taken off the study within 48 hours, because their pneumocystis had progressed until it was no longer considered mild enough for inhaled medication to reach the lungs properly. The researchers concluded that inhaled pentamidine deserves more study.

Note: in San Francisco at least, many leading physicians have much interest in nebulized pentamidine, both as a preventive and as a treatment for pneumocystis. Primary-care physicians do not need to obtain the equipment required or learn how to administer the treatment themselves; instead they can prescribe preventive doses for patients at risk, such as those who have already had pneumocystis, those with low or rapidly falling T-helper counts, and those beginning certain kinds of chemotherapy. Several other preventives for pneumocystis are also in use; no one knows for sure which is most effective. The advantage of nebulized pentamidine is that virtually no side effects have been found, even from the much larger doses used to treat the disease after it has already started.

Unfortunately this treatment is not available in most parts of the country. In some cities patients have organized a successful effort to convince physicians in private practice or in a hospital to learn how to administer it. Since patients receive the preventive dose only once every two weeks, they may find it practical to travel some distance for it if necessary. At least one home-care service (Caremark, in Hayward, California) can administer preventive doses at home, when prescribed by the primary-care physician.

For more information on aerosol pentamidine, see "A Breakthrough in Treating Pneumocystis" (Issue Number 23).

AL 721. One talk and one poster session at the Conference were devoted to AL 721. In addition, Yehuda Skornick, M.D. of Tel Aviv, Israel presented results of treating 28 patients; his data wasn't ready until after the Conference deadline, so he spoke at an unofficial meeting in a church across the street.

No surprises came out of these meetings; instead they strengthened what we already knew. Usually AL 721 does not raise T-helper counts significantly, at least not for several months. Apparently it stops further decline although we don't have scientific proof. However, mitogen skin tests, as well as HIV reverse-transcriptase assays, improved dramatically in most patients, though not in all.

Dr. Skornick's report concerned the nine of his 28 patients who had been on AL 721 for five months or longer. Platelets improved in all of them, in one case going from 16,000 to 110,000 in a month. In most, white blood cell counts improved. Temperature improved after 20 days. The only side effect was mild diarrhea in some. Dr. Skornick noted that several of his patients had started with very advanced AIDS or ARC, and that even cases considered terminal had been reversed.

Avarol and avarone. These naturally-occurring substances from a marine sponge have shown good results against the AIDS virus in the test tube, and have low toxicity in mice. They do cross the blood-brain barrier. A clinical trial with AIDS patients is being planned.

Bestatin. This immune modulator has been used with cancer patients. A double-blind trial on 22 HIV-positive patients apparently did not show any benefit in immunological tests in the doses used.

Castanospermine. This substance found in an Australian chestnut inhibits the AIDS virus in the test tube, by acting against the enzyme glucosidase I. No human tests have been done. The researchers (from Harvard Medical School, Harvard School of Public Health, and the University of Washington in Seattle) are now conducting laboratory tests to find out if castanospermine is synergistic with other antivirals.

Diethylcarbamazine citrate. A study at the Harvard School of Public Health showed some success with this drug in treating feline leukemia in cats. The researcher suggested that these results "may have implications" for the treatment of AIDS and ARC.

This poster session, presented on the first day of the Conference, would have attracted more attention if scheduled later. For a major talk on the second day of the Conference focused almost entirely on feline leukemia ("Vaccination Against Retroviruses," W.F.H. Jarrett, University of Glasgow, Glasgow, Scotland, available on audiotape from InfoMedix—see Appendix B—tape number T205-T6). This talk pointed out that the disease in cats is very similar to AIDS; what it causes is not really leukemia but rather an immune suppression.

D-Penicillamine. Two poster sessions reported on the use of this antiviral in patients with lymphadenopathy or ARC. The drug clearly can suppress HIV in patients, but the doses needed to be effective often reduce T-cell numbers or cause other serious side effects.

The researchers do seem to be finding dosage schedules which can suppress HIV in patients without causing serious problems. One protocol completely suppressed HIV replication in three of five patients—for as long as 24 weeks after treatment was stopped. The published abstracts do not report whether the patients' overall clinical condition improved.

This work is important because D-penicillamine has long been used, in high doses, for treating other diseases such as rheumatoid arthritis. It is readily and cheaply available by prescription. Side effects are serious, but they are well known, at least for persons without HIV. The drug deserves prompt study to see whether it can be clinically useful—as well as to discover its mechanism of action (chelation?) and see whether variations of the molecule, or other drugs which produce some of the same effects, could be more valuable.

For background information on D-penicillamine, contact Project Inform (see Appendix B).

DTC (Imuthiol). This immune modulator now looks very good. A poster session at the Conference reported a double-blind, placebo controlled study of 90 patients with ARC or lymphadenopathy at five different medical centers in France; 80 of the 90 patients had completed four months of the study and their results were reported. Impressive improvements occurred in almost every measurement taken, with no significant side effects. For example:

• In overall clinical condition, 18 of the treated patients improved after the four months, 20 were stable, one was worse. In the placebo group, two improved, 35 were stable, three were worse. The odds of getting results this good by chance are less than one in ten thousand.

- Three of the 40 placebo patients progressed to AIDS; one died. None of the treated patients progressed to AIDS or died.

- T-helper cells in the treatment group started at an average 393 and increased by 169. In the placebo group, the average started at 398 and increased by 38. (The increase in the placebo group was not explained. Possibly some patients obtained their own DTC on the side.)

- DTC also has some antiviral properties. The new T-helper cells do not become targets for the virus.

- The number of ARC symptoms decreased, from an average of 2.5 before treatment to 1.7 after. Meanwhile, in the placebo group the number went from 2.3 to 2.1.

- After stopping DTC, the benefits were progressively lost. This treatment appears to help in the management of HIV infection, but it is not a cure.

- Trials at six U.S. medical centers, as well as in France and in Germany, are now studying the effect of DTC on survival of AIDS patients, optimization of dosage, and combinations of DTC with antiviral drugs.

Note: At this time DTC compares very well with other possible treatments for AIDS and ARC. We now have much better information about it than about other experimental treatments which are getting more attention (such as Ampligen and DDC). DTC appears to be completely safe, is taken orally, costs almost nothing to manufacture, has shown major clinical benefit in a well-controlled trial, and would probably work even better if combined with antivirals.

But without initiative from the AIDS, medical, gay, and/or other affected communities, DTC will not become widely available soon. This treatment, developed by Institut Merieux, a French pharmaceutical company, does not have the political clout of AZT or DDC. Notice that the preliminary report of the French study—a double-blind trial of 90 patients at five medical centers—rated only a poster session at the Conference in Washington, easily overlooked among a thousand other poster sessions. Also notice that the U.S. government is not helping to finance even the trial at six medical centers within the U.S., apparently because Merieux chose not to apply for U.S. funding. DTC hardly has the inside track so necessary in the U.S. drug-approval process.

How can we help to make DTC available? At least three strategies deserve to be considered:

(1) New FDA rules allowing more liberal access to experimental drugs—providing the manufacturer is willing to make them available for compassionate use. DTC appears to be an ideal test case. Physicians who want to get the drug may need the help of an advocacy organization or a skilled staff person or volunteer, to help them through paperwork or bureaucratic logjams.

(2) A grassroots movement could distribute DTC—probably on the model of the DNCB "guerrilla clinics," which have provided DNCB to about 4,000 people. DTC is fairly easy to buy, or to make in a laboratory. It appears to be both safer and more effective than DNCB; certainly we have more scientific information about it from scientific trials.

Only one bottleneck has held back DTC so far: the difficulty of administration. The official studies use "enteric coated" capsules, which pass through the stomach and release DTC in the intestines. DTC would be destroyed by the acidity of the stomach, and might produce toxic byproducts.

Four means of homemade administration have been proposed; at least two are in use:

(A) Enteric-coated capsules. These are quite difficult to make, but it has been done. There have been some reports of stomach irritation from these capsules.

(B) Administration by enema. This writer has heard of four persons using DTC this way; all report good or very good results. The effects seemed to start rapidly, with people feeling better within one day. Only one enema per week is used.

(C) DMSO. This readily available solvent carries other chemicals through the skin. But one expert thought that DTC would break down too rapidly for this method to work.

(D) Disulfiram (Antabuse). This prescription drug, given to alcoholics to prevent them from drinking by making them sick if they do, is very similar to DTC. Apparently the two chemicals exist in equilibrium in the body, meaning that if either one is taken, a portion of it will turn into the other. For this reason, some physicians suggest that taking disulfiram could be a way to use DTC. If so, the availability and administration problems would be largely solved. But we have not yet heard of anyone trying disulfiram as an AIDS/ARC treatment yet.

The key to the development of a guerilla-clinic movement is the existence of instructions which enable people to use the treatment successfully. We would need a few people who would keep the instructions up to date.

Project Inform in San Francisco (see Appendix B for phone numbers and address) is preparing an information packet on DTC.

(3) One or more organizations could start tracking the development, approval process, and accessibility of DTC, AL 721, and other drugs which deserve far more attention and official support than they are getting. Such efforts could model themselves on environmental organizations, which study the details of natural habitats, corporate plans, and government regulations and procedures, in order to intervene with publicity, litigation, legislation, or private purchase as appropriate, to prevent environmental destruction. With thousands of lives already lost, and major logjams clearly visible in drug development and approval, it is surprising that no one has yet given AIDS treatments the same kind of attention and advocacy commonly received by forests, seashores, and wildlife.

Note: *AIDS Treatment News* previously reported on DTC in Issue Number 29, before the new results above were available. In that article we reported that patients in the clinical trial at San Francisco General Hospital were told not to use aspirin or nonsteroidal anti-inflammatory agents while they were using DTC. Since then we have heard from several sources that this restriction was not required for medical reasons. Apparently the purpose of excluding these drugs was to improve the data.

Issue Number 36
July 17, 1987

"GENERIC AL 721" AVAILABILITY

The egg-yolk lecithin product distributed by the PWA Health Group in New York can now be ordered from the distributor, who will ship individual kilograms, hopefully within a few days of receiving a money order. The total price is $250 per kilogram including shipping and handling. As far as we know, this product is the closest to AL 721 generally available now (mid July 1987), without having to wait several weeks or pick up the product locally. The situation is changing rapidly, however, and other products will soon become available. For information about ordering egg yolk lecithin, you can call American Rolland Chemical Corporation (reference deleted by editor as out of date; this text is retained here for historical purposes). Naturally the distributor cannot discuss medical claims.

THE WASHINGTON AIDS CONFERENCE: PART III

This article concludes the discussion of HIV treatment papers presented at the III International Conference on AIDS, Washington D.C., June 1–5, 1987. Note that the writeups below only summarize information presented at this particular conference. We have not had time to prepare a full background report on any of these treatments. For the earlier articles in this series, see AIDS Treatment News, *Issues Number 33 and 34. The reference numbers in the text of this article refer to the* Volume of Abstracts *of Conference papers; to obtain the abstracts discussed here, see below.*

Foscarnet. Several papers reported successful treatment of CMV pneumonitis, CMV retinitis, and HIV itself in persons with AIDS and ARC.

Foscarnet (chemical name trisodium phosphonoformate hexahydrate), an antiviral developed in Sweden by ASTRA Pharmaceuticals, has shown activity against HIV,

CMV, and all the herpes viruses. Side effects are usually small or moderate and they are reversible, although sometimes they are severe enough to require discontinuation of the drug. The main drawback of Foscarnet is that it needs to be administered continuously by intravenous infusion.

The results on CMV pneumonitis (THP 237) may be most important, because of the difficulty of treating this infection by other means. This study by researchers at hospitals in England treated eight CMV pneumonitis patients with Foscarnet for between eight and 26 days. All of the patients improved, and seven left the hospital.

In the CMV retinitis study (session number Th 8.1, reported here from the abstract prepared before the Conference), Foscarnet was given to 10 patients, nine with AIDS and one with severe ARC. In five of the patients the retinitis resolved completely; in the others it improved or stabilized. But after the drug was stopped, retinitis returned in six of the eight surviving patients. In three of them, it responded to subsequent use of the drug; the abstract does not say whether the other patients failed to respond to Foscarnet the second time, or whether other treatments were used instead.

Two HIV studies (THP 13 and THP 238), one with eight patients and the other with 14, reported a decrease in the ability to isolate HIV after Foscarnet treatment. One of these abstracts also reported clinical improvement; the other said nothing about clinical status.

Glycosylation inhibitors.   This paper (TP 23) reported a successful laboratory test of an approach to preventing the virus from initially attaching to the cell, by blocking the expression of glycoproteins on the envelope of the virus. The glycosylation inhibitor used in this test was 2-deoxy-D-glucose. The authors, at universities in Philadelphia, Wilmington, Delaware, and Brussels, Belgium, suggested that glycosylation inhibitors might prove useful in treating AIDS.

GM–CSF (Granulocyte-Macrophage Colony Stimulating Factor).   This substance, produced by genetic engineering, increased the white blood count in a test of four different dosage levels on a total of 16 AIDS patients (MP 222). The counts returned to near their original levels two to 10 days after the drug was discontinued. The authors suggested that GM CSF might be useful either alone, or in combination with antivirals.

Note: According to a report published after the Conference, GM CSF might cause the AIDS virus to replicate. Anyone considering using the treatment should investigate this serious risk. See "Cytokines Alter AIDS Virus Production," *Science* (June 26, 1987), page 1627.

HPA-23.   Two studies, one in Paris and one in New York, had little remarkable to report (WP 216 and WP 218). Both found moderate side effects, especially decreases in the number of platelets, but these effects were reversible when the treatment was discontinued. The French study found some success in HIV inhibition, but did not state whether there had been any clinical improvement. The New York study only reported on side effects in the abstract reviewed here.

Imreg 1.   Two poster sessions by the same authors (MP 218 and THP 241) reported on this substance, which is extracted from normal human white blood cells. One of the reports summarized the results of 50 patients with AIDS or ARC who have been treated repeatedly with Imreg 1 for over several months.

T-helper cells increased or did not fall in 23 of 48 patients followed for at least three months. Delayed hypersensitivity returned in 60 percent of the patients. Some patients showed clinical improvement such as weight gain, but the abstract did not report how many benefitted. The best results were found in persons starting with T-helper counts of 100 or more. A new study will enroll 150 patients with ARC or recent-onset KS.

Isoprinosine. This immune modulator is widely used in dozens of countries, but has long been out of fashion in the U.S., for reasons unclear. Persons with AIDS and ARC in this country have for several years obtained supplies from Mexico, often for use in combination with ribavirin.

One poster session at the Conference (MP 132) reported a study of Isoprinosine by researchers at Mount Sinai School of Medicine in New York. The study consisted of complex laboratory tests of blood from ARC and AIDS patients who were using Isoprinosine. The highly technical abstract concluded that Isoprinosine "initiated a cascade of cellular interactions leading to restoration of cell-mediated immune responses. These interferences with the defective helper/suppressor regulatory pathways may have important therapeutic implications."

Milk from hyperimmune cows. This treatment for chronic intestinal cryptosporidiosis was tried on three patients with AIDS, at the St. Luke's-Roosevelt Hospital Center in New York (THP 148). All three improved, and in the two who were tested, the organism disappeared from the stools.

The treatment consisted of proteins extracted from the milk of cows vaccinated with a preparation of human intestinal bacteria. The milk was specially pasteurized to avoid destroying the antibodies.

The researcher concluded that "While preliminary, the results strongly suggest that a large molecular weight fraction in cow's milk effectively suppresses cryptosporidiosis in patients with AIDS." This study is important because cryptosporidiosis, which causes chronic diarrhea, has resisted treatment with available drugs.

Naltrexone. A poster session at the Conference (WP 227) released more information from the same research project described in our article, "Naltrexone for AIDS/ARC," (Issue Number 16). Naltrexone, a prescription drug normally used to keep opiate addicts off drugs by blocking opiate receptors so that narcotics will have no effect, is taken in very small doses before bedtime by persons with AIDS or ARC, to stimulate the pituitary to produce more endorphins, the body's "natural opiates." The result seems to enhance the immune system; in fact, endorphins may be the mechanism by which exercise or good morale can be helpful.

The abstract presented at the Conference reported a double-blind placebo-controlled study with 39 patients, 38 with CDC-defined AIDS and one with ARC. Those getting the naltrexone showed a significant drop in a form of alpha interferon which is usually too high in these patients. After three months, the placebo study was ended and all patients received the naltrexone.

Of the 39 patients on naltrexone, 23 showed a large decline in alpha interferon over a one-year period; 16 failed to respond. There were far more opportunistic infections and deaths in the non-responder group. As of December 1986, 81 percent of the non-responders had died, compared to 17 percent of the responders.

No side effects were seen.

These results support the earlier impression that naltrexone appears to be helpful to some people, and appears to have no drawbacks.

Phosphorothioate analogs of oligodeoxynucleotides. This laboratory study by researchers at the U.S. National Cancer Institute and Food and Drug Administration tested what may become a new class of antiviral agents (T 4.4). Different chemicals of this class were effective in different degrees against HIV in laboratory tests. At least one worked synergistically with dideoxyadenosine (DDA), an experimental antiviral related to AZT or DDC.

Rifabutin (ansamycin). A study found that this drug, used to treat the opportunistic infection MAI but which also can inhibit HIV in larger doses, does cross the blood-brain barrier, thereby fulfilling one requirement of an HIV treatment. The drug had been given orally for several weeks. The abstract (THP 228) does not state whether any clinical benefits or side effects were found.

A related study (THP 233)—also by researchers at SUNY in Stony Brook, New York, Long Island Jewish Medical Center in New Hyde Park, New York, and the U.S. Centers for Disease Control in Atlanta, Georgia—is giving increasing doses of rifabutin to patients until either antiviral or toxic effects are found. The published abstract, written before the Conference, reported neither effect at 600 mg. New information may have become available later. Incidentally, the researchers chose rifabutin because it inhibits HIV in the laboratory, has low toxicity when used to treat MAI, crosses the blood-brain barrier, and is given orally.

Tumor necrosis factor. This abstract (T 4.5) reported that tumor necrosis factor and alpha interferon worked together to protect cells against HIV in the laboratory.

Vaccines. Vaccine development has become a major area of AIDS research; we cannot summarize it here. Note that some of the potential vaccines being developed for AIDS are also treatments; they might work after persons have been infected with the AIDS virus, or even after they have become ill.

Issue Number 37
July 31, 1987

BEE PROPOLIS FOR THRUSH, FUNGUS, OR LEUKOPLAKIA?

Update 1988: We have continued to hear good results from persons using propolis for leukoplakia. In many cases it seems to be the best treatment available. The cost is almost nothing. The propolis usually sold in health-food stores is too weak to be effective. The right kind is either the raw form described in this article, or, if that cannot be obtained, a very strong tincture such as the one available from Herb-Pharm (see below). It would be very easy to test propolis for leukoplakia in a scientific trial, since when it works it shows dramatic results within a few days. Needless to say, however, no such trial has been done in the nine months since this article appeared. There is no institutional interest in such a trial.

Last week we first heard word of mouth reports that propolis, sold in health-food stores, may be helpful in treating thrush, fungal infections, and even hairy leukoplakia. We interviewed two persons with ARC who have used it; both are known personally to this writer. We have not heard of any others with HIV who have used propolis. But the results for these two were dramatic enough to suggest that this treatment might be useful for others.

Background on Propolis

Propolis, a waxy, resinous substance gathered by bees from buds of trees and used as a cement in the hive, has been scientifically studied as an antifungal, antibacterial, and antiviral treatment in the Soviet Union, Eastern Europe, and China. But U.S. medicine has ignored propolis so completely that the word does not even appear in any of three major medical dictionaries in common use. Health-food stores have long carried propolis, both in its raw form and in tinctures and capsules.

The published work on propolis, mostly from Eastern Europe and the Soviet Union, consists of highly technical laboratory studies, along with largely anecdotal clinical reports, usually of treatment for infections. Apparently there has not been a major effort to prove the effectiveness of propolis with controlled clinical trials, as is done with new drug products from Western pharmaceutical companies. Such trials would be expensive, and it is hard to see a motive for them in countries where physicians and lay persons alike already use the treatment as part of traditional practice. Nor would a U.S. pharmaceutical company be likely to spend the millions of dollars required to gain marketing approval under our system of medicine, for a product already cheaply available through the health-products industry. So propolis simply dropped out of the U.S. medical system. Only the patients might have cared, and they have had no voice for systematic research or advocacy on such matters.

Some of the more interesting clinical studies of propolis are a Soviet report on its use with 460 patients with infections (Tsarev *et al.*, 1985), and a Romanian paper on promising herpes treatments (Esanu, 1981), which mentioned propolis, garlic, and marine algae as promising antivirals. Other reports concerned propolis for treatment of various conditions, including 45 cases of oral leukoplakia, probably not AIDS related, in China (Pang and Chen, 1985).

For information on propolis use in the U.S. we asked a well-known herbalist, Ed Smith of Herb-Pharm in Williams, Oregon. He sells propolis (among other products), and described it as a very strong antifungal. He said that quality varies, as there are no marketing standards, although most of the products are good or excellent. Propolis also varies depending on the area from which it comes, because the bees gather resin from whatever kinds of trees are available.

Smith sells only a little propolis—several gallons a year—and is more interested in another product for thrush, a mixture of herbs which his company has formulated. (The herbs are: spilanthes; usnea, also called "old man's beard;" oregano; and pau de arco.)

Smith prefers either raw propolis, or the tincture. The tincture can be applied better for uses such as nailbed fungal infections. No one we talked to recommended propolis in capsules.

Safety

Propolis is not totally harmless; some people become allergic to it and develop skin rashes where it is applied. A number of articles mention this "contact dermatitis" from propolis, but most report just a handful of cases (Trevisan and Kokelj, 1987; Young, 1987).

One paper reported 22 cases (Rudzki and Grzywa, 1983), but 18 of them had dermatitis before exposure to propolis. Of the other four, whose dermatitis was primarily evoked by propolis, only two remembered the details of their exposure, and these suggested excessive use—such as applying 40 percent propolis in lanolin for ten days, or drinking propolis extract for fourteen days and rubbing it into one's fingers for the last four of those days, at which time the rash appeared.

The two persons with ARC interviewed by the writer used propolis only as necessary, and they had no problems.

Use By Persons With ARC

This writer hears many reports of proposed treatments for HIV-related conditions, and usually waits for more evidence than just two cases before writing a report. Here it seemed appropriate to go ahead because:

* I personally know both the persons with ARC reported below who used propolis. Neither has any commercial or other ulterior motive to promote this or any other treatment. They spoke only because they believe their experience may be valuable to others.

* Medical research in Eastern Europe and Asia, as well as folk medicine in many parts of the world, support use of propolis for fungal and other infections.

* It is reasonable to suspect that propolis may contain one or more natural antibiotics, as it is not destroyed by fungus or other microorganisms in the hive. Many plants produce anti-microbial substances for protection; and many antibiotics used in Western medicine come from these sources, such as penicillin from mold.

* Propolis is readily available, inexpensive, relatively safe, and quickly and easily tested to see whether it is working for someone. The harm which would be caused by raising a false alarm if it turns out that propolis doesn't work is much less than the cost of being wrong the other way.

* The results reported below were decisive enough that it seems unlikely they were coincidental.

Jim

Jim first brought propolis to my attention. He had been treating thrush for a month with Mycelex. This medicine worked at first, but the thrush became more aggressive until even Mycelex five times a day did not stop it. And even when the treatment was working, the thrush would come back the next day if it was stopped.

Jim used propolis only three times, and in one day the thrush was gone. Then he stopped the treatment to see how long it would take for the thrush to return. It has not come back in the week and a half which has elapsed until the time of this writing.

One complication in this case, however, is that Jim started using AZT one week before using the propolis. It is possible that AZT and not propolis was responsible for the result. That possibility seems unlikely, however, as AZT usually takes longer than a week to show any benefit. Here the improvement happened very quickly and dramatically, coinciding exactly with use of propolis. Jim is convinced that the AZT had nothing to do with it.

Jim used raw propolis, only a small amount and only when necessary. Twice a day he used a cube about a quarter inch on each side, and chewed it for half an hour. As reported above, only three uses were necessary. The expense was minimal, a few dollars for a small bottle which could last for weeks or months.

Bob

Bob has reason to believe that he had hairy leukoplakia four years ago, but the disease had not been recognized at that time, and the spot on his tongue was diagnosed as thrush.

But it did not respond to nystatin or other thrush medicines, even for several months, so Bob consulted a nutritionist, Denise Buzbuzian of Au Naturel health-products store in San Francisco, who suggested trying propolis. He used it for three days in the raw form, and the problem disappeared and did not recur for almost four years.

Then a few months ago, Bob had a severe case of poison oak which was treated with prednisone, a drug which can suppress the immune response. The spot on the tongue reappeared in the same place. This time it was biopsied and diagnosed as both hairy leukoplakia and thrush. The biopsy removed the entire spot, but two weeks later it returned, and Bob used propolis again. After three days the spot was gone, so Bob stopped the propolis. The hairy leukoplakia has not returned in the three months since, even without further propolis treatment.

Bob's physician explained that it was very important that the leukoplakia was gone, because when it was present Epstein-Barr virus was active. Scientists now believe that viruses such as Epstein-Barr and herpes stimulate the growth of the AIDS virus by increasing activation of the immune system. They may be important cofactors in the development of AIDS. If propolis stops the hairy leukoplakia, it may prevent this activation and help prevent progression to AIDS.

Bob's T-helper cells went from 490 four years ago to 860 recently. During this time he used ten to 15 grams of vitamin C orally per day, and also selenium, acidophilus, zinc, l-lysine, vitamin E, and multi-vitamins, in addition to using propolis only as needed. He stressed that people with hairy leukoplakia should not despair, as there are things they can do to help prevent the development of AIDS—including at least one experimental medical treatment for the leukoplakia.

Bob urges people to network back to the community with any information about successful or unsuccessful treatments. If something does or does not work for you, let others know.

Incidentally, Bob told Jim about propolis. Bob does not know anyone else who is using it at this time for any AIDS-related condition.

Let Us Know

If you have any experience with propolis for an HIV-related condition, please contact us so we can publish follow-ups on this article.

Acknowledgements

We wish to thank Jim and Bob, and Ed Smith of Herb-Pharm, for helping us with this article. Also thanks to herbalist Paul Lee of Santa Cruz, who referred us to Mr. Smith.

For information about Herb-Pharm products, you can call them (see Appendix B). They have a retail catalog for ordering products by mail.

Denise Buzbuzian of Au Naturel in San Francisco, who first mentioned propolis to Bob, may be the first person to have brought this treatment to the attention of the AIDS community—and the first person anywhere to have found a successful treatment for hairy leukoplakia.

REFERENCES

Esanu, V., "Recent Advances in the Chemotherapy of Herpes Virus Infections," *Virologie* 32(1) (January–March 1981), pp. 57–77. In English, although published in Rumania.

Pang, J.F. and S.S. Chen, "Treatment of Oral Leukoplakia with Propolis: Report of 45 Cases," *Chung Hsi I Chieh Ho Tsa Chih* 5(8) (August 1985), pp. 485–6 and 452–3.

Rudzki, E. and Z. Grzywa, "Dermatitis From Propolis," *Contact Dermatitis* 9 (January 1983), pp. 40–5.

Trevisan, G. and F. Kokelj, "Contact Dermatitis from Propolis: Role of Gastrointestinal Absorption," *Contact Dermatitis* 16(1) (January 1987), p. 48.

Tsarev, N.I., E.V. Petrik, and V.I. Aleksandrova, "Use of Propolis in the Treatment of Local Suppurative Infection," *Vestn Khir* 134(5) (May 1985), pp. 119–22.

Young, E., "Sensitivity to Propolis," *Contact Dermatitis* 16(1) (January 1987), pp. 49–50.

AIDS TREATMENT NOTES

Fake AL 721 on the Way?

Industry sources tell us to expect that one or more companies will start selling powdered egg yolk as "egg lecithin." The product, commercially called "dried egg yolk solids," is normally used in cake mixes, breads, milkshakes, and other processed foods. Cheap and readily available, it can be sold at an enormous markup and still undercut legitimate "generic AL 721" type products. It is no closer to AL 721 than egg yolks from a grocery store.

The best defense will be community-run organizations such as buyers clubs, which can do laboratory testing when necessary to expose bad products and select good ones.

Danger: AZT and Tylenol Don't Mix

Update 1989: Recent results have questioned the earlier conclusion that combining AZT and acetaminophen is dangerous.

Anyone using AZT should know that combining it with acetaminophen (the active ingredient in Tylenol and some other pain-killers) can seriously increase the hematologic damage which is the worst side effect of AZT.

The package insert on Retrovir (AZT), supplied to physicians by Burroughs-Wellcome, warns several times against combining AZT and acetaminophen (March 1987 version). Yet even in San Francisco we are finding that many patients using AZT have never heard this warning.

A number of other drugs might also be dangerous if combined with AZT. Patients using AZT should make sure they are advised by their physicians about possible drug interactions.

AIDS/ARC/HIV-Positive Affinity Groups

We received the following notice from Gary Babcock in Berkeley, California, who is facilitating the development of HIV-positive affinity groups. You can call him for more information. We highly recommend this effort.

"Some persons who are HIV positive or who have ARC or AIDS are forming their own affinity groups of eight to 12 people. These groups meet regularly, usually once a week, to discuss the latest news about therapies, drug trials, availability of different treatments, and so on. Another function served by such groups is to buy nutritional supplements or drugs (such as AL 721) in bulk, thereby reducing members' cost.

"Activities often associated with traditional support groups are also undertaken by HIV positive affinity groups. Readings are often assigned from books on self-healing, and are discussed at subsequent meetings. Doctors or other experts sometimes speak before the group to share their information and advice. Group meditations are often undertaken, and sometimes meetings are simply occasions at which people may express concern and support for their fellow group members.

"There is no known larger organization of such affinity groups; there probably should be. Those who are interested in forming their own group, or a larger umbrella organization of such groups, and in learning what some already existing groups have found helpful, are invited to call Gary Babcock evenings before 9:30 PM (see Appendix B).

Issue Number 38
August 14, 1987

WHERE TO GIVE MONEY FOR AIDS RESEARCH

Update 1989: At this time we would also add other worthy treatment-advocacy organizations, such as ACT UP, Lambda Legal Defense, and community-based research organizations in many cities.

Several people have asked this writer to suggest where they could contribute to AIDS research in order to do the most good. The answer depends on your perspective and what you want to do.

This article outlines some options by giving examples which the writer recommends. The options are extremely diverse, as you will see. And no such listing could be comprehensive; many equally important possibilities do not appear here.

Those who prefer to make anonymous contributions can do so by using postal money orders.

The AIDS-Research Problem

Already the Federal government spends hundreds of millions of dollars on medical research relevant to AIDS. Most of this funding does go to worthwhile projects. But the money gets distributed through an intensely political process—a process reflecting the interests of the biggest drug companies, old-boy networks of scientists who want high-tech, glamorous projects, and a national political administration fundamentally hostile to AIDS research. Almost no one represents the interests of persons with AIDS or ARC when these funding decisions are made. The result is that only a narrow range of research ideas—mainly those related to AZT and similar drugs such as DDC—get serious mainstream attention. The current system does fund worthwhile projects, but it also leaves gaping holes of neglect.

The real decisions on AIDS research are made outside of public view—sometimes because of corporate secrecy, but mainly because of the inattention of AIDS service organizations and of the press. This lack of public attention has made it hard for individuals to make independent funding decisions which bypass the politics of AIDS treatment research.

Fortunately there are some attractive organizations which either give money to AIDS research, or are directly involved themselves. You can contribute through them and let their scientific committees evaluate specific proposals. Or you may want to contribute to advocacy, investigative, or political groups working to improve public policy on AIDS research.

Direct Support of Research

The American Foundation for AIDS Research (AmFAR). By far the largest and most established non-profit AIDS research group, AmFAR gave about four million dollars last year, mostly for laboratory biomedical studies. AmFAR also publishes the excellent *AmFAR Directory of Experimental Treatments for AIDS & ARC,* available from their New York office (see Appendix B).

At least 70 percent of money received goes directly into laboratory and clinical investigation, to accelerate the development of a vaccine and effective therapy for AIDS. In addition, AmFAR gives grants for educational, ethical, legal, and behavioral research, and conducts in-house projects such as the Directory, and the preparation of public-service announcements.

AmFAR can fund projects much faster than the U.S. National Institutes of Health— approximately two to three months, compared to 12 to 18 months for Federal funding. However, researchers who apply need to fit into AmFAR's twice-yearly funding cycle. The application process first starts with a letter of intent; if that is accepted, a formal application will be sent. AmFAR does not have the flexibility to award, say, a few thousand dollars to a scientist next week for a quick test of a promising idea.

The 32-member scientific advisory committee, which makes the funding decisions, includes some of the best-known people in AIDS research. Some of the familiar names are Robert Gallo and Samuel Broder of the National Cancer Institute, Jay Levy and Paul Volberding in San Francisco, and Mathilde Krim, a medical researcher and well-known advocate for faster development of and access to treatments. The board also includes physicians known for their work with AL 721 and other experimental treatments at St. Luke's/Roosevelt Hospital Center in New York. AmFAR's president is Mervyn Silverman, and its national chairman is Elizabeth Taylor. The founding co-chairs are Mathilde Krim, Ph.D., and Michael S. Gottlieb, M.D.

Typical studies funded in the current year include "Analysis of AIDS Retrovirus Envelope Gene" ($60,000), "Studies Towards the Development of an AIDS Virus Vaccine" ($47,500), and "Increasing T-Cell Resistance to Primary Infection by HIV" ($50,000).

Tax-deductible contributions can be sent directly to AmFAR (see Appendix B).

Community Research Initiative (CRI). This research organization originates from the AIDS community, and has obtained legal status as an Institutional Review Board (IRB) to conduct rapid, low-cost clinical trials of promising AIDS/ARC treatments, in cooperation with private physicians and their patients. The CRI is a subsidiary of the People With AIDS Coalition, Inc., in New York.

Most IRBs exist in hospital research centers. Unfortunately, it costs so much to do anything in that setting that little can happen without the initiative of a major pharmaceutical company. If a drug is unpatentable or otherwise doesn't fit into corporate business plans, it is unlikely to ever get tested, regardless of its medical promise.

The Community Research Initiative, with its IRB and associated Scientific Advisory Committee, can organize testing through private physicians at far less than the usual cost. Therefore, it can raise enough money in the community to do trials that should be done, even for treatments not commercially attractive. It will also work with pharmaceutical companies to test their products when appropriate.

The CRI is already setting a healthy example by designing studies without placebos, trials not arranged to sacrifice one group of patients in order to prove that the drug received by the others is effective. One example of such a trial is a design to test aerosol pentamidine in two different doses, both equally reasonable according to all current knowledge, in order to see which dose works best.

The scientific committee, which decides which tests to do, includes Dr. Bernard Bihari (developer of the naltrexone treatment for ARC/AIDS), Michael Lange (of Columbia University, currently conducting trials of AL 721 at St. Luke's-Roosevelt Hospital Center), Dr. Donald Armstrong (Chief of Infectious Diseases at Memorial Sloan-Kettering Cancer Center), and 12 other physicians. The IRB itself, which functions primarily to assure the welfare of patients in the trials, has 16 members including Dr. Bihari, Michael Callen (a founding member of the National Association of People With AIDS and ARC), Dr. Mathilde Krim (also with AmFAR), Ms. Carol Levine of The Hastings Center Institute of Society, Ethics, and the Life Sciences, Dr. Nathaniel Pier (who has a large AIDS/ARC practice in New York and has long urged proper testing of lentinan), and Dr. Joseph Sonnabend, one of the principal organizers of the Community Research Initiative. The IRB first met in March of this year.

The Community Research Initiative is now considering clinical trials with aerosol pentamidine pneumocystis prophylaxis, AL 721, DHPG for early intervention in AIDS, DNCB, naltrexone, transfusion therapy, large-dose penicillin, and a hyperimmune milk treatment for cryptosporidiosis. It is investigating the feasibility of a computerized database for treatment information and rapid communication among physicians. In addition, it plans to review research at other institutions and to publish critiques.

If there is one place where money could do the most good in the direct support of clinical AIDS research, it is probably the CRI. The low-budget clinical research makes donated funds go a long way. The organization has first-rate physicians and scientists, and it is fast, flexible, open-minded, and responsive to the AIDS/ARC community.

For information on contributing to the Community Research Initiative, call them in New York (see Appendix B). Contributions are tax deductible.

Changing Public Policy:
Advocacy, Investigative, Political, and Other Groups

Your contribution might accomplish more for AIDS research by changing public policy than by paying for the research directly.

AIDS is a major public emergency which has not been handled in a responsible manner. Part of the problem stems from homophobia. But an equal part stems from lack of advocacy—something easier for us to remedy.

The U.S. government runs on pressure groups. Yet almost all AIDS, medical, and gay organizations have refused even to look at public policy concerning the management or direction of treatment research, ethics in the conduct of clinical trials, or compassionate access to drugs not yet fully approved for massive commercial promotion and marketing.

The groups below are some of the exceptions. These low-budget organizations rely almost solely on individual contributions. Just a few hundred dollars can be a major part of a monthly budget and make a visible impact on some of the most important AIDS work now being done. These groups seldom get any of the money from the major AIDS fundraising appeals; individual donors need to inform themselves and make their own allocations.

The list below includes only San Francisco-based organizations, because those are the ones this writer is most qualified to recommend. Many equally important organizations are working elsewhere.

Mobilization Against AIDS (MAA). In existence since 1984, Mobilization Against AIDS has consistently fought for huge increases in funding for research on the Federal level. It focuses especially on the House Budget Committee, which sets the high ceiling mark for Federal expenditures for AIDS research. It has been very effective in organizing constituents in Congressional districts around the country, especially for members of the House Budget Committee and other key persons in Congress.

Last year, MAA fought for 500 million dollars for Federal AIDS research, despite criticism from other lobbying groups which said such an amount was impossible. MAA got diverse groups to use 500 million as their high figure in discussions—instead of a much lower ceiling—probably resulting in far more money being appropriated in the final compromise than otherwise would have been the case. This year, MAA is asking for one billion dollars for research—an amount also recommended in the National Academy of Sciences report on AIDS.

In addition to its work on research funding, MAA organizes the world-wide candlelight vigils on Memorial Day. In California, it has also taken major leadership roles in the fight against attacks on civil liberties, such as the LaRouche Initiative, or the current efforts of State Senator John Doolittle to force much of the LaRouche policy through the California legislature.

Mobilization Against AIDS does not receive, nor would it accept, funding from any government agency. It receives very little help from foundations and relies almost entirely on member and other contributions.

You can contribute to the Mobilization Against AIDS by sending a check—or anonymous money order if you prefer—to them (see Appendix B for address and phone number).

Project Inform. This organization is one of the few which is willing to give information on treatments not already approved by the Food and Drug Administration. It runs a toll-free hotline (see Appendix B), trains volunteers, and answers about 400 phone calls and mails about 250 information packets per week. It has conducted its own research surveys of reports from users of experimental treatments, including ribavirin and isoprinosine, and AL 721.

For background information on Project Inform, see *AIDS Treatment News,* Issue Number 27.

Project Inform is supported primarily by individual donations, although recently it has received some foundation support, and last year it received a research grant from ICN Pharmaceuticals, the manufacturer of ribavirin. It needs more donations to maintain the toll-free hotline, the special telephone equipment required for the high volume of calls, and the paid staff of two.

For information on contributing to Project Inform, call them on their toll-free hotlines (see Appendix B).

Guerilla Clinics. In July of last year, a leading U.S. dermatologist was scheduled to begin a clinical trial with DNCB in the treatment of AIDS/ARC, at the University of California San Francisco Medical Center. This chemical is painted on the skin where it causes a reaction very much like poison oak. It also increases the number of T-cells in most patients. Considerable anecdotal evidence suggests that this treatment may be helpful for many people with KS or other forms of HIV infection. (For background information on DNCB, see *AIDS Treatment News,* Issue Number 14.)

But the study kept being postponed, due to funding and other problems; to this day it is still being postponed. Meanwhile a grassroots "guerila clinic" movement came into being and distributed DNCB to an estimate four to five thousand people, who have used it under a physician's supervision when possible, otherwise without.

A center of this movement has been Jim Henry, who established a national DNCB information phone (see Appendix B) and sends out about 20 free packets of DNCB information per day.

We asked him about the concern of some physicians that DNCB might increase growth of the virus, either by providing more T-helper cells to infect, or by causing inflammation, which recent indications suggest might itself stimulate growth of HIV. He replied that most people using DNCB today are combining it with an antiviral. Until recently most had been using ribavirin, but now many are switching to AL 721, primarily because of the prohibitive cost of ribavirin. Some are using AZT. Mr. Henry has seen that most people whose T-helpers are not too low to begin with can sustain an increase in T-cells by using the DNCB/antiviral combination.

We asked about indications that DTC (Imuthiol) may be better than DNCB in every way—safer, more effective, not leading to increased viral growth despite increase of T-helper cells, and now supported with much better data than DNCB. Jim Henry replied that the guerilla clinics do indeed have an interest in DTC, but right now their hands are full maintaining what they are already doing.

Mr. Henry and other leaders of the guerilla clinic movement are approaching burnout due to the heavy commitments of time and money required, and lack of sufficient support from the community. Jim Henry works 40 hours a week to support himself and the clinics, and an additional 40 hours a week on DNCB. Donations haven't paid all the bills, so he must contribute his own money in addition. He needs enough support to cover postage and printing expenses, and to either hire someone to help with the work or to enable him to devote full time to it.

Chances are excellent that people looking back on the epidemic will realize that the guerilla clinic movement saved dozens if not hundreds of lives. To discuss how you can contribute to this important effort, call Jim Henry (see Appendix B).

Citizens For Medical Justice (CMJ).   *Update: Citizens for Medical Justice was superceded by the AIDS Action Pledge, which became ACT UP/San Francisco (see Appendix B), and by the continuing work of the AIDS/ARC Vigil (see Appendix B).*

This group (CMJ) conducts protests to publicize the issues around AIDS research, affordability of treatments, and civil liberties violations. Recent demonstrations focused on red tape in AIDS research and access to treatments, and major delay in the development and operation of AIDS Treatment Evaluation Units, the Federal program for testing drugs for AIDS and ARC. Other demonstrations have focused on the Governor's veto of a California bill to protect persons with AIDS/ARC against discrimination, on the exorbitant cost of AZT, and on mandatory testing of applicants for the Job Corps—and exclusion of those testing positive.

CMJ has also taken a major role in organizing protests against the Doolittle bills in the California legislature.

Some of the demonstrations involve legal picketing and communication only. Others involve civil disobedience and arrest. CMJ specializes in thorough, very strict non-violence training, to avoid any behavior which would antagonize or harass persons working at the demonstration site; instead, all action is focused on publicizing the issues. CMJ has also specialized in conducting fast-paced public meetings, at which representatives from different constituencies can reach consensus on major goals and on specific demonstrations or other actions to achieve them.

Citizens for Medical Justice consists of a core group of about ten people, plus others who join in some of the projects. It operates on a low budget, about $1500 per month in expenses, mostly contributed from the pockets of the organizers.

National Gay Rights Advocates.   This public-interest law firm specializes in litigation which can have a broad impact on public policy. It has been highly effective in opposing insurance discrimination, quarantine, and other civil-liberties violations.

In June of this year NGRA filed a class action lawsuit against the U.S. Department of Health and Human Services, the Food and Drug Administration, and the National Institutes of Health, concerning mismanagement of treatment research and access to treatment by persons with AIDS and ARC. NGRA will be able to use subpoena powers to obtain and make public previously hidden information from government records and from the testimony of government officials concerning AIDS treatment research and how it has been conducted. If you have specific information about conflict of interest or other improper actions by Federal officials in AIDS research, contact Leonard Graff, the attorney in charge of the lawsuit, at the address or phone number given in Appendix B.

Donations to NGRA are tax deductible. They can be directed to the class action lawsuit on AIDS treatments, or given for the general work of the organization. For more information, contact NGRA at the address or phone number given in Appendix B.

MAJOR NEW BOOK: *LIVING WITH AIDS: REACHING OUT*

San Francisco AIDS activist Tom O'Connor has had ARC for seven years and was seriously ill in 1982 and 1983. Then he began a systematic study and practice of many forms of AIDS/ARC treatments and healthy ways of living, centered around nutrition. Recently he has done extensive organizing work with groups such as the Gay Macrobiotic Network, the AIDS Healing Alliance, and the Healing Alternatives Buyers Club. And with Ahmed Gonzalez-Nunez he has put together an excellent survey book on all kinds of nutritional, holistic, and conventional medical treatments for AIDS and ARC.

The authors designed the book for "people who want to do something about their disease but don't know where to start; who see a need to take responsibility over their lives, no matter where they are; and who are willing to participate actively in their healing." The book presents the authors' excellent and wide-ranging research in a style remarkable coherent and easy to read. The book is scientifically literate, and maintains a solid, common-sense perspective from the point of view of the person with AIDS or ARC.

Some of the major topics include background on the immune system and on health and nutrition, choosing and dealing with physicians and other health practitioners, background and specifics on nutrition and diet, and problems such as food allergies, alcohol and recreational drugs, and likely cofactors in the development of AIDS such as herpes viruses and intestinal parasites. The book also discusses dozens of specific treatments, such as AL 721, DNCB, naltrexone, vitamin C, other vitamins, garlic, herbs, acupuncture, homeopathy and others. Included are many conventional medical treatments such as chemotherapy, antibiotics such as Bactrim and fungal treatments, and others. The authors see conventional medicine as an essential and major part of a treatment program, although they criticize certain excesses, and certain blind spots such as nutrition.

Extensive appendices include a comprehensive psychosocial and nutritional treatment approach by Keith Barton, M.D., a very extensive list of conventional and experimental drugs, information on vitamin C, food additives, food allergies and elimination diets, the use of herbs in AIDS and ARC, and macrobiotics. A resource directory includes addresses and phone numbers of dozens of information sources, from acupuncture to people with AIDS organizations to physicians sympathetic to complementary therapies (conventional Western medicine plus holistic approaches such as diet, herbs, orthomolecular treatment, and healthy living).

Living With AIDS: Reaching Out is being widely distributed to bookstores and can be ordered at most bookstores if they don't have it in stock. Copies may also be ordered from Corwin Publishers (see Appendix B). The retail price is $18.95, or, if you're ordering the book from within the United States, Corwin will sell at a discount price of $16. California residents need to add sales tax ($1.23 on the full $18.95 price or $1.04 on the discounted $16 price).

Issue Number 39
August 28, 1987

AL 721 SURVEY RESULTS: PRELIMINARY REPORT

Last month this writer mailed a questionnaire on AL 721 and other treatments to all subscribers to *AIDS Treatment News*. We asked people who have used any form of AL 721 to report on their personal experiences with it, as well as with any other AIDS/ARC treatments which were important to them. We received 147 completed questionnaires, with information not only on AL 721 but also on AZT, vitamin C, homeopathic treatments, Chinese herbs, lysine, DNCB, zinc, diet, spiritual practices, and many other treatment approaches. We are now analyzing the information; this article is the first published report.

We believe that this study will add important new knowledge about the effectiveness of AL 721—as well as some other experimental and alternative treatments, many of which have never received formal clinical investigation.

Goals and Design of the Study

We started with several questions. First, how many of the people who are using AL 721, etc. are getting good results? Are some of the versions proving better than others? What other treatments are people combining with it? Which patients are most likely to benefit? What improvements do they report—improvements others could watch for to see if the treatment is working for them?

And aside from AL 721, this study asked which treatments of any kind are proving most valuable.

We chose to use open-ended questions, to let people answer in their own words instead of giving multiple-choice responses. Open-ended questions take longer to analyze, but they let people tell us what is happening even if it doesn't match any of our preconceptions. We asked respondents to ignore our questions if necessary; several did so and wrote long letters instead.

How does one analyze such open-ended replies? Our basic approach was first to use certain questions or other information provided by the respondents to divide the set of questionnaires into subsets. One breakdown, for example, would divide the questionnaires into those from people who believed AL 721 helped them, those who found no benefit, and those who were uncertain. Other breakdowns could be those who used egg-derived vs. soy-derived products, those who used AZT vs. those who didn't, those who did or did not have KS, etc. After each division or subdivision, we cover each subset journalistically, reporting what those people have to say and how their experience differs from that of the others.

By analyzing the questionnaires this way we can use all the information people provided, whether or not they followed the formats we suggested. (This preliminary report gives mainly tabulations, however, due to time constraints.)

This survey could not rely on any standardized treatments, protocols, laboratory tests, or data collection. So we designed it as a study of peoples' beliefs about their treatments—admittedly subjective—rather than attempting to make it a scientific study of the treatments themselves. We asked people to tell us what they believed and to back up their beliefs with any evidence available, such as laboratory tests, symptoms, or how they feel overall.

Beliefs are not the same as proof; placebo effects and medical treatment fads illustrate errors the human mind does make. Those who consider patients' beliefs irrelevant will find nothing of interest in this study. But we think that people's beliefs about what works for their health are worthy of respect, and are valuable guidelines in the absence of perfect knowledge. It is better to face the danger of error by educating ourselves about how these errors happen, than by refusing to listen in order to protect ourselves from being misled.

How do we answer the criticism that any good results about AL 721 might be false "artifacts," because people who think the treatment is helpful might be more eager to tell us about it, biasing the statistics?

First, we tried to minimize such biases. We carefully worded the questions in a neutral way, and emphasized that we wanted to hear from everyone who used any form of AL 721, whether it worked or not. To increase the response rate, so that we wouldn't hear only from the most committed, we included a self-addressed stamped envelope with the questionnaire, set an early deadline for its return, and later sent a reminder with a short extension of the deadline. Almost all of the responses arrived on the forms and in the envelopes we provided—a protection against any possibility of a malicious attempt to "pack" the study, and also against well-meaning efforts of enthusiasts to get other enthusiasts involved. We found no indication of any such problems.

Second, this study has generated many results, often unexpected and unpredictable, which do fit together into coherent pictures or patterns. Attributing the whole outcome to errors and artifacts would require belabored, contorted explanations.

Ultimately, however, this study is descriptive; it does not claim to show conclusive or scientific proof that any treatment works. This survey cannot substitute for clinical trials. But it provides the clearest picture we could obtain of what peoples' experience has been.

Early Results

Exhibit II below summarizes the results so far:

How much success are people having with AL 721?   Of the 147 persons who returned the questionnaire, 110 had used AL 721 or a substitute for at least three weeks, a cut-off point which we chose before starting this analysis. Half of the 110 (50 percent) found it helpful, 15 percent found it not helpful, and 35 percent were uncertain. No one found the treatment harmful.

The actual picture is considerably brighter than these figures suggest. See other results and discussion below.

Does the version matter?   Few Americans can obtain the "real" official AL 721; only three of the 110 reported above had done so. But various substitutes have come into use. This study confirmed that only two of the substitutes had been widely available before August of 1987: the "home formula" made with PC-55™, a commercially available soy lecithin concentrate, and the egg-lecithin lipids from the PWA Health Group, a non-profit buyers' club in New York. Sixty-nine of the 110 (63%) had used the home formula, 33 (30%) used the Health Group version, and 8 (7%) used other versions, including the three who obtained the official one.

The version does matter. Of those who used the soy formula, only 43 percent reported it helpful, vs. 22 percent not helpful. Of those who used the egg version (from the PWA Health Group), 58 percent reported it helpful and only 9 percent not helpful. These percentages were computed from numbers given in Exhibit II, below.

These numbers are conservative because the questionnaires made it easy to get into the large "uncertain" category. The 33 percent uncertain about the egg formula (100 minus 58 minus 9) and 35 percent about the soy include several different groups of people. Some checked "uncertain" on the questionnaire, or expressed uncertainty in their own words. Others had improved but were using many treatments and could not know what benefits if any to attribute to AL 721. Others did not answer Question IV at all but left it blank without explanation. Others had been healthy throughout—such as those who were asymptomatic HIV positive—and therefore had no basis of comparison about whether any treatment worked.

If we consider only those who answered the question and had an opinion, then 67 percent of those using the soy version, and 86 percent using the egg, reported benefits. So the real fraction reporting benefit seems to be between 43 and 67 percent for the "home formula" soy version, and 58 to 86 percent for the egg version.

Future Reports

Analysis not yet completed includes what improvements, side effects, or other changes people found while using AL 721, etc., and which patients were most or least likely to benefit.

We will also analyze the dozens of other treatments reported—especially those volunteered in response to Question III, "What treatments—of any sort—seem to have been most valuable to you?" For each treatment in common use, we can also compute the proportion of its users who listed it as "most valuable," to obtain an index of the value of a treatment independent of its prevalence or popularity. For this analysis we will use all the questionnaires, not only those reporting use of AL 721.

We will also look at particular groups of patients, such as those with KS, to see what treatments they reported as most valuable.

Exhibit I: The Questionnaire

The following questionnaire was mailed to the 898 subscribers to *AIDS Treatment News*, on July 8. About two-thirds of these subscribers have AIDS or ARC.

The text below is identical to the form which was mailed, except that blank spaces for replies have been deleted.

AL 721 Survey

AIDS Treatment News is conducting a survey of AL 721 (and substitute or related treatments such as the "home formula"). The results, to be published here and elsewhere, will provide much-needed information which may help people make better treatment decisions.

If you have used AL 721 or any substitute, whether it helped you or not, or if you have cared for anyone who has, you can participate by returning this survey before July 20.

Answer in your own words. Use the back of this sheet or other paper if necessary to continue. Don't hesitate to change or ignore our questions; just tell us what matters. We will read and consider everything you have to say.

I. *What version(s)* of AL 721 (or substitutes) have you used? What daily doses and schedule? For how many weeks? (You can identify the version by telling us where it came from. If you are using an unusual product, tell us whether it comes from egg or soy lecithin.)

II. *What other treatments* have you used during this time? How long have you been using each one?

III. *What treatments*—of any sort—seem to have been *most valuable* to you?

IV. Do you believe that AL 721 has been *very helpful?; somewhat helpful?; no noticeable change?; harmful?* Are you very confident of this belief, somewhat confident, or uncertain?

V. *What changes* in symptoms, overall condition, or laboratory tests have you noticed while using AL 721?

VI. *Diagnosis.* Have you been diagnosed with AIDS? KS? ARC? Lymphadenopathy? Low helper T-cells but no symptoms? HIV-positive but no symptoms? No medical diagnosis but suspect you may have been exposed? Or are you using AL 721 or substitute for a condition unrelated to AIDS? How long have you had each diagnosis?

VII. Any other thoughts or comments?

Include your name, and phone or address, if we may contact you if we have questions (optional). *It's okay to remain anonymous if you prefer.* Return this survey to: John S. James, *AIDS Treatment News*.

Exhibit II: Preliminary Tabulations

One-hundred forty-seven (16%) of the 898 questionnaires were returned by the August 1 deadline. Of these 147:

- 110 had used AL 721 or substitute for three weeks or more.
- 18 had used it, but didn't say how long.
- 7 had used it less than three weeks.
- 1 was sent by a physician reporting on four patients.
- 11 had not used AL 721.

Of the 110 who had used AL 721 or substitute for 3 weeks or more:

- 55 (50%) found the treatment either somewhat helpful, helpful, or very helpful; and they did not check "uncertain" or otherwise express uncertainty about this estimate.
- 17 (15%) found the treatment not helpful.
- 38 (35%) either checked "uncertain," said it was too early to tell, or otherwise expressed uncertainty, or left the question blank.
- No one rated the treatment harmful.

Effect of different versions of AL 721, etc:

- Only two versions, the "home formula" using the PC-55™ soy lecithin concentrate (PC), and the all-egg version from the PWA Health Group in New York (HG), were reported often enough to give reliable information. The tabulation below shows that the egg-lecithin version gave better results.

RESULT	PC (soy)	HG (egg)	OTHER
Helpful	30	19	6
Uncertain	24	11	2
Not helpful	15	3	0

This table shows that 43% of the users of the soy formula rated it helpful, 22% found it not helpful. But 58% of the users of the egg formula found it helpful, and only 9% not helpful.

Those who started with one version and then switched to another were tabulated as using the later version, unless it could be determined that they had used it less than three weeks.

Continuing AL 721 Study

The AL 721 survey reported here is a one-time study; we are not sending out more questionnaires. However, Project Inform in San Francisco is conducting an ongoing AL 721 study. They want to hear from people using AL 721 or similar treatments, especially from people who can report over time and keep in touch for followup later.

To participate in the Project Inform study, call them and ask for their questionnaire. See Appendix B for their phone numbers.

Issue Number 40
September 11, 1987

AEROSOLIZED PENTAMIDINE

Update 1989: Aerosolized pentamidine was fully approved by the FDA in June 1989.

Last week physicians at San Francisco General Hospital and the University of California, San Francisco Medical Center published the first article on aerosolized pentamidine inhalation therapy to appear in a medical journal (*The Lancet,* August 29, 1987). We interviewed A. Bruce Montgomery, M.D., a principal investigator in this study, in order to answer some widespread questions about this anti-pneumocystis treatment which is already well known in the community.

Pneumocystis usually infects only the air sacs of the lungs. Physicians have long injected pentamidine as a standard pneumocystis treatment, but when given this way the drug causes severe side effects and often must be discontinued. Scientists found that very little of the injected pentamidine went to the lungs, where it was useful; most went elsewhere in the body where it did no good and could be harmful. But when made into a fine mist and inhaled, almost all of the medicine went to the lungs and stayed there, greatly reducing the side effects.

The Lancet article reports the results of treating 15 patients who had already developed mild to moderate pneumocystis. Aerosolized pentamidine in large doses was the sole treatment for 21 days. In 13 of the 15 patients the treatment was successful; of the other two, one died and one was switched to other pneumocystis treatments and recovered. Except for coughing, no one had any side effects attributed to the treatment.

In addition to the 15 patients in the study, three others were also given the aerosol because they could not tolerate other pneumocystis treatments. All three recovered.

Aerosolized pentamidine also reduced the average length of hospital stay to eight days, from two to three weeks for comparable patients treated with standard therapies.

Use for Prevention

The Lancet article does not discuss preventive use of aerosolized pentamidine—which uses much smaller doses, given every two to four weeks. Another team at San Francisco General is conducting a separate preventive study, expected to enroll up to 400 patients. Meanwhile physicians especially in New York and San Francisco are already prescribing the preventive treatment for their patients.

(Editor's note: the following paragraphs on dosage are including for historical interest; as of late 1989, the standard preventive dose is 300 mg, once every four weeks.)

For preventive use, many different doses are being tried—30 mg, 45, 60, 90, even 150, at different schedules varying from once a week to once every four weeks. We asked Dr. Montgomery, an expert in inhalation therapy, to help resolve the confusion about doses common among patients and physicians. He made the following points:

• Most importantly, doses cannot be compared across different nebulizers (the machines which make the aerosol mist). The size of the droplets produced is more important in determining the effective dose than the amount of pentamidine in the nebulizer.

• Most nebulizers in common use do not make a fine enough spray. Most make droplets about five microns in diameter. However, animal studies in San Francisco have shown that pentamidine is three times as effective if the droplets are reduced to less than two microns. Most of the large droplets are deposited in the airways of the lung rather than the air sacs, where the pneumocystis organism lives. And large doses with the wrong droplet size could cause severe coughing or possibly asthma-type reactions, because the form of pentamidine currently available was not prepared for inhalation use.

• The most convenient nebulizers are ultrasonic, often hand-held and battery-powered. But the ones in use today do not produce small enough droplets.

Ultrasonic nebulizers use a piezoelectric crystal—a crystal which vibrates at the frequency of an electric current which is applied. The droplet size depends on the electrical frequency. Unfortunately the ultrasonic nebulizers available today were designed to produce larger droplets for delivering asthma medicines to the air passages of the lung, not to the air sacs. Presumably it would be easy to use a higher frequency to make smaller droplets, but no one is manufacturing such a machine at this time.

So the San Francisco team designed its own nebulizer, which uses a gas jet to produce the droplets and a baffle to filter out most of the larger ones. This nebulizer is less convenient than the ultrasonic machines because it needs a source of compressed air or oxygen.

• *The Lancet* article tells physicians everything they need to know to use aerosolized pentamidine with the correct droplet size—including where to get the nebulizer.

• In San Francisco, a large community-based study of preventive use of aerosolized pentamidine is testing three different doses. If physicians find any dose to be less effective than the others, they will stop using that dose immediately. But it will take much longer to prove efficacy for the preventive treatment than for therapy given to persons who are already ill.

AIDS FRAUD TASK FORCE

The California Attorney General's AIDS Fraud Task Force, the first effort of its kind in the nation, held its initial meeting on August 18. This group of 24 persons from law enforcement, medicine, and AIDS organizations was formed to protect persons with AIDS or related conditions from unorthodox remedies considered to be "quack" or fraudulent.

This writer is a member of the Task Force. I accepted the invitation to join despite misgivings. For example:

• It is hard to distinguish legitimate unconventional treatment attempts from fraudulent ones when so much is unknown.

• AIDS quackery is less prevalent than people are eager to believe, as the community is highly skeptical of claims and inclined to discuss them with peers and physicians before buying.

• A legal crackdown would threaten the openness and communication which allows rational grassroots experimentation and cumulative development of treatment knowledge in the AIDS/ARC community.

But the Task Force will exist with or without my presence. Being involved allows me to bring to its attention certain information which otherwise would not be considered—and to report on its doings to the community.

Readers outside of California will not be directly affected, but may be interested because other states are likely to organize similar efforts.

Government Powers

The first meeting, by telephone conference among three locations in San Francisco, Los Angeles, and San Diego, was largely devoted to explaining the enforcement powers available under California and Federal law. Those of us involved in alternative treatments may need to become aware of these powers and laws. The specific citations below apply to California; you can easily look up the text of the laws, together with helpful annotations, in a public library.

• Deceptive advertising. It is unlawful to make statements which the person knows or should know are false or misleading, with the intent to sell goods or services. The statements need not actually be false to violate the law, nor made with intent to defraud. Violations are punishable by up to six months in jail and fines up to $2500 per violation—which could become hundreds of thousands of dollars since every person solicited by the advertisement could be considered a separate violation. (Business and Professions Code 17500, Health and Safety Code 26460)

• Unfair competition. This extremely broad law covers deceptive advertising and much, much more. Any business practice which violates any public policy may be included. Basically the law applies if the prosecutor can convince the judge that something isn't right. (Business and Professions Code 17200)

Unfair competition is not a crime in California, but the law provides extraordinarily powerful civil remedies. The court can place the business under supervision, and order corrective advertisements or other restitution, etc.

- California's Sherman Food, Drug and Cosmetic Act prohibits selling or giving away any new "drug" which has not been approved. "Drug" is defined to include "any article which is used or intended for use in the diagnosis, cure, medication, treatment, or prevention of disease. . ." Technically this language would outlaw almost all of the health-food and vitamin industries; it hasn't been used that way because of political constraints.

- The State can bring felony or misdemeanor charges of intent to defraud. It can remove any dangerous product from sale, and seize and destroy it at the site. It can order local health departments to remove a product from sale if the product is a health concern.

- California law prohibits any advertisement—false or otherwise—that any drug or device can have any effect on any of 37 specific diseases, from appendicitis to whooping cough (the list is in alphabetical order). AIDS is not listed, but the Task Force is following up on a suggestion to ask the legislature to add it to the list. The only exceptions are advertisements distributed only to medical professionals, or claims specifically allowed by State health authorities. (Health and Safety Code 26463)

- Special California laws make it a crime to offer, sell, or give anything to be used to treat cancer, unless officially approved in advance. This law applies even to medical doctors, even if the treatment is given away free, and even if it does in fact work. Only certain faith healing is exempt. (Health and Safety Code 1707.1, 1709, 1715)

At least one member of the Task Force is trying to get this cancer law amended to apply also to AIDS and related conditions. Such legislation would apparently criminalize all unofficial, alternative treatments, such as AL 721 or DNCB, or vitamins, nutritional supplements, herbs, acupuncture, etc. when used for AIDS—even by a medical doctor. Anyone who helped a friend obtain such treatments could be prosecuted. The legal choices would be AZT or nothing. Yet this critical policy change could slip through the legislature, unknown to the AIDS community and even to the legislators who voted for it, because only a few lines of text would be needed to amend the existing cancer law. This small section could be buried in other legislation. Without competent, ongoing community vigilance this nightmare could easily happen.

- There are other government powers, too. Any district attorney can require advertisers to provide evidence to support certain claims—and obtain court orders if they don't respond or if officials have reason to believe the advertising is false. (Business and Professions Code 17508) The Task Force plans to make extensive use of this provision, partly to educate itself about unconventional AIDS/ARC treatments.

Practitioners of unapproved treatments could be prosecuted for grand or petty theft. The Board of Medical Quality Assurance can revoke the licenses of physicians. The U. S. Post Office can cut off the mail of a business, or prosecute for mail fraud. The FDA can seize goods, bring injunctions, or prosecute criminally. California can prosecute violation of Federal laws, guidelines, and regulations, as being "unfair competition" under California law. State prosecutors can be deputized to assist in Federal cases when the Federal agencies have greater powers.

Though not mentioned by the Task Force, persons involved in unapproved treatments could be charged with "conspiracy" to violate any of the above laws or others—a felony even if the alleged violations are misdemeanors, and even if in fact they never occurred.

California enforcement officials are now examining traditional ethnic medical practices, translating medicine labels from Spanish, Chinese and other languages to judge them according to U.S. and California laws. They have been watching the gay press, and are now increasing this surveillance.

Restraints on Powers

• The main limitation on all these powers is the First Amendment in the Bill of Rights. Citizens have the freedom to discuss unorthodox medical ideas in books or articles, on talk shows, etc. However, government agencies may prepare guidelines for media, which publishers may voluntarily use, making it harder for unapproved ideas to reach large audiences.

• Most official attention focuses on false or unsupported medical claims. It's much harder to prosecute someone who doesn't make any claims.

Sometimes this system works well, allowing the community to make its own judgments free of commercially motivated misinformation or distortion. Persons who have informed themselves can then buy the necessary products from individuals, organizations, or companies whose sole business is to supply those products, not to promote their use or persuade anyone to buy. By contrast, the quick-buck artist is usually an outsider who cannot operate without advertising.

Medical frauds have almost always been promoted by someone with a commercial interest in them. By contrast, with unapproved AIDS/ARC treatments, the manufacturers, distributors, retailers and anyone else with a commercial interest in the treatment are often the last to know about its relevance to AIDS. The initiative normally comes from persons with AIDS or ARC, not from the seller.

• Law enforcement is far less efficient in detecting and stopping one-on-one "quackery" than the publicly advertised variety, because there is no good system of surveillance for detecting the former.

• Members of the Task Force are concerned about "not losing the public relations war," as they perceived happened in an earlier crusade against laetrile, an unapproved cancer remedy made from apricot pits.

This concern appears, for example, to have protected the "guerrilla clinics" so far. A central principle of the guerrilla clinic movement is never to charge money, to give away everything for free. Prosecution would be perceived as an attack against persons with AIDS who were trying to save their lives—not as an attack against unscrupulous promoters preying on those persons' desperation.

Since the many overlapping laws are broad enough to prosecute virtually any involvement with any AIDS treatment not already officially approved, public relations in all its facets may be our only solid defense. The laws embody a paternalistic, experts-know-best philosophy; yet for years the public has turned away from this approach, toward more personal knowledge and involvement in one's health care. Thousands of Americans with diseases other than AIDS know that they are being denied necessary pharmaceuticals readily available in Europe or Japan, purely by red tape and officials' turf protection, unsupported by any scientific or medical justification. Probably millions of others are being denied proper treatment although they don't know it yet. We can work in coalitions to support public policies which are more rational and humane.

• The Task Force is making a sincere attempt to target clearly unjustified or exploitative practices, without depriving people with AIDS of treatment options. The law-enforcement staff wants to focus its resources on those cases which represent major financial or health risks to patients. The dangers arise from difficulties in defining the task, not from ill will. It is easier to conduct a legal arms race than to deal with the central ambiguities of what the Task Force seeks to accomplish.

How can you distinguish treatments which are worthless from those which in fact are promising though they are not yet accepted by the mainstream—a distinction which by definition the doctors and scientists closest to the matter are not able to make? How can you stop the seller without also restricting the buyer? How can you apply enough heat to scare off the would-be frauds—often professionally skilled in the use of legal loopholes—without also chilling the information flow which is essential for the health of the community? How can you avoid a frontal attack on hope when mainstream medicine has so little of it to offer? How can the public rely on good intentions of prosecutors, when these could change overnight with a new political climate or new personnel? The growing war against AIDS fraud will have fundamental problems until these questions have clear answers. The answers are not in sight.

(Note: The Attorney General's staff particularly wants to hear about any AIDS treatment practices which you believe are fraudulent or otherwise improper. You can reach the Attorney General's AIDS Fraud Task Force through Michael R. Botwin at the Attorney General's Office; see "AIDS Fraud Task Force" listing in Appendix B for address and phone number.)

DTC (IMUTHIOL)

Project Inform has just published a fact sheet on DTC, including instructions on how to obtain and use it. For a copy, call them (see Appendix B).

For additional background on DTC, see *AIDS Treatment News,* Issues Number 29 and 35. This immune modulator, developed in France, is now being tested at San Francisco General Hospital and several other U.S. medical centers. Results of a double-blind trial with 80 ARC patients at five French medical centers were released at the "III International Conference on AIDS," June 1–5, 1987, in Washington, D.C. The drug showed clear benefit in both blood tests and clinical improvement, with almost no side effects when used properly.

The Project Inform fact sheet omits the names of companies where you can buy DTC, a common industrial chemical. According to Project Inform, the FDA has warned suppliers not to sell DTC to persons with AIDS, since it has not been approved for human use. Such approval will probably take years. Meanwhile, you usually have to be a business with an appropriate reason to buy DTC. For most people, the only workable way to obtain such unapproved treatments will be through affinity or support groups (see section on "Unapproved Treatments" below, page XXX). DTC costs almost nothing to use and could easily be distributed free once anyone in the group obtained a supply.

One drawback to underground use is the difficulty of making the "enteric coating" required to protect the chemical against stomach acid—and the potential danger of making the coating improperly. Because of this difficulty, the most successful route of administration so far has been rectal, described in the Project Inform fact sheet. But few people have used DTC this way, so there could be problems which have not appeared yet.

An alternative to underground use of DTC is disulfiram (Antabuse), a readily available prescription drug usually used for alcoholics. Disulfiram turns into DTC inside the body. We have heard that four persons in an unrelated drug trial did notably better than the others, and physicians who examined their medical records found that they were being given disulfiram for alcoholism. At this time a number of persons with AIDS or ARC, in San Francisco at least, are receiving disulfiram through their physicians, in amounts somewhat smaller than commonly used for alcoholics. We will publish more information as it becomes available.

DEXTRAN SULFATE

Japanese research published in *The Lancet* (June 13, 1987, p. 1379) suggests that this antiviral could have major importance.

• In the laboratory, dextran sulfate (sometimes spelled "sulphate") worked as well as AZT against the AIDS virus. But the combination of dextran sulfate and AZT together worked much better than either one alone.

• In humans, dextran sulfate has been used for more than 20 years in Japan, mainly for arteriosclerosis. Side effects have been small. It is sold without a prescription, and taken orally. The cost is small, about $1 a day.

• The researchers strongly suggest that dextran sulfate be studied as a treatment for persons with AIDS and ARC. San Francisco General Hospital and other medical centers are or will be conducting clinical trials.

This writer knows one person who has used dextran sulfate for three weeks after obtaining it through family connections in Japan. He is enthusiastic about the results so far.

One possible drawback: researchers suspect that this drug may not cross the blood-brain barrier. But even if not, it could have important uses, perhaps in combination with other treatments.

The researchers do not know the mechanism of the antiviral action. There are indications that it may inhibit reverse transcriptase.

We will publish more information as it becomes available.

Note: Our earlier article on dextran sulfate ("Japanese Antiviral Discovery," AIDS Treatment News, Issue Number 32) reported laboratory work by a different researcher on dextran sulfate in combination with heparin. The research reviewed above is more relevant to human use.

UNAPPROVED TREATMENTS

Delays in Federal new-drug approval have become so serious that "over 70 percent of the drugs eventually approved for use in this country are on the market elsewhere long before Americans can buy them," according to California Attorney General John Van de Kamp, speaking to the Harvey Milk Democratic Club in San Francisco, May 21, 1987.

Even this figure understates the case, because many important drugs never even get submitted for U.S. approval because their manufacturers choose to give up the U.S. market rather than face the delay, difficulty, and expense required. U.S. citizens can never buy these drugs, and they don't count in the 70 percent figure above.

The much-publicized new FDA rules, intended to liberalize access to drugs urgently needed for life-threatening conditions, have so far had no effect on any drug. Last we heard, not even a single application has been filed under these rules.

Most unapproved drugs cost very little—for at least two reasons. First, the treatment underground must usually stay away from brand-new, high-tech medicines—the ones which are most difficult, dangerous, and expensive. And second, pharmaceutical companies have not yet jacked up the price to what Americans or their insurance will bear.

The first and most important step toward increasing your medical options is to get involved with a treatment-oriented support or affinity group—or start one. Such groups may be even more important for sharing information, referrals to physicians, etc. than for obtaining treatments themselves. They can empower the community to take care of itself when the government and the medical system fail to do their job.

For information on forming AIDS/ARC/HIV-positive affinity groups, you can call Gary Babcock in Berkeley, California (see Appendix B).

In San Francisco, an excellent resource for learning about treatments is the Healing Alternatives Buyers Club (HABC) (see Appendix B for address and phone number). At this time the HABC is most interested in egg lecithin lipids (related to AL 721), and aloe vera juice (related to Carrisyn). The group needs volunteers to help organize projects, for example laboratory testing of commercial products for consumer education and protection.

Issue Number 41
September 25, 1987

FLUCONAZOLE: A MAJOR ADVANCE FOR CRYPTOCOCCAL MENINGITIS AND OTHER SYSTEMIC FUNGAL INFECTIONS?

Update 1989: Fluconazole is still not approved in the United States.

Fluconazole is an experimental broad-spectrum antifungal taken orally once per day. About 150 persons have received this drug for serious or life-threatening systemic fungal infections related to AIDS; over a thousand others (mostly in Europe) have used smaller doses orally for less serious fungal infections. But despite this widespread and successful use, most physicians know little about fluconazole. They can often obtain the drug if necessary in an emergency, but they have not known to ask for it.

Fluconazole appears to be effective for cryptococcal meningitis, other systemic cryptococcal infections, systemic candidiasis, histoplasmosis, coccidioidomycosis (also called valley fever or San Joaquin fever), and other fungal infections.

We first heard of fluconazole several weeks ago, when a friend of a person with cryptococcal meningitis called to urge us to look into it. He told us it had been a wonder drug, giving all the benefit of the standard treatment, amphotericin B, without the side effects. The patient no longer had to spend half of each day for months or longer in the hospital for the hours-long intravenous infusion of amphotericin B (often called "amphoterrible" by patients); instead he took the fluconazole capsules once per day.

We asked two leading AIDS physicians about the drug; both had heard of it and knew what it was used for, but neither had much more information. A computer database search found several animal studies. We couldn't find more until last week, when a personal friend happened to mention that he knew someone with cryptococcal meningitis, and we told him about fluconazole. Our friend has contacts at medical research centers, and he was able to learn that the physicians working with the drug are enthusiastic about it. They are hoping for cure of cryptococcal meningitis, not only control, as they have been unable to find the organism in the cerebrospinal fluid after treatment in some cases, although other patients still have the disease-causing organism and continue to require preventive or maintenance medication. There has been little if any trouble with side effects. And preventive use simply requires taking the capsules once a day or less, not the repeated trips to the hospital for amphotericin B.

Most importantly, many people have been unable to tolerate enough amphotericin B to treat cryptococcal meningitis successfully. As a result, the disease has had a high fatality rate despite the standard treatment. Many of these deaths may be avoidable if a less toxic treatment can be used.

Another computer search found the only report yet published on human use of fluconazole: a letter from two physicians at the Pasteur Institute in Paris (Dupont and Drouhet, 1987) reporting successful treatment of cryptococcal meningitis. We also found published statements from the chairman of the manufacturer, Pfizer Inc., to financial analysts. Then we interviewed a spokesperson for Pfizer Central Research in Groton, Connecticut, to complete the research for this article.

Background

Fluconazole is known chemically as an azole compound, in the same class as ketoconazole (Nizoral), an antifungal in common use. It differs from ketoconazole in crossing the blood-brain barrier, and also in being effective in far smaller doses. In some animal studies, doses ten to a hundred times less than the ketoconazole dose had the same antifungal effect. Typical human doses are 200 to 400 mg for ketoconazole and 100 to 150 mg or possibly more for fluconazole. Most of the fluconazole taken is excreted unchanged in the urine.

No human studies comparing fluconazole with amphotericin B have yet been done; these should begin soon. Animal studies have given varying results (see references). Sometimes amphotericin B has been more effective, sometimes fluconazole has been, and sometimes they have been equivalent.

In the U.S., the main interest in fluconazole is for major, life-threatening fungal infections usually resulting from AIDS or other immune deficiencies. In Europe, a different branch of Pfizer Central Research, in Sandwich, England, has studied fluconazole mainly for less serious infections such as vaginal candidiasis or fungal skin infections. In Europe the drug is better known and more widely used than in the U.S.

The only published report of human use, at least for the serious systemic infections, is the letter in the May 1987 *Annals of Internal Medicine* from physicians at the Pasteur Institute (Dupont and Drouhet, 1987). An HIV-positive patient with cryptococcal meningitis had been treated for two and a half months with amphotericin B and flucytosine, but toxic effects required that the treatment be stopped.

Several months later the meningitis returned, and because of the previous toxicity with standard treatments, the physicians tried fluconazole. Temperature decreased by the fourth day, and by the tenth day the headache was gone and the patient was able to walk around in his bedroom. In one month, the organism could not be cultured from cerebrospinal fluid. Still the physicians are keeping the patient on the long-term maintenance recommended for persons with AIDS; they are using 150 mg of fluconazole twice per week.

The two physicians summarized the results as follows: "The patient is being followed at regular intervals and is asymptomatic and in excellent general condition five months after the end of daily treatment. Clinical tolerance of fluconazole is excellent; hematologic, renal, and hepatic characteristics show no abnormalities."

This letter reported only one case. For more information, we called the press office at Pfizer Inc., which referred us to one of Pfizer's researchers. He told us that fluconazole has been used with an estimated 150 to 200 patients with serious systemic fungal infections (as well as many others with less serious conditions). They have not seen any serious toxicity with fluconazole; very few side effects have either been definitely related to the drug, or serious enough to cause treatment to be interrupted. Side effects may be similar to those of ketoconazole, which in rare cases can cause serious liver toxicity, so the physicians conducting the clinical trials are carefully testing for any liver problems.

The researcher we spoke with explained that early trials have emphasized cryptococcal meningitis because it is immediately life-threatening, much more common with AIDS than most other fungal infections, and easily diagnosed from the cerebrospinal fluid, allowing a quick test to determine how well the drug is working. But he explained that other infections are expected to increase as AIDS moves into areas of the country where these fungal diseases are endemic, such as coccidioidomycosis in the Southwest and histoplasmosis in the Midwest. Pfizer plans to watch for increases in these infections and design new trials for them. Some trials have already accepted patients with serious fungal infections other than cryptococcal meningitis.

Public Policy Concerns—And Three Recommendations

The example of fluconazole illustrates serious problems in the drug-development system in the United States. Lives have been lost and are continuing to be lost unnecessarily, because the system fails to deliver medical care in the best interest of the patients.

We should point out that Pfizer Inc. has handled fluconazole much better than many other companies have typically handled AIDS treatments entrusted to their care. Pfizer has made a serious effort to develop and test fluconazole, an effort costing several million dollars already. By contrast, many companies appear to be using their potential AIDS treatments for stock manipulation—although it is almost impossible to get proof as we cannot know the intentions of their directors. Other companies have apparently engaged in speculation, buying the rights or options to promising but unproven substances on the cheap and holding these rights in case they become hot later, meanwhile neither developing the drugs nor letting anyone else do so.

Pfizer has also been open to compassionate use of fluconazole in emergencies; many others have not. This compassionate policy, however, has only affected those whose physicians have heard about fluconazole and are willing to try an experimental, non-approved treatment. While exact figures are not known, the available numbers suggest that most of those whose cryptococcal meningitis or other severe fungal infections cannot be treated successfully with standard therapies have been left to die without fluconazole being tried or considered.

Most of all, the example of fluconazole illustrates a lack of communication among physicians and others concerned with AIDS treatments. By the end of last year, 1986, over two thousand people had used fluconazole orally as an antifungal—mostly in Europe and in the smaller 50 mg doses and for less serious infections. Yet now in

September 1987, few U.S. physicians even among AIDS specialists know enough about fluconazole to consider using it.

What should be done to correct this problem for the future? In our opinion, three things need to happen:

• Medical ethicists must examine the barriers to treatment development and to professional communication, and speak out when necessary. With fluconazole the biggest problem may have been requirements of professional secrecy. The protocols describing the clinical trials are trade secrets of the manufacturer. The results of the trials belong to the researchers, who will publish them, but medical journals usually insist that they not be published elsewhere first. Peer-reviewed journals often take months or longer between receipt and publication of an article; some have greatly reduced this time for AIDS studies. But researchers themselves are busy, and naturally they want their articles to be perfect before they are submitted to journals, because once published an article remains public forever and cannot be changed. Usually researchers will share vital information with other physicians before publication, but these physicians must first know to ask.

Other AIDS treatments have suffered worse problems, such as being used primarily for stock manipulation or for speculation; companies have acquired the rights and then sat on these drugs, allowing essentially no research to proceed.

There is no legal recourse in these cases, because U.S. law allows a corporation to acquire exclusive proprietary rights to a drug and then refuse to develop it or allow anyone else to do so, for any reason or no reason as it sees fit. But medical ethics is becoming a small industry in this country. If ethicists would investigate these problems and speak out about them, then at least the most grievous abuses could become universally unacceptable in the professional community. Few companies would ignore such a consensus.

• Practicing physicians seldom have time to keep up with research. Many learn about new treatments primarily from drug-company salespersons—who are forbidden to say anything about drugs or uses of drugs not already approved by the FDA. Such approval often lags several years behind the time researchers are confident that the treatment is valuable. And the expense of U.S. new-drug approval, usually estimated at about 80 million dollars per drug, deters many companies from ever starting the process in the first place.

Physicians who specialize in complex diseases like AIDS or cancer might consider doing what a few in private practice have already done: have a research person on their staff. This person, perhaps a research nurse, can spend full time keeping up with the published literature, as well as telephoning researchers to learn what is and is not working, in order to keep the physician informed on current developments. In addition, this information can help the physician evaluate drug-company claims.

• AIDS organizations need to pay attention to treatments and develop in-house expertise, in order to advocate in the interests of their clients. If service organizations put as much effort into making sure promising treatments were properly researched and made available as they now put into teaching people to die, much of the dying would be unnecessary. Organizations should consider hiring a research nurse or physician to follow research full time and keep them informed.

Effective patient advocacy could force ethicists and other professionals to re-examine the whole issue of medical decisions which are not in the interest of the patient, but instead serve the purposes of drug companies or other organized professionals. We need a new look at widely and unthinkingly accepted procedures, such as withholding access to unapproved treatments in order to force patients into clinical trials, or requiring those in trials to give up all other treatments or otherwise accept substandard care which gets them sicker faster, reducing the cost of conducting the trials and proving efficacy. Even double-blind trials can and should be designed so that patients do not need to be desperate to accept them.

Whenever patients and their physicians are removed from decision making about their own care, we can reasonably suspect that someone else's interests are being served. No one can stop powerful forces such as the pharmaceutical industry or the Federal drug bureaucracy from acting in their own behalf. But let's stop pretending that they represent the patient's interest too.

Information for Physicians

Physicians can obtain fluconazole for compassionate use in an emergency, if amphotericin B has failed or cannot be used because of toxicity. For more information, physicians only should call Pfizer Central Research, Groton, Connecticut (see Appendix B).

Pfizer Inc. plans to increase its clinical testing of fluconazole, adding several hundred more patients. The National Institutes of Health through its AIDS Treatment Evaluation Units plans to begin its own study soon on cryptococcal meningitis and expects to enroll 200 patients. Trials will take place in many cities, including San Francisco, New York, Los Angeles, and Miami, but none of these trials is recruiting at this time (September 1987). They may begin doing so in the coming weeks. Many of these studies will be double blind, comparing fluconazole with amphotericin B (no placebo will be used), so patients cannot enter if any condition would rule out their use of amphotericin B. Those patients should qualify for compassionate use instead.

Pfizer does not expect to be able to apply for permission to market fluconazole as a prescription drug in the United States until 1989. At that time Pfizer will present its data to the U.S. Food and Drug Administration, which must then make its decision. No one knows when fluconazole will become generally available. But physicians can obtain it now for life-threatening infections, when standard treatments cannot be used.

REFERENCES

Dupont, B., M.D., and E. Drouhet, M.D., "Cryptococcal Meningitis and Fluconazole," *Annals of Internal Medicine* 106(5) (May, 1987), p. 778.

Seventeen other technical references, mostly animal and laboratory studies, can be found by a Medline computer search. The European database Excerpta Medica contains 25 references at this time.

DDC DANGER

Some persons have obtained "underground" dideoxycytidine, or DDC (not to be confused with DTC, Imuthiol, an entirely different treatment). In scientific tests dideoxycytidine has caused severe side effects which may be irreversible—especially neuropathy and pain in the feet. Scientists are still looking for a way to use DDC, but clearly it is much too dangerous to be taken without expert supervision.

Information on the toxicity of DDC has long circulated in the treatment underground. It appeared in print in the *Wall Street Journal* (September 18, 1987), page 36.

NEW TREATMENT NEWSLETTER
FROM GAY MEN'S HEALTH CRISIS

The Gay Men's Health Crisis is preparing to offer its own newsletter on experimental and alternative AIDS treatments, edited by Barry Gingell, M.D. It will primarily feature in-depth drug analysis, while also covering other issues pertinent to AIDS research.

The monthly newsletter will seek to make new data available in laymen's terms to PWAs and others who are touched by AIDS. Technical information will also be included but will be set apart for reading ease. The first issue of the newsletter will be available in the coming weeks.

For more information, contact the Gay Men's Health Crisis (see Appendix B).

Issue Number 42
October 9, 1987

AL 721 TODAY

AL 721, also called "egg lecithin lipids" or just "lipids," may be getting more public and professional attention today than any other alternative or experimental treatment for AIDS and ARC. Many people want to know what this treatment is, what evidence supports its use, and how can they obtain it and try it.

We have published several articles on AL 721 since April of last year. Here we summarize its status as of early October 1987, report recent developments, and answer the questions most often asked.

A Note on the Name "AL 721"

(1) The name "AL-721" is a trademark of Ethigen Corp. in Los Angeles (formerly Praxis Pharmaceuticals), and technically refers only to the proprietary product of that company.

The current popular interest in AL 721 developed entirely independently of Ethigen, and probably against its wishes, mainly through PWA organizations mostly in and around New York City. The people in this AIDS treatment movement generally use "AL 721" as a generic term, but acknowledge that technically it refers only to the proprietary product and that "egg lecithin lipids," "lipids," or "AL 721 substitute" would be more correct.

The phrase "AL 721" has been used in the medical literature at least since 1985 (Sarin *et al.*, 1985); "AL" and "active-lipid," other names for the same substance, have been used at least since 1982 (Heron *et al.*, 1982). We will use "AL 721" and "egg lecithin lipids" interchangeably.

Background

AL 721 was developed at the Weizmann Institute of Science, Rehovot, Israel, by a team led by Meir Shinitzky, Ph.D., a cancer researcher there. It consists entirely of three ingredients, all of which are found in ordinary egg yolks. The first formal human trial was a successful test to correct a certain immune deficiency (diminished lymphocyte proliferative response) in elderly persons, all of whom were over 75 years old. The problem returned when the treatment was stopped.

AL 721 does cross the blood-brain barrier.

Other early medical interests in AL 721 (before any antiviral properties were known) were for treating cystic fibrosis, and also for reducing the symptoms of alcohol or opiate withdrawal in order to help people quit using these drugs. These possibilities still look promising.

Theory suggests that AL 721 may also be useful with other lipid-coated viruses, such as Epstein-Barr. We are hearing anecdotal reports of successful use for treating chronic fatigue syndrome.

The first public notice of any connection between AL 721 and AIDS came in a letter published in the *New England Journal of Medicine* (November 14, 1985) by several scientists including Robert Gallo, M.D. of the U.S. National Cancer Institute, one of the world's leading AIDS researchers. The letter reported that AL 721 clearly inhibited AIDS virus infection of human white blood cells in the laboratory. It also mentioned that oral doses had been well tolerated in the preliminary tests on elderly persons mentioned above, and that these doses had indeed shown a medicinal effect comparable to what would be expected from laboratory data.

The fact that a treatment inhibits the AIDS virus in the laboratory certainly does not prove that it will work in people. But AL 721 not only worked in the laboratory. It had already been given to people with no sign of any toxicity. (And it consists entirely of food substances, further reducing the risk.) In addition, it had already demonstrated pharmacological benefit when taken orally for a non-viral immune deficiency. The oral medicine had indeed reached the bloodstream, and had shown the expected effect on white blood cells in the human body.

All this was published two years ago, in a letter in the most prestigious medical journal in the United States. Why not simply try AL 721 for treatment of AIDS or ARC?

In the two years since publication of that information, only eight persons with any AIDS-related condition have received AL 721 in scientific tests. This trial with eight people, sponsored by Praxis Pharmaceuticals (now Ethigen), was conducted at St. Luke's/Roosevelt Hospital Center (affiliated with Columbia University) in New York. It found encouraging results, especially a large reduction in reverse transcriptase, a measure of viral activity. But despite this success, presented at a scientific meeting in the Fall of 1986, no other clinical trials have begun in the last year.

A few days ago the U.S. National Institutes of Health had planned to begin its own clinical trials—almost two years after the *New England Journal of Medicine* publication—but these trials were placed on hold, for reasons unknown to the NIH press office. We called the FDA, which said it placed the hold because Ethigen had changed its supplier—the company with which it had contracted to manufacture the AL 721—but that now Ethigen had agreed to use the original supplier, the hold had been released and the trials could start.

The new manufacturer for Ethigen was to have been Abbott Laboratories, surely capable of making AL 721 properly. This incident illustrates the kinds of delays holding up treatment research.

Unfortunately the trials now supposed to begin will be "phase I" (dosage and toxicity) studies, apparently repeating the work of the last two years. They will have room for very few people. Beth Israel Medical Center in New York, which plans to conduct NIH trials of AL 721, is not recruiting at this time.

Except for the eight persons at the St. Luke's/Roosevelt study, no one with AIDS or ARC has received AL 721 in scientific trials anywhere in the U.S.—or anywhere else except Israel (see below).

The problem isn't lack of volunteers. There are widespread reports that hundreds of persons with AIDS or ARC are now on a waiting list for a larger study which was supposed to start at St. Luke's/Roosevelt, and that researchers there are despondent about not being able to let these people begin. We called St. Luke's/Roosevelt to confirm or deny these reports, but were unable to get the permission required to discuss the matter with their researchers before press time.

Scientists looking for in-depth background on the laboratory work which led to the development of AL 721 should see *Physiology of Membrane Fluidity*, edited by Meir Shinitzky, Ph.D.—the principal developer of AL 721—and published by CRC Press, Boca Raton, Florida. This two-volume book, by Shinitzky and 19 other scientists, is a model of thoroughness and careful workmanship. Shinitzky's article, "Membrane Fluidity and Cellular Functions," has over 300 references to relevant scientific papers.

Researchers should also note that the Medline computerized database, produced by the U.S. National Library of Medicine, has over 1,800 articles indexed under "membrane fluidity," the concept on which AL 721 is based.

New Israeli Results

The Baltimore Jewish Times, in a story on AL 721 scheduled for publication today, obtained recent information on the use of this treatment in Israel through its correspondent there:

> Of the 60 AIDS victims (sic) who have been treated with AL 721 in the past year, 48 have shown very considerable improvement in their general well being, sometimes within days of embarking on the treatment. They have lost much of the lassitude associated with AIDS, fevers have been reduced, other symptoms have diminished, and they have suffered no side effects. Three patients who were considered terminal are now in remission. More importantly, clinical tests show that in a phase of the treatment, the deadly virus loses much of its infectivity, in other words its power to spread from one cell to another (*Baltimore Jewish Times,* October 9, 1987).

Despite these good results, Yehuda Skornick, M.D., one of one of several Israeli physicians using AL 721 to treat AIDS and ARC, emphasized that this treatment is not a cure. "There is as yet no cure for AIDS, and it would be wicked and irresponsible to claim otherwise."

We called Dr. Skornick before going to press; he told us that 52 of the 60 are now showing improvement.

Underground Medicine

For the first 14 months after publication of the *New England Journal of Medicine* article, AL 721 was completely unavailable in the U.S.; a handful of Americans were treated secretly in Israel. Only in January of 1987 did the first good substitute reach the United States—the "home formula" made from concentrated soy lecithin (see discussion and formula below). Several months later, in May of 1987, the first all-egg version became available, in New York City only, through PWA organizations there. Today people can buy several different all-egg versions, through buyers clubs in some cities, at health-food stores in many areas, or from several different suppliers by mail.

Thousands of people are using one or another of these AL 721 substitutes at this time. Three independent surveys have questioned hundreds of these users and are finding exactly the same result—that a large majority report substantial benefits or better. Many users have reported dramatic improvement in their health, even some near death when they started, and have attributed their recovery to AL 721.

The original eight-patient study at St. Luke's/Roosevelt did not find any consistent change in T-cell counts. Others have used AL 721 and found that counts did increase, although slowly. T-cell improvement is not a strong point of AL 721; therefore some physicians suspect that the treatment might work especially well in combination with DTC, an immune modulator which is very good at improving T-helper counts, but no trials have been done. Israeli scientists are reportedly developing treatments which combine AL 721 with thymus hormones.

AL 721 seems to be most helpful in improving overall clinical condition. People report more energy, reduced or eliminated night sweats, clearing of skin conditions, and improved sense of well being. Skin mitogen tests as well as viral assays improve.

We do know that AL 721 is not a cure; it needs to be continued indefinitely. It does not help everybody; maybe ten to 20 percent of those who try it report that it does nothing for them.

We also know that AL 721 is harmless—although there may be a dangerous "rebound effect" if someone with AIDS or ARC stops taking it suddenly. See discussion of side effects below.

The overwhelming weight of available evidence indicates that AL 721 is a significant benefit to most people who use it—and decisive for many. All the information points in the same direction. But we don't have conclusive proof of efficacy because no one has done the clinical research necessary to know for sure.

It is almost impossible that Federal approval for general use of AL 721 could happen before 1989—the year after next—if it even happens then. Meanwhile, thousands of people have build a grassroots movement to obtain this treatment for themselves and their friends.

What Went Wrong?

If AL 721 really is good, why has it had to develop as underground medicine? Why has mainstream, official research done so little with it in the U.S.? The answer is that AL 721 (and most other promising treatments) have fallen through many cracks in the current AIDS research system.

Despite the highly touted advances in AIDS research, almost all of the work has been in high-tech studies which could not possibly lead to useful treatments in the near future. Such projects stimulate professional and commercial interest because they generate elegant science, will probably produce Nobel prizes, and tie into the vast economic potential of commercial biotechnology. But for many reasons it takes years to go from a challenging scientific idea to a practical medicine in widespread use. These high-tech studies produce fundamental knowledge of inestimable value, and may lead to an eventual cure for AIDS; certainly they are worth doing.

But they are unlikely to save the lives of those now ill. For that we need competent, speedy testing of a number of treatments already available and supported by all existing evidence, but largely dropped from official research because no major institution cares enough to push them through the 50 to 80 million dollar process of new-drug approval.

And despite the Wall Street feeding frenzy around AIDS research, most of the commercial interest isn't in treatments at all but in new HIV tests—much easier to develop, gain Federal approval for, and bring to market. And the treatments which do receive financial attention are again the high-tech ones which will take years to be ready for widespread use. Companies can get a better return on their investment by manipulating their stock prices with public relations, than by actually trying to develop and market a treatment for AIDS.

Why haven't physicians insisted on studies of AL 721? First, because the great majority of physicians do not treat anyone with AIDS, so they are not involved—and neither are their professional associations. Most physicians are too busy treating patients to keep up with research. And the medical literature has carried almost nothing about AL 721—understandably, since the research hasn't been done so there is nothing to publish.

Because AL 721 is patented (U.S. patent #4,474,773, "Lipid Fraction for Treating Disease," October 2, 1984) and unavailable from the patent holder, physicians cannot be involved without bending or breaking the rules—unless they happen to be working in the only existing official trial, with the handful of patients at St. Luke's/ Roosevelt. Physicians don't advance professionally by bending or breaking rules, nor by spending their time learning how, when, and why to do so. They have every professional incentive to simply ignore the matter.

Because of the patent and Federal restrictions, nothing can happen unless the patent holder, the FDA, and a number of other parties including investors, institutional review boards, physicians, and patients can all work together. One problem anywhere can stop all clinical research on a drug.

And no one has investigated or articulated these problems. Until recently, the mainstream press blacked out almost all stories about AL 721 and similar treatments. It didn't want to raise false hope, or risk being used in possible quackeries or scams. So newspapers and other media did not allow their reporters to cover medical stories at all until they were published in a professional forum or appeared in official press releases—and the science which should have been done but wasn't will never appear in these ways.

Even today, most investigative reporting on AIDS treatments is looking very hard for fraud—not because of any great evidence or problem of fraud, but because journalists don't feel safe reporting that an unapproved treatment might possibly be good.

These media policies, predilections, and restraints make it almost impossible for journalists to cover AIDS research in any critical fashion. Instead, the major media has covered treatment research almost exclusively by rewriting official press releases.

For both similar and different reasons, most AIDS activists and organizations, especially those which receive public funds, have completely abandoned treatment and research as issues. They have refused to develop expertise or provide critique or scrutiny. They have refused to support persons with AIDS in any involvement with unapproved treatments. They have left treatment and research—the only way to save the lives of those already infected—solely to the experts and professionals, as they would never do with issues of testing, education, social services, or civil liberties. They have placed the FDA, the NIH, and the research departments of drug companies into an Olympus above criticism, by anyone except the very experts whose professional constraints and dependencies prevent them from speaking freely.

But medical research does not occupy a magic pedestal above the mismanagement, opportunism, and defective national commitment seen elsewhere in the U.S. response to AIDS. Even doctors and scientists with the highest personal motives must make accommodations to national policy—deeply flawed in this case—in order to operate at all.

We have today a near-complete abandonment of persons with AIDS or ARC who are actually trying to save their lives with anything other than the one approved treatment, AZT. Many thousands of people are now building their own treatment movements from scratch because the AIDS, the gay, the medical, the religious and ethical, the political, and all other institutions of our society have refused to support or assist, refused to cooperate, refused to become informed, refused to even discuss the issues. Promising treatments like AL 721 will continue to be underground medicine until physicians, activists, and others have the courage and commitment to look at the evidence, make informed, independent decisions, and speak and act accordingly.

To Be Continued.   Part II of this article will tell how to use AL 721, what different versions are available, and where to obtain them, including a list of buyers clubs in different cities. It will address common questions such as the rebound effect, and how to use AL 721 while traveling when refrigeration is not available. It will summarize four different survey studies of persons using AL 721 for AIDS or ARC. It will include technical background and references, including citations to several double-blind clinical studies—largely unknown in the U.S.—which used the main active ingredient of AL 721 successfully for treating several different forms of viral hepatitis.

COMMON ANTIBIOTIC MAY STOP AIDS VIRUS

Update April 1988: Fusidic acid does not look useful at this time. We do not have the latest information, but from what we are hearing it appears not to be effective, and to cause an unpleasant rash in many people.

This apparent failure as an AIDS drug, however, should not mask the outstanding success of the research which followed up on the first indications that fusidic acid might be useful. Small clinical trials in Denmark and England—with about ten to 20 patients—quickly determined what we needed to know.

Fusidin (fusidic acid), a cheap and readily available antibiotic marketed since 1962, has shown very promising results in early human tests for persons with AIDS. Two October 9 dispatches by Reuters, an international wire service, carried the story, which first appeared in a Danish newspaper.

About ten people in Denmark have received Fusidin for treatment of AIDS or ARC, and other tests are starting in England. The news stories had only a sketchy report of results from one patient, who had taken Fusidin tablets three times a day for several months. He regained 10 kilograms of the 16 kilograms weight that he had lost, with no side effects. We do not know what dose was used.

Fusidin seems to work by preventing the virus from entering healthy cells. Scientists do not know whether it kills the virus or only suppresses it.

We checked medical files for non-AIDS uses of Fusidin, and for side effects. This antibiotic is used for many kinds of infections. There seem to be few side effects of Fusidin given orally, although some patients develop jaundice which clears up when the medicine is stopped.

Unfortunately Fusidin is not marketed in the United States at this time. Apparently it is used in Canada, in Europe, and in many other countries.

Scientists studying Fusidin for AIDS/ARC include Professor Viggo Faber of the National Hospital in Copenhagen, and British virologist Angus Dalgleish of the Northwick Park Hospital in Harrow, England. The manufacturer is Loevens Kemiske Fabrik, in Denmark. The British Medical Council will meet next week to consider how extensive the British trials should be.

We will continue to follow this important research. Let us know if you hear more about Fusidin.

FANSIDAR WARNING

Fansidar, a drug usually used to prevent or treat malaria, is also being used as a preventive for pneumocystis. Physicians and patients should be aware of rare but sometimes fatal side effects, and of the need to stop using Fansidar immediately in case a skin rash develops or in certain other situations. Recently we heard from the lover of someone who died from a reaction to the drug.

The 1987 *Physician's Desk Reference* includes the following in bold text in a separate box—reproduced twice on the same page for additional emphasis:

> Fatalities associated with the administration of fansidar have occurred due to severe reactions, including Stevens-Johnson syndrome and toxic epidermal necrolysis. Fansidar prophylaxis should be discontinued at the first appearance of skin rash, if a significant reduction in the count of any formed blood elements is noted, or upon the occurrence of active bacterial or fungal infections.

A long list of additional warnings and precautions urges that:

> patients should be warned that at the first appearance of a skin rash, they should stop the use of Fansidar and seek medical attention immediately. Adequate fluid intake must be maintained in order to prevent crystalluria and stone formation. Patients should also be warned that the appearance of sore throat, fever, pallor,

purpura, jaundice or glossitis may be early indications of serious disorders which require prophylactic treatment to be stopped and medical treatment to be sought."

The fatal reaction described above is extremely rare; and fansidar also has important benefits. Our next issue will include more information on weighing the risks and benefits.

You can look up prescription drugs yourself in the *Physician's Desk Reference;* most public libraries have it, or you can buy it in bookstores (the 1987 edition cost $32.95). A new edition comes out each March. Note that this book emphasizes dangers and problems; the texts are written by pharmaceutical manufacturers which must cover themselves legally, and some of the drug descriptions may be unduly alarming. The value is that if side effects do occur, patients will know to consider the drug as a possible cause, and take appropriate precautions.

A number of other drug reference books, including some written for the general public, may also serve this purpose.

A CALL FOR VOLUNTEERS INTERESTED IN ALTERNATIVE TREATMENTS

The AIDS Treatment Library is a new service being developed in San Francisco that will utilize a cluster concept to help inform people with AIDS about treatment options. A series of self-contained mini libraries, each offering a range of information about both conventional and alternative treatments for AIDS, will be placed in bookstores, AIDS service organizations, cafes, etc.

I have been involved from the beginning of the planning process, and *AIDS Treatment News* will be included as part of the library's resources. The goal is to assure that people with AIDS are receiving the information they need to make informed decisions about available treatments.

The project requires committed, energetic volunteers, with a considerable degree of initiative, to serve as coordinators for the project. The role involves helping to identify and approach appropriate sites to house the mini libraries; to regularly check on the condition of the libraries; and to bring updated information to the libraries as new findings emerge.

If you would like to become involved, send a letter including a statement about your interest in the project, and an estimate of the number of hours per month you are able to contribute, to: AIDS Treatment Library, c/o The Healing Alternatives Foundation in San Francisco (see Appendix B for address/phone).

Issue Number 43
October 23, 1987

AL 721 TODAY, PART II:
WHERE TO GET IT, HOW TO USE IT

Part I of this article on AL 721 today (*AIDS Treatment News*, Issue Number 42) gave an overview of the experimental AIDS treatment AL 721, also called egg lecithin lipids. Part II answers specific questions such as how to use AL 721, and where to find buyers clubs or distributors. Part III includes more technical information, and references.

The Buyers Club Movement

The HIV-positive buyers clubs are typically nonprofit organizations set up by persons with AIDS, ARC, or a positive antibody status, in order to buy nutritional products at wholesale prices, especially products not readily available in health-food stores. These organizations also help in consumer protection, by making more sophisticated product selection and purchasing decisions than individuals would be likely to do on their own, negotiating better prices with vendors, and often sending samples of products to commercial laboratories for independent testing. Most of the buyers clubs work together well, sharing information and negotiating as a unit when necessary, so they provide the power of a national network created and controlled by HIV-positive persons and entirely dedicated to making the best treatments available.

In practice, buyers clubs vary widely. Some of the smaller ones skip the considerable paperwork of incorporating as a nonprofit, so technically they are for-profit businesses even if they were not set up to make money. Some clubs will ship products by mail; others are not set up to handle mail order, so customers must pick up their orders locally. Some need to collect money in advance and then place orders, requiring a wait; others have stock on hand.

Besides organizing group buys of products, buyers clubs can also serve as treatment-oriented support groups. People share information not only about products handled by the group, but about whatever has or has not worked for them, including local physicians and clinics, and all kinds of conventional, experimental, or alternative treatments. These grassroots groups fill the gap left by major AIDS support organizations, which have usually refused to allow their support groups to focus on treatment information.

You don't need to buy from the clubs. Egg lecithin lipids are now also available from distributors or mail order outlets. You may want to go through the clubs because of the information network they provide. Also, the clubs may have the best products, because manufacturing quality can vary from batch to batch, and sometimes clubs do their own testing in order to reject all but the best batches.

Most of the buyers clubs started in the last few months. The biggest impetus to the growth of this movement was the fact that until recently it was the only way to obtain all-egg generic AL 721. These organizations—especially the PWA Health Group in New York, the largest and most experienced of them—sought out industrial sources of supply, and arranged bulk purchases to make the products available to the public.

Buyers Club List

For this volume of collected *AIDS Treatment News,* we have listed buyers clubs in Appendix C, at the back of the book, along with listings for PWA coalition groups, ACT NOW chapters, and ACT UP affiliates. The reason for listing these groups at the back of the book is that, over time, we will be able to update these listings periodically as this volume is reprinted. Please see Appendix C, page 500.

Different AL 721-Like Products

The official AL 721 is not available. The patent licensee, Ethigen Corp. (formerly Praxis Pharmaceuticals) is seeking FDA approval to market AL 721 as a drug, a process which may take several more years. Meanwhile Ethigen could legally market the material as a nutritional supplement without medical claims, but the company has not done so.

Meanwhile a number of generic products more or less close to AL 721 have become available, through the buyers clubs and otherwise. A confusing and sometimes bitter debate has arisen over which is best. Here is how we see the current situation.

The "home formula," made from concentrated soy lecithin (usually PC-55™, a product of Twin Laboratories), has shown good results, and it costs about a quarter as much as the others.

But now we also have several all-egg generic versions which are closer to the official AL 721, and the consensus is that these are better than the soy-lecithin substitute. The interest today is in the all-egg versions, although some people still prefer the soy home formula because it has worked well for them.

Several powder and/or capsule egg lecithin products have also appeared on the market. These are not close to AL 721—even if they advertise as egg lecithin with a 7:2:1 ratio—and we don't recommend them as an AL 721 substitute.

Four different all-egg versions are available today. We believe that all of them are acceptable, but none is completely satisfactory. Here is an annotated list, in alphabetical order of the names by which they are most commonly known.

American Rolland. This product was first distributed in May of this year, by the PWA Health Group in New York. It is the only one which has been used long enough by enough people to have much information available from surveys of users; and the survey results, as well as informal word of mouth, have been very favorable. Disadvantages are that (as with most of the other products) the ratio of the ingredients is not ideal; it has about seven percent PE (phosphatidylethanolamine), instead of the 10 percent which would be preferred. Also it is not packaged in a convenient form, so it needs to be thoroughly mixed and then separated into individual doses by the user.

EggsAct. This is the only one available now which can keep for a reasonable time without refrigeration—an important feature for travelers—in sealed individual-dose packages. (Refrigeration or freezing is recommended when possible.) It is extracted from fresh egg yolk with food-grade ethyl alcohol. EggsAct is sold in over three hundred health-food stores, making it more convenient to buy but also more expensive than the others. The PE is lower than we would want, like most of the others.

Jarrow. This product has convenient packaging and a low price. The PE has been low, about seven percent like the others, but the last two batches have improved to about 8.5.

Levine. Manufactured by a new process co-designed by Stephen Levine of Allergy Research Group/Nutricology, which distributes the product, and Abco Laboratories of Concord, California, which manufactures it, this product is the first to get the right PE level, about 9.5—the closest to the Israeli formula yet available. It does not have the convenient packaging, however, and has a taste and smell which some people object to.

Some in the buyers clubs have assumed that the Levine product is clearly the best because it has a PE level closest to the original AL 721. My own feeling is to reserve judgment and avoid picking any one as best at this time. Much is still unknown; for example, the different products look and taste different, and have different consistencies, for reasons that nobody has fully explained.

The Levine product is the first one to be custom made with the PE level the buyers clubs wanted. The other three are off the shelf from large companies which have produced and sold them for some time for other purposes; these companies have been reluctant to custom manufacture a modified version for our use. But on the other hand, the designers and the manufacturer of the Levine product are new to the lecithin business, so they are at an earlier point on the learning curve. And the product is so new that we don't yet have much reporting on results. We choose to list all four of these versions as acceptable, instead of naming one as clearly best.

Recently the buyers clubs have learned that Houba Inc. in Culver, Indiana, the company which has manufactured official AL 721 for Ethigen beginning in 1983, will enter the market with its own egg lipid product, probably by December 1. Houba is considering simultaneously conducting its own research which could lead to FDA approval for certain medical claims, while selling the same product as a food supplement in the meantime. The food product will be manufactured with the same standards of quality control used for pharmaceuticals.

The buyers clubs are especially interested as this company has much more experience than the others in manufacturing what they want.

Houba will market this product through Rachelle Laboratories, Inc., an ethical pharmaceutical company which is a Houba subsidiary.

Prices

Most of the all-egg AL 721 substitutes are selling for about $150 to $200 per kilogram—a one- to three-month supply depending on the dose used. For those using an average dose the cost comes to about $3 or $4 per day. Prices have been dropping.

The soy "home formula" costs about $1 per day for the same dose.

How to Use AL 721

Your doctor should know what treatments you are using. But if you ask whether you should use AL 721, it is hard for physicians to say yes, because this treatment has not been officially approved. Instead, patients usually ask if there is any reason not to use it. If your physician is entirely intolerant of non-approved treatments, then it is your decision whether or not to find another doctor.

One dosage schedule has been 20 grams per day (10 grams in the morning and 10 grams in the evening) for the first month, then 10 per day after that. Many people continue the 20 grams per day instead of cutting back to ten. The study at St. Luke's/Roosevelt Medical Center in New York is now using 30 grams per day, 15 in the morning and 15 at night.

To be effective, AL 721 must be taken on an empty stomach. No fats, and preferably no other food, should be taken for at least two hours before and two hours after. A fat-free breakfast one hour or more after the morning dose may be okay. People usually take AL 721 before going to bed at night, and early in the morning.

The experts believe that AL 721 will be most effective if thoroughly dispersed in water, as with a blender. (The St. Luke's study uses 10 ounces of chilled orange juice, which may be better than plain water.) Use the blender at least until no lumps remain. If you use warm water to soften the lipids first so that they can be mixed more easily, keep the temperature below 115 degrees F, as higher temperatures may affect the material.

What we have found most convenient is a pocket-size battery powered drink mixer, such as the one from VitaMinder in Laguna Niguel, California, sold for about $7 in health-food stores. It mixes one glass at a time, is easy to clean, and is much quieter than regular blenders so it doesn't wake housemates if used at night. Others prefer a larger, plug-in appliance such as the Braun hand blender, which costs about $25; it also can mix a drink in a large glass and is easy to clean.

AL 721 spoils rapidly after it has been mixed with juice or water, so it should be used immediately, and never later than half an hour after mixing.

Dividing the Bulk Product

If you get AL 721 in bulk, usually in a kilogram jar, you need to divide it into doses. It might not work just to scrape some of the frozen material out of the jar (1 tablespoon equals 12 to 13 grams), because some products tend to separate while being frozen, so the top and bottom of the jar could be different. Follow the manufacturer's suggestions.

If you do need to divide the product, read whatever instructions came with it. The lipids will have to be warmed enough so they can be thoroughly mixed and poured; avoid getting air into the mixture. Most people pour the kilogram into a cake or cookie pan, re-freeze with the pan covered and level in the freezer, then cut the frozen lipids into individual doses with a knife, and wrap each dose in aluminum foil or plastic like Saran Wrap™. For example, one kilogram carefully divided into ten rows and ten columns gives 100 equal doses, of ten grams each.

Possible Side Effects

There is no known toxicity of AL 721. And since this substance consists entirely of ingredients found in ordinary egg yolk, toxicity would be unlikely.

The only serious concern is the possibility of a "rebound effect" if the treatment is stopped suddenly. In the St. Luke's study, three of eight patients progressed from serious lymphadenopathy to AIDS within 20 weeks of stopping AL 721. Physicians feared that the treatment may have held the disease in check, so that suddenly withdrawing it could allow the condition to get worse for a time than it would have been without the treatment. Physicians now recommend that people not start AL 721 unless they plan to continue until more is known or a better treatment is available.

There are no known problems in combining AL 721 with other drugs, but persons should check with their physicians. There has been some concern that AL 721 might interfere with AZT, making the latter less effective. Two physicians debated this question in a recent issue of the *PWA Newsline* (July/August, 1987 issue, available from the PWA Coalition in New York; see Appendix B for their phone number). A number of people are using both treatments together, and we have not heard of any problems.

Too much lecithin can cause minor side effects such as nausea or diarrhea, and possibly mental depression; these go away if the dose is reduced. A review of possible dangers as well as medicinal uses of lecithin (Wood and Allison, 1982) concluded that lasting health hazards were unlikely, as the unpleasant side effects of excessive use would cause people to stop before serious harm was done. (However, animal studies have indicated that large amounts of lecithin taken by pregnant women may be harmful to the fetus; see Bell and Lundberg, 1985.)

A Book on AL 721—How You Can Help

Arthur Kahn, a retired classics professor in New York, is writing a book about AL 721 and wants to hear from anybody with first-hand knowledge of it, especially about it's history and development. He is doing an excellent job of research, and has already traveled to Israel and elsewhere to interview leading scientists.

You can call him at (reference deleted by editor; at press time, we have heard that Professor Kahn has completed his manuscript).

FANSIDAR WARNING: ANOTHER VIEW, AND A RETRACTION

The last issue of *AIDS Treatment News* (Issue Number 42) reported a case of a fatal reaction to the drug fansidar, being used for prevention of pneumocystis. We wrote that we heard from the patient's lover that the physician prescribing the drug had failed to warn the patient to stop using it if a skin rash developed. We received this report shortly before press time and ran it without checking with the physician first.

We have since heard from the physician that he did indeed tell the patient to stop all medication after the rash occurred—and also that discontinuing the drug would not have prevented the death in this case.

Clearly there was a misunderstanding somewhere, as the patient kept using fansidar. But the facts do not justify our statement that the physician failed to warn the patient, or that there was negligence in this case. We retract these statements, and offer our apology to the physician, and to anyone else affected.

The physician also provided us with another view on fansidar. This case is the first fatality from the reaction (toxic epidermal necrolysis) caused by fansidar when used to prevent pneumocystis; five such fatalities have been reported among persons using fansidar to prevent malaria. The risk should be weighed against the benefit; the chance of death from pneumocystis is one in ten, compared to one in several thousand from using fansidar. This danger could be greater for persons with AIDS or ARC, because of the greater prevalence of allergy to sulfa drugs; physicians are accordingly reconsidering their use of fansidar for prevention of pneumocystis.

Issue Number 44
November 6, 1987

DHPG BLINDNESS DRUG THREATENED?

Update 1989: DHPG (ganciclovir) was approved by the FDA in June of this year.

Update 1988: Despite the FDA committee action, the manufacturer of DHPG has continued to make it available without charge on a compassionate basis, at great expense to the company, preventing thousands of cases of imminent blindness or death. We do not know how long this situation can continue. The committee's decision continues to be widely criticized and unpopular in medical circles.

On October 26, the FDA's Anti-infective Drug Advisory Committee voted 11 to 2 to recommend against approval of DHPG (also called Cytovene, or ganciclovir), on the grounds that the Committee did not have enough data to prove the drug effective for CMV retinitis. The FDA itself is not bound by the recommendations of such panels, but usually follows them. A final decision may be made in as little as two to three weeks.

Tests in thousands of persons, many published in medical journals, have shown beyond any doubt that DHPG is helpful in treating CMV retinitis, as well as CMV colitis and probably other systemic cytomegalovirus infections. No other drug has been approved for CMV retinitis. According to a Reuters news report on the controversy, CMV affects up to 98 percent of persons with AIDS, and if untreated will cause blindness or death in up to 25 percent of them. According to Syntex Corporation of Palo Alto, California, the manufacturer of DHPG, untreated CMV retinitis inevitably leads to blindness.

Syntex has provided DHPG free to over 2,500 patients in a compassionate-use program, at a cost to the company of about 25 million dollars, and submitted the resulting data to the FDA. Because of serious side effects, mainly hematologic toxicity, the drug has been limited to those who urgently need it. It is usually given intravenously, but an experimental oral form has now been developed.

The Advisory Committee wants dose-response data on DHPG from prospectively controlled trials. It will probably take years to fund, set up, conduct and analyze this research, and gain approval for the result. Meanwhile Syntex will presumably be allowed to continue compassionate use of the DHPG. But there is fear in the PWA community that the drug could become more restricted or even unavailable, resulting in thousands of cases of unnecessary blindness or death.

Comment

DHPG has long been in a regulatory limbo. It is so certainly effective that it would be grossly unethical to do a placebo study to prove it. Yet it is very hard to gain FDA approval without a double-blind study, which would usually require a placebo if no substitute drug is available. DHPG has become close to a de facto standard therapy on an experimental, compassionate basis, a situation enormously expensive to Syntex, the manufacturer, which may not be able to bear the burden indefinitely. The result is a catch-22 in which the drug cannot be approved just because it so clearly works and has no substitute.

The FDA's Anti-infective Drug Advisory Committee, a group of outside scientists not employed by the FDA but selected and instructed by the agency, did not ask for placebo trials. It wants prospectively controlled dose ranging trials, presumably meaning that patients must be randomly assigned to different doses in a standardized procedure not always responsive to the physician's judgment of what is best for the patient. Such trials may mean further restricting access to the drug in order to force persons to volunteer.

Analyzing and reporting the results of compassionate use of the drug in over 2,500 patients—results also published in a number of medical journals—was not good enough, despite the fact that this experience showed beyond any doubt whatever that the drug is in fact effective.

The rejection of DHPG (like the similar rejection in May 1987 of TPA, a major advance in treating heart attacks after they have already begun) tells the pharmaceutical industry that the FDA disfavors compassionate use and will largely ignore any information gained from such practical experience. This policy will make it even harder to get manufacturers to make their drugs available to desperately ill patients. Compassionate use is already very expensive for drug companies, because of the Federal paperwork required. If they cannot use the resulting data toward gaining FDA approval, then they have no incentive to be involved.

Discouraging compassionate use and refusing to consider knowledge gained from it will also slow the development of new knowledge by tightening the most critical bottleneck in AIDS research—clinical testing to learn exactly when and how to use the many drugs already well known to science and medicine which appear very likely to be useful in the treatment of AIDS or ARC but are not being tested or brought into use.

One physician who has used DHPG pointed out that over 80 percent of patients treated with it improved or stabilized, compared to under five percent of those left untreated. CMV in the urine became negative in over 90 percent. As for side effects, he has treated dozens of patients and never had to discontinue the drug permanently; sometimes he had to stop temporarily when certain blood counts became low. He also noted that today many more AIDS patients are outside of major medical centers, making it much harder for them to obtain treatment by compassionate use. The costs of taking care of these people will greatly increase, he pointed out, if we let them go blind. He also noted that the Advisory Committee's request for dose-response data is in fact a political euphemism for a placebo trial, as some of the doses would presumably be small enough to be ineffective; otherwise there would be no point in the study.

If the recommendation against approval was really so bad, why did the committee of experts vote for it? There seem to be several reasons. First, the clinical information available on DHPG is admittedly not clean or elegant science, because it comes from case reports, not from a controlled study designed in advance. Second, the FDA's regulations require two prospectively designed controlled studies, unless there are very compelling reasons not to have them; with DHPG, for ethical reasons, there were none. Third, most of the panelists were not experienced with DHPG or eye diseases. For example, one suggestion was to use visual acuity tests to make sure DHPG worked. But in fact such tests would not be appropriate, because with CMV retinitis visual acuity depends entirely on whether the part of the retina destroyed happens to include the macula, the small spot most important for vision; a visual field test should be used instead. The two votes for approval were from ophthalmologists familiar with DHPG. We don't know why the others put the letter of the law ahead of the views of those panelists with experience in the matter being decided.

There is no appeal from an FDA decision. And the public does not realize what is happening because those close enough to know are afraid to speak publicly. They fear with good reason that if they alienate the officials on whose decisions they depend, they will no longer be effective in accomplishing the goals they believe are important— whether gaining approval for a drug they are championing, or furthering any other project.

This situation will persist until Congressional committees, media, and private organizations realize that they will learn what is going on only through long-term commitment to this investigation, with private, off the record conversations in which scientists, physicians, and officials explain what is happening and what the problems are—without the well-founded fear of damaging or destroying their work.

AL 721 TODAY, PART III:
SURVEYS, TECHNICAL, REFERENCES

Part I of this report (see *AIDS Treatment News,* Issue Number 42) gave an overview of the experimental AIDS treatment AL 721, also called egg lecithin lipids. Part II answered specific questions such as how to use AL 721, and where to find buyers clubs or distributors. Part III gives technical information and references.

Surveys of AL 721 Users

Three surveys have asked persons who are using AL 721 about their experience with it. All are finding comparable results.

AIDS Treatment News mailed a questionnaire to its 898 subscribers in July 1987, and published results in Issue Number 39, August 28, 1987. Of the 147 completed questionnaires we received, 110 were from persons who had used some form of AL 721 for at least three weeks. Only the soy-based "home formula" and the all-egg product distributed by New York's PWA Health Group had enough users to allow meaningful statistics. Of those using the soy version, 43 percent found it helpful and 22 percent not helpful; with the egg version the percentages were 58 percent helpful and 8 percent not helpful. The remaining persons in both categories were those who checked "uncertain" or otherwise expressed uncertainty, said it was too early to tell, or left the question blank. For more information on this survey, see *AIDS Treatment News,* Issue Number 39.

The PWA Health Group in New York did a telephone survey of 168 randomly-selected purchasers who had used the lipids for two or more months; it summarized the results in a two-page breakdown dated September 22, 1987. Forty-two percent of the 168 described themselves as better, 43 percent as the same; 12 percent said they were worse (or were reported to have died). Four percent had discontinued the lipids. The percentages total 101 instead of 100 because of rounding approximations.

Eighty-eight of the 168 people had AIDS. 43 percent of those with AIDS reported that they were better, 39 percent the same, and 18 percent worse. Forty-five people had ARC; 36 percent said they were better, 42 percent the same, 9 percent worse, and 13 percent had discontinued the lipids. Of the 35 people who were HIV positive but described as healthy and asymptomatic, 46 percent described themselves as better and 54 percent as the same; no one said they were worse or had discontinued the lipids. For more information, contact the PWA Health Group in New York.

The third survey is keeping track of about 40 clients of the AIDS Assessment Clinic of the Community Health Project in New York—about 20 using lipids and 20 not. As of early October the study had been going for three months. Results were not yet available, but the impression of those doing this survey is that it is confirming the other ones: persons on the lipids feel better, and objectively improve.

A fourth survey is an ongoing study conducted by Project Inform. We don't have results yet, but mention this study because it is the only one still open for participation.

Technical Background

AL 721, a form of lecithin, consists entirely of a mixture of three substances, all of them extracted from ordinary egg yolk. These ingredients are phosphatidylcholine (abbreviated PC), phosphatidylethanolamine (PE), and neutral lipids (NL), which are ordinary fats similar to those found in butter or olive oil, but from egg yolk instead. AL 721 consists of a 7:2:1 ratio, 70 percent NL, 20 percent PC, and 10 percent PE. (Hence the name; "AL" stands for "active lipid.")

AL 721 is a brown, viscous liquid at room temperature. It readily disperses but does not dissolve in water.

Laboratory tests by the Israeli developers of the mixture found that the 7:2:1 ratio had a much greater effect on human white blood cells than other ratios tested. AL 721 removed cholesterol from the cell membranes, increasing the "fluidity" of the membrane, the degree to which protein molecules there can move freely.

AL 721 is believed to make it harder for lipid-coated viruses (a group which includes HIV, herpes, Epstein-Barr, and CMV) to attach themselves to the T-4 receptor site on the cell. Unless the virus can attach to this molecule, it cannot enter the cell. AL 721 does not kill the virus, but may make it less able to infect healthy cells, probably by removing cholesterol from the lipid coat of the virus.

When dispersed in water, AL 721 forms tiny spheres visible with an electron microscope. These spheres are believed to have the neutral lipid in the center, and a layer of PC and PE one molecule thick on the surface. In the laboratory, this spherical structure works especially well for removing cholesterol from cell membranes, changing the fluidity of cell membranes toward the more-fluid end of its normal range.

What happens when AL 721 is eaten and digested? Most physicians believe that the spheres would be broken up, and the three ingredients absorbed separately into the bloodstream. Many think that AL 721 could not possibly work, because it would be separated into its three components and treated by the body like ordinary food. But the fate of ingested AL 721 is poorly understood; it may get into the bloodstream as the spheres, or it may work anyway even if it doesn't. The theory which says that AL 721 could not work is far from infallible. But it seems to have kept many physicians and scientists from giving this treatment the attention it would otherwise have received.

Some professionals suspect that another reason mainstream scientists have been slow to pay attention to AL 721 is that its developers are not microbiologists. They are experts in cell membranes, not viruses, and their laboratories are not equipped to work with HIV. The link to viruses comes from the work of a few virologists such as R.R. Wagner, on reducing the infectivity of lipid-coated viruses by removing cholesterol from the coat. Apparently other virologists have been slow to recognize the importance of this work, so the developers of AL 721 were placed in the politically difficult role of outsiders telling other scientists that they had overlooked the importance of work in their own field.

For more technical information on AL 721, see the references below.

Hepatitis and Phosphatidylcholine

In the U.S., persons with hepatitis are usually told that there is no specific treatment. But in Europe and elsewhere a number of published studies, including double-blind trials with dozens of patients, have shown that phosphatidylcholine, one of the ingredients of AL 721, is clearly useful in treating several kinds of hepatitis, including acute hepatitis A and B, and HBsAg negative chronic active hepatitis. Few of these studies have been published in English; they seem to be largely unknown in this country.

Most of these trials have used "Essential Phospholipid" ("Essential Forte," Nattermann, Germany), which contains several common vitamins, mostly B vitamins, in addition to phosphatidylcholine. The dose used was about three grams per day, sometimes less. The studies found improvement in clinical condition, laboratory parameters, and absence of relapses in patients receiving the phospholipid, compared to controls.

We don't know how the polyunsaturated phosphatidylcholine in the Nattermann preparation compares to the kind of phosphatidylcholine in AL 721, or to the kind in ordinary soy lecithin. ("Phosphatidylcholine" refers to a class of closely related substances, not to a single chemical.)

These studies do not prove that AL 721 could be helpful for persons with hepatitis, although they suggest that it might. But their results do strengthen the case for AL 721 by showing that orally administered phosphatidylcholine can be effective as a treatment for a viral disease, as shown by controlled, double-blind trials. We are not aware of any studies which failed to show efficacy.

Four clinical studies are cited in the references below (Atoba *et al.*, 1985; Jenkins *et al.*, 1982; Kosina *et al.*, 1981; and Visco, 1985). Several other animal and clinical studies of phospholipids and liver diseases have been published recently.

The Home Formula

This soy-lecithin preparation, easily made in a kitchen, was the best AL 721 substitute we had until the all-egg versions became available. A widespread consensus of persons using these materials is that this soy formula does work, but the egg products are better. Many people still use the soy substitute because it costs a quarter as much, can be easier to obtain, and may work as well as the egg version for some people.

Steve Gavin developed this formula. It was first distributed in January 1987, at PWA meetings in New York. *AIDS Treatment News* reprinted it on January 30 (see Issue Number 24). We don't know how many people have used the formula by this time, but there are reasons to believe there have been thousands.

> PC-55™ is a high-strength lecithin concentrate made by Twin Laboratories, Inc., of Ronkonkoma, New York, and sold in health-food stores. It contains two of the three ingredients of AL 721; they are in a 5:2 ratio, close to the 2:1 used in AL 721. Neutral lipids can be added to PC-55™ making it a membrane fluidizer comparable to AL 721. This material is a food nutrient, it is not a drug. It is safe.
>
> Combine five tablespoons of PC-55™ and 12 tablespoons of water in a bowl, and whip with an electric mixer or blender. Slowly add 6 tablespoons plus one teaspoon of butter (6⅓ tablespoons butter) which has been melted (measure the butter before melting). Whip thoroughly three to five minutes. This mixture divided into ten even doses gives slightly over 10 grams of the lipids per dose. Each dose should weigh about 30.4 grams or 1.06 ounces.
>
> The individual doses can be placed into plastic sandwich bags for freezing. If you don't have a scale, you can measure out two tablespoons to each bag, then add a much smaller amount to divide the remainder. One person separates the doses in an ice-cube tray. Move each dose from the freezer to the refrigerator a few hours before use. This preparation spoils very rapidly at room temperature; it must be frozen unless used immediately.
>
> (An earlier version of this formula used cooking oil instead of butter. The proportions are 5 tablespoons PC-55™, 5 tablespoons + 1 teaspoon oil, and 10 Tbsp water.)
>
> The material is best eaten in the morning, spread on fat-free bread or mixed with fruit juice. The user should eat a fat-free breakfast which might consist of fat-free cereals, skim milk, fruits, or vegetables. There are no restrictions on lunch or dinner. An additional dose might be taken before going to bed. Patients treated in Israel are given two doses a day for about four weeks, then single doses indefinitely. Some people with AIDS might experience diarrhea with this membrane fluidizer, especially with the additional dose. Eat brown rice and other solid foods.
>
> You can help others and yourself by keeping a record of your experience—doses, dates, and any resulting effects.

REFERENCES

Atoba, M.A., E.A. Ayoola, and O. Ogunseyinde, "Effect of Essential Phospholipid Choline on the Course of Acute Hepatitis-B Infection," *Tropical Gastroenterology* 6(2) (April–June 1985), pp. 96–9.

Bell, J.M., and P.K. Lundberg, "Effects of Commercial Soy Lecithin Preparation of Development of Sensorimotor Behavior and Brain Biochemistry in the Rat," *Developmental Psychobiology* 18(1) (1985), pp. 59–66.

Davis, H., "AIDS Patients Flock to Israel for Experimental Egg Yolk Drug," *Baltimore Jewish Times* (October 9, 1987).

Heron, D., M. Shinitzky, and D. Samuel, "Alleviation of Drug Withdrawal Symptoms by Treatment with a Potent Mixture of Natural Lipids," *European Journal of Pharmacology* 83 (1982), pp. 253–61.

Jenkins, P.J., B.P. Portmann, A.L.W.F. Eddleston, and R. Williams, "Use of Polyunsaturated Phosphatidyl Choline in HBsAg Negative Chronic Active Hepatitis: Results of Prospective Double-blind Controlled Trial," *Liver* 2 (1982), pp. 77–81.

Kosina, F., K. Budka, Z. Kolouch, D. Lazarova, and D. Truksova, "Essential Cholinephospholipids in the Treatment of Virus Hepatitis" (English translation of title), *Casopis Lekaru Ceskych* 120 (31–32) (August 13, 1981), pp. 957–60.

Lyte, M., and M. Shinitzky, "A Special Lipid Mixture for Membrane Fluidization," *Biochimica et Biophysica Acta* 812 (1985), pp. 133–8.

Ma, Wen-Chao, "A Cytopathological Study of Acute and Chronic Morphinism in the Albino Rat," *Chinese Journal of Physiology* 5 (1931), pp. 251–74. (This study, overlooked for 50 years, suggested use of lecithin for treating drug addiction.)

Moore, N.F., E.J. Patzer, J.M. Shaw, T.E. Thompson, and R.R. Wagner, "Interaction of Vesicular Stomatitis Virus with Lipid Vesicles: Depletion of Cholesterol and Effect on Virion Membrane Fluidity and Infectivity," *Journal of Virology* 27 (2) (August 1978), pp. 320–9.

Rivnay, B., S. Bergman, M. Shinitzky, and A. Globerson, "Correlations Between Membrane Viscosity, Serum Cholesterol, Lymphocyte Activation and Ageing in Man," *Mechanisms of Ageing Development* 12(2) (February 1980), pp. 119–26.

Sarin, P.S., R.C. Gallo, D.I. Scheer, F. Crews, and A.S. Lippa, "Effects of a Novel Compound (AL 721) on HTLV-III Infectivity In Vitro," *New England Journal of Medicine* 313 (November 14, 1985), pp. 1289–90.

Shinitzky, M., (ed), *Physiology of Membrane Fluidity,* Volumes 1 and 2 (Boca Raton, Florida: CRC Press, 1984).

Shinitzky, M., M. Lyte, D.S. Heron, and D. Samuel, "Intervention in Membrane Aging—The Development and Application of Active Lipid," IN *Intervention in the Aging Process, Part B: Basic Research and Preclinical Screening,* pp. 175–86. (New York: Alan R Liss, Inc., 1983).

Skornick, Y., I. Yust, V. Zakuth, and M. Shinitzky, "Treatment of AIDS Patients with AL 721 in an Open Trial," Paper from M. Shinitzky, Department of Membrane Research, The Weizmann Institute of Science, Rehovot, Israel (1987).

Visco, G., "Polyunsaturated Phosphatidylcholine in Association with Vitamin B Complex in the Treatment of Acute Viral Hepatitis B: Results of a randomized double-blind study" (English translation of title), *Clinica Terapeutica* 114 (3) (August 15, 1985), pp. 183–8.

Wood, J.L. and R.G. Allison, "Effects of Consumption of Choline and Lecithin on Neurological and Cardiovascular Systems," *Federation Proceedings* 41 (1982), pp. 3015–21.

For those who want more information, the Medline database produced by the National Library of Medicine has over 1800 scientific papers indexed under "membrane fluidity." Those interested in the relevance of these concepts to viruses should check the work of R.R. Wagner, who has authored or co-authored over 100 scientific papers.

AIDS TREATMENT NEWS PUBLISHER
TO SPEAK IN NEW YORK

John S. James, editor and publisher of *AIDS Treatment News,* will participate in panels on treatments in New York, November 17 and 18.

The November 17 panel is a symposium of the Columbia Gay Health Advocacy Project, "AIDS: Improving the Odds—Care and Treatment for Currently Healthy People Who are HIV Infected or at High Risk." Other panelists who have agreed to participate are Donald Armstrong, M.D., Bernard Bihari, M.D., Michael Callen, Barry Gingell, M.D., Richard Keeling, M.D., Donald Kotler, M.D., Michael Lange, M.D., Jeffrey Laurence, M.D., Joseph Sonnabend, M.D., and Daniel William, M.D. The discussion is scheduled in the Columbia Law School Building, Rooms A and B, northeast corner of 116th St. and Amsterdam Avenue, one block east of Broadway (across the campus). Space is limited.

The November 18 meeting will be a PWA Coalition Public Forum on promising interventions, at the Gay and Lesbian Community Center, 208 West 13th Street, just west of 7th Avenue.

Issue Number 45
November 20, 1987

NEW OPTIMISM ON TREATMENT

We have heard from New York physicians treating persons with AIDS and ARC that they are having far fewer deaths this year than last, and fewer serious complications requiring hospitalization, even though they have more patients. And in San Francisco, median survival time after an AIDS diagnosis increased unexpectedly, from ten months to 14, after staying the same for five years. Meanwhile, the most comprehensive study yet of AIDS outcome found long-term survival much better than expected, and found that the evidence does not show that AIDS is always fatal.

Many physicians now see a reasonable chance that AIDS could become usually a manageable disease within the next year or two. No cure is on the horizon at this time, but the hope is that most people could become healthy and remain that way indefinitely, even without a cure.

We are preparing a review of this information, probably for the next issue of *AIDS Treatment News*.

NEWSLETTER ON AIDS TREATMENTS FROM GAY MEN'S HEALTH CRISIS

The first issue of *Treatment Issues,* a new monthly newsletter on AIDS treatments edited by Barry Gingell, M.D., is now available without charge from the Gay Men's Health Crisis in New York.

Treatment Issues, Volume 1, Number 1 (November 10, 1987) has articles on nutrition and AIDS, a discussion on whether persons with AIDS should receive routine immunizations for influenza and pneumococcal pneumonia, and an update on aerosol and intravenous pentamidine for treating pneumocystis.

Treatment Issues is somewhat more conservative than *AIDS Treatment News,* but still it is full of useful information. For example, the nutrition article recommends lots

216

of protein, including animal protein; for reasons discussed, it recommends against a strictly vegetarian diet. Instead it suggests using certified organically grown meats to avoid unwanted antibiotics, hormones, pesticides, and other chemicals often used in commercial meat production. It urges that cured meats (such as bacon, salami, or corned beef) be avoided, because they contain immunosuppressive chemicals such as nitrites. It tells where to get good-quality organically grown poultry in New York.

A discussion of zinc supplements provides another example of practical information. The article suggests doses, and tells why too much is harmful.

The newsletter is written primarily for persons with AIDS or ARC. But it has numerous references to the medical literature for physicians and researchers.

To get on the mailing list to receive *Treatment Issues* without charge, write with your name and address to the Gay Men's Health Crisis in New York (see Appendix B for their address).

NEWS FROM THE COMMUNITY RESEARCH INITIATIVE

The Community Research Initiative (CRI), a project of the PWA Coalition in New York, continues to do some of the best work anywhere in furthering AIDS research. (For background on the CRI, see *AIDS Treatment News,* Issue Number 38).

The CRI now has a $300,000 contract with LyphoMed, the manufacturer of pentamidine, to conduct a 200-patient study of aerosol pentamidine. The protocol for this research was revised to support the FDA-approved design used in San Francisco General Hospital, so that the CRI study can contribute toward FDA approval of aerosol pentamidine, which will make it more accessible for patients.

The CRI has also received $51,000 from People Taking Action Against AIDS, a new fund-raising organization, for a study of egg lecithin lipids (generic AL 721) as an AIDS/ARC treatment. A parallel arm of the study, funded separately, will use an injectable form of the lipids. Dr. Jeffrey Askenazi will be the principal investigator in this study, with Dr. Joseph Sonnabend as co-investigator.

Study design and funding negotiations are also proceeding for studies on: Ampligen, Erythropoietin, Cryptosporidium Milk—Immune Globulin, Methionine Enkephalin (MEK), DHPG as CMV prophylaxis, and an Antabuse/Imuthiol Monitoring Project.

POLIO VACCINE FOR AIDS TREATMENT?

Twelve persons with ARC and one with AIDS have been treated by repeated injections of killed-virus polio vaccine three to seven times per week. All have show major improvement or complete remission of symptoms, usually within two months, and T-cell counts have also improved. Results of one case have been published (Pitts and Allen, *Clinical Immunology and Immunopathology* 43, 1987, pp. 277–80). A report on the next four cases is in press, and a complete report will be published later.

The physicians tried polio vaccine because they had already had good results with one case of acute lymphocytic leukemia, believed to be caused by a retrovirus related to HIV. In this case, a child who was not expected to live was given the vaccine for several years, and tested for eight years to confirm the remission of the leukemia. He has now been healthy for 20 years after the treatment began.

That child's physician had tried the vaccine in desperation, after learning that new leukemia cases decreased in areas which had a polio outbreak. This decrease suggested that there might be a cross immunity between polio and the retrovirus—perhaps because mammals had evolved an ability to produce antibodies to a certain groups of disease-causing organisms when exposed to only one of them.

The first HIV patient was a physician with KS, thrush, fatigue, weight loss of 60 pounds, and a T-cell count of 40. Improvements started within six weeks; by ten weeks the KS, thrush, and most of the other symptoms had disappeared. He still had severe mental depression, however, and stopped the treatment in favor of another experimental therapy, and was lost to follow-up.

The next four patients treated were gay men with ARC; an article on this phase of the study will appear in *Clinical Immunology and Immunopathology.* Three of these patients started with relatively high T-cell counts averaging over 400; their symptoms resolved completely within two to seven months. The fourth did not have an initial T-cell count available; his lymphadenopathy resolved completely, but some fatigue remained after 11 months of treatment.

The killed-virus (Salk) polio vaccine used is believed to be entirely safe, and is commonly used for persons with immune deficiencies who cannot use the Sabin live-virus vaccine. However, there has been some controversy about whether persons with AIDS or ARC should receive any immunization, because of fear that increasing activation of the immune system could stimulate the growth of HIV. Last week we spoke with Dr. Pitts, one of the authors of the paper cited above; he is convinced that the benefits far outweigh any risk.

He has now treated 12 persons with ARC, and every one treated long enough to evaluate has shown resolution of symptoms. They are able to work and entirely healthy. T-cells have increased by at least 67 percent, and sometimes much more.

The polio vaccine trial has met skepticism from some immunologists, who say that polio immunization would not work for AIDS because it is a different virus. Immunologists are currently emphasizing the specificity of the immune response. Dr. Pitts points out that although the polio virus and HIV are in different families and reproduce differently, they are similar in structure in some ways. And there are many examples of common antibodies among different viruses, going all the way back to the first vaccination, which used cowpox virus to prevent smallpox.

Dr. Pitts is board certified in both psychiatry and pediatrics. He has studied the effects of viruses in the brain's limbic system (which controls mood)—including possible viral causes of depression. He became interested in retroviral diseases because the child whose case is described above is his son.

The polio vaccine trial has IRB (institutional review board) approval to enroll 100 patients; since only 12 are enrolled so far, places are open for others. Dr. Pitts will consider persons with AIDS as well as ARC for the study. Only one person with AIDS has been treated so far, however, and it is not known whether the vaccine will be effective if the illness is very far advanced.

Dr. Pitts is also recruiting physicians to work with him in testing this treatment. Physicians could of course use the treatment anywhere.

Issue Number 46
December 4, 1987

GOOD NEWS ON AIDS SURVIVAL, AND TREATMENTS

Recent studies in San Francisco and New York have found major, unexpected improvement in median survival after an AIDS diagnosis, and in long-term survival. And many physicians with large AIDS caseloads are having far fewer deaths this year than last, and fewer complications serious enough to require hospitalization, even though they have more patients.

This article examines the statistical evidence on survival in San Francisco and New York, and in the United States as a whole. It looks at why the improved survival figures may be even more important than they first seem.

We also interviewed Nathaniel Pier, M.D., a New York physician in private practice with about 300 AIDS/ARC patients, on the much lower death rate he and his colleagues are seeing this year, on current ethical issues in AIDS, and on what medical approaches seem to be making a difference. (More on this interview will appear in a later issue.) And we asked Michael Callen, a founding member of the PWA Coalition in New York, about his current interview study of long-term survivors diagnosed with AIDS for over three years.

San Francisco Survival Study

Since 1981 the San Francisco Department of Public Health has kept track of the median length of survival of persons diagnosed with AIDS each year. (The median is not the average, but the middle of the range of length of life after diagnosis.) For the first five years median survival was unchanged, about ten months. But in 1986 it unexpectedly jumped to about 14 months.

This improved survival resulted from better outlook for persons with diagnosed with pneumocystis. Survival for KS did not improve last year, but it has always been much better than for pneumocystis.

The *San Francisco Examiner* interviewed Dr. George Lemp, an epidemiologist with the Department of Public Health, and reported this increasing survival on November 6 (page A4); so far there has been little notice of these results outside of San Francisco. No one knows for sure why persons are suddenly living longer after an AIDS diagnosis, but San Francisco epidemiologists suspect that it may be due to prevention and better treatment of pneumocystis, and/or to use of AZT.

We asked Dr. Lemp for more details on the new findings, and on how the research was conducted. Information on what treatments people used was not recorded. This is an epidemiological study not a clinical one, and keeping track of all the different diagnoses and treatments would have been difficult. In June of this year the epidemiologists did start asking what antiviral drugs each person used, so by early to mid 1988 they will be able to start checking on correlation of survival with use of AZT.

How were the annual medians derived? Dr. Lemp explained that, for purposes of analysis only, all patients diagnosed with AIDS within a given calendar year were followed as a cohort. Because persons with AIDS often survive for a long time, the median survival cannot be estimated accurately until well after the year has ended. For example, the "1986" data includes followup through August of 1987. For this reason it is too early to know 1987 results yet. But very early indications are that 1987 looks better than 1986.

No one knows for sure why the median survival time increased in 1986, when it had not done so before. But it seems reasonable to guess that the improved survival is due to treatments. We do not have scientific proof. But it is hard to devise any other plausible explanation.

Few new treatments were widely used in 1986, the year of diagnosis for the cohort which survived longer; AZT, aerosol pentamidine, and AL 721, for example, had only reached a few. But since the 1986 survival data actually includes what happened as late as August 1987, treatments received in 1987 could also have had an effect.

Before August 1987, both AZT and aerosol pentamidine had become widely used in San Francisco. Less publicized improvements in clinical treatment for pneumocystis and other infections were also being used on enough patients that they might have affected the survival statistics.

What about alternative treatments? On AL 721, the all-egg generic versions arrived here in late summer, probably too late to affect the 1986 survival median; the soy-based "home formula" arrived in January 1986, however, so it might have had an effect. It would be worth checking whether other treatments, such as ribavirin, DNCB, megadose vitamin C, or certain herbal treatments, first became widely used during the time when they might have contributed to improved survival of the 1986 San Francisco cohort.

If it is true that one or more treatments are responsible for the 1986 improvement, they would probably be adding much more than the four months of additional survival seen in the median figures. For only a minority of persons in San Francisco had access to new treatments and chose to use them by early 1987. And those diagnosed in early 1986 were largely affected by 1986 treatment anyway. For both these reasons, the four-month figure includes the majority which was not treated and presumably did not survive longer than those diagnosed in previous years. Therefore, the minority which did get new treatments and presumably accounted for the four-month increase in the median survival must have had much more than a four-month improvement.

New York Survival Study

The most detailed study yet on AIDS survival was published in the *New England Journal of Medicine* (November 19, 1987), and widely reported in the press at that time.

This study by the U.S. Centers for Disease Control of over five thousand persons diagnosed with AIDS in New York City found as many as 15 percent surviving up to five years. Although the researchers admitted that they may have missed some deaths, they concluded that the general impression that AIDS is always fatal cannot be supported. The existing evidence does not rule out the possibility that some people could live indefinitely with AIDS, or could recover.

This New York study included only patients diagnosed through December 1985. Therefore its findings would not reflect the improvement (presumably due to new treatments) shown in the 1986 San Francisco cohort discussed above. For this reason, survival today may be even better than shown by this study.

National Survival Study

Seemingly contradictory and much more pessimistic results of a smaller study at the Centers for Disease Control (CDC) were released at a conference on October 5, 1987 and widely reported in the press the next day.

This study, by researcher Ann Hardy, was designed to check the reliability of the official CDC estimate that 15 percent of persons with AIDS survive three years, by verifying that the people on whom that statistic was based were indeed still alive. Only two to five percent had been determined to be alive, and the news stories which went out listed the three-year U.S. survival rate as only two to five percent. This figure differs greatly from the New York and San Francisco findings.

We spoke with Ms. Hardy, who pointed out that San Francisco might have longer survival times than elsewhere in the country because more persons with AIDS here have KS, and those with only KS survive much longer than others, on the average. She did not know why the New York results differed so greatly from hers, and referred us to the researchers who conducted that study. We reached one of the researchers, but were unable to get the permission required for an interview by press time.

Ms. Hardy's study only involved persons diagnosed with AIDS in December 1983 or before. Therefore it has no bearing on the major San Francisco result, the large increase in survival for those diagnosed in 1986 compared to any previous time.

Long-Term Survivor Interviews

Michael Callen, a founding member of the PWA Coalition in New York and himself a long-term survivor diagnosed in 1982, is interviewing persons who have survived with an AIDS diagnosis for over three years. So far he has interviewed 17 persons. Results will appear in an article and probably in a book. Meanwhile, Mr. Callen told us of some of the early, often surprising findings so far.

Here are some of his preliminary observations. Be careful in interpreting them. The fact that these survivors made certain choices three or more years ago, when their options were very different from the options today, does not necessarily imply that people should make the same choices today.

- Persons can survive far longer with KS than many have been led to believe. Persons can lead a long and happy life with KS.

- Only three of the 17 used aggressive chemotherapy. One of these was in a suramin trial, and almost died. The other used HPA-23. A third is now on AZT (see below).

- Mr. Callen at first had trouble finding persons who had survived three years after a pneumocystis diagnosis (a diagnosis made three or more years ago, before improved treatments were available). But eventually he did find persons who have survived for four years, and for four and a half years, after the diagnosis.

- Only one of the long-term survivors is on AZT. Others said if it wasn't broke, don't fix it. They had done well before AZT became available, and didn't want to rock the boat.

- All of them had dabbled in alternative approaches. With KS, there were several striking stories of success with macrobiotic or vegetarian diets. About half of the long-term survivors had made major diet changes. And the rest paid more attention to their diets.

- Most or all had used approaches such as shiatsu massage, acupuncture, or visualization. A clear majority were involved with groups such as Louise Hay, or AIDS Mastery.

- All but two found solace in religion—about half in the religion of their childhood. Others did not seek organized religion, but spoke of spirituality, or a sense of oneness. None became Bible-thumping fundamentalists. All who did become involved in churches were critical of some aspects of organized religion.

- All said they needed hope to survive. Each had to deal in some way with the media's repeated message that everyone dies. Some found it important to know survivors; many knew each other. All but two are aggressively involved in the AIDS movement, or working with PWAs; many are in the forefront.

- They are fighters, often difficult patients, not passive. Most used a group of physicians to coordinate their care, not just one. A majority have fired a physician, or ordered one out of their hospital room.

- Several had moving, near-death experiences.

- There was no magic bullet, no single treatment used by all the survivors. Not all of them used lipids, or macrobiotics, or ribavirin, or anything else. Their experience suggests that AIDS is not one disease, with one substance which will work for everyone.

Mr. Callen is continuing this study. Results will appear in the *Village Voice*, and probably in book form also.

To Be Continued. Later articles will examine the experience of AIDS physicians who have had fewer deaths and serious infections this year than last, despite having more patients. We will examine physicians' views of what does and does not work in AIDS treatments and care, and in the development and application of new drugs.

AZT AND ACYCLOVIR COMBINATION

Acyclovir (Zovirax), a readily available prescription drug, appears to work synergistically with AZT, meaning that the combination may be a better AIDS treatment than either one alone. Several studies of this combination are now going on; for a list of the studies, see *AmFAR Directory of Experimental Treatments for AIDS & ARC,* published by the American Foundation for AIDS Research (see Appendix B). Trials are planned or underway in France, Italy, Sweden, Germany, Belgium, Switzerland, United Kingdom, Denmark, Australia, and the U.S.

Meanwhile a number of physicians and patients are using this drug combination—sometimes as a half dose of AZT combined with a full dose of acyclovir—but few physicians are willing to speak publicly about it, because the combination has not been approved and, according to the October 1987 edition of the *AmFAR Directory,* no confirmatory data is available.

AIDS Treatment News hereby releases what may be the first published data on the use of this combination in the treatment of AIDS and ARC.

Project Inform, in San Francisco, California, filed a Freedom of Information Act request and obtained extensive internal documentation of the large double-blind placebo-controlled AZT trial with 282 patients. One paragraph of this documentation concerned the combination of AZT and acyclovir. We reproduce the paragraph here:

> Seventy of the 282 patients enrolled in this trial (25%) received acyclovir (ACV) in addition to their study medication. Thirty-four were patients randomized to receive AZT . . . no evidence of increased hematologic toxicity. . . . Only 2 of the 34 patients (6%) who received ACV in addition to AZT developed opportunistic infections over the course of the trial compared to 22 of 111 (20%) of the AZT recipients who did not receive ACV during the study.

Researchers should consider the possibility that the benefit of including acyclovir with AZT in the treatment of AIDS or ARC may be even greater than the above figures suggest. For the AZT patients who also received acyclovir presumably had an infection which the acyclovir was being used to treat, so as a group they were probably sicker to begin with than the AZT patients who did not receive acyclovir. Even so, they did much better.

It is too early to know for sure that the combination is useful. We will report more information as it becomes available.

PAYING FOR AZT

James Palazzolo, who is writing an article on AZT, brought the following to our attention:

(1) Family Pharmaceuticals in South Carolina, a company which specializes in low prices for expensive prescription drugs for chronic diseases, sells AZT at what is reported to be one of the lowest prices in the U.S. In early December 1987 (before the 20 percent price reduction announced in mid December by Burroughs-Wellcome) it quoted $204.85 per 100, about $6000 per year for a full dose, two capsules every

four hours. For the current price or for more information, call Family Pharmaceuticals (see Appendix B).

(2)   The Federal AIDS Drug Reimbursement Program appropriated $30,000,000 to pay for AZT for persons who cannot afford it. Unfortunately, however, some states are not yet ready to disburse the money.

This program, traded off in Senate deal-making for AIDS testing of immigrants, pays only for FDA-approved anti-HIV agents, meaning only AZT.

Income eligibility is about $11,000 per year for family of one.

This program only applies to those who meet the official FDA guidelines for use of AZT. Basically, persons must either have had pneumocystis, or have under 200 T-helper cells and be symptomatic.

The money is given to each state, based on its number of AIDS patients.

In San Francisco, the Health Department will issue a press release when California sets up an office to administer the program. At that time the San Francisco AIDS Foundation hotline will have information on how to apply.

FANSIDAR DANGER, AGAIN

In Issues Number 42 and 43 we discussed the dangers and benefits of fansidar, one of several preventive treatments for pneumocystis. Recently we heard of two more cases of serious reactions to this drug. One happened to a friend of this writer, who used fansidar because he was unable to obtain aerosol pentamidine in San Diego. He had not realized that fansidar must be stopped if a skin rash occurs, and almost died as a result.

We repeat the following warning from the *Physician's Desk Reference,* which also includes other precautions. This part of the warning is printed twice in all caps, and set off in separate boxes for additional emphasis:

> FATALITIES ASSOCIATED WITH THE ADMINISTRATION OF FANSIDAR HAVE OCCURRED DUE TO SEVERE REACTIONS, INCLUDING STEVENS-JOHNSON SYNDROME AND TOXIC EPIDERMAL NECROLYSIS. FANSIDAR PROPHYLAXIS SHOULD BE DISCONTINUED AT THE FIRST APPEARANCE OF SKIN RASH, IF A SIGNIFICANT REDUCTION IN THE COUNT OF ANY FORMED BLOOD ELEMENTS IS NOTED, OR UPON THE OCCURRENCE OF ACTIVE BACTERIAL OR FUNGAL INFECTIONS.

Persons with AIDS or ARC may be more likely to have these reactions than other people. (Fansidar is usually used as a preventive for malaria.)

Use of this drug may be justified in some cases. But patients should make sure to get the warnings from their physicians—or look them up themselves in the *Physician's Desk Reference,* usually available in public libraries.

Fansidar seems to be used infrequently in San Francisco, as aerosol pentamidine prophylaxis is more available here.

IMPORTANT ARTICLES
FROM PROJECT INFORM

The October 1987 issue of *PI Perspectives,* the newsletter of Project Inform, has two articles which are proving influential.

"Evaluating New Treatment Alternatives" urges a cautious approach to proposed treatments. It provides checklists of questions for rationally evaluating the available evidence of efficacy, when there isn't full scientific proof. No available drug, mainstream or alternative, gets a perfect score. The point is not to reject them all, but rather to weigh the evidence properly.

"False Hope: Smoke and Mirrors From the FDA" reviews the new rules approved by the FDA in June of this year, rules supposed to provide easier access to experimental treatments which were safe and probably effective, although they had not yet achieved full mass-market approval. The article analyzes why these rules have failed to work.

A section titled "Questions for the FDA" caused annoyance at that agency, as reporters from around the county have found that the FDA is indeed unable to answer eight simple questions which Project Inform suggested. Some of the questions are:

- What is the procedure by which a physician may apply to receive an experimental drug for a life-threatened AIDS or ARC patient? Where can we get the forms?

- Are there any drugs for AIDS or ARC, immunomodulators or antivirals, that the FDA feels would currently be eligible for release under the new regulations?

- What criteria will be used to determine the effectiveness of a drug so that it can be released under the new regulations Where are those criteria spelled out?

- What, if any, role is there for the private physician under the new regulations?

To obtain the October issue of *PI Perspectives,* and to get on the mailing list for future issues, contact Project Inform (see Appendix B).

NEW BOOK:
STRATEGIES FOR SURVIVAL

This book, by three authors including the two founders of Project Inform, gives workbook-like checklists and exercises concerning strategies for one's own health, and for the health of the gay community. It also has annotated lists of community services, as well as relevant books, articles, and videotapes. The authors designed the book not to tell to reader what to do, but to provide information on ways to assess one's situations and make one's own choices.

The authors made major efforts to keep the price down; the book has 310 8½ by 11 pages and sells retail for $10.95. It is available in bookstores, or from St. Martin's Press, New York, NY.

COLUMBIA SYMPOSIUM TAPES, TRANSCRIPT AVAILABLE

Tapes and transcripts are now available from the Columbia Gay Health Advocacy Project panel on treatments for antibody-positive persons, which took place on November 17. The panel included nine medical doctors experienced in treating AIDS, and two other persons including this writer. For more information see *AIDS Treatment News*, Issue Number 44.

This panel could only begin in its main purpose: finding consensus among knowledgeable physicians about recommendations for preventing the development of AIDS or ARC by early treatment of antibody-positive persons, even before symptoms appear. The main bottleneck is the reluctance of physicians to recommend treatments without final proof of effectiveness—proof which will take many years to obtain because of the slow speed with which the disease develops. However, much useful information about treatments in general did come out of the meeting.

Tapes and transcripts can be ordered from the Columbia Gay Health Advocacy Project (see Appendix B). The videotape is $100, audiotape $25, transcript $20. PWAs with problems paying can call and discuss—or see if the local AIDS service organization can order the material.

Issue Number 47
January 1, 1988

TREATMENT OPTIMISM AND RESEARCH ETHICS: INTERVIEW WITH NATHANIEL PIER, M.D.

Nathaniel Pier, M.D. has about 300 AIDS/ARC patients in his private practice in New York. He also works with New York's Community Research Initiative (CRI), a project of the PWA Coalition. The CRI has obtained State and Federal approval to design and conduct clinical drug trials, providing unique opportunities for persons with AIDS to have input into clinical drug research.

We have spoken with Dr. Pier several times in the last two months, about the growing optimism on AIDS treatments, and about problems in research policy. We recorded and transcribed parts of these conversations and interviews.

We have learned that physicians in private practice are more free to speak openly if they want to, than scientists who usually need permission to make public statements, and who dare not offend the institutions which control research funding.

Growing Optimism On AIDS Treatments

"The point we've reached in late 1987 is really quite an optimistic one. A year ago when we were just starting out with AZT we could say that whether or not AZT works there's a profound change here, which is that we do have a tool which is a first step in treating people. And it forced the government and Otis Bowen at the meetings in June (the III International Conference on AIDS, in Washington, D.C.) to admit that people who are already affected by AIDS should not be thrown on the dunghill of humanity, that it was worth trying to save them, that in fact medications could be developed or should be developed that would treat them. And that's led to a profound change in the way people approach AIDS.

"Part of the optimism here is that we're beginning to bias the process in favor of good news. We're beginning to have more than one option. It's not just AZT now, it's AZT plus a number other drugs that are in phase II testing that may work.

"This perspective must be brought out. Patients must hear that although they have a serious problem that may result in them getting very ill or even dying, it's equally reasonable for them to hear that scientific progress has advanced significantly to the point where we can now introduce variables into the course of their disease that may mean they will not die. That, coupled with the fact that it is clear that there are long-term survivors, and that this is not a universally fatal, 100-percent-everybody-dies disease, makes it from a medical person's point of view a much more manageable disease. If you look at the 30- to 35-year-old age group who have Kaposi's, one in three is living more than five years. This is better statistics than many cancers. And somebody who presents in that fashion should not be told that they have a universally fatal illness.

"We must appeal to other physicians to stop the gloom and doom stuff. I know people are dying of AIDS, but when you're talking to an individual patient who is perhaps being diagnosed for the first time...they shouldn't necessarily feel that they're obligated to get sick and die to prove the CDC correct, or the *New York Times* for that matter.

"As far as practical things, if you ask the doctors in New York City about mortality rates, most of them, in fact everyone I talk to will tell you that the mortality rates have gone down considerably, partly because of AZT, some believe, partly because we're getting better at treating diseases that occur in AIDS, partly because of pneumocystis prophylaxis. But it is clear that AIDS is not the profoundly, 'Oh, shit, the patient's got six months to live' kind of thing that it was a year or two ago. And it's clear that physicians who are very skilled at dealing with AIDS do not lose patients in the kind of numbers that the same physicians did two years ago, or that other physicians who are not very skilled at dealing with AIDS are losing their patients."

The Wrong Way To Treat AIDS

"Recently some Harvard-trained physicians visited me to look at my practice and see how I deal with AIDS, because I've had so few deaths. They were astonished. What I do they do not do. They never heard of resources like *AIDS Treatment News* or Project Inform. And as a consequence their patients don't get the full spectrum of counseling, their opportunities for choosing their therapies are limited, and they don't do as well.

"It should be clear to the medical community that if you make a concerted effort with each individual to discuss therapeutic options that may be appropriate for them, such as participating in a trial of an experimental drug, or trying alternative therapies, they may do better, and survive longer and in better shape with a better quality of life. That's the message that's being lost. If you ask the infectious disease specialist, who may be the typical doctor that is asked to consult on an AIDS patient, what to do, it's AZT or nothing. That's a disaster. They don't take a look at what options the patients have, they don't counsel the patients as to what other alternatives there are, and if the patient doesn't do well on AZT they don't offer them anything else.

"If you look at medical literature you see statistics like 80 to 90 percent of AIDS patients develop dementia. These reports come from a skewed population. These papers are written by neurologists who see end-stage AIDS patients in tertiary care centers. They don't see what I see or what the usual clinical doctor sees. I have 300 patients with AIDS or ARC in my practice, and maybe one of them has dementia. And why? Because I see the healthy group of AIDS patients. The people who write papers in tertiary care centers see a biased population. They see the disasters, they see the ones who haven't done well. And so naturally they publish these horrendous statistics of how poorly AIDS patients do. But if they come and they see my practice and they see what I see week after week, of basically healthy people who are out there in society, who are working, who are not demented, who don't have severe peripheral neuropathies, who very occasionally have problems that are AIDS related but are basically doing okay, they would write very different papers. There's a serious bias in the medical literature also as to what is being reported, and it's giving people a distorted picture of what is going on with AIDS. They're not seeing the people who are doing well, the people who are surviving long, the people who have good quality of life, because those people don't go to those centers and therefore they don't get papers written about them.

"The bottom line is that if a physician takes the time to look at each individual and talk about what their options are, in terms of taking standard orthodox therapy, in terms of enrolling in an experimental treatment program, or in terms of looking at alternative therapies that may in fact have some value, like AL 721 or naltrexone, you can not only treat a patient and get them into a state where they can have some hope and some idea that there's something to do besides wait for the bomb to drop, that in fact if one of these therapies works, you've done an enormous good."

Research Policy and Ethics:
Pneumocystis, DHPG, Ampligen, Lentinan

"The people who are affected by the research, by the disease, are demanding to know what the timetable is, and they want explanations.

"AIDS has forced the American medical scene to look at aspects it's never looked at. Like the bioethics of drug testing. Is scientific data proprietary? Should the private drug companies, which the FDA constantly points to as being in partnership with the government, should they have proprietary interest over scientific data, like do their drugs work, or should the people who are actually paying for the government have the right to demand that these companies make their scientific data public? What about the degree of time it takes to get scientific data published?

"A good example of that is pneumocystis prophylaxis. In New York we've been using pneumocystis prophylaxis for a year, some have been using it for 18 months or longer. And in June when we spoke with Dr. Anthony Fauci (of NIH) about pneumocystis prophylaxis, people from ACT-UP and the PWA Coalition, he told them that they were fools, that there was no study that showed that pneumocystis prophylaxis was of any value and that we might be putting people in danger by doing it. In fact, five months later the *New England Journal of Medicine* published an editorial which essentially states that prophylaxis for pneumocystis should be standard therapy for people with AIDS. If we were wrong it would have done little harm. But we were right and therefore many people's lives were saved.

"If a therapy is generally deemed safe and we employ it, if we're wrong we haven't lost much, but if we're right we've done a great good. In drug therapies where there is a track record in human beings of safety, we needn't wait for efficacy to be proved before we give the individual the opportunity to choose to use or not use such a therapy. This doesn't mean that good rigorous studies couldn't or shouldn't be done; it's just that the number of people affected is so large and the time so precious that we need to construct a system whereby both the needs of the individual to choose therapies is acknowledged and accepted as well as the need for researchers to do rigorous science.

"If DHPG has clearly been demonstrated to help people with CMV retinitis, it seems completely illogical not to approve it for use, even though the studies haven't been done. And to punish people, to punish the patients by letting them go blind or die, in order to make the companies do the tests right, is just not logical or humane, and it should call into question why this decision is made and who is making it.

"I know of a patient in a small town who went blind in one eye and was told by an ophthalmologist who diagnosed him as having CMV retinitis that there was nothing to do about it. In fact within a few hours of his getting me on the phone he was in an appropriate hospital in Miami receiving DHPG therapy. It's disturbing to me that the medical establishment feels it has no responsibility to offer to people with no other options therapies that have at least shown some efficacy. One can't exactly say that this ophthalmologist was committing malpractice, but certainly in the name of humanity, in the name of this man's vision, he should have known that in fact there was something to do besides letting him go blind.

"The FDA continues to say that the DHPG rejection was an advisory committee decision that has nothing to do with whether the FDA will or will not approve it. What the FDA hasn't done is put down a set of guidelines or rules that will allow persons who are interested to determine whether or not a drug will be approved. Exactly how many trials need to be done, what kind of trials, how many patients, etc.? In a meeting with FDA Commissioner Frank Young that a number of concerned people had a couple of weeks ago, what he said is that it was completely up to his judgment, that there were no hard and fast rules; all you could say is that if a company wanted the drug to be approved, it would just have to apply and the FDA would use its judgment. But he refused or was unable to give out any guidelines. Of course if he did that it would allow people with AIDS to determine whether and how the FDA was influencing research policy.

"A good example is that the Ampligen study that's being done now in New York City at St. Luke's/Roosevelt Hospital apparently forbids any pneumocystis prophylaxis. This is a major ethical point; if you have a therapy that is of accepted benefit, is it ethical to deny this therapy to people at risk, because it might interfere with your endpoint for drug tests? This is an major question, and I asked the fellow who spoke about the Ampligen study who designed this protocol, and was there any input into this protocol by persons with the disease, did they voluntarily say yes, we will agree not to take this life-preserving therapy in order to advance science?

"It is clear that if the FDA has decided that, say, the endpoint for the efficacy of a drug that is designed to prevent people from going on to develop full-blown AIDS is whether or not they develop PCP, and therefore pneumocystis prophylaxis cannot be given, this is an major ethical question. I don't think that most people who are in genuine risk of developing PCP would in fact agree that this is an acceptable endpoint. And since Ampligen is one of the most hopeful drugs that we have, the exclusion of the ability to prevent PCP and the exclusiveness of Ampligen, the lack of number of slots in the trial, is coercive, is basically saying to a patient, 'You do what we say, or die.'

"I would still like to know why lentinan hasn't been tried. I would still like to find out what goes on in the AIDS drug selection committee, why they meet so infrequently, why the minutes of their meetings aren't published, and why people aren't watchdogging them from Congress or other public agencies, and why they don't allow proprietary data that's submitted to them by private companies to be examined if it's relevant to the health and well being of people. Like the studies of lentinan, why Bristol Labs does not allow them to be published, it's completely unethical. And I think that people with AIDS should rise up en masse, and say that you can't do this to us anymore.

"These questions of ethics in human research are profound, and it's a service to humanity that the community of people with AIDS is performing by calling them into question and forcing the medical establishment to examine them. And we can be proud of the fact, and look forward to the resolution of some of these issues in favor of the people who are suffering. This would include not only AIDS, but also other grave illnesses like cancer and multiple sclerosis. It's always the case that in war like this, episodes of heroism and rapid progress occur even in the face of disasters. In this war the people who are suffering most are also offering the most and making the profound changes that will benefit everybody.

"This is not just a call for expressing anger, but a call to organize behind dramatic change in the way that medical research is done, and organize behind a further dethroning of the cult of medicine. The medical authorities must also be asked to be responsible to the public that benefits from their efforts and also pays for their work. We're asking that these people acknowledge the fact that the consuming public does have the right to do this, even though they might not have the knowledge to make medical judgement. We don't want to condemn the sincerity of any individual's efforts to combat AIDS. What we're asking for is a two-way street."

SEROPOSITIVE CLINIC OPENS IN SAN FRANCISCO

(Editor's Note: "Positive Action Healthcare" discontinued its practice under that name in 1989, but Dr. Levin remains a practicing physician in San Francisco. To contact him, see his listing under "Levin, Alan, S." in Appendix B. We retain this article for the historical record.)

On January 1, Alan S. Levin, M.D., an immunologist in private practice in San Francisco, will open Positive Action Healthcare, one of the first outpatient clinics focused on treating healthy seropositive persons to attempt to prevent progression to AIDS or ARC.

Typical patients will be HIV-positive persons usually with some T-cell or other immunological deficiency, but either asymptomatic or only mildly ill. While Dr. Levin is willing to treat persons more seriously ill with AIDS or ARC, he believes that other physicians are better equipped to do so and will refer such patients to them.

Dr. Levin is best known for his work with "transfer factor"—a substance prepared from human white blood cells of healthy donors and used to confer certain immunities to patients. But he emphasizes that Positive Action Healthcare will not be a transfer-factor clinic.

Dr. Levin has developed a protocol for seropositive persons, including transfer factor, AZT, acyclovir, and intravenous gamma globulin. But he is willing to modify the protocol in cooperation with the patient, including using experimental treatments as they become available. For example, four patients are already using dextran sulfate.

The clinic will also publish a monthly newsletter for patients and others. And it will offer evening support groups, run by mental-health professionals.

And Positive Action Healthcare has hired an attorney who is also a physician, to go after insurance companies which try to evade reimbursing patients. This service will be available at no cost to the patient.

Comments

This writer cannot evaluate the medical merits of the treatment protocol planned for Positive Action Healthcare; readers may want to discuss it with a physician they trust. But we believe that this clinic can contribute toward a national model for care of seroposi-tive persons, in several ways:

• Willingness to treat healthy seropositive persons with both conventional and experimental treatments—and to be public about it.

Official FDA guidelines do not recommend any treatment for seropositive but healthy persons. Yet current information indicates that without treatment, over 70 percent of these people will eventually become ill with AIDS or ARC. And many physicians strongly suspect that treatments given early are both safer and more effective than if they are delayed until after serious illness develops.

But there is no proof that any specific treatment will help prevent progression to AIDS or ARC. The disease progresses so slowly that it will take years to run the trials to get such proof. And the medical profession has developed a cautious approach—which usually served well before AIDS—of strongly preferring in theory at least to use only procedures which have been tested and proven to work. Physicians are reluctant to recommend treatments based only on the best possible inferences from available information, when there has never been an actual test to show that the treatment works in fact, not only in theory. And here the tests will take years, time the patients don't have.

The result of this situation is that many leading physicians provide very different treatment to their own patients than they are willing to recommend publicly. (For an overview of some of the issues involved, see the page-one story in the *New York Times*, "Doctors Stretching Rules on AIDS Drug," December 21, 1987.) The big problem we see with this situation, one not discussed in the *Times* article, is the lack of development of a professional consensus because leading physicians are reluctant or unwilling to give their colleagues in public the benefit of the same best judgment they give their patients in private. As a result, most patients end up getting treatment by the book which is in fact second-rate care.

By being open and high-profile about what it is doing, even to the point of working with a public relations firm and planning a press conference later in January, Positive Action Healthcare may help to bring the huge but largely silent issue of treatment for seropositive persons to the much-needed forefront of national attention.

• Willingness of leading non-gay physicians to get involved in AIDS. A tiny minority of physicians now treat most of the patients with AIDS or ARC. Unwillingness of many physicians to treat persons with AIDS threatens to become a serious problem. Dr. Levin already has an allergy practice of about a thousand patients; he could easily have chosen to stay away from AIDS. But he has excellent qualifications to get involved.

Dr. Levin has been an M.D. for over 20 years and is board certified in both immunology and pathology. He has published dozens of articles in major medical and scientific journals. In addition to private practice he has academic experience, and is currently Adjunct Associate Professor of Immunology at the University of California, San Francisco Medical Center.

Dr. Levin has little experience in treating AIDS or ARC; that is why he refers the more seriously ill patients elsewhere. But no one has much experience in treating healthy seropositive persons to prevent progression of the illness—especially since it is too early to see much of the results of such treatment—and here Dr. Levin's academic and research background stands out.

Incidentally Dr. Levin's wife, Vera Byers, M.D., an immunologist who also has a Ph.D., has also published dozens of medical and scientific articles on immunology.

Dr. Levin's resume also includes a paragraph-long listing of military honors, awarded during his service as a flight surgeon in Vietnam. In recent years he has been a leading witness in the lawsuit by Vietnam veterans seeking government assistance and compensation for injuries suffered from exposure to Agent Orange, a chemical defoliant used by the U.S. military during the Vietnam War.

• A collaborative relationship with patients. Dr. Levin is willing to work with patients to devise an individual program which they want to pursue, which may include experimental treatments.

We talked to one patient on another matter and found that he is very happy with Dr. Levin. John Athey of San Francisco, a long-time survivor who was diagnosed in January 1984 and who is active in helping other persons with AIDS, has been a patient of Dr. Levin since September 1984. He liked the reassurance that if one treatment didn't work it wasn't the end, there were others to try.

"Dr. Levin said, 'Don't worry, John, we'll keep you alive until they find a cure. And by we I mean you and I working together.'

"If you go in and you have questions, he'll take time, he'll answer them, he'll write all over the table, he'll get books out and pile books up on the examining table, he's just incredible. I'll ask a question and he'll say, 'Well, here's how it works,' and he writes all over, and he gets out books, and he hands me articles and I give him articles.

"He really cares, he listens, he gets excited, and he fights."

• Openness to community input and cooperation. One of the partners in Positive Action Healthcare is Fred Ponder, a patient of Dr. Levin, who works professionally doing business development projects. Mr. Ponder has been active for years in the

National Gay Rights Advocates, and is currently chairman of the board. Recently he also joined the board of Project Inform.

The third partner in Positive Action Healthcare is Richard White, the chief operations officer. He is the one whom persons are most likely to talk to first when they call the clinic for information.

Incidentally, fees are comparable to those of other physicians. For example, the initial visit includes a two-hour physical and costs $225; the routine monthly followup is $60. Transfer factor is expensive, costing $170 every two weeks for an injection. AZT will of course be the major cost when it is used.

The good news on costs is that Positive Action Healthcare plans to go to great lengths to help patients obtain reimbursement for their treatment from their insurance.

• Prompt reporting of usable results. Dr. Levin is now treating 20 HIV-positive patients. He plans to publish frequently, and also report informally in the clinic's newsletter to patients. He made available to this writer T-cell statistics of the ten patients treated long enough for data to be obtained.

These results so far, of five patients who started treatment in 1987 and five who started in earlier years, are interesting but not spectacular. Overall, helper T-cells increased in three of these ten, and decreased in seven. Seven of the ten are using transfer factor and had before and after T-helper values; of these seven, the counts increased after transfer factor in four and declined in three. None of the 20 patients has progressed to AIDS or ARC.

These early tabulations do not prove anything. But we are impressed that Dr. Levin is willing to put them on the table, letting outsiders see raw data immediately, both good results and otherwise. Unfortunately most physicians do not collect or report data suitable for research; and most research projects take years from conception through proposal, funding, running the trial, analysis, and final publication of edited results. By contrast, Positive Action Healthcare plans monthly or even biweekly reporting of raw data, organized in a way which makes outside analysis possible.

No one knows for sure what treatments may slow or prevent progression from seropositive status to AIDS or ARC. What interests us about Positive Action Heathcare is not any specific treatments—physicians must evaluate those—but the contribution toward an open, community-based model of treatment and research which may greatly speed the process of finding out what works.

For More Information

For more information about Dr. Levin's work, contact him at his San Francisco office (see Appendix B).

CORRECTION: PAYING FOR AZT

A note in our last issue on a Federal program to help persons pay for AZT erroneously stated that the only medical qualification required was a valid prescription from one's doctor. The correct information is that persons will have to meet the FDA guidelines for use of AZT, which generally means either having had pneumocystis, or having T-helper cells under 200 and having ARC symptoms.

The person who brought the story to our attention had heard the wrong information from a California state office; he was the first of several to inform us of the correction. We have heard that the confusion resulted from the fact that the Federal law itself does not require the FDA guidelines. But states have the right to insist on them, and they will do so in order to protect themselves from possible lawsuits.

For an overview on the different medical practices on the use of AZT, see "Doctors Stretching Rules on AIDS Drug," *New York Times* (December 21, 1987), p. 1.

Issue Number 48
January 15, 1988

DHEA: MYSTERY AIDS TREATMENT

DHEA, a hormone already present in the human body and related to the male hormone testosterone, has been tested secretly for several months with a few AIDS patients in Paris. Word of the study leaked out; but those who know the most are not talking, and an aura of intrigue and confusion surrounds the research. No other reporting in *AIDS Treatment News* has presented more ethical ambiguities and difficulties than DHEA.

On the plus side, the few persons with AIDS who have used DHEA are happy with it, and there is some scientific basis to believe the treatment might be helpful. In addition, recent epidemiological statistics showing much worse survival rates for women than men after an AIDS diagnosis—apparently because of hormonal differences between the sexes—suggests that DHEA may be a new class of treatment, working by means now unknown. If so, it could open doors to important advances in treatment development.

On the down side, only a few AIDS patients have used the drug; we have only partial, sketchy information from the Paris trial. So there is no proof that DHEA is helpful. And while experts consider the substance safe for short-term use, long-term effects are unknown, and they could possibly include increased risk of certain cancers. The treatment for AIDS requires large doses for long periods of time.

DHEA is a prescription drug in some countries, including Canada. In the U.S., it used to be sold by health-food distributors as an aid in losing weight, but the FDA forced the vendors to remove it from the market. (In a press release dated April 9, 1985, the agency said, "FDA has few adverse reaction reports on the drug, but said the risks from long-term use are unknown.") Today DHEA is widely used in research and is available through chemical supply channels; there are also natural sources. While individuals cannot readily purchase DHEA in the U.S. at least, it is clear that the AIDS community could obtain supplies if it wants to.

For the community, the bottom line on DHEA does seem clear. It would be a mistake to ignore this treatment possibility and just walk away. And it would also be foolish to rush into it.

For several weeks we have gathered information about DHEA. Many of our sources spoke off the record and cannot be named. This article presents what we have learned so far.

What Is DHEA?

DHEA, or dehydroepiandrosterone, is a steroid secreted by the adrenal gland and excreted in large amounts in the urine. The substance is well known to science—over four thousand published scientific or medical papers refer to it in some way—but no one clearly understands its role in the body.

DHEA can be taken by mouth, and researchers are investigating it as a possible treatment for aplastic anemia, diabetes, and breast cancer in women. Animal studies have found that DHEA prevents obesity in breeds which are normally fat. It also seems to extend the lifespan of animals.

Relatively few studies of human use have been published. Experts agree that DHEA seems safe for men, although women may have troublesome side effects from large doses. Results of long-term use are unknown. The drug has weak testosterone-like effects, and may have the same risks as testosterone.

DHEA seems to have gone through something of a "miracle-drug" phase several years ago (Kent, 1982); also there has been much excitement among some scientists (Kahn, 1985). Most of the published studies of human use in clinical trials came out several years ago, however, and this published record presents a confusing picture of scattered, miscellaneous attempts to treat various obscure diseases, with mixed results.

Now there has been a sudden burst of excitement about DHEA as a possible AIDS treatment, among the few persons so far who know about the small clinical trial in France. We looked behind this excitement to find solid evidence on which it is based, and we could find only a little at this time. The drug does seem to be helpful to some people. And there may be more to it than meets the eye.

The Paris Study—And Controversy

A small research project in Paris has tested DHEA for several months with at least ten subjects, including five Americans. We have spoken with four of them, including one whom this writer knew personally before he became involved in the study. These four were able to tell us about the results with six of the people in the trial; we have heard nothing about the other four or more subjects.

Much intrigue has surrounded this research, and what you hear depends on whom you talk to. Those involved do seem to agree:

•   That the two principals currently working with DHEA as a possible AIDS treatment, Irish microbiologist Patrick Prendergast and the Irish company Elan Corp., appear to be fighting over the direction of the project.

•   That Prendergast both initiated and financed the research, then went to Elan to negotiate an agreement for them to distribute the drug.

Beyond this, viewpoints vary greatly. At least some of subjects in the Paris trial, who talk mainly to Prendergast, believe that he wants to move quickly to get the benefits of DHEA out to people with AIDS, whereas Elan wants to conceal the discovery until it can create a variation of the drug which is patentable and could have commercial value. (DHEA itself is already in common use and therefore largely unpatentable.) Elan has allegedly obtained a court order forbidding Prendergast from speaking with anyone about the matter—even with the subjects using the drug in Paris.

Prendergast himself did not return our calls. He would have been legally forbidden to do so.

We did speak to J.G. Masterson, M.D., the President and Chief Operations Officer of Elan Corporation. He said that Elan had licensed EL-10 (Elan's code name for the project) from Prendergast, and that the substance was in laboratory investigation in the United States. He said no controlled clinical trials had been done to date, there was no scientific evidence of efficacy, and that this was an extremely sensitive subject and it was premature to talk about it at all.

Dr. Masterson said that Elan's goal was to speed orderly, non-sensational, scientifically acceptable development if the product had any merit. But he was going to the Irish High Court today (January 11) and therefore it would be inappropriate to talk to a newspaper. He said that there was no scientifically acceptable clinical evidence (of efficacy of the drug), and that as soon as they had that, we would be the first to know.

Asked about the Paris study, Masterson suggested I talk to Prendergast; he said that Elan was not conducting any clinical trial. He asked how I knew about the matter, and especially wanted to know how I knew about the existence of a legal dispute.

We did not think to ask why Elan would license a drug without credible evidence of efficacy.

Complicating the picture is the fact that Elan's stock suffered greatly during the October crash. A public run on this stock, of the sort which has often occurred on rumors of hot AIDS developments, could be worth tens of millions if not hundreds of millions of dollars to the stockholders.

For additional information on the politics surrounding this trial, see Keith Griffith's article, "New Hope and New Intrigue: Top Secret AIDS Study," published last week by *AIDS Action Call* (Griffith, 1988).

Paris Study Results: What We Know

All four of the people we spoke to who were using DHEA in the small trial in Paris were convinced that the drug had been helpful to them and to everyone else in the study.

Of six persons in that DHEA study on whom we can find any information, at least five have AIDS. All were healthy enough before using DHEA to travel to Paris and live there in a hotel during the trial. Here is what we have learned about their response to the treatment:

• One has had T-helper cells improve from 248 to 641; his KS lesions seem to be lightening, although some new lesions have appeared.

• Another has had only slight improvement in T-helper cells, which are still under 100, but his other blood values which had been somewhat low have all improved and moved into the normal range. All of his fungal infections have cleared up, as has his leukoplakia. Besides the DHEA, he no longer needs to take any medications whatever for these infections, nor follow dietary restrictions to avoid thrush.

- Another had T-cells go up significantly, from under 300 (with a low of 186) to 560. His fungal problems diminished.

- Another who had had pneumocystis but was overweight at the start of the study has lost the unwanted weight, and has far more energy now.

- The fifth person started doing very well, but was depressed and decided to leave the study. We don't know how he has done since.

- The sixth had not seemed to be doing well, but then he improved dramatically after receiving a transfusion of platelets—so dramatically that the investigators want to give platelets to another subject also, to see if there is a synergistic effect.

Most or all of the six men were fairly healthy when they started the trial. They used large doses, always by mouth, up to 500 mg per day (100 mg five times a day, preferably taken just before a meal). They started with smaller doses, 200 to 300 mg per day, and increased the amount gradually; at least one person increased the dose by 100 mg each week until the 500 mg maximum dose was reached.

At least one patient also tried another treatment, DNCB, which may have contributed to his improvement.

Asked how long a person should try DHEA to see if it was working for them, one patient suggested three months. Presumably there should be unmistakable improvement in that time if the treatment is working.

This is all we know about the results of using DHEA with AIDS, ARC, or any HIV-related condition.

An Expert Evaluation

One physician who is very experienced with AIDS spoke with us off the record. He also talked to three scientists who are experts on DHEA, and with one of the patients in Paris, to help us put this information into better perspective. Here is our summary of his report:

Possible Scientific Basis. DHEA has protected rats against the immune-suppressing effects of severe stress (Kahn, 1985, p. 258). The stressed rats without the drug showed severe immune depression, atrophy of the thymus, marked reduction in lymphocytes, and increased disease and death. DHEA protected the animals against this outcome. How it did so is not clear.

Another possible mechanism might account for benefit from the drug for persons with AIDS or ARC. DHEA stimulates the bone marrow and increases production of all bone-marrow elements, including red cells, platelets, monocytes, macrophages, and lymphocytes. Apparently it acts on the stem cells themselves, before they are infected by HIV, and therefore it should be safer than some of the colony-stimulating factors, which some researchers fear might stimulate growth of the virus.

Even though T-helper cells are most impaired in AIDS and ARC, other blood elements are likely to be low, too. For example, a healthy seropositive person may be about 20 percent low on hemoglobin, platelets, and white count, and 60 to 80 percent low in T-helper cells. DHEA may help by bringing all the blood elements up toward the normal range.

Safety. All three experts agreed that short-term use at least was very safe for men. But women could have masculinizing side effects comparable to those of testosterone, such as loss of menstrual period, changing of the voice, and growth of facial hair. Women who choose to use DHEA should be counseled about these possible problems.

Little is known about risks of long-term use; people have not used DHEA long enough. There is a theoretical risk that it could increase the danger of prostate cancer. Also, one breed of rats developed pituitary tumors after extended use of DHEA. (Many animals seem to have benefitted from long-term use, however, living longer and in better health than normal untreated animals.) Another theoretical risk should be considered. DHEA is effective against obesity because it causes more of the digested carbohydrates to be used for immediate energy, and less to be used to provide building blocks of fats and proteins. Therefore DHEA might make it harder to gain weight, which some persons with AIDS need to do. No one had this problem in the Paris study, but as far as we know nobody was underweight to begin with.

Another physician suggested testing liver function as a precaution when using DHEA, because the drug is processed by the liver.

Form and Method of Intake. The experts said plain DHEA would be absorbed better by the body than DHEA sulfate or other variants of the chemical. (Incidentally, we do know that the Paris study used DHEA itself, not the sulfate form or any other variant.)

Two of the three experts suggested taking DHEA rectally. They felt that taking it by mouth would be unreliable, since the circulating blood goes directly from the stomach to the liver, which destroys most of the drug.

Another physician feared that rectal use might be dangerous, however, since it bypasses many of the body's defenses, and there seems to be no human experience using DHEA this way. This physician, who has used DHEA in smaller amounts for other conditions, suggested staying with the oral administration which was tested in Paris, even though it is not an efficient way to administer the drug.

Physician's Overall Evaluation. The physician we interviewed sees DHEA as having relatively little toxicity. But he also notes that we have little hard evidence for its effectiveness for AIDS or ARC at this time. We only have anecdotal stories of a handful of patients who improved. He believes that DHEA might have value, but does not want hundreds of people to start using it on the basis of the little evidence we have now.

Miscellaneous

• A recent study found that AIDS seems to be worse in women than in men; women in several cities had a much shorter survival time after diagnosis, for reasons that do not seem explainable by differences in quality of care. Biochemical differences between the sexes seem to be responsible. (For more information see *New York Times,* October 18, 1987.)

DHEA is related to the male hormone testosterone. A common mechanism may explain its action and also the different survival times for men and women. If so, DHEA may open the door to a whole new approach to the treatment of AIDS and related conditions.

• There are reasons to suspect that the DHEA normally present in the body may be abnormally low in persons with AIDS. If so, use of DHEA may help by replacing the levels which should be there. It is easy to measure DHEA concentrations; apparently no one has done so in persons with AIDS or ARC because scientists did not suspect that DHEA had any relationship to this disease until now.

• DHEA may have a direct antiviral effect. In the Paris study, researchers expected that there would be an initial drop in T-helper cells as the DHEA caused the killing of infected cells. They did find a large drop immediately in most of the patients— although not in one person who started with a very low T-helper count.

The researchers also hope that DHEA can attack HIV infection in the macrophages, an important reservoir of HIV infection in the body. At this time we have no evidence to either support or contradict this theory.

At least two leading U.S. research centers are doing laboratory tests in conjunction with the Paris DHEA study. Apparently the researchers cannot talk, but we have learned that one found some antiviral effect but nothing spectacular in laboratory tests.

• In the Paris study, improvement was often gradual. For example, the person who went from a low of 186 to over 500 T-helper cells had been taking DHEA for five months, and described his improvement as very slow. T-helper cell counts kept fluctuating, but both the low and the high values kept improving.

• The people in the Paris study were fairly healthy to start with, even though almost all of them had AIDS. Apparently no one has yet tried DHEA when they were acutely ill.

• DHEA has two different names in common use: "dehydroepiandrosterone" and "dehydroisoandrosterone." These are two different names for the same chemical. The latter name is used more often in Europe.

Availability

DHEA cannot be sold as a drug in the United States. Chemical supply houses do carry it, but they are unlikely to sell to individuals without the credentials to convince them that the material will be used only for research and not for human use.

The wholesale chemical cost for the largest dose (500 mg per day) can be as low as 50 cents a day. Retail prices may be much higher.

DHEA is available by prescription in Canada, and it is also used as a drug in Italy. It is used all over the world and presumably is readily available in many countries, sold either as a drug and/or in quantity as a chemical. But we do not know which countries at this time.

Alan S. Levin, M.D., a San Francisco immunologist who has previously prescribed DHEA for other purposes, is considering setting up a small study of its use with AIDS and ARC. (See our article about Dr. Levin in *AIDS Treatment News,* Issue Number 47.) Clearly the AIDS/ARC community will be able to obtain DHEA if it wants to;

some are already taking steps to do so. But since this drug may not be harmless, and hard evidence of effectiveness is thin at this time, it may be best to wait and see what the pioneers report, rather than rushing too quickly into widespread use.

REFERENCES

Griffith, Keith, "New Hope and New Intrigue: Top Secret AIDS Study," *AIDS Action Call* (January, 1988). (*AIDS Action Call* is the newsletter of AIDS Action Pledge. For a copy, call them (see Appendix B), or send a self-addressed stamped envelope to them (see Appendix B).

Kahn, Carol, *Beyond the Helix: DNA and the Quest for Longevity* (New York: Times Books, 1985).

Kent, Saul,"DHEA: 'Miracle' Drug?," *Geriatrics* 37(9) (September 1982), p.157.

NEW TREATMENT APPROVED FOR ITP— ALSO USED FOR KS

The FDA has recently approved the marketing of a device for filtering the blood and removing unwanted antibodies in the treatment of ITP. The same treatment may also help for KS and possibly other AIDS-related conditions, but these uses have not been approved at this time.

The device, called the Prosorba Column, uses a disposable filter to treat the blood outside the body. Blood is removed, treated, and put back. In a study done by the manufacturer, persons with ITP received four to eight treatments over a four to six week period. Fifty-five percent showed a significant rise in platelets; most maintained the benefit over an average followup period of eight months.

In addition, 17 patients with KS who were HIV positive were treated as part of a larger study of persons with cancer, and their progress was rated in the standard categories used in evaluating cancer therapy. Six showed a "partial regression," meaning at least a fifty percent reduction of tumor size for at least 30 days. Two showed "less than partial regression," a 25 to 50 percent reduction. Eight showed "stabilization," meaning less than 25 percent increase or decrease. Only one continued with progressive disease. We do not know the condition of these patients before the therapy, nor what outcome would be expected in the absence of treatment.

About half those treated had some side effects, usually chills and fever—effects expected with any blood-handling procedure.

Unfortunately the treatment is expensive, since each filter can only be used once and costs $650—meaning that the complete course of treatment costs several thousand dollars. But since it is approved by the FDA, insurance may pay for it.

Unfortunately also, the approval of the Prosorba Column does not show that the FDA has streamlined its approval process for drugs for serious or life-threatening conditions. This treatment obtained approval as a device—much easier to get than approval for a new drug.

(Incidentally, we have learned that as of today, six months after the publication of the FDA's new "treatment IND" rules which are supposed to allow easier access to experimental drugs before full approval for persons with serious or life-threatening illness, not a single person has received a single drug for any AIDS-related condition under these rules.)

For more information about the Prosorba Column, physicians or patients can call customer service at IMRE Corporation in Seattle, Washington (see Appendix B). The company cannot refer patients to physicians, but it can refer physicians to other physicians who are experienced with this treatment.

The *Wall Street Journal* ran an informative article on December 28, 1987.

PROTEST MARCH ON BURROUGHS-WELLCOME

The AIDS Action Pledge, a new political group in San Francisco, will hold a protest march on January 24 from San Francisco to the Burroughs-Wellcome western regional office in Burlingame, a nearby suburb. On January 25 there will be a rally and civil disobedience at the Burroughs-Wellcome site.

According to a statement from the organization, "The AIDS Action Pledge is demanding accountability from Burroughs-Wellcome about the prohibitive cost of AZT, whether people have been misled about the drug's effectiveness, and evidence that some important research has been blocked into possible treatments that could compete with AZT."

IN MEMORIAM: TOM JEFFERSON

(The following note was written by Martin Delaney, co-founder of Project Inform and a long-time colleague and friend of Tom.)

Tom Jefferson, one of the founders of the alternative treatments movement, passed away on Saturday, December 26. Since 1983, Tom had devoted his life to helping make HIV infection a manageable, chronic illness. In the early years of the epidemic, Tom served as the Special Projects Coordinator at the San Diego AIDS Project. After developing serious complications of HIV in 1984, including lymphoma, Tom made a remarkable recovery treating himself with unapproved drugs. He became a pioneer in the use of combined anti-viral and immune boosting therapy and shared his knowledge with countless others who passed through San Diego seeking treatments across the Mexican border. Through his role as a media spokesman, Tom became a symbol of hope for people across the country. The key players in nearly every AIDS organization and healing group came to know and respect him. Many believe that the guidance he extended them helped save their lives. In 1986, Tom joined Project Inform to set up its hotline service and help the group grow from a small local organization into a national resource serving thousands of callers each month.

After returning to San Diego in last October, Tom sought access to aerosol pentamidine as a preventative against pneumocystis. Researchers at the San Diego ATEU, however, were skeptical of the San Francisco studies and offered no help. Later, Tom was refused access to the treatment by the San Diego Veterans Administration Hospital—despite the fact that other VA hospitals were already using it. While he continued to struggle with VA bureaucracy, researchers at the ATEU put

Tom on fansidar, reportedly without warning him of the potential consequences described in a recent column in *AIDS Treatment News*. In less than a week, Tom came down with the dreaded fansidar side effect called Stevens-Johnsons disease. Over the next two weeks, this led to treatment with massive doses of Prednisone, which shut the rash down, and his entire immune system along with it. A few days after beginning with the Prednisone, Tom came down with pneumonia, in particular Legionnaire's disease. His physician believed that the organism wouldn't have affected him at all if he had not been on the Prednisone. He was placed on a respirator for about a week. When he came off life support, still in a very serious condition, Tom was too tired to go on fighting the bureaucracy and the arrogance of competing researchers, and instead chose to go home for Christmas with his loved ones. He knew well the consequences of his decision, and yet reveled in that fact that what would happen would be his own choice—not someone else's. Completely at peace with his decision, and satisfied with what he had accomplished in the last years of his life, Tom enjoyed Christmas at home and passed away quietly with a smile on his face on Saturday, the 26th.

It is a great irony that after successfully managing his own illness, Tom finally succumbed not to HIV, but to complications of treatment with a drug he was forced to use against his will. In his final days, it became very important to Tom that people understand how he died, lest his death be seen as a statement of hopelessness about treatment and the values he believed in. Unfortunately, mainstream press reports have condescendingly reported his death as evidence of the terrible and all-powerful grip of AIDS. The real story of his death is one of bureaucratic obstinance and competitive behavior between researchers.

His death raises questions our community must face, perhaps as Tom's final legacy. First, why is this barbaric drug, fansidar, still being used in some parts of the country? Project Inform has now received 3 reports of death from the drug in the last 3 months. Fansidar's potential for deadly side effects is well documented in healthy people. Yet, it is given to gay men with deeply compromised health— despite the availability of better and safer treatments. There is no justification for continued use of fansidar. Will it take a malpractice suit before the message is heard throughout the country?

A second issue raised is the quality of care in the VA system. Tom's experience is hardly unique, as he and others had already been contemplating complaining to Congress about the poor quality of care being given to AIDS patients by the VA.

Finally, Tom's experience can't help but make us wonder how many of our brothers' deaths, attributed to HIV, really occurred when a patient was caught in a whirlpool of causes and effects set off by one false move, one bureaucratic stall, one act of ego or medical arrogance? How much does the life expectancy of AIDS patients depend upon on where and from whom they are getting their treatment?

In Tom's memory, let's stop the use of fansidar. And let's begin to report on the stories of others who may have died unnecessarily, whose deaths are being swept under the rug of AIDS.

Tom asked that donations be made in his name to Project Inform, where a special account has been set up in his name. Its funds will be used to promote the causes which mattered most dearly to this brave and giving man.

Issue Number 49
January 28, 1988

CRYPTOSPORIDIOSIS, AND TREATMENT LEADS: PRELIMINARY REPORT

Cryptosporidiosis is a serious, sometimes fatal opportunistic infection which causes severe diarrhea. Persons with a normal immune system can get the disease, which seems to be responsible for many cases of ordinary diarrhea, but they recover in a few days or at most about two weeks. Persons with a serious immune deficiency may not recover, however; and at least 20 drugs expected to be effective against this organism have been tried but they largely failed to work. No one knows why the parasite which causes the illness is so resistant to available antibiotics.

Some people with AIDS do recover spontaneously from cryptosporidiosis, however, and at least one drug does seem to cure or control the disease in some people.

This article cannot offer a complete or authoritative coverage of cryptosporidiosis. Instead, we called physicians, alternative practitioners, and persons with AIDS, to collect leads about treatments they may have found helpful or have reason to believe might offer promise. We didn't find confirmed cures, of course, but several treatments are clearly worth more investigation. These are listed after the "background" section below.

Readers should be warned that we have not been able to check out these treatments—their dangers or supporting evidence—as much as we usually do. The leads presented here are only options to consider and explore with one's physician. We hope this article will help researchers by highlighting a wide range of treatment options worthy of investigation.

Background

An authoritative review of the published literature, covering what was known about cryptosporidiosis as of July 1987, appears in "Cryptosporidiosis: Overview, Epidemiology, Microbiology and Pathogenesis," by Constance Wofsy, M.D. This article was published on AIDS Knowledge Base, a computerized collection of AIDS articles written mainly for physicians. We summarize some of the information here; our comments are in parentheses:

• The organism cryptosporidium, a protozoan (single-cell animal), was first discovered in animals in 1907, and in humans in 1975. It is an intestinal parasite which later was found to cause many cases of ordinary diarrhea. (Presumably it has long been a common infection in humans, but was not recognized until recently because it was hard to diagnose.)

The organism is related to the protozoan which causes toxoplasmosis.

• Infection can be diagnosed by bowel biopsy, or by examination of stools, but special techniques must be used for the stool examination, since otherwise the protozoan looks like yeast and can easily be missed.

• The disease can spread from person to person or from animals to persons, probably by feces to mouth transmission. The incubation period is five to 14 days.

• Even in severe cases, cryptosporidiosis causes little structural damage to the intestines. This finding suggests that the organism may cause the diarrhea by secreting a toxin, as cholera does. (It also suggests that full recovery should be possible even after severe illness, if the organism could be eliminated or if the effect of the toxin could be blocked.)

• Cryptosporidiosis usually appears late in AIDS, but nevertheless it is now officially part of the definition of AIDS. About four percent of AIDS cases are diagnosed this way, with cryptosporidiosis as the presenting infection.

(The disease seems less common than we had feared. Many physicians and other practitioners we spoke to who treat AIDS patients had seen few or no cases.)

• Cryptosporidium can sometimes spread outside the digestive tract, to infect the gall bladder or respiratory system, but it has not been found to infect other organs.

• In an animal study, 25 drugs which were tried failed to treat cryptosporidiosis effectively. In humans only one drug, spiramycin, seemed to cure or control the disease in some cases.

Spiramycin, an antibiotic with little toxicity, is manufactured by Rhone Poulenc and used in Canada and Europe to treat a number of infections, including toxoplasmosis. In 1982, the U.S. Centers for Disease Control reported that the drug showed benefit in some cases of cryptosporidiosis. But today (over five years later) the drug is still available in the U.S. only for investigational use.

(Today at least one placebo-controlled trial is being conducted in the U.S., apparently required as part of the FDA approval process. Meanwhile we don't know how many U.S. patients are or are not able to get spiramycin when medically indicated.)

• Besides spiramycin, most medical treatment for cryptosporidiosis has been supportive, such as fluid and electrolyte replacement, antidiarrheals, and sometimes total parenteral nutrition (intravenous feeding) if the patient cannot absorb food.

Additional Background

We interviewed a gastroenterologist who has treated a number of cases of cryptosporidiosis, and he added the following information:

- The disease can vary greatly in severity. If the infection is in the lower bowel only, the persons can still absorb food. The disease is worse if it also affects the small intestines and the stomach.

- In some patients, as in persons with cholera, the intestines expel water, as if a pump were turned on by a biochemical switch. This mechanism apparently requires certain prostaglandins, and sometimes the switch can be turned off by drugs like indocin which inhibit prostaglandin synthesis. The patient still has the more usual diarrhea, however.

(Note: There are other indications that one kind of prostaglandin is involved in causing damage in AIDS. Some physicians have used nonsteroidal anti-inflammatory drugs like indocin to mitigate this damage, but word of this treatment possibility has not spread widely among physicians. Some non-prescription drugs such as ibuprofen or even ordinary aspirin might also have a similar beneficial effect, but prescription drugs seem to be preferred by knowledgeable physicians.)

- This physician thought that somatostatin might be a valuable treatment for controlling the diarrhea in some cases. However, it has not yet been tried for cryptosporidiosis.

Treatment Leads

We only have sketchy information about most of these treatment possibilities, and list them here as leads for further research. We arranged this list more or less in order starting with the more conventional—not necessarily more or less powerful, or better or worse. This list resulted from only a few days' research and is certainly incomplete. And we have largely omitted the many routine supportive therapies.

Spiramycin. See discussion above.

Hyperimmune Milk. This treatment, developed by Donald Kotler, M.D., of Columbia University St. Luke's/Roosevelt Hospital Center, extracts antibodies from milk of cows exposed to cryptosporidiosis. An ongoing study will need more volunteers; at this time, however, the project cannot get enough supplies of the milk extract. For information about the study, call Anita in Dr. Kotler's office (see "Kotler," Appendix B).

An Australian team is also studying this treatment, but for children with a congenital immune deficiency, not with AIDS.

Trimetrexate with Leucovorin. This new treatment for pneumocystis looks very good theoretically. But we do not know of any human test for cryptosporidiosis at this time.

Trimetrexate, an experimental drug used in cancer treatment, is given in toxic doses for treating pneumocystis. Leucovorin is an antidote which rescues human cells from the trimetrexate. Protozoa cannot use the leucovorin, however, so the trimetrexate kills them without killing the human cells. Physicians are interested in trying the treatment for cryptosporidiosis, also caused by a protozoan.

As a pneumocystis treatment, trimetrexate with leucovorin has had very few side effects (Allegra *et al.*, 1987); it had to be discontinued in only one of 49 pneumocystis patients in this trial, reported last October in the *New England Journal of Medicine*. This therapy should be available for cases when other pneumocystis treatments do not work or cannot be used, as it was found to save the lives of over two-thirds of pneumocystis patients when standard drugs had failed. Laboratory studies have also suggested possible promise for toxoplasmosis.

We will continue to follow trimetrexate with leucovorin as a treatment for pneumocystis, and possibly for cryptosporidiosis and other protozoal diseases.

Bovine Transfer Factor. We don't have details of this research at this time.

AZT. There have been reports of cryptosporidiosis improving or clearing up entirely in some persons when they were treated with AZT. At this time we have little information. For one published report, see the letter in *American Journal of Medicine* (July 1987), p. 187.

Artemisia Annua. This herb, a close relative of wormwood, is used in China to treat malaria, and appears to be clearly effective against malaria which has become resistant to antibiotics. Malaria, like cryptosporidiosis, is caused by a protozoan.

We have heard a report that at least one U.S. physician has obtained Artemisia Annua from China and used it successfully to treat cryptosporidiosis, but we have not yet been able to contact anyone with first-hand experience.

Garlic. Garlic appears to have some effectiveness against many microorganisms. For example, it has been used in China to treat cryptococcal meningitis.

While this disease is apparently unrelated to cryptosporidiosis, this indication that an active ingredient in garlic crossed the blood-brain barrier led John Athey, a well-known person with AIDS in San Francisco, to try large amounts of garlic for controlling his toxoplasmosis. According to his report at a seminar organized by Tom O'Connor (the author of *Living With AIDS: Reaching Out*), a large amount of garlic has clearly worked every time for him—not to cure the disease, but to control it and stop the symptoms. Toxoplasmosis is caused by a protozoan related to the one which causes cryptosporidiosis.

However, we did not find anyone who had used garlic for cryptosporidiosis, or who knew anyone who had. And the gastroenterologist we interviewed (above) doubted that it would work.

Acidophilus. Acidophilus, commonly sold in health-food stores, consists of billions of living beneficial microorganisms which may help crowd out the disease-causing ones. There are great variations in types of acidophilus, and in the quality of the products. We heard good reports about the Jarro-Dophilus brand, and also about a brand from West Germany called Eugalan Forte.

Hydrogen Peroxide. We talked to one person who was convinced that drinking dilute hydrogen peroxide helped him recover from cryptosporidiosis; he was also using an aloe vera preparation and acidophilus. But there is much controversy about hydrogen peroxide. People disagree greatly about its possible benefits and dangers. We are looking for more information about this treatment, but don't have a clear picture at this time.

REFERENCES

Allegra, C.J. *et al.*, "Trimetrexate For the Treatment of Pneumocystis Carinii Pneumonia in Patients with the Acquired Immunodeficiency Syndrome," *New England Journal of Medicine* (October 15, 1987), pp. 978–85.

Horn, Bill, *Bibliography on AIDS and Nutrition, Gastrointestinal Tract Lesions, Physiology and Organ Function* (San Jose, CA: Nutrition Services).

Klayman, D.L., "Qinghaosu (Artemisinin): An Antimalarial Drug From China," *Science* (May 31, 1985), p. 1049–55.

Wofsy, C., "Cryptosporidiosis: Overview, Epidemiology, Microbiology and Pathogenesis," ON AIDS Knowledge Base computer system (Access through BRS Colleague; see Appendix B).

MORE SEMINARS BY TOM O'CONNOR

Tom O'Connor, author of the excellent book *Living With AIDS: Reaching Out* (available in most gay bookstores) is continuing his one-day seminars in San Francisco:

- February 20: Being Educated and in Control when Using Doctors and Hospitals
- February 27: Putting into Place Quickly All the Resources Available to Persons with Low Income
- March 5: Drugs, Nutrition, and Stress Reduction
- March 12: Nutrition and Supplements for Building the Immune System

TREATMENT ISSUES REVIEWS CARRISYN, DEXTRAN SULFATE

Treatment Issues, the Gay Men's Health Crisis newsletter of experimental AIDS therapies, reviewed both Carrisyn/aloe juice, and dextran sulfate, in its second issue, December 31, 1987. Both received very favorable reports.

Barry Gingell, M.D., the editor of *Treatment Issues,* has studied Carrisyn in depth during the last several months—including visiting physicians in Dallas and studying detailed medical records. Therefore we have waited for his article instead of writing our own. Now his report is available.

The same issue has a short but important writeup on dextran sulfate, one of the most promising antivirals being tested today. We will cover dextran sulfate in a future issue.

Both of these treatments are more or less available. The issue also has an update on Fusidin (fusidic acid), which does *not* look good at this time, although it has not been ruled out.

For more information, contact GMHC, Department of Medical Information (see Appendix B). GMHC distributes *Treatment Issues* at no charge; you can get on their mailing list for future issues.

AIDS ORGANIZATION AND HOTLINE DIRECTORY

KPIX Channel 5, which together with the *San Francisco Examiner* co-sponsored the unveiling of The Names Project quilt in San Francisco's Moscone Center, has published *AIDS Lifeline,* an excellent San Francisco/Northern California annotated directory "of organizations and agencies who use volunteers in their services to people with AIDS and their loved ones." Over 50 organizations are listed. To obtain a copy of this short directory, write or call KPIX Channel 5, Public Relations Department (see Appendix B) and ask for the *AIDS Lifeline Directory.*

An extensive national directory of hotlines and organizations listed by state was published in *Medical Times* (September 1987), pp. 91–98. And a list of PWA (People With AIDS) organizations is published by NAPWA (see Appendix B).

DHEA SAFETY NOTE

DHEA (covered in *AIDS Treatment News,* Issue Number 48) is sold by a number of suppliers all over the world. But some of these products are not intended for human use and may contain toxic hormones or other harmful byproducts of the manufacturing process.

The best way to assure that a product is safe is to use pharmaceutical grade, intended for human use. Other grades might be safe, but they might not be, and expert advice would be essential in determining their safety if pharmaceutical grade cannot be obtained.

Unfortunately there is no simple test to tell whether a given sample of DHEA is fit for human use. DHEA can be synthesized (or extracted from natural sources) in many different ways. A chemist testing a sample must know how that product was manufactured, in order to know what impurities to look for.

Issue Number 50
February 12, 1988

DEXTRAN SULFATE: NEW PROMISING ANTIVIRAL

DISCLAIMER: We interviewed several physicians in researching this article, but were unable to get them a draft copy to review before press time. Any mistakes are our responsibility, not theirs. We must also emphasize that information is changing rapidly and this article may soon become obsolete—and in any case cannot be relied on for medical advice.

Dextran sulfate, a drug used for 20 years in Japan and available there without a prescription, has become an important AIDS treatment possibility. While it is still too early to be sure the drug will be useful, preliminary experience is good and a number of people are already obtaining and using the substance, especially in Los Angeles, New York, and San Francisco.

Briefly the case for dextran sulfate is:

• In the laboratory it works about as well as AZT in inhibiting HIV, at concentrations which can be achieved in the blood by oral use, yet it has very little toxicity (Ueno and Kuno, June 1987).

In addition it seems to be synergistic with AZT; in the laboratory the combination works much better against the virus than either drug alone (Ueno and Kuno, June 1987; Ueno and Kuno, October 1987; disputed by Berenbaum, 1987).

Besides inhibiting reverse transcriptase, dextran sulfate blocks the formation of giant syncytial cells in the laboratory—important because healthy cells are trapped and destroyed when syncytial cells form. Dextran sulfate may be the first drug which can stop this cell-to-cell spread of the virus.

• Dextran sulfate is safe enough to be available without a prescription in Japan, where it is used for arteriosclerosis. Because of its 20-year history of human use, much safety information is known.

Persons with AIDS or ARC are using doses two to three times larger than commonly used in Japan; however these larger doses have been tested in humans without problems. Persons with AIDS or ARC can show unexpected toxicities to drugs; but so far over fifty persons have used dextran sulfate under the close observation of private-practice physicians we have contacted, apparently without any serious problems. A common side effect is loss of appetite and a feeling of fullness; occasionally there is a minor rash.

Even persons allergic to sulfa drugs can apparently use dextran sulfate (Gingell, 1987).

• Dextran sulfate is being studied by Donald Abrams, M.D. at San Francisco General Hospital—the only official trial anywhere of dextran sulfate for persons with AIDS or ARC—and recently was put in the highest priority category for research by NIH. Abrams' study has not reported on efficacy, as it is a "phase I" dosage and toxicity trial, but it has not had any safety problems yet, even at doses higher than people are using for AIDS or ARC.

• The limited, anecdotal information we have on use of dextran sulfate for AIDS or ARC looks very good at this time.

• The drug is taken by mouth, and is not expensive.

• It is more or less available today.

The case against dextran sulfate is:

• The fact that something works in the laboratory does not mean it works in humans.

• No formal clinical trial has yet been done to prove whether or not dextran sulfate works.

• We only have anecdotal information on a few people who have used the drug long enough to see results. The benefits found may have been coincidence; and even if they were real, they might not be lasting.

• We do know that dextran sulfate is not the whole answer or the answer for everybody. We know of one person who died of AIDS complications despite having used the treatment for several weeks at least.

AIDS/ARC Experience So Far

Michael J. Scolaro, M.D., a Los Angeles physician very experienced in treating AIDS and ARC, has been following over 30 patients who have obtained dextran sulfate. About 15 of them have used it for at least two months, long enough for results to be seen.

These patients have also used other antivirals, especially low-dose AZT, acyclovir, and AL 721 substitutes. None of the patients on dextran sulfate is using the full dose of AZT. A handful are using only dextran sulfate and acyclovir, because they cannot afford AL 721 and cannot tolerate AZT; they are also doing well.

Dr. Scolaro has found that at least 60 percent of the patients who have used dextran sulfate for at least two months have shown dramatic improvement in laboratory tests and clinical well being. Often T-helper cells have doubled, from 300 to 700 or more, from 400 or 450 to 900.

For patients with less than 100 T-helper cells, however, he has not seen increases in the numbers, so he counsels these persons not to look only at numbers but also look at clinical effectiveness. Are they feeling well, avoiding new opportunistic infections, and responding well to treatment for pre-existing ones?

Dr. Scolaro's first patient who used dextran sulfate, seen in August of 1987, "was literally preterminal, with advanced neuropathy, mycobacterium avium, CMV retinitis, and he was semicomatose." He was on a number of drugs, including large doses of acyclovir, glucocorticoids, and several anti-MAI treatments, but not including AZT. "He is now not only alive and walking and talking, he walks with a walker, he had almost a complete regression of his peripheral neuropathy, a magnificent return of cerebral function, has gained about 65 pounds." Dr. Scolaro explained that he could not necessarily attribute the improvement to dextran sulfate, but that he and another physician on the case were impressed and felt that this drug may have been the key element that made a difference, in combination with the other drugs.

Recently Dr. Scolaro had another case much like this one. But despite great improvement so far it is still too early to be sure the second person will survive.

Dr. Scolaro does not see dextran sulfate as proven. "It's exciting, I think it's promising, I think it's premature to be able to say that it's going to be the answer. I don't know that it works *in vivo* by itself; the *in vitro* studies showed that Ueno's compound did not suppress HIV by 100 percent; the exciting thing was the synergistic effect...

"I have to say that from my perspective and my observation now over the last four to five years, that I have not found a compound that seems to thus far be doing things so quickly. Not even AZT did that. I had very few patients who had a dramatic rise in T-4 counts. And even when there was a rise it was not sustained. In fairness to what we're doing now, I don't know that the rises in cell counts are going to be sustained with dextran."

We talked to Fred Ponder, a partner and business manager of Dr. Alan Levin's Positive Action Healthcare in San Francisco (see *AIDS Treatment News*, Issue Number 47); Mr. Ponder has computerized the patient data. About 20 patients at the clinic are using dextran sulfate now, five of them for two months. These five are also using transfer factor; four of them are asymptomatic seropositive, one has AIDS. Only one of the five is on AZT.

All five who have used dextran sulfate for at least two months have improved. One went from 500 T-helper cells and falling to over 800; he was negative for P-24 antigen all along. Another went negative on the P-24 antigen, after being a high positive for several months. Two others had improved T-cell counts. The person with AIDS went to over 400 T-helper cells for the first time in a year.

Another clinical researcher, however, failed to get results with dextran sulfate. He tested only three patients, one with ARC and two asymptomatic seropositive. He found no change in the P-24 antigen or in reverse transcriptase levels. But he used less than the usual dose—1600 mg per day vs. the more common 2100 mg for a person of average weight. And he had to stop the study after only a month, apparently because of pressure from his institution.

Our impression from interviews so far is that most of the people who are getting good results are using frequent doses of dextran sulfate—usually every four hours. Some do and some do not include the middle of the night dose. Almost all are combining dextran sulfate with other antivirals, especially acyclovir, and often low-dose AZT and/or AL 721 in addition.

Precautions and Safety

The usual anti-AIDS dose is two to three times higher than the standard clinical dose in Japan. But animal studies suggest that there is a large safety range, with the lethal dose over one hundred times the AIDS dose (see below). And long-term studies have found no harm in human use of the doses commonly used for AIDS (Gingell, 1987).

Dextran sulfate has an anticoagulant effect so theoretically it could cause bleeding problems; we have not heard of any problems, however, and some studies have failed to find any effect on coagulation. But to be safe, the literature for physicians recommends coagulation tests. (See other precautions below.) The clinical trial at San Francisco General Hospital requires subjects to have acceptable values on various blood, kidney, liver, and other tests, and to avoid aspirin during the trial, presumably to help guard against any bleeding problems. There are many exclusion criteria and restrictions; some may be for safety, others to make it easier to interpret the results of the trial.

An anonymous "underground" instruction sheet has the following safety section:

> Cautions/Side Effects: Before starting dextran sulfate, make sure from your doctor that your kidneys and platelets are okay. Otherwise there could be some very extreme problems with bleeding.
> There are two nuisance side effects which can occur with dextran sulfate. One is a mild loss of appetite, the other is mild diarrhea..."
> ("Dear Dextran User," unsigned.)

The section below entitled "Dextran Sulfate Information from the Japanese Equivalent of *Physician's Desk Reference*" (page 255) gives recommended safety precautions, but it was written for other uses, not treatment for AIDS or ARC.

Note that this article (including the section translated from the Japanese) does *not* contain complete safety precautions, nor instructions for use. The dextran sulfate situation is moving so rapidly that any detailed instructions could be obsolete very quickly. Instructions for use, including safety precautions, will continue to evolve as more information becomes available. Check with treatment organizations such as buyers' clubs or Project Inform (see Appendices B and C), or with any source from which you obtain dextran sulfate, to get the latest information. And let your physician know about any treatment you plan to use, in case he or she knows about any new dangers or precautions.

Availability

So far most people have obtained dextran sulfate by going to Japan, or knowing someone who lives there or travels there. But more convenient sources are developing.

The interest in this treatment is so new and growing so rapidly that we can give few specifics, as information changes as soon as it is written. To find out about getting dextran sulfate, we suggest the following:

• Your physician might be able to help—although few are familiar with dextran sulfate at this time.

• Check with friends, support groups, or buyers clubs.

• If you cannot find information locally, check with Project Inform in San Francisco (see Appendix B).

In Canada, dextran sulfate is available from Dextran Products Limited (a subsidiary of Polydex Pharmaceuticals), near Toronto. It is sold for investigational use. Persons must pick it up in Toronto, as the company cannot ship it to the U.S.; the minimum order is $500. For more information call George Usher or Mr. Patel at the Dextran Products Limited (see Appendix B).

Dextran sulfate may also be available from a Mexican company, Medicina Del Futuro (reference deleted by editor; no longer viable). It is our understanding that the company was unable to arrange purchase from Japan, and may have the product manufactured in Mexico instead.

Nutricology, Inc., of San Leandro, California may carry the Polydex product; for more information call them (see Appendix B).

Quality Control

There are many different forms of the chemical "dextran sulfate." The right kind has a molecular weight of 7000 to 8000 and a sulfur content of 17 to 20 percent (Ueno and Kuno, June 1987).

For use by mouth, dextran sulfate must be "enteric coated," prepared so that it will pass through the stomach and dissolve in the intestines, because the stomach acidity would destroy it. Most dextran sulfate for human use comes as coated tablets; but some has been enteric coated as individual granules, which can be placed in ordinary capsules for use.

Japan appears to be the only country where dextran sulfate has been used as a drug. Because it has been available there without a prescription for 20 years, companies have much experience in manufacturing it for human use. Fifteen different Japanese suppliers are listed below. As far as we know, all of them supply the right kind of dextran sulfate, with good quality control. So far, most people have been using the Kowa tablets.

The Canadian company has much experience in making dextran sulfate, but has not provided enteric coating until now. On the Mexican product, we do not yet have information on quality because we do not know who is doing the manufacturing.

All the knowledgeable people we have talked to trust the Japanese products. But most think there should be independent testing of any others before they come into widespread use. The HIV-positive buyers clubs have experience in testing other products, such as AL 721 substitutes, and some of them are investigating how to test dextran sulfate properly.

DEXTRAN SULFATE INFORMATION FROM THE JAPANESE EQUIVALENT OF *PHYSICIAN'S DESK REFERENCE*

(NOTE: We have translated the main points, not the full text. Our comments are in parentheses.)

Indication: Hyperlipidemia

Caution:

- While using, administer coagulation tests.
- Don't use on anyone with a tendency to hemorrhage.
- Don't use if severe renal problems.
- Note synergistic effect with mitomycin, a cancer drug.

Interactions with other drugs:

- Administer very carefully when other anticoagulants used.
- Note caution on mitomycin, above.

Side effects:

- Loss of appetite or feeling of bloating (most common side effect, found in 3.5 percent of patients in one study).
- Diarrhea.
- Occasional skin rash.
- In IV injections, dizziness can occur.
- In IV injections, shock can occur; stop therapy.

Dose (antilipemic) 450–900 mg per day in 3–4 doses.
(Note that HIV doses are higher, about 30 mg per kilogram per day—somewhat more than 2000 mg for a person of average weight.) The IV form is available from Kowa for when the oral form cannot be administered or is not effective.

Store at room temperature below 25 degrees C, in low humidity, away from light.

Actions:

- Antilipemic
- Anticoagulant
- Antiplatelet activity
- Effective for arteriosclerosis in humans

Toxicity tests:

- Lethal dose in animals, about 4300 mg/Kg—(about 140 times the AIDS/ARC dose).
- Long-term toxicity test in rats at 1019–1209 mg/Kg found higher rate of growths in mucosal lining of lower intestines and rectum than controls.

Absorption, distribution, and elimination:

- Short half life, 25 minutes when injected in marmots. (Presumably the medicine would last longer in oral use, due to time taken for absorption.)

- Studies with radioactive markers showed distribution primarily in the liver, lungs, bone marrow, muscles, and brain.

The Japanese PDR includes technical details on many of the points listed above.

Brand Names and Suppliers

The Kowa product comes in two forms: "MDS Kowa T" and "MDS Kowa A." The "T" form is correct; the "A" form (ampules prepared for intravenous use) has the wrong sulfur content, three to six percent.)

BRAND NAME	TABLET SIZE, mg	PHARMACEUTICAL COMPANY
Asuro	150	Nippon Kayaku
Emstlan	300	Towa Yakuhin
MDS	150, 300	Kowa
Colyonal	300	Mochida
Shanbird	150	Tsuruhara
Smedon	150	Meiji
DSS	150	Fujimoto
Dexpepe	150, 300	Toho
Dexul	150, 300	Sawai
Destromyde	150, 300	Kanebo
Tokistornin	150	Mekuto
Dolomezan	150, 300	Taiyo Yakuhin
Bicibon	150, 300	Toyama Kagaku
Maleton	150	Takeza
Ripoferol	300	Nichii

(Usually the brand name, above, appears once in Roman letters on the box or in the package insert which comes with it. The molecular weight and sulfur content should also be legible to those who do not read Japanese.)

ACKNOWLEDGEMENT: Jim Palazzolo, a professional Japanese translator in San Francisco, obtained the Japanese PDR section on dextran sulfate and translated this information for us.

REFERENCES

Berenbaum, Morris C., "Anti-HIV Synergy Between Dextran Sulphate and Zidovudine," *The Lancet* (August 22, 1987), p. 461.

Gingell, Barry, "Dextran Sulfate—an Exciting New Drug," *Treatment Issues* (GMHC) (December 31, 1987) p. 5.

Ito, M. *et al.*, "Inhibitory Effect of Dextran Sulfate and Heparin on the Replication of Human Immunodeficiency Virus (HIV) In Vitro, *Antiviral Research* (July 1987), pp. 361-7.

Ueno, R. and S. Kuno, "Dextran Sulphate, a Potent Anti-HIV Agent In Vitro Having Synergism With Zidovudine," *The Lancet* (June 13, 1987), p. 1379.

————, "Anti-HIV Synergism between Dextran Sulphate and Zidovudine," *The Lancet* (October 3, 1987), pp. 796–7.

For More Information

For an information sheet about dextran sulfate, persons can contact Project Inform (see Appendix B). Also, check with local buyers' clubs, such as Healing Alternatives Foundation in San Francisco (see Appendix B), or the PWA Health Group in New York (see Appendix B).

ERRONEOUS NEWS REPORT THAT KOOP BELIEVES THERE WILL NEVER BE A CURE

On January 27, U.S. Surgeon General C. Everett Koop was widely quoted as saying that he didn't believe a cure for AIDS would ever be found. Koop was speaking at a London conference of health officials from 148 nations.

We called Koop's office to find out what information that report was based on, and learned instead that the report was erroneous, that is not Koop's position. Koop meant to say that some people believe there would never be a cure because the HIV virus integrates itself into the genetic information of the cells it infects. But he himself remains optimistic, because there are ways to interfere with the activities of the virus.

Unfortunately the error went all over the world but correction received little publicity.

The day after the initial report, leading AIDS expert Robert Gallo, M.D. replied that no one could safely predict what would happen in the next five years. He added that he would not be working on the problem if he did not think it could be solved.

We could add that many scientists are working on the approach of killing the infected cells—probably by forcing the latent virus to express itself and then killing the cell when it does. The virus infects few cells at any one time, and the body could easily spare those. Many immunologists believe that full recovery would occur if the virus could be entirely stopped.

Even targeting the virus while it is latent in the DNA of the cell may not be forever impossible. A new technology called hybridons uses short, manufactured strands of DNA to attach to specific genes and block them. Hybridons have already shown partial success against the AIDS virus in laboratory tests (*Breakthrough* newsletter, published by Boardroom Reports, Boulder, Colorado, January 1987).

Although a complete cure seems far away at this time, it may instead be possible to control the disease indefinitely with continued treatment—keeping people alive and healthy throughout their normal lifespans or until a cure is found.

Issue Number 51
February 26, 1988

AIDS TREATMENT ACCESS: A WISH LIST, SOME PROBLEMS, AND RECOMMENDATIONS

Testimony of John S. James
Before the Presidential Commission on the HIV Epidemic New York City, New York, February 20, 1988

The biweekly newsletter *AIDS Treatment News* began as volunteer research and writing for an AIDS archiving organization in San Francisco. In little over a year it has grown to a circulation of over 3,500 almost entirely by word of mouth—an unexpected public response which illustrates the critical dearth of practical treatment information felt by patients and physicians alike. Researching treatment articles for *AIDS Treatment News* has provided an unusual opportunity to hear what this community would like to see happen, and where it sees the obstacles now.

People react to an AIDS diagnosis in different ways. Some resign themselves to dying and begin to prepare for death. Others ask their doctors to make the medical decisions for them, without their personal involvement. I do not have contact with these people and do not know what they feel about treatment research and access issues.

But very many persons with AIDS or other HIV infections choose to involve themselves in decisions about their health care. They often become experts in the disease and potential treatments.

And most of these people come to feel abandoned and betrayed by society. They believe that many physicians, researchers, and officials have been quick to write them off as already all but dead—despite all the unknowns about this disease which make it impossible for anyone to be sure that death is inevitable. The projected deaths of at least a quarter of a million Americans seem to have been accepted with surprising equanimity and surprisingly little sense of crisis or mobilization.

Oddly enough there seems to have been no professionally-conducted survey asking the persons most directly affected by AIDS what they thought about the issues

259

of treatment research and access now before this Commission. Certainly the people I know have never been asked how they see the situation, what problems they find in the institutional response to the epidemic, and what improvements they would suggest.

A Wish List

Since we have no scientific survey information on what people with AIDS would most like to see done, we did the next best thing and interviewed Nathaniel Pier M.D., a physician with a large AIDS practice in New York City. We have found his statements about what is needed to be as close as anyone's to the beliefs of the persons with AIDS with whom we have communicated while writing *AIDS Treatment News*.

Dr. Pier proposed above all "That anybody diagnosed with HIV-related disease or immunodeficiency be given a full assessment of their situation and be allowed to choose to receive a therapeutic regimen or decline it. Theoretically, all five hundred thousand persons infected in New York should be allowed access to some form of therapy if they wished. To satisfy scientific needs, they could be enrolled in formal protocols. Otherwise clinicians should be allowed to use empirical regimens, with patients properly monitored.

"This way everybody would be given the optimal chance to save their lives and nobody would be allowed to twist in the wind. Furthermore, we could look at the results—and get a sense of what works much more rapidly than under the current system.

"Persons could use single drug treatments, or rational combinations based on the best judgment of experienced physicians.

"What we propose here is what is already done with cancer patients. Almost no one diagnosed in the United States today with cancer is denied an opportunity to participate in potentially lifesaving therapy. There is in place a widely accepted system for providing these experimental and established therapies to cancer patients. This system advances our knowledge of the treatments for this disease but is also a humane and compassionate way of caring for patients.

"To the argument that there are no AIDS treatments except AZT because no others have proven effective, we would answer that we are currently capable of choosing safe, rational approaches to therapies. In addition, people are using therapies anyway. Our proposal would allow them to do so under supervision, so this can be done safely and the data developed can be critically evaluated and thereby be helpful to others instead of remaining anecdotal."

Some Problems

"It is clear that the best hope for people with immune deficiency or at risk for the illness is the rapid development and dissemination of safe and effective therapies. Until this goal is achieved, the most humane approach to dealing with AIDS and AIDS-related problems is to give people access to supervised therapeutic protocols. The main problem, therefore, is to develop such a system—a system that would allow rigorous scientific analysis of therapies and still incorporate anyone wishing to try to help themselves with experimental therapies.

"The present system for developing AIDS therapies has been painfully slow in starting. Access is so severely limited that the majority of people affected by this disorder are left without intelligent recourse.

"In addition it is unclear where the leadership for determining priorities in therapy development is coming from. It is also unclear how the decisions for prioritizing the various therapeutic approaches are being made. For people with AIDS it is unclear who is setting the timetable and who is supervising the large-scale effort to develop therapies.

"For the individual who must make decisions there is no centralized method of gaining access to the information that will allow him or her to choose the best course of action.

"How does the present system work? As an example, we submit correspondence relating to a potential therapy for AIDS which first was recognized in 1984. In spite of prominent AIDS researchers acknowledging the potential benefit of this therapy, no clinical trials on humans with HIV infection have been initiated since then. In addition, you will see that letters to the people vested with protecting the public health have gone ignored and unanswered. This has left the impression that they are inefficiently and callously dealing with this very important issue. We do not believe that this is truly the case. Nevertheless the letters have gone unanswered and the trials have not materialized."

Other Concerns

Lentinan. Dr. Pier's statement above concerns his two-year attempt to get this drug considered. We should point out that lentinan has long been used for cancer treatment in Japan, with complete safety. And a letter to *The Lancet* (October 20, 1984), signed by seven scientists including Robert Gallo M.D. describes its use in the successful treatment of two patients with retroviral infections (one with HIV, the other with HTLV-I).

In four years nothing has been done. Examination of Dr. Pier's correspondence with governmental authorities clearly illustrates the frustration and difficulty he experienced in attempting to get this potential treatment considered on its merits. Now we have heard that NIH has put lentinan into its highest priority category for investigation—without major new information, essentially on the basis of what was known four years ago. However the drug-selection process is secret so we only have hearsay and have not been able to confirm that lentinan has been placed into the high priority category, or that it was done without new information.

AL 721. The unhappy story of the repeated failures to test this drug properly and make benefits available is presented at length in the back issues of *AIDS Treatment News,* submitted into the record of this hearing.

In yesterday's hearings one of the Commissioners asked FDA Commissioner Dr. Frank E. Young if a therapy might be developed to help overcome drug abuse, which is becoming so important in the spread of AIDS. AL 721 was in fact first developed primarily for that purpose. Theory, laboratory, and animal studies have suggested that it might be effective in reducing the symptoms of opiate or alcohol withdrawal, thus helping abusers to overcome their habits permanently. However to our knowledge no human study has been done—not even a small, quick, inexpensive pilot study which would give some sense of whether it was worth proceeding with this potential medical intervention against drug abuse.

Trimetrexate.　The important news about the approval of the first AIDS-related treatment IND has failed to acknowledge a major concern. Theory and laboratory studies suggest that the trimetrexate with leucovorin therapy now approved for pneumocystis pneumonia (when standard therapies have failed) would very likely also work against cryptosporidiosis, a severe and often fatal diarrheal illness of persons with AIDS. Cryptosporidiosis presently has no satisfactory treatment.

We have heard that even a leading gastroenterologist has been unable to obtain trimetrexate for compassionate use for treating cryptosporidiosis. We have also learned that the manufacturer, Warner Lambert, has no plans to develop the drug for this condition.

The result is that this drug, already proven so safe in persons with AIDS that almost none of the (pneumocystis) patients had to have the therapy terminated, will never be tested for cryptosporidiosis under the current system, despite the immense benefit the discovery of a successful therapy for this opportunistic infection might bring.

Salk Polio Vaccine.　The "old" Salk killed-virus polio vaccine (not to be confused with Salk's current work on an HIV vaccine) has recently been tried as a possible ARC or AIDS treatment. Although it is far too early to be sure it is effective, this therapy has generated considerable excitement among the physicians who have seen the results. In addition, according to an overview article which appeared in *The Wall Street Journal* on January 27, 1988, this possible therapy has also attracted unusual attention from some NIH scientists, who have determined that persons receiving repeated treatments with this vaccine have produced neutralizing antibodies against the AIDS virus. We have heard that Dr. Pitts is now collaborating with a university and a county board of health on a formal study, approved by his IRB—but that Dr. Pitts and a colleague must pay for the vaccine out of their own pockets.

We have also heard two reports that Connaught Laboratories Inc., the only company able to sell the Salk polio vaccine in the United States, has recently made it difficult for physicians to obtain supplies for use in treating AIDS—even though it is perfectly legal for physicians to use it for that purpose. One internist told us that the company refused to ship the vaccine unless he signed an affidavit that it would only be used to immunize against polio. And we also heard that Dr. Pitts' group had to threaten a lawsuit in order to obtain supplies for the study cited above.

We have been unable to confirm these reports because Connaught has refused to discuss them.

It is widely believed in the AIDS community that companies do not on their own resist the development of new markets for their products. It is generally presumed that these cases reflect fear by the company of making enemies at the FDA, which may fear damage to the regulatory process from the development of a public demand for a drug outside of normal channels. Bureaucratic interests may be best served if the usefulness of a valid AIDS treatment is never discovered in the first place. Patients' interests differ. All this is conjecture, of course, as in these cases no one talks, and unless an insider reveals information nothing can be proved.

The polio-vaccine case is not at all unusual. In case after case, too numerous to list here, deliberate roadblocks and obstacles have impeded patients in obtaining treatments, and prevented research which could serve as early pilot studies to indicate whether or not an idea deserved further, more formal trials.

Recommendations

1. That either the Commission or another body investigate the problems cited above, and dozens of similar ones which we can bring forward, to find out what did happen, if there are indeed roadblocks to treatment and treatment research, and how these roadblocks could be overcome.

2. That the Commission arrange for a survey to ask persons with AIDS, ARC, and asymptomatic HIV infection what they think about current public policies regarding the epidemic, and how those policies might be improved.

3. That the Commission ask the FDA to provide guidelines to researchers outlining what studies would be required to qualify a drug for treatment IND or for approval. These guidelines should specify when it is and is not ethical to use placebos in persons with life-threatening disease, or to withhold use of previously-proven therapies such as pneumocystis prophylaxis.

4. That the Commission recommend the creation of a public, computerized and printed registry of all human trials for treating AIDS and related disorders. This registry should include pertinent information about each drug, and the protocols, in language that can be understood by a lay person. Registration in this database should be required for all government-funded protocols, and voluntary registry of all others should be encouraged.

5. That the Commission recommend steps to make access to therapeutic trials equally available to all qualified persons. A system must be established for insuring fair access to everyone in need. A lottery might be suggested.

6. That the Commission suggest the creation of a confidential, voluntary registry of individuals affected by AIDS and related disorders, whereby these individuals can be notified automatically when there are new trials for which they can qualify. (This system could also help researchers recruit for their trials.)

7. That the Commission recommend the immediate expansion of funding for experimental trials organized and run at the community level, using the resources of private and community physicians, such as the Community Research Initiative in New York, and the County Community Consortium in San Francisco.

8. That the Commission encourage the current attempts to share and disseminate reagents, materials, and scientific data within the scientific community, to speed the discovery of safe and effective therapies for AIDS.

9. That the Commission recommend the development of a system such as compulsory licensing which would prevent proprietary restrictions on data and access to drugs from impeding development of AIDS treatments.

10. We urge the Commission to recommend that individual patients and their physicians be allowed to choose to use safe experimental therapies under supervision, even before efficacy has been confirmed, if informed consent is obtained.

COMMENT ON THE PRESIDENTIAL COMMISSION

It has been widely reported that the Presidential Commission on the HIV Epidemic has greatly improved after getting off to a bad start. We agree with this assessment. The current chairman, retired admiral James D. Watkins, is very good at running this kind of commission, and has approached the task without preconceptions. Typical commissions write reports which mostly gather dust; the HIV commission has already implemented public-policy improvements even before its report is written.

Recently the Commission held three days of hearings on AIDS treatment development in New York, February 18–20; see our testimony above. Although these hearings were open to the public—as is everything this Commission does—surprisingly few people attended. The auditorium had seats for 700 people but only once was it even half full.

We cannot review the three days in this short space, but here are some impressions of the highlights.

The NIH (National Institutes of Health) scientists who testified looked almost entirely at long-term projects. The slogan of the day was that there is no quick fix. They asked for "bricks and mortar"—more laboratory facilities—as well as money to train more Ph.D.s and postdoctoral researchers. They also asked for more independence for scientists to choose their own projects, instead of merely fulfilling preconceived research contracts as they have all too often had to do in the past. NIH wants more than year-to-year spending authority, so that administrators could make balanced long-term plans, and it wants permission to award grants faster to scientists.

We strongly support these requests to strengthen the often-neglected infrastructure of U.S. medical research. But we question the excessive control of old-boy networks and the resulting narrow focus on AZT-type drugs or long-term solutions only. This problem is less the fault of the scientists than of the pervasive lack of national mobilization to save the lives of those who are already ill. Scientists today depend so heavily on access to money, equipment, permissions, and prestige journals that they can only study what others approve. Even within their own fields they must follow national policy, seldom lead it.

The FDA also wants more money, to be able to evaluate the greater numbers of AIDS drugs which increased research funding will produce. The FDA, like the NIH, usually insists on time frames too long to be useful to those now ill.

The Commission avoided asking pointed questions, and considerable self-congratulation, aggrandizement, and fluff crept into the testimony. There seems to have been a deliberate policy of keeping the witnesses comfortable so they could say more than if they had been on the defensive. The NIH, the FDA, and the alternative-treatment movement all got a good reception and left happy. Perhaps the Commission decided that there isn't time now to reform the agencies, that a better way to fight the epidemic is to mobilize existing forces by giving them what they need to operate.

MEMO TO THE WAR CONFERENCE, FEBRUARY 26–28, 1988

AIDS Treatment Research and Care Issues: The Need for Advocacy

During the last two years I have published 50 articles on experimental AIDS treatments and the public policy issues around AIDS research. This work has illuminated critical gaps in advocacy for medical, research, and treatment-access concerns of persons with AIDS, ARC, or asymptomatic HIV.

Many "AIDS deaths" are in fact unnecessary. For example, even in San Francisco many people known to be at risk for pneumocystis die of it without having had any preventive treatment—despite an editorial in the *New England Journal of Medicine* (October 15, 1987) that persons at risk should receive such treatment. And an article in the same issue of the *New England Journal* showed that a "salvage" therapy with two experimental drugs (trimetrexate and leucovorin) saved the lives of over two-thirds of the patients for whom the standard drugs had failed. This new treatment has almost no side effects. Yet how many persons with pneumocystis have access to it if needed?

Apparently two-thirds or more of the deaths from pneumocystis could now be prevented if safe, effective (though officially experimental) treatments were used when appropriate. The basic problem is the lack of uniform standards of care. And there has been *almost no advocacy* from gay political organizations (or from AIDS service groups or even gay physicians' organizations) on such matters. We have relied almost solely on the pharmaceutical companies to do our advocacy for us—and their interests get pushed, not ours. Horror stories like the example of pneumocystis above are common because necessary treatments remain "experimental" for years after they are known to work, and physicians are discouraged from considering them no matter what the facts of the cases in their care.

The gay movement has understandably deferred such issues to the physicians. So has the national media. The physicians have deferred to the scientists. And the scientists have deferred to the White House—to the tone and undercurrents of national policy which scientists do not flout if they want their careers to prosper. And Reagan's White House has proved highly agreeable to forces with mixed feelings to say the least about saving the lives of those now ill or infected with AIDS.

The United States government controls much of the money for AIDS research—not only in the U.S. itself, but around the world. (Few of the large pharmaceutical companies even have an antiviral research program, let alone an AIDS program.) And in the U.S. itself, Federal agencies also control an immense network of interlocking permissions necessary if any project, even in the private sector, is going to move. No wonder scientists are notoriously afraid to speak to the press on the record—unless they are acting as official spokespersons for their institutions. Pharmaceutical corporations are even more afraid to speak out, because their lifeblood is FDA approvals which can be denied at any time with no reason given.

The result is that practically every public statement from a "credible" source about AIDS research is loaded with institutional self interest. It may not represent the speaker's (or anyone else's) real beliefs about what is wrong in AIDS treatment research and what should be done about it.

And we cannot rely on the media to challenge medical and scientific experts, as they challenge other public and private officials. The media simply defers to scientific expertise, and refuses to question what government experts say. The media has come to feel that in order to avoid raising false hope, in order to avoid being used in unethical promotions of false remedies, it will not report medical information except from official sources. That's understandable—but results in coverage which is little more than rewrites of official press releases.

With the exception of AZT, almost all of the money in AIDS research has gone into basic-science projects which couldn't possibly come into widespread use for several years or more. Scientists have a bias toward elegant research based on attractive theories, the kind of work that wins Nobel prizes. They don't like to do what the AIDS treatment underground is doing—searching the world for safe treatment options which seem to have something going for them (under any theory—or perhaps none at all because no one knows how they may work) and trying them out. We are not arguing against careful, theory-based basic research—just that there should be empirical research too.

Look at the example of dextran sulfate, an antiviral now being studied at San Francisco General Hospital. It took a year to get this study going, as the FDA was concerned about safety. (The drug has been used in Japan for 20 years and is safe enough to be available there without a prescription. Antiviral effects were described in published papers as far back as 1964.) And this study—the only official clinical trial in the world of dextran sulfate for AIDS or ARC—is only a "phase I" dosage and toxicity trial. When it is finished, there will be more years for "phase II" (efficacy) and "phase III" (comparison with other drugs). (The "new rules" of the FDA, supposed to liberalize access to experimental drugs, only come into effect well into phase II, and then only if the Commissioner of the FDA wants them to; no standards for how a drug can qualify have ever been released. And no person has yet received any treatment for AIDS or ARC under these rules.)

Meanwhile hundreds of people have obtained dextran sulfate underground and used it, usually under their doctor's supervision. We have been told that the medical records of over 300 people are now being entered into a computer in an underground research project. Everyone agrees that it is too early to be sure—several more months of experience will be needed—but most of the doctors who are using (whoops, monitoring patients who are using) dextran sulfate in combination with other antivirals are saying that they have never seen so much early promise, from AZT or anything else. And this drug has the advantage over AZT of having little toxicity.

In short, the *practical* work (for saving lives) of several years of official treatment research is being condensed into a few months—and with no funding at all. The key to the great effectiveness of this kind of research is that it works together with people's efforts to save their own lives.

Yet the official research establishment has little use for this kind of directly practical research. It prefers to test individual drugs for years before testing treatment combinations which have been suggested by the best judgment of experienced practicing physicians. This academic research approach reflects the interests of scientists in producing elegant work, based in state-of-the-art theory, impervious to criticism—and the interests of pharmaceutical companies, which want their new drug approved—but not the interests of patients, who need straightforward, competent testing of treatments potentially ready now.

Official research has often displayed an arrogance which considers only its own ideas, initiatives, and procedures; which refuses to cooperate with patients' attempts to save their lives; and which belittles and ignores the practical knowledge and experience developed by thousands of peoples' long-term, committed, and often highly informed and intelligent efforts to find and use treatments for themselves.

What Can Be Done?

On these kinds of issues—illustrated by the examples of pneumocystis or of dextran sulfate—we have to advocate to save our lives; the system will not do it for us.

How far would the environmental movement have come if it had no independent expertise and could not evaluate ecological or conservation issues on their merits, but had to rely solely on government and corporate experts for its definition of reality? It would be limited to replanting trees, caring for injured animals, etc., and could almost never go to the courts, the legislatures, or to the media and public opinion, as an equal player at least as well informed on its issues as are the representatives of the corporations or government agencies.

And that is where the gay movement is today on the life-and-death issues surrounding AIDS treatment research, development, access to treatments, and standards of medical care for persons with AIDS. We can only support people through the dying process, and have not touched the very addressable issues that determine life or death.

How many medical or scientific experts do all of the organizations represented at The War Conference together have on their staffs? Full-time, paid, that is, so they don't have to depend on grants or salaries from anyone else, and can formulate independent views.

We have assumed that on something so serious as AIDS treatments and research, everyone is working together, and therefore we can accept the official experts' views as delivered, we don't need independent analysis or advocacy. Nothing could be further from the truth. We obviously need advocacy on civil liberties issues surrounding AIDS. We need it just as truly on the medical and scientific issues reflecting research and patient care.

Notes:

(1)   A few AIDS organizations like AmFAR already have access to scientific and medical experts. AmFAR does excellent work, but it funds laboratory science, seldom or never clinical studies. And AmFAR is unlikely to advocate, lobby and litigate for changes in medical or regulatory practices, such as improved standards of care for persons at risk for pneumocystis, or immediate trials of promising combination therapies without years of preliminaries with single drugs.

(2)   Today the FDA approved trimetrexate/leucovorin therapy discussed above for pneumocystis, under the new rules for "treatment IND" (Investigational New Drug), in cases where standard drugs could not be used. This is the first approval of any AIDS drug under these rules, which were intended to speed access to new drugs for serious or life-threatening diseases—over six months after the rules were published.

We could interpret this approval as proof that the FDA is doing its job and we don't need to be involved. Or we could ask about the dozens of other drugs (such as fluconazole for cryptococcal meningitis) which clearly should be more available. We could ask why trimetrexate wasn't made available last October when data clearly supporting it was published (reference above); was the announcement timed to correspond with an AMA-sponsored conference on access to new drugs, and the Presidential Commission's hearings on AIDS drugs, which both occurred in the same week as the announcement?

We could ask if trimetrexate can finally be tried for cryptosporidiosis, where it would very likely be effective. And above all we could monitor how many persons with pneumocystis who need trimetrexate and have no other option but death actually have access to it in the future.

Three Recommendations

(1)   Improve liaison and communication between gay political organizations and treatment-oriented organizations such as AmFAR, Community Research Initiative, Project Inform, and gay physicians' organizations. The War Conference should set up a task force to facilitate such communication.

(2)   Create an advisory board of scientists and physicians as a resource on scientific and medical issues for gay political organizations. Choose members able and willing to break with established views when appropriate.

(3)   When funding permits, the gay political community needs a research and advocacy organization which includes scientists and physicians on its staff.

Issue Number 52
March 11, 1988

FDA MOVES AGAINST
EGG LIPID COMPANY

(March 15) On March 2 the U.S. Food and Drug Administration ordered Houba, Inc. of Culver, Indiana to stop manufacturing and selling its lipid product EL 1020 (which some have compared to AL 721). The letter said that ". . . promotional activities which accompanied the initial shipment of EL 1020 suggested that the article was intended for use in the treatment of acquired immunodeficiency syndrome (AIDS). Because such promotional activities included statements which represented and suggested that this article was intended to be used in the cure, mitigation, treatment, or prevention of disease, or was intended to affect the structure or any function of the body of man, this product is a drug within the meaning of Section 201(g) of the Federal Food, Drug, and Cosmetic Act." The letter also said that the product was "misbranded in that its labeling does not contain adequate directions for use as this term is defined in 21 CFR 201.5 since the conditions for which it is offered are not amenable to self diagnosis and treatment by the laity; therefore adequate directions cannot be written under which the layman can use this drug safely and for the purposes for which it is intended." The letter gave Houba ten days to answer detailed questions concerning how it was going to discontinue its manufacturing and marketing of EL 1020.

No one has alleged that there is anything harmful about the product; the dispute concerns how it was marketed.

This FDA action caused great concern in the AIDS community, as nobody knows exactly why Houba was singled out, and whether the FDA will try to cut off all supplies of egg lipids, which are used by thousands of people. In the week since the FDA action became known, AIDS advocates have conveyed community concerns to high officials in the FDA. Fears have eased somewhat, although the final outcome is still unknown.

Background on Houba

Houba differs from all other suppliers of egg lipid products in several ways:

• Its subsidiary, Rachelle Laboratories, Inc., which manufactures and sells the EL 1020, is a pharmaceutical company which deals routinely with the FDA.

• Until last year, Houba had manufactured the official AL 721 for Ethigen Corporation (formerly Praxis Pharmaceuticals), which holds worldwide licensing rights acquired from the Weizmann Institute of Science in Israel, which developed the product, and also holds the copyright on the term "AL 721." Houba's new product provides the egg lipids in a syrup form which differs from AL 721.

• Houba planned to sell its product primarily or exclusively through HIV-positive buyers clubs, such as the PWA Health Group in New York, or the Healing Alternatives Buyers Club (HABC) in San Francisco. (The New York group has sold one of two forms of EL 1020; the San Francisco-based HABC has not carried either.)

• At about the same time as the three-month FDA investigation of Houba, the company was subjected to sensationalized newspaper articles in a South Bend, Indiana paper. The first article said that Houba was doing secret AIDS research, and that a resident of Culver, Indiana, where the factory is located, was concerned that there may be a health hazard from materials used. A source within Houba told us that this article raised such panic that the AIDS virus may be on the premises that there was fear that the factory could be burned down.

To avert possible violence Houba gave the newspaper information on what they were in fact doing, which had nothing to do with the AIDS virus. The publication of this information reduced the panic, but it may also have constituted some or all of the "statements which represented and suggested" that the product was to be used for AIDS. The newspaper followed up with a headline and story that Houba's "AIDS drug" lacked FDA approval. According to a source within Houba, the newspaper later learned about the FDA order against Houba before the company itself did.

AIDS Community Concerns

Official approval of AL 721 is one to several years away. Almost no progress has been made toward approval in the last two years. Meanwhile, several thousand people with AIDS or ARC have started using egg lipid food products; the current generation first became available in April of last year. Many are convinced that these have been a major help to them, while others have found no effect.

So far the FDA has avoided direct attacks against the AIDS treatment community, so the first concern about the Houba action was whether this policy was changing. A war between the FDA and persons with AIDS could seriously harm both. The AIDS community fears increased difficulty in access to treatments, and diversion of energy which should go to better use in the AIDS crisis. The FDA fears bad publicity, as it knows that Congress can enact laws to take some of its powers away, as it has done at least once in the past (when the FDA tried to make vitamin pills exceeding government-recommended dosages into prescription drugs). Both sides have strong incentives to compromise.

The AIDS community is also concerned about what precedent this case sets. The FDA has the power to declare that a product is a drug (when it would otherwise be a food) even in the absence of any medical claims by the manufacturer—if the manufacturer's marketing targets a specific group such as persons likely to use the product as a drug. This means that the mere fact that a manufacturer sells a product to AIDS treatment organizations could be used against it—setting up a new kind of AIDS discrimination, government inspired or even government required, whereby private manufacturers are forced to boycott AIDS groups and cut off supplies of potential treatments.

The same situation could apply to persons with other diseases. But with AIDS at least, this problem is far from academic; it has already had serious consequences. The availability of egg lipid products was delayed last year, probably for several weeks, when the first manufacturer found to have a suitable product refused to sell to anyone involved with persons with AIDS. And today, the only company in the world which makes the old Salk polio vaccine is refusing to sell it to physicians who want to try it as an AIDS treatment, despite serious scientific interest in this possibility and good early results. The FDA, which may *not* be responsible for the problem in this case, has no legal right to stop physicians from using an approved drug for a non-approved use, which physicians can legally do; but a private company can refuse to sell its product to anyone, even physicians engaged in the completely legitimate practice of medicine, even when it is the world's sole supplier. The history of the AIDS epidemic is loaded with obstacles to treatment access and prompt treatment research. The AIDS treatment community wants to handle these problems in ways that avoid unnecessary fighting on the one hand, and compromises embodying destructive precedents on the other.

We interviewed two AIDS treatment advocates who are FDA experts and have been in close touch with FDA officials in the week since they learned about the Houba case. Both have different views of a murky situation. It is clear that the outcome has not yet been determined.

To Martin Delaney, co-founder of Project Inform in San Francisco, the key issue is whether the FDA pursues the case against Houba only on the basis of statements made by Houba—facts which apply to that immediate case and do not spill over to involve the larger AIDS treatment community. But if the FDA chooses to prosecute Houba because it sold its product largely or exclusively to HIV-positive buyers clubs, the precedent would contribute to discrimination by telling suppliers that their products could be classified as drugs and banned if they sold them to AIDS groups, even though the identical products would remain foods if sold in health-food stores or otherwise to the public in general.

At this time Delaney has heard that the FDA has weighed the various considerations and chosen not to use the sales to buyers clubs against Houba in this case.

Another FDA expert, Jay Lipner, a volunteer attorney who works with Lambda Legal Defense in New York and has worked closely with Martin Delaney on this issue, sees the outcome as still to be determined. He sees only that some progress has been made in clarifying for the FDA what the viewpoint is of some members of the gay community.

"The facts and the law remain complex and confusing," said Lipner. "The one clear message so far is that the AIDS community must have long-term, ongoing, professionally assisted advocacy on treatment and research issues. Otherwise even the most basic interests of persons with AIDS will not be protected."

RIBAVIRIN AND MORTALITY: NEW INFORMATION

This reporter obtained previously-unpublished information comparing persons with ARC who chose to use or not use ribavirin after finishing major clinical trials conducted at four medical centers in 1987. The numbers look very good, but they are not conclusive because of the way self-selection worked in this case.

After the patients completed a double-blind placebo study of ribavirin, they were entitled to obtain the drug free if they wanted it, in return for their participation in the study. A total of 116 patients (from both the ribavirin and placebo groups) did choose to use the drug in this "open-label" phase of the study; 74 chose not to. In the 116 who did use ribavirin there were 6 deaths (5 percent), but in the 74 who did not use ribavirin there were 25 deaths, or 34 percent. Some of these patients had been on ribavirin for as long as 80 weeks; others, in the placebo group in the original study, had been using the drug for less time.

These figures look conclusive, but they could have happened by self selection. Suppose ribavirin didn't do anything. The patients who happened to be doing well while on ribavirin in the study would be likely to want to stay on the drug, since it would have seemed to be working for them. But those patients who happened to be doing poorly would be likely to drop the drug in order to switch to AZT, which cannot be combined with ribavirin. The result is that those who were doing well would tend to put themselves into the ribavirin group, while those doing poorly would go into the other group. This self selection of healthier patients into the ribavirin group during the open-label phase of the study could have caused a difference in death rates, even without any effect from the drug.

It may be possible to analyze the patient records to see how much of the difference in death rate could be attributed to self selection and how much to the drug. This analysis will almost certainly require subjective judgments. And ribavirin has become so politicized that it will be hard to trust this judgment to any researchers not truly independent of both the drug's manufacturer and the FDA. We don't know how such a study could be arranged.

In the absence of better information, it seems unlikely to us that this large difference in death rate could be explained solely by self selection—especially since all patients entering the trial had to meet medical inclusion criteria designed to give a fairly homogeneous group for the study. Instead, this information seems to fit with anecdotal reports that some persons have stopped using ribavirin and quickly deteriorated, whereas others stopped it and had no change. It is possible that ribavirin delays certain stages of progression of HIV infection, while having little or no effect at other stages. It may be possible to study this question by using newer diagnostic tools, such as the P-24 antigen test.

Ribavirin Update

On January 15 we published a short article, "Ribavirin Available By Prescription?". We have since heard from Robert S. Smith, a director of ICN Pharmaceuticals (the manufacturer of ribavirin), and of Viratek (the ICN subsidiary which developed the drug). He asked us to make it clear that ICN had nothing to do with the plans described in the article, and that to the best of his knowledge their product was not being used.

Ribavirin By Prescription?

Ribavirin has been available in the U.S. by prescription for some time, but the only FDA-approved use has been for aerosol treatment of respiratory syncytial virus in infants. Physicians are, however, allowed to use an approved drug for other than approved uses. (An excellent discussion of this issue appeared in the *FDA Drug Bulletin*, Volume 12, Number 1, April 1982. It points out that gaining FDA approval for legitimate medical advances "may take time and, without the initiative of the drug manufacturer whose product is involved, may never occur. For that reason, accepted medical practice often includes drug use that is not reflected in approved drug labeling." You can get the *FDA Drug Bulletin* from a Federal depository library—which can be found in most cities.)

Recently we heard from a pharmacist that he could fill prescriptions for ribavirin if the physician specified that it be used "as directed." This would be the official ribavirin, not an imitation product.

However we have not heard from anyone who has actually obtained and used the drug in this way. And according to Martin Delaney of Project Inform, ribavirin is sold only through hospitals, since the aerosol treatment for infants is not suitable for home use.

If a pharmacy does have the drug, we suspect that the words "as directed" get the pharmacist off the hook, leaving the issue of prescribing ribavirin for treatment of AIDS or ARC between the physician and the FDA. And physicians as a group have long been protective of their right to practice medicine as they see fit; they have considerable political power when they use it, and when the laws were written they were careful to guard their professional sphere against intrusions. Pharmacists in this country do not have the same protections. The phrase "as directed" apparently works its magic by not giving notice to the pharmacist of the non-approved use.

Ribavirin is of course a special case, in that a state of war has developed between ICN, the manufacturer, and the FDA. ICN has not always played by the rules—rules of a game which has grown to be rigged against small to medium companies like ICN, in favor of giants like Burroughs-Wellcome. We don't know who will win this war, but tragically we do know who will lose it. No one knows for sure whether ribavirin does any good for persons with ARC or AIDS, but few could have confidence in the system currently in place for finding out.

We should add that ICN had nothing to do with our comments here, and knew nothing about them in advance. While physicians are allowed to prescribe approved drugs for non-approved uses, drug manufacturers are strictly forbidden to do anything to encourage them to do so.

And physicians have been reluctant to exercise or even discuss the rights they have—possibly from fear of losing professional flexibility if the issue came to a head. Physicians have already lost influence and freedom in the face of Federal efforts to control medical costs. The big money in medicine, which so enriched U.S. allopathic physicians by legislating rival systems out of existence earlier in the twentieth century, may turn against its beneficiaries now that bigger money is involved.

TRIMETREXATE WITH LEUCOVORIN: DECISIONS THAT SAVE LIVES, DECISIONS THAT KILL

On February 16, the FDA and the National Institute of Allergy and Infectious Diseases (NIAID) approved the first-ever "treatment IND" for early release of an AIDS treatment—trimetrexate with leucovorin for pneumocystis. The AIDS community rightly welcomed this step forward—the first AIDS use of the FDA's widely-publicized "new rules" intended to allow physicians to use promising drugs before full approval for commercial sale, in cases of serious or life-threatening illnesses. If it works as intended, the new approval should save many lives.

Unfortunately the trimetrexate ruling also contains a tragic flaw which will almost certainly result in many deaths of others who could be saved.

Background

On October 15, 1987, *The New England Journal of Medicine* published a major article on a new treatment for pneumocystis (Allegra *et al.*, 1987). Trimetrexate, an experimental anticancer drug, had been found to be 1500 times more powerful than trimethoprim, part of a standard treatment, for inhibiting an enzyme obtained from the protozoa which cause pneumocystis.

The dose of trimetrexate required to treat pneumocystis is potentially lethal; but an antidote, leucovorin, can be used to rescue human cells. Protozoa, such as pneumocystis, cannot use leucovorin.

A trial of the trimetrexate/leucovorin combination with 49 patients found clearly better survival than would have been expected for those patients with standard treatments. And the new drug combination had very few side effects; only one of the 49 patients had drug intolerance serious enough to require discontinuing the treatment. Most significantly, the trimetrexate treatment saved 11 of the 16 patients who could not use either of the standard therapies (intravenous bactrim or pentamidine), either because they had severe side effects or because they had been ineffective.

The New Approval: Who Can, Who Cannot Qualify

Under the new approval announced February 16, the NIAID will provide trimetrexate only for patients who have shown "a severe or life-threatening adverse reaction to the approved therapies" (quote from FDA/NIAID press release). The drug, available only from the NIAID, will *not* be provided for patients for whom standard therapies have merely proven ineffective—but not caused severe or life-threatening toxicities. These patients will be left to die.

This ruling flies in the face of the recommendation of the eleven physicians who wrote the October 15 article in *The New England Journal of Medicine*. Their abstract concludes "that the combination of trimetrexate and leucovorin is safe and effective for the initial treatment of pneumocystis pneumonia in patients with AIDS and for the treatment of patients with intolerance or lack of response to standard therapies."

A spokesman for Warner Lambert, the manufacturer of trimetrexate, said that the restriction (against using the drug when all standard treatments had failed to work, though they had not caused a severe or life-threatening reaction) was an FDA decision; it had been explained to him once but he didn't recall the rationale. A spokesman for the FDA gave two reasons. First, the drug had not been approved; clinical tests had not been completed. Second, it is not a drug to be used lightly, as it was potentially lethal unless leucovorin was also administered. When we asked how these reasons applied when the only alternative was the death of the patient—and the trimetrexate/leucovorin combination almost never had side effects severe enough to cause its use to be discontinued—he had no meaningful answer but suggested we talk to the NIAID, which developed the protocol (with the help of the FDA, which approved it). He did say that individual cases might be considered under an emergency treatment IND—an option we believe unlikely to happen in actual hospital practice, especially since physicians would be applying for something explicitly not allowed in the new NIAID/FDA protocol. He also said that the question of whether to expand the conditions under which physicians could use the drug was now being considered by NIAID.

NIAID said, however, that the exclusion of patients for whom all standard treatments failed was an FDA decision. NIAID is now working on "protocol 30," which is designed for these patients; we have not seen protocol 30 since it has not yet been released, but it is part of a series of protocols designed for scientific use, not treatment access, so presumably it will have selection criteria which exclude many patients for whom trimetrexate treatment would be medically indicated.

We do not know why these patients were excluded from the treatment IND (which is designed for treatment access), since no one involved will take responsibility for this decision. The best guess is that the reason for it was to force a selected group of the patients affected into protocol 30. Most of the others will end up in the morgue.

The public had no input this decision, hidden in the fine print of the first AIDS-related treatment IND, which was announced by surprise at the time of two major meetings where it was important for the FDA to look good. Persons with AIDS, and as far as we know their physicians, also had no input. Unless compelling new information has developed since last October—information unknown to the press offices of either the drug manufacturer or the FDA—this access restriction could only be called a ghoulish decision to deny trimetrexate to pneumocystis patients for whom all other available treatments have failed—despite the clear recommendation of the world's leading experts on the trimetrexate treatment, based on their published evidence. The press, which usually only rewrites official news releases on medical-treatment stories, largely missed what happened here.

The February 16 NIAID/FDA press release saw the matter as follows:

> 'Today's action reaffirms FDA's commitment to broaden early patient access to promising experimental treatments for AIDS, AIDS-associated conditions and other life-threatening diseases,' said FDA Commissioner Dr. Frank E. Young, PhD. 'Thanks to this effort with NIAID, trimetrexate's increased availability to those people with AIDS who could potentially benefit from it brings us another step forward in treating one of the most devastating infections seen in AIDS.'
>
> NIAID Director Dr. Anthony S. Fauci said, 'This treatment IND will allow us to offer an important treatment alternative to severely ill patients who cannot tolerate the standard therapy. It is also an example of how NIH is meeting one of its major goals—enabling community physicians to select the most appropriate therapies for their patients with AIDS.'

(Note: We should add that aerosol pentamidine treatment—also highly safe and effective, though not yet approved—should be another treatment option. But even at San Francisco General Hospital, which developed the treatment and knows it better than anyone else, red tape and institutional fears of using a non-approved treatment have kept it out of reach of many patients. The October article on trimetrexate did not discuss aerosol pentamidine.)

Physicians who want details on this distribution of trimetrexate/leucovorin can call an NIAID hotline, between 8AM and 8PM EST, Monday through Friday (see Appendix B). We asked at FDA whether physicians should start paperwork in advance, as the drug might be needed in an emergency. We were advised that the most important thing was to keep patient records up to date, as physicians must prove that there had been severe or life-threatening reactions to the standard treatments before obtaining the trimetrexate.

REFERENCES

Allegra, Carmen J., M.D., Bruce A. Chabner, M.D., Carmletia U. Tuazon, M.D., Debra Ogata-Arakaki, R.N., Barbara Baird, R.N., James C. Drake, B.S., J. Thayer Simmons, M.D., Ernest E. Lack, M.D., James H. Shelhamer, M.D., Frank Balis, M.D., Robert Walker, M.D., Joseph A Kovacs, M.D., H. Clifford Lane, M.D., and Henry Masur, M.D., "Trimetrexate for the Treatment of Pneumocystis Carinii Pneumonia in Patients with the Acquired Immunodeficiency Syndrome," *The New England Journal of Medicine* 317 (October 15, 1987), pp. 978–85.

NALTREXONE SAFETY NOTE: DOSAGE ERROR

A typographical error in the October 1987 *AmFAR Directory of Experimental Treatments for AIDS and ARC* caused the recommended dose of naltrexone to be listed erroneously as "1.75 mg/kg". The intended dose was 1.75 mg per day. The erroneous dose was over 50 times too large and is potentially harmful.

A photocopy of the section containing the error also went out (together with correct information) with material from Project Inform.

Meanwhile Bernard Bihari, M.D., the developer of the naltrexone AIDS/ARC treatment, has increased the recommended dose from 1.75 mg per day to 2.75 mg per day.

For complete instructions including all the corrections, contact Project Inform (see Appendix B).

Issue Number 53
March 25, 1988

TOP SAN FRANCISCO HEALTH OFFICIAL
URGES FASTER DRUG TRIALS

San Francisco's Director of Health, David Werdegar, M.D., M.P.H., departed from his prepared testimony to the Presidential Commission on the Human Immunodeficiency Virus Epidemic to call for much faster clinical trials of drugs to reduce illness and death from HIV infection, at hearings on March 25 in San Francisco.

The oral testimony, on the fourth of six recommendations to the Commission, was as follows:

> I believe in greatly accelerated clinical trials. When you look at our projections to 1993 you can see that the clock is ticking. The current national cooperative drug trial system is cumbersome and unduly long; it just won't produce the results fast enough.
>
> And there are other approaches. We could do community-based trials in high-prevalence areas. We'd be perfectly happy to do it here in San Francisco under Health Department auspices. We can get clinical trials, large scale, with controls, going tomorrow. The current clinical trials, I'm afraid, are just leaden-footed.

The prepared text reads as follows:

> Greatly accelerated clinical trials of potentially useful drugs to reduce the morbidity and mortality of HIV infection. The national cooperative drug trial approach is unduly long and cumbersome. It should be supplemented by speedier mechanisms. As our own projections show only too well, time is of the essence.
>
> Community-based trials in high prevalence areas is one such approach. The Health Department in San Francisco, for example, would welcome the opportunity to conduct large scale clinical trials locally, utilizing the San Francisco General Hospital, the Public Health Hospital, community hospitals and practitioners, and the University of California Health Science Center. These could get under way promptly.

The other five recommendations concerned a comprehensive national plan; Federal block grants for education, prevention, and treatment, directly to the health departments of cities seriously affected by the AIDS epidemic; financial incentives for the development and support of long-term care services; continued support of anonymous and confidential testing programs; and legislation to prevent discrimination in jobs, housing, and health insurance.

We find the research recommendation particularly noteworthy, as it is one of the very few times that any government official has broken with the official line that we're moving as fast as we can, science can't be rushed, there is no faster way—and too bad about those now infected.

Dr. Werdegar's statement also hints that the central issue in treatment research is *not* financial. What we need most—quick, practical trials which could be integrated with ongoing patient care—would cost relatively little, much less than the ineffectual research programs now in place, and far, far less than the cost of care of perhaps hundreds of thousands of cases of unnecessary terminal illness.

HIV CLINICAL CARE PROGRAM OPENED BY COLUMBIA UNIVERSITY STUDENT HEALTH SERVICES

A new program at Columbia University for care for HIV-positive students could provide a model for universities and other institutions as well.

The clinic will offer anonymous antibody testing and counseling. Lab work for the antibody test will be done by New York City; counseling by the Gay Health Advocacy Project, which is assisting the University's health service in setting up the program. All costs will be included in existing student health coverage; the program is designed to keep costs low.

At the initial visit, HIV-positive students will be given a standard medical workup, including an anergy panel and lymphocyte subset, to be repeated every three or six months. Those who show a drop in T4 cells, or HIV symptoms, will be referred for consultation to an AIDS expert at St. Luke's/Roosevelt Hospital, which is affiliated with Columbia University. Students will also be referred to a seropositive support group, to meet periodically.

To start the project, a nurse-practitioner from Community Health Project of the Gay and Lesbian Community Center, which has much experience working with people with AIDS, will see patients and also train one physician and two nurse practitioners at Columbia's Student Health Services.

This project, starting on an experiment with an evaluation after six months, will open March 30. For more information, call Columbia University Student Health Services (see Appendix B).

NATIONWIDE AIDS DEMONSTRATIONS, APRIL 29–MAY 7

A network of AIDS advocacy organizations including ACT UP (AIDS Coalition To Unleash Power—chapters in New York, Boston, Los Angeles, San Diego, Rochester, Philadelphia, New Jersey, New Orleans, and elsewhere) and similar organizations such as AIDS Action Pledge and the ARC/AIDS Vigil (San Francisco), MASS ACT OUT (Boston), OUT (Washington, DC), C-FAR (Chicago), and several chapters of the National Association of People With AIDS will conduct coordinated demonstrations and other actions in over 30 cities to focus public attention on the need for effective action on AIDS. Some of these actions will include nonviolent civil disobedience; others will be educational forums, fundraisers, etc. Persons who want to help out in AIDS advocacy could use this organizing effort to meet others in their area.

A coordinating group called ACT NOW (AIDS Coalition to Network, Organize, and Win), set up by these groups, organized communication for this effort, which is called Spring AIDS Actions '88. Each local group has determined and planned its own actions.

For more information, write or call the ACT NOW or ACT UP organization closest to you. See Appendix C for a listing of these organizations by state.

IMMUNOTOXIN TREATMENT FOR AIDS?

A San Francisco immunologist has proposed using immunotoxins, a technology already tested in humans as an experimental cancer treatment, in the treatment of AIDS and ARC. Alan S. Levin, M.D. of Positive Action Healthcare in San Francisco, who is presenting the idea this week at a meeting of the AIDS Medical Resource Center Physicians Association in Chicago, based the proposal on a model (theory) of the development of AIDS, a model he derived from recently published work of a number of researchers. (For background on Dr. Levin and Positive Action Healthcare, see *AIDS Treatment News*, Issue Number 47).

Even though the proposed AIDS treatment has not yet been synthesized—let alone have any clinical data supporting it—we are interested in the proposal for several reasons:

• The technology of immunotoxins has developed far enough that creating one for AIDS would be almost routine; according to Dr. Levin it could probably be ready for human testing within six months, if unforeseen problems do not intervene. We do not know of any other researchers developing an AIDS treatment based on immunotoxins; a computer search of the literature turned up only one reference, a published letter which suggested this approach in 1986.

• Dr. Levin is in an excellent position to develop the treatment. His wife, Vera S. Byers, Ph.D., M.D., is an expert in making monoclonal antibodies and immunotoxins. Dr. Levin has already started to assemble a scientific team for the project.

• Aside from a treatment possibility, the theory itself summarizes what a number of leading researchers are now learning about AIDS, and addresses several troubling questions such as how HIV can cause AIDS when it only infects a tiny fraction of

T-helper cells (an issue raised by retrovirologist Dr. Peter Duesberg, who has argued that HIV could not cause AIDS). Levin's model also explains why no animals get AIDS, even if they can be infected with HIV; this question could be important for developing strategies for future research, for example by suggesting more emphasis on human immunology rather than animal models.

The Theory

We interviewed Dr. Levin for this article but explained the theory in our own words; any errors are our own responsibility. This explanation is complex because the theory depends on several concepts from immunology; readers who find it confusing can skip to the "Proposed Treatment" section, below.

The central element of Dr. Levin's theory is that part of the protein of HIV imitates part of a *human* protein which has a key role in the immune system. (Proteins consist of sequences of simpler chemicals known as amino acids; a virus may happen to have the same amino acid sequence within one of its proteins as is found in a human protein.) This unfortunate coincidence not only enables HIV to infect human T-helper and certain other cells; it also explains—according to the theory presented here—how later immune dysfunctions develop, through mechanisms well known to immunologists. And fortunately this explanation suggests several approaches to treatment.

The theory arose from a question. AIDS depletes the T-helper cells, but HIV infects very few of them at any one time, less than one in ten thousand. The body could easily replace these cells. Therefore if HIV is causing the damage (and there is much evidence that HIV is the *sine qua non* of AIDS, whether or not it is the sole cause or may also require cofactors) it must be depleting the cells by some means other than directly infecting and killing them.

Levin's model is not new research but rather a coherent summary of a number of findings of others. His theory proposes that HIV does its damage primarily by causing cells to produce an AIDS-virus protein, called gp 110 (or gp 120, another name used for the same substance), which circulates in the blood. Gp 110 (gp 120) includes the sequence which allows HIV to attach to the CD4 molecule—which is the receptor site on the T-helper (T-4) group of white blood cells.

This sequence causes the gp 110 (gp 120) protein to attach to T-helper cells, just as HIV does when it infects the cells. This protein cannot reproduce, as it is not the whole HIV virus, only part of it. But it causes damage in other ways.

The gp 110 (gp 120) molecule can attach itself to more than one cell, causing clumps of T-helper cells to fuse together into giant clusters called syncytia. These cells stop working and soon die. In this way, a single cell which is infected by HIV and secreting the gp 110 (gp 120) protein can cause the destruction of many healthy T-helper cells elsewhere in the body.

In addition, the immune system recognizes gp 110 (gp 120) as a foreign protein, and forms antibodies against it. Presumably these antibodies do help to reduce its concentration.

But since gp 110 (gp 120) contains the sequence by which HIV matches the CD4 molecule (the receptor on the T-helper cell), an antibody against this AIDS-virus protein can also act against the human protein sequence which normally uses the

CD4 receptor site. As a result, communication between T-helper cells and certain other cells, such as macrophages (see below), becomes disrupted.

(It might be helpful in understanding this process to visualize an antibody and its corresponding antigen as a key which fits the lock. Like the key and the lock, the antibody and antigen fit because the shapes match exactly. When the body is invaded by a foreign organism—the lock—it produces an antibody (the key) which precisely fits the protein from that organism—and usually no other. But unfortunately the AIDS-virus protein gp 110/gp 120—the lock—happens to fit a key which is already in normal use in the body—the CD4 molecule, which is the T-helper receptor site to which the AIDS virus attaches itself in order to enter and infect the cell. Therefore when the immune system makes new antibodies to gp 110/gp 120, these new keys not only fit this AIDS-virus protein, as intended. They also fit the "lock"—found on other cells such as macrophages—which was intended to use the "key" on the T-helper cell. Therefore these antibodies intended to attack the AIDS-virus protein also attack the normal cells such as macrophages, interfering with communication between the macrophages and T-helper cells and perhaps doing other damage as well.)

Normally macrophages, which are large immune-system cells which can circulate in the blood or remain in various organs of the body, engulf foreign organisms such as bacteria or fungi. Later they present the foreign proteins to T-helper cells, which instruct other cells to make antibodies specifically targeted against the invading organisms. The antibodies which the immune system produces against gp 110 (gp 120) interfere with this process.

After the macrophages present antigen to the T-helper cells, these cells in turn secrete chemicals called growth factors (such as colony-stimulating factors, abbreviated CSF), which cause the maturation of new T-cells and other cells. When the antibodies to gp 110 (gp 120) interfere with the macrophages, these chemicals are not secreted in the normal amounts, resulting in further depletion as the new cells which should have matured do not do so. (One new treatment, called GM-CSF, is being tested for a deficiency of white blood cells often found in AIDS, especially after treatments with certain drugs such as AZT. GM-CSF is a colony stimulating factor given to correct for a shortage of this substance, a shortage which could be caused by the mechanism outlined above.)

Besides the damage described above, the AIDS-virus protein gp 110 (gp 120) causes harm indirectly in still another way. Normally after the immune system makes antibodies, it makes antibodies against the antibodies themselves. These, called antiidiotype antibodies, help to turn the immune response off.

But this AIDS-virus protein contains the sequence which matches the CD4 molecule on the T-helper cell. Therefore its antiidiotype antibody can also act against the T-helper cell—further interfering with the normal functioning of the immune system.

All of these forms of damage come about because the HIV virus—and its gp 110 (gp 120) protein—has a sequence which mimics a key human protein in the immune system.

And according to this theory, the reason animals do not develop AIDS from HIV is that they have different proteins, which HIV does not mimic.

Proposed Treatment: An Immunotoxin

An immunotoxin consists of an antibody chemically attached to a toxin—a preparation intended to kill specific cells. The antibody targets the right kind of cells and binds to them, but the antibody itself does not kill the cell. The toxin kills the cell; the antibody is custom made to bring the toxin only to a specific group of cells, a group which must be immunologically distinct in some way.

For AIDS, the proposed treatment will use an antibody which seeks out the gp 110 (gp 120) protein but not any normal human protein. This antibody will carry a toxin to the HIV-infected cells which are producing gp 110 (gp 120); these cells can be recognized because they have this protein on their surface. The immunotoxin will kill these infected cells, greatly reducing the amount of gp 110 (gp 120) being produced. Dr. Levin believes that it should be possible to reduce the level of this AIDS-virus protein by 100 times through the use of an immunotoxin.

This treatment will not be a complete cure; it would not eliminate the virus entirely, as some cells infected with HIV show no outside evidence of infection. And of course there may be unforseen difficulties in creating a practical drug. But the approach, already in use for cancer, certainly deserves serious attention for AIDS.

NEW MAI (MYCOBACTERIUM AVIUM INTRACELLULARE) TREATMENTS

A friend of ours who is a medical professional (not a physician) recently called a number of physicians and research centers to find out about treatments for MAI, for his lover who has AIDS. He suggested that we pass on what he learned to our readers.

He heard that a year ago there were no good treatments, but today there are at least two treatment protocols, each of which combines a new drug with traditional anti-tuberculosis drugs. But physicians differ greatly in their approach to MAI; for example, those on the East Coast are more likely to treat it than those on the West. Most physicians believe that MAI is not life threatening, but a few believe that it kills many people.

Persons with normal immunity can occasionally get pulmonary MAI, but persons with AIDS usually have a systemic infection in the bloodstream; it must be diagnosed by culturing the organisms from the blood. MAI can also affect the bone marrow and cause anemia.

Symptoms include night sweats, high spiking fevers, cough, loss of appetite, and general fatigue. The illness may be misdiagnosed as flu. Often no one suspects MAI until the blood culture is done. Because the organisms grow slowly, the culture takes from two to six weeks.

One treatment now being tested at several California universities combines a new drug, ciprofloxacin, recently made available by prescription, with three older TB drugs: rifampin, ethambutol, and amikacin. The disadvantage of this combination is that amikacin is toxic, and must be given intravenously for a month.

Another treatment combines an experimental drug ansamycin (also called rifabutine, or rifabutin) with ethambutol and clofazimine. This regimen has the advantages of less toxicity, plus the fact that ansamycin may have anti-HIV activity. The disadvantage is that ansamycin must be obtained specially from the Centers for Disease Control; it can take two weeks for delivery, and only a month's supply is sent at one time, so planning is necessary to avoid running out; make sure your physician reorders two weeks in advance each month. (Incidentally we have been hearing good things about ansamycin; it is a drug to watch.)

These treatments do not always work, as there are different organisms which cause MAI, and not all are susceptible to any one drug. Even when the drugs do work, they usually do not kill the organisms completely but reduce their level in the blood. Physicians recommend that treatment be continued indefinitely; unfortunately MAI treatments can sometimes interfere with AZT therapy.

Better treatments for MAI are expected, as a new generation of mycobacteria drugs is now being developed. Meanwhile this disease will become a more serious problem, mainly because fewer people are dying of pneumocystis. MAI develops slowly, and usually occurs, if at all, late in the course of AIDS, often about a year after the first attack of pneumocystis.

Incidentally our friend responded well to the ansamycin (rifabutin) treatment, after six weeks.

For more information about MAI treatments, physicians should check through professional contacts. Also, a number of articles have been published about all of the above drugs in the treatment of MAI or related diseases.

Issue Number 54
April 8, 1988

CONVERSATION WITH DONALD ABRAMS, M.D.

Donald Abrams, M.D., is Assistant Director of the AIDS Division at San Francisco General Hospital, and Assistant Clinical Professor at the Cancer Research Institute, University of California, San Francisco. He also chairs the County Community Consortium, a group of about 80 San Francisco physicians treating persons with AIDS. At times he has been controversial in the AIDS community, where some see him as a leading opponent of alternative treatments.

Originally we asked for this interview in order to give our readers the widest range of opinions, by presenting a viewpoint which we thought would be opposite of our own. But we found that the differences were not as great as we had expected. Much of the controversy has stemmed from lack of information and communication rather than from fundamental disagreements.

Recently representatives of both parties—AIDS researchers at San Francisco General, and persons with AIDS who have chosen to take an active part in their health care—have made major efforts to improve communication so that each can understand and address the others' concerns. This interview is part of that process.

We asked Dr. Abrams to discuss whatever he wanted. The conversation included several areas: the activities and plans of the County Community Consortium, and background on clinical trials, including how the Imuthiol (DTC) results had been delayed. We edited and rearranged the questions and replies, with Dr. Abrams' permission.

JJ: What can you tell us about the Consortium, and its future plans?

DA: The County Community Consortium was set up in March of 1985 at the request of Mayor Feinstein, who felt that there should be some mechanism to maintain open communications between physicians here at the "County" hospital, San Francisco General, and physicians in the "community" who were caring for people with AIDS. Originally Paul Volberding called a meeting of the dozen or so physicians who were

284

caring for AIDS patients predominantly at that time (1985), and started a series of now monthly meetings. I became the chairman of the Consortium shortly after it was formed and have been involved in shaping its direction; and I'm certainly gratified by the progress and the enthusiasm around the Consortium.

Initial goals of the County Community Consortium were to inform physicians in the community as to what protocols were ongoing here at SFGH so that they could refer patients; to update physicians on information that we may have heard that they didn't hear about yet—pre-publication from research going on here as well as elsewhere; and also to maintain lines of communication so that patients' care could be transferred most effectively from here to private physicians when necessary.

After a while it became clear as the group became more cohesive that the physicians in the community didn't just want to sit and listen to the clinical investigations that we're doing here. They wanted to participate as well. And they wanted to participate with their patients in their practices without sending them over here. So we said, okay, let's think about something we can do. And in the beginning of 1986 we spent six months together working on a protocol to try to evaluate the best way to prevent pneumocystis from coming back in people who have a previous episode.

Every physician in the community had their own pet way to prophylax. I used to give no treatment in patients who had had pneumocystis once. I would say, "Let's wait till you get it again, then we can treat it again," because I didn't have any evidence that prophylaxis really prolonged survival. Other physicians were giving septra, others were giving pentamidine on a monthly basis, some people were using dapsone at various dosages on a daily basis, or twice a week, and some were giving fansidar once a month. So we decided to organize and do a real study, because we were not collecting data and this information which was potentially very important, not only for us but around the country where physicians didn't have all the experience we had here, was going up in smoke.

So we as a group of physicians worked out a protocol and got it approved by the various Committees on Human Research at the hospitals around San Francisco. And we initiated a four-arm pneumocystis prophylaxis trial in July of 1986.

But then in September of 1986 AZT became available for the same group of patients, people who have had pneumocystis. The stipulation then was that they couldn't take another medicine, so although we put 25 patients on our study very quickly, the study came to a halt because all those people who were eligible for pneumocystis prophylaxis wanted AZT at that time.

So next we decided to set up a mechanism to collect information on patients who were going to be given AZT. But that never caught on, the physicians didn't really want to participate because that study lacked the drama and glory of doing a randomized trial; just collecting information is not as exciting.

But during that time the community began, on the basis of information trickling in from New York, to become more interested in aerosolized pentamidine. A number of respiratory care centers in the community, as you know, began treating patients with aerosolized pentamidine—again, without any attempt to collect data systematically, without any attempt to standardize the dose or the delivery of the drug. So again, the Consortium, with the collaboration of Bruce Montgomery here in San Francisco General, and Gifford Leoung, decided to run a three-arm study of aerosolized pentamidine.

We decided to include not only people who have had an episode of pneumocystis, but also patients at risk to develop pneumocystis, those with KS and those with ARC. So in July of 1987 we opened this study for enrollment. This was a most gratifying experience—we actually had 440 patients onto that trial within two months through the participation of physicians at 20 different centers not only in San Francisco but in the East Bay, Sonoma, Sacramento, a truly regional study.

Extending clinical trials into the community physicians' offices is a fabulous thing and I think it's obvious through the enthusiasm of the Consortium—every month our meetings have about 70 to 80 physicians. Our mailing list has grown from 12 to 125 physicians who are caring for people with AIDS and coming to the Consortium meetings because they're interested in this community-based clinical research.

It can be quite draining for physicians dealing with AIDS all day in their offices—they're all alone with their office staff and seeing patients all day, and sometimes they ask what am I really doing to help? By putting patients on clinical trials, the physician feels like he's doing something not only potentially for that patient but for the people that are coming down the road. It really lifts some of the burden off the health-care provider, and provides an increased sense of satisfaction.

JJ: I hear everywhere that this is the direction things are moving today, toward clinical trials through physicians' private practices.

DA: There are problems, however. Physicians in their private practices, or at medical centers, care about their patients predominantly, and want to provide what they believe is optimal care. When you design a study by committee, it's harder to get everybody to believe that the study is valid. So, for example, on the first pneumocystis prophylaxis trial physicians used to call up and randomize a patient, and they would hear that their patient was randomized to either fansidar or dapsone or pentamidine or no treatment. But after calling up to put the patient on the trial, if they were told that their patient was on the "no treatment" arm, the physician would say that they didn't want this patient on the study then. And so they withdrew.

That's not how one does clinical research. So there is a little bit of a tension in the community health-care provider between doing clinical investigation and providing first-rate care.

And now in the aerosol pentamidine study we're seeing potential jeopardy of all the valuable data we could get, because patients in the community and their physicians feel that one particular dose is inferior to the other. That's the point of doing the study, to determine that. That's the whole purpose, and we have not even begun to really look at the data because it hasn't matured yet to a point were we feel that any significant information can be gained. But because of the activism of the patient community as well as the conflict that some of the physicians have between providing optimal care and doing clinical investigation, our current study is threatened. And that's one of the problems I see in doing clinical studies in the community where some of the community physicians might not really have all their heart into doing the investigation.

(Dr. Abrams explained that a separate team is monitoring the results as they occur, so that if any dose turns out to be clearly inferior, that arm of the study will be stopped and the patients will be put onto the other doses. There is no placebo in this study; everybody gets some dose of the drug. Dr. Abrams also explained that during the treatment with aerosol pentamidine persons should take a deep breath every 30 seconds to every minute, to help the medicine get to all parts of the lungs.)

JJ: It seems that an extra amount of creativity and prior thought is necessary to bring these two values into harmony.

DA: You're absolutely right and that's what we're trying to do now. Do you have to work out some sort of a contract with physicians who say, "Yes, I want to participate in this study." Should they sign something saying that if they do participate in the study they will carry out this agreement?

JJ: But also they should have some input into the study.

DA: Oh yes, they are designing it. Now we have on the burner about five different studies. We have one monthly meeting for physicians in the community; that's our business meeting where we discuss the protocols and the studies that we want to do and the studies that we are doing; also we have guest speakers. We've had Project Inform, we're having Dr. Ellen Cooper (the head of the AIDS division of the FDA) to our next meeting.

JJ: What kinds of studies are you planning for the Consortium in the future?

DA: I think that some studies, such as testing a brand new drug, an antiviral or immune modulator, need to be done in a medical center that has the necessary research support to collect the information in a standardized, carefully controlled, quality assured manner, as opposed to having 15 or 20 different physicians trying to do it in their offices. Private physicians don't have time to do a lot of paperwork and extra studies; I think some things really need to be done at a single center.

Our goal in Consortium trials is to evaluate some of the treatments to prevent infections; to lessen the toxicity of AZT; to perhaps improve nutrition—studies that are not using the high-tech, brand-new antiviral or immune modulator. We'll need to continue to do those here at SFGH, on a pilot level.

The CRI (Community Research Initiative) in New York is being a little more aggressive, in trying to obtain drugs for early private-practice trials. That might be a little more than we can do well at this time and obtain quality data. I think there's a need for centralization of some studies at the AIDS center, if you will, and then other studies certainly are much more important to decentralize and do out in the community.

Now we are certainly aware that the AIDS Clinic at San Francisco General and the physicians in the community are not the only people who are prescribing therapies, that patients themselves have taken it into their own hands to self-medicate. And this is a constant question that we've been discussing within the Consortium for a long time. What should, what can we do, to monitor that group of people? Can we collect any valuable information if 14 different people are taking 12 different dosages of six different preparations of AL 721, can we obtain any useful information? Can we validate any of the testimonial claims by collecting their T-cells or their clinical status? Can we have a registry that physicians in their offices can fill out for consenting patients, and get honest information from the person on what they are really taking, get all that data and see if a computer can sort any of it out?

JJ: What I hear from talking to people around the CRI in New York is that for such a registry to work, they will need employees who visit the physicians' offices and collect the information.

DA: Right, and that was our model. That's the grant I wrote, to have itinerant nurse practitioners who would be the research nurses who would help, because the physicians don't have time to do that, so that's what we applied for government funding for, but we didn't get it.

Just last weekend I wrote the protocol to set up a registry so that we can collect this data because so much information out there is just going up in smoke. We're still talking about it in the Consortium because this registry idea hasn't met with overwhelming approval. But that's the beauty of the Consortium, that physicians who are interested in participating in a study can choose to do so, can offer it to their patients.

(Part II of this interview appears in issue number 56, page 300.)

URGENT: CALIFORNIA AIDS RESEARCH INITIATIVE NEEDS HELP

Persons living anywhere can help make available $180 million additional money for AIDS research. But you must act in the next four weeks.

The AIDS Tax Credit Initiative will allow a California tax credit of up to $25 per year for contributions to a new state AIDS-research fund ($5000 each for corporations, trusts, and estates). Virtually certain to pass in November if it gets on the ballot, this initiative is expected to raise $180,000,000 for AIDS research over the next three years. The money will be especially valuable because California law allows researchers to bypass the U.S. Food and Drug Administration and obtain state approval instead. (See "Why AIDS Treatment Delay?", below.)

Although the initiative applies only to California taxpayers and finances research within this state, the knowledge and treatments developed will of course benefit people everywhere. Persons with other diseases will benefit too, since new understanding of the immune system promises treatment breakthroughs against many other conditions.

The problem is that to get on the ballot, the AIDS Tax Credit Initiative needs over 400,000 valid signatures of registered voters before May 20—less than five weeks away— and it has less than half of them so far. To get the rest in time, the campaign for the initiative must use paid petition circulators. It must raise $300,000 within the next four weeks to have a comfortable margin.

This AIDS tax credit proposal passed both houses of the California legislature unanimously—but Governor George Deukmejian vetoed it, and Republican legislators refused to help override the Republican governor's veto. Legislation to place the measure on the ballot has been stalled, making the signature campaign necessary. Lack of $300,000 now will lose $180,000,000 for AIDS research.

TREATMENT ISSUES ON DEXTRAN SULFATE, IMUTHIOL/ANTABUSE, AND "GERMAN ENZYMES"

We continue to recommend *Treatment Issues,* a newsletter published by the Gay Men's Health Crisis and edited by Barry Gingell, M.D. The current issue (Volume 2, Number 2) includes a short update on dextran sulfate, and a long article on Imuthiol (DTC) and Antabuse.

The article "German Enzyme Therapy" may be particularly interesting. This treatment, used in Germany for several diseases including AIDS, is believed to reduce excessive levels of circulating immune complexes, which may cause much of the damage in certain autoimmune conditions. Comparable preparations are available in the United States as health supplements. For more information, see the article in *Treatment Issues.*

To subscribe to *Treatment Issues,* send your name and address to: GMHC, Department of Medical Information (see Appendix B for address of Gay Men's Health Crisis).

WHY AIDS TREATMENT DELAY?

ACT UP Los Angeles newsletter asked us for this article. It is appearing simultaneously in *ACT UP Los Angeles* and in *AIDS Treatment News.*

Today we *know* that hundreds of thousands of people will die of AIDS in the United States alone over the next several years—unless effective treatments become available. Yet government, business, the general public, and the AIDS community alike have failed to mobilize to assure that solid treatment leads get prompt attention and research, and become accessible to patients when they should be. Far more attention has gone to supporting the dying process than to making it unnecessary.

Dozens of serious, promising treatment possibilities exist. For almost all of them, virtually nothing effective is being done. We won't be any closer next year than now to knowing if and when they work.

A look at the promising treatments of two years ago—such as ribavirin, isoprinosine, AL 721, DNCB, foscarnet, HPA-23, lentinan, gamma globulin, plasmapheresis, AZT—shows that in two years nothing decisive has happened, except for AZT. The rest are still in the same limbo they were then, still on the same promising-treatment list two years later, still neither in nor out. Some have suffered vituperation or neglect in the shifting political winds, but none has been rejected (or accepted either) on rational grounds based on evidence. The research just was not done.

And it isn't being done today. The much-touted spectacular progress in "AIDS research" concerns high-tech, basic science which could not possibly produce practical treatments for years.

Treatment research *can* be done right. For example, some European physicians noticed spectacular improvement in one AIDS patient treated with an antibiotic, fusidic acid. Small trials with ten to twenty patients each were quickly started in Denmark and England; apparently they showed that the drug is ineffective. Although the drug failed, the research which tested it succeeded excellently. It showed how *practical* trials can be done.

Similar immediate, no-nonsense trials could test not only single drugs, but drug combinations, in fact any reasonable therapeutic plan or protocol. Recently the head of San Francisco's Department of Public Health offered to start trials immediately in City facilities; he called the current clinical trials "leaden-footed."

Virtually never has quick but workable testing of any other AIDS treatment possibility (besides fusidic acid) been carried out. In the United States, the rules of the Food and Drug Administration would not allow it. These rules often require, for example, "phase I" dosage and toxicity tests even for drugs in common use for years and well known to be safe. Even such well-known drugs can take a year or more of negotiations and paperwork just to crank up a phase I trial even after financing has become available—as it almost never does unless the drug happens to fit into the commercial plans or scientific preconceptions of the day. "Phase II"—efficacy testing—takes years longer.

AIDS experts have agreed for years that drug *combinations* will probably be necessary for treatment. But the FDA refuses to allow human testing of combinations of two or more unapproved drugs. Except for combinations with AZT—which is approved, but unsuitable for many patients—this rule alone adds several years delay before testing can even begin on any promising AIDS therapy.

U.S. rules and procedures also delay drug trials abroad in Europe and elsewhere, even if privately financed by foreign companies with no U.S. support. How can the U.S. government affect AIDS research conducted elsewhere without U.S. funding? The answer is that the U.S. AIDS market so dwarfs all others that pharmaceutical companies fear doing anything anywhere in the world, until the FDA has given its blessing to their research plans.

We have heard that a handful of people at the FDA—one report said only two, both young physicians recently out of training—constitute the bottleneck which all proposed AIDS drugs must go through. Almost every AIDS drug trial anywhere in the world waits in line for permission at this door.

U.S. medical planners can confidently predict hundreds of thousands of deaths, because there is no way an effective drug could get through this system in time. The FDA's much touted "new rules"—supposed to allow faster access to treatments for serious or life-threatening diseases—apply only late in phase II, have no constituency within the FDA, and have had practically no effect on AIDS treatment availability in almost a year of their existence.

The official U.S. drug-research system may find a cure in five to ten years, but meanwhile it has nothing to offer but death.

An alternative-treatment movement is growing explosively and doing some of the most useful AIDS-treatment research—the only AIDS research in the United States at least designed to get quick results. Now it faces increasing attacks through government, corporate, and even international sabotage—actions taken solely to deny treatment access to persons with AIDS, or to harass research efforts by private physicians. For example, at least fifteen companies in Japan sell dextran sulfate—available there as a *non*-prescription drug for 20 years, and now one of the most promising experimental AIDS treatments—but within the last two months every one of these companies started refusing to sell it to Americans. And when the old Salk killed-virus polio vaccine showed good results as an AIDS/ARC treatment, the only company in the world which manufactures it refused to sell it to physicians for that purpose. We don't yet know where the pressures came from, or why. But no one involved has even pretended that concern for patients' safety or welfare led to these decisions.

For the first six years of the epidemic, practically every AIDS organization slept on treatment and research issues, refusing to inform itself or have anything to do with the matter. This utter lack of treatment advocacy allowed horrors like those outlined above to come into being. Now the community is awakening. The faster it awakens, the more lives will be saved.

Issue Number 55
April 22, 1988

DEXTRAN SULFATE: SAN FRANCISCO RESEARCHER REPORTS EARLY RESULTS

On April 20, Donald Abrams, M.D. presented early results from the world's only clinical trial of dextran sulfate as a potential HIV treatment to the County Community Consortium, a group of several dozen physicians in San Francisco. The same data had already been presented to the Federal government's AIDS Clinical Treatment Group in Bethesda, Maryland, at the end of March.

This "phase I" (dosage and toxicity) study conducted at San Francisco General Hospital found that patients were able to tolerate all six dosage levels (900 mg per day, 1800, 2700, 3600, 4500, and 5400) for the two-month trial. However, four of the 30 patients were dropped from the study, and six others had their doses reduced, due to reactions which may have been side effects of the drug (see "Dextran Sulfate: Monitoring and Safety," below).

This ongoing study did not find evidence of efficacy in patient data analyzed from the first three doses. T-cells showed only an insignificant rise. Only one of several patients who were P24 antigen positive (indicating viral activity) at the start of the trial went negative; and one of several who started negative became positive. This lack of improvement in T4 numbers and viral antigen level does not necessarily mean that the drug does not work, because:

• This study was not designed for efficacy. And only 15 patients have been tested so far.

• Only the lower three of the six doses have been analyzed, as the eight weeks of blood work has not been completed for the other patients. The blood work for these patients on the higher doses is being batched for a single run, to be done soon.

• Two months may not have been long enough to show clear changes on the blood tests.

- We do know that patients felt better with the drug. However there was not enough time to register clinical improvement as studies usually measure it, by reduced numbers of opportunistic infections or other incidents.

- These patients used dextran sulfate alone, and the drug may need to be combined with other treatments to be effective.

- The information has not been formally analyzed for this early report. For example, we know that P24 antigen went negative for only one patient, but we do not know if it decreased for the others.

Dr. Abrams has already written a protocol for "phase II," a study designed to test for efficacy. It will select only patients who are P24 antigen positive to start, use dose ranges but no placebo, and follow patients long enough to see if improvements occur.

The phase II study, like the phase I, will test dextran sulfate alone. But Dr. Abrams has also written another protocol for a trial of dextran sulfate combined with AZT. Theory as well as laboratory evidence suggest that this combination may be more effective than either drug alone. Combined toxicities are unknown at this time.

Private physicians monitoring patients using dextran sulfate (not part of Abrams' study) have reported encouraging results. Usually these patients are combining dextran sulfate with low-dose AZT (generally half dose or less), high dose acyclovir, and often an AL 721 substitute. Usually T-helper cells have shown large increases for those starting with 200 or more; for those with less than 200, T-cell results are inconsistent. Patients also report feeling better, for example having more energy, and have gained weight. But their physicians believe it is too early to tell whether benefits will be sustained beyond the five to six months for which data is available.

Dextran sulfate remains a promising treatment possibility—especially in combination with other drugs—but at this time nobody can be sure whether or not it will prove helpful. Dextran sulfate stops HIV in the laboratory at concentrations which can be achieved in the bloodstream, suggesting that it might work as a treatment—but not proving that it will.

DEXTRAN SULFATE: MONITORING AND SAFETY

Anyone using dextran sulfate should be monitored by a physician. While the drug has been used in Japan for 20 years and is available there without a prescription, the doses being tried for AIDS and ARC—usually 1800 to 3600 mg per day—are larger than the 900 per day commonly used in Japan.

No one has been harmed by dextran sulfate so far as we know. But there have been minor side effects, and changes in blood tests which might lead to serious problems if not caught early. Until more is known, it makes sense to err on the side of safety.

What we have heard as effects to watch for are:

- High transaminase levels, which could indicate liver toxicity. Most physicians are only seeing these at higher doses, and are not worried by small changes.

- Serious drops in white blood count, or in platelets. We have only heard of this problem in one or two patients. These changes may not have been due to dextran sulfate; but just in case, these values should be monitored.

- Some patients report a bloated feeling, or diarrhea, especially when starting the treatment.

- We have heard one report of a nosebleed. However, the San Francisco General trial has not found any coagulation problems.

- Especially at very large doses, some patients in the San Francisco test reported feeling "speedy."

The Japanese equivalent of the *Physician's Desk Reference* lists other precautions. These are translated in *AIDS Treatment News,* Issue Number 50.

For more information on dextran sulfate, including availability, call Project Inform (see Appendix B).

AL 721 DEVELOPER SPEAKS

The experimental AIDS treatment AL 721 continues to be controversial. Recently we spoke with the principal developer of AL 721, Meir Shinitzky, Ph.D., a cancer researcher and Professor in the Department of Membrane Research at the Weizmann Institute of Science in Rehovot, Israel. Dr. Shinitzky gave us new information about two trials of AL 721 in Israel, and an additional study beginning in France to compare AL 721 with AZT.

We tape recorded part of the conversation, but we chose to quote most of the material indirectly rather than word for word, as we could not get back to Shinitzky by press time to verify the changes which would have been necessary to make our discussion clear to readers unfamiliar with AL 721. We used verbatim quotes when we could. "AL 721" is a trademark of Ethigen Corporation, Los Angeles.

The Compassionate Study in Israel

Shinitzky told us that there were two clinical trials now ongoing in Israel. The first is a compassionate trial started by Yehuda Skornick, M.D. This trial (now being conducted by other physicians because Dr. Skornick is working in the U.S.) has treated about 60 patients so far.

But this compassionate trial, Shinitzky explained, was not organized for obtaining scientific data; and therefore "the medical community will never accept such a trial for documentation."

A major problem has been the difficulty in followup. About 80 percent of the patients are from abroad. After laboratory work and diagnosis, they were given AL 721; the physicians asked them to send back data after they returned home. But most didn't comply and disappeared after they left Israel.

"We have data on only 12 of them. It's hard to make any real statement. But out of this 12 there was a clear-cut positive effect."

A Scientific Trial

Shinitzky explained that in addition to this compassionate trial, Israeli researchers at the Tel Aviv Medical Center started a more scientific study with 16 patients about one year ago; the principal investigator is Dr. Yust. Unlike most U.S. studies, which try to select a more uniform groups of patients, this trial included persons with AIDS, persons with ARC, and asymptomatic seropositives within the group of 16.

Nine of the 16 were P24 antigen positive when they started; all 16 were HIV antibody positive of course. "In these nine, five showed clear-cut reduction to the basal detectable level" (apparently meaning they became antigen negative) on the Pasteur test kit used. Shinitzky noted that this result seemed compatible with the result of the only U.S. clinical trial of AL 721 completed so far, the St. Luke's/Roosevelt study in New York, in which about 60 percent of the patients showed a large reduction in reverse transcriptase (an earlier measure of viral activity, used before the P24 antigen test was available).

We asked how often the P24 antigen went negative without any treatment. Shinitzky said such cases were rare and would never happen five times out of nine.

For two of the other four patients who did not respond to AL 721, the researchers started AZT in addition to AL 721. These patients had a marked decrease in antigen; one, however, had a brain infection and died in two weeks. The other is alive and doing well. Shinitzky noted that while two cases could certainly not provide proof, it seemed that the drugs might be synergistic, working much better in combination than separately. Shinitzky also thought that the AL 721 might be reducing the side effects of the AZT.

The other two patients did not respond at all. Both of them had AIDS.

Of the five who did become antigen negative, three were asymptomatic, one had lymphadenopathy, and the other had KS, which has since disappeared. All of them feel far better than when they started.

We asked about the other seven of the 16, who had been P24 antigen negative at the start of the trial. Shinitzky said that all responded well to the treatment, but that it was hard to evaluate these cases because there was no biochemical measure to follow.

We asked if these results would be presented at the Stockholm AIDS conference in June. Shinitzky said the work had been submitted; if it is accepted the researchers will present it formally, otherwise they will finalize it for scientific publication elsewhere as soon as possible.

French Study Planned

We asked Shinitzky about reports of an AL 721 study which has just begun in France. Here is his response:

> The French researchers, in particularly Dr. Montagnier of the Pasteur Institute, who is the key figure in AIDS research today probably in all of Europe, expressed his willingness to participate in such as study. As you know the French won't do it unless they are quite convinced.
>
> The head of the Israeli AIDS Association went to Dr. Montagnier's lab to learn the latest in antigen monitoring and so on. They developed good relations and together designed a protocol that later was given to other groups, including one from Marseilles. The study has just started.

In this particular study a well defined group of people—100 to 200, I don't have the exact number—will be divided into equivalent groups. One will be given AZT for three months, the other will be given AL 721, and then there will be a crossover. With this design we avoid using a placebo for a control group. The results can be analyzed as a comparative study.

Since AZT is already approved as an effective drug, if you find that our material is as effective or even further, of course it has the advantage of being nontoxic.

And after this study is finished, both groups will be kept on AL 721. Some of them will also be given a thymus hormone, assuming that the virus has been reduced.

In those people in whom the virus has been reduced after six months of the trial, all will be kept on AL 721, and some of them will be given a thymus hormone; the one selected was THF, thymus humoral factor, which has been analyzed and characterized at the Weizmann Institute by Dr. Trainin. So it will be a combined-treatment study, even though the beginning and the most substantial part of the study will be our compound.

AL 721 VS. "WORKALIKE" PRODUCTS— BACKGROUND NOTE

AL 721 has looked promising for almost three years, and safety has never been an issue. Nevertheless for most of this time persons with AIDS or ARC have been unable to obtain the treatment, as it was tied up in the process of seeking approval from the FDA as a drug—a process originally expected to take four years, but which will probably take longer than that (even if AL 721 is in fact effective). Both Ethigen Corporation (the company which holds worldwide rights to AL 721, under license from the Weizmann Institute), and the FDA, can make a case that the delays are not their fault. Meanwhile the treatment, known to be safe and widely suspected to be significantly helpful to many people, remained unavailable.

During the last 15 months, especially the last year, self-help groups of persons with AIDS and ARC have found sources of comparable products through food-processing and pharmaceutical companies. This treatment underground has grown almost overnight until now thousands of people are using these products, commonly called "egg lecithin lipids," or just "lipids." Several informal surveys, including one which this writer conducted of over 100 users of AL 721 workalike products, have all found comparable results: roughly half of those who have used them are convinced they are helping, less than a quarter are convinced they are not, and the others are uncertain. (For our survey results, see *AIDS Treatment News*, Issue Number 39.)

We asked Dr. Shinitzky what he thought about how these products compared to the official AL 721 as he made it in Israel. The question puts him in a difficult position, as his institution licensed exclusive worldwide rights to AL 721, and he didn't have a simple answer. He did indicate that some of the "generic" products he has seen are considerably closer than others. But the only product named in our conversation, an egg-lecithin capsule sold in health-food stores, was a "straw man" as no one considers it an AL 721 equivalent.

Shinitzky has examined the manufacturing and quality control now used for the "official" AL 721, and is happy with it.

We asked what we should look at when comparing the generic products with AL 721. He answered:

> There are two important factors that contribute to the activity of this compound. The first one is obvious: the correct ratio, 7:2:1. But even if you have separate components hypothetically and you mix them together to get the ratio 7:2:1, it won't necessarily be as potent as the original AL, because the process of production of AL, the acetone extraction, is critical, in my view.
>
> There is a chemical rationale. The reason we started with acetone extraction is that if you take lecithin and dissolve it in acetone, and cool it, you get separation between two components; one precipitates and the other stays in solution. We collect just one of them, this is the part that is included in the 7:2:1. Other extractions do not discriminate. I didn't realize this could be a big difference between the materials, but it turns out it's indeed so. So both the composition and the process of manufacturing are critical.

Shinitzky warned that acetone extraction can be dangerous because this solvent is highly flammable.

(At least one of the "workalike" products—the "Nutri PE9+" from Nutricology, Inc. in San Leandro, California—does use an acetone extraction step in its manufacturing process.)

Preparing AL 721

We asked Shinitzky if it was true that AL 721 may work better if well mixed with water or orange juice, as with a blender.

Shinitzky said that there were still unanswered questions about how AL 721 is absorbed from the small intestines. But he does think that mixing the substance well in liquid (orange juice or water are often used) may make it easier to absorb. He thought that one minute in a blender would be plenty—and that one can see a change visually when the lipids are mixed well, as the mixture takes on a lighter, milkier appearance.

NOTE ON AL 721 TECHNICAL CONTROVERSY

Many U.S. physicians and scientists believe that AL 721 could not work, because it would be digested and not have any effect except as a nutrient. Shortly before going to press we found published information bearing on this question. We could not reach Shinitzky for his comments, however.

In the laboratory, according to Shinitzky's published papers, AL 721 forms "chylomicron-like" assemblies, visible under an electron microscope. These are believed to consist of a spherical core of "neutral lipids" (one of the ingredients of AL 721) with a thin layer of phospholipids (the other two ingredients) around the surface. Most U.S. physicians who have considered the matter have dismissed AL 721, saying that the chylomicrons would be broken up during digestion, and the product would therefore be ineffective.

Recently we found a discussion of blood lipids in a standard medical reference work, *The Pharmacological Basis of Therapeutics* (1985 edition, pages 827–829). It lists chylomicrons as one of six classes of blood lipids. It also lists the source of the neutral-lipid core of these chylomicrons as dietary fats absorbed from the small intestines during digestion.

The chylomicrons this book referred to have the same neutral-lipid core, but different molecules on their surface (not phospholipids as in AL 721). In both cases, however, the surface molecules have electrical charges which predispose them to form chylomicron structures. And it is generally accepted that the phospholipids in AL 721 do enter the bloodstream in a biologically active form; dozens of articles in medical journals describe trials using these food substances alone as experimental treatments for a variety of conditions, with mixed results.

No one has studied the digestion and absorption of AL 721, therefore no one knows if chylomicrons of AL 721 are found in the blood after oral use of the substance. The information cited above certainly suggests that they might be.

As far as we know, those who have said that AL 721 could not possibly work because it would be digested have never cited any facts or arguments to support their assertion. The hasty dismissal of this potential treatment seems not to accord with available information, but to contradict it.

SHINITZKY INTERVIEW IN *NEW YORK NATIVE*

In a wide-ranging interview in the *New York Native* (April 25, 1988), Meir Shinitzky used examples from the history of AL 721 to examine the state of AIDS research. That article, full of specifics and details, includes some of the strongest criticism ever made of the mismanagement of AIDS treatment development in the United States.

For a copy of the April 25 issue, send $3 to the *New York Native*, Back Issues Department (see Appendix B).

Issue Number 56
May 6, 1988

AEROSOL PENTAMIDINE, DEXTRAN SULFATE DELAYED BY LACK OF STAFF

On April 28 and 29, Representives Ted Weiss, Nancy Pelosi, and others on the House Subcommittee on Human Resources grilled Federal officials on AIDS treatment research delays. *The New York Times* reported in a page-one story (April 30) that Dr. Anthony Fauci, director of the National Institute of Allergy and Infectious Diseases (NIAID), admitted that lack of staff had delayed some of the most promising drugs for up to a year. Examples given were dextran sulfate and aerosol pentamidine—the latter still not in Federal trials for over a year after receiving high-priority status at NIAID. Of 24 drugs assigned high priority status by a NIAID committee, only 13 are now in Federal clinical trials.

Fauci said that lack of a single full-time person to "chaperone" aerosol pentamidine through the many bureaucratic obstacles to testing and approval had caused the year-long delay in Federal trials and subsequent FDA approval. (We could add that this delay is almost certainly responsible for many hundreds of deaths, as many physicians refuse to consider using treatments not approved by the FDA, regardless of circumstances.)

Fauci also said that if he had pneumocystis, he would probably try to get the treatment wherever he could.

We were not at the hearings, which took place in Washington, D.C.; but Martin Delaney of Project Inform, who testified April 28, told us that Representatives Weiss and Pelosi were very well prepared, and very aggressive in representing the patients' point of view.

Quote

"Future historians will decide whether AIDS was an epidemic that was allowed to happen in America or an example of the biomedical community's ability to respond promptly to a crisis. Perhaps both are true." (From Howard M. Termin, M.D., in "An Academic's Perspective On AIDS Research," *Issues In Science and Technology,* published by the Institute of Medicine, National Academy of Sciences, Winter 1988. Dr. Termin's article is a commentary on Dr. Anthony Fauci's "The Scientific Agenda for AIDS," in the same issue.)

AEROSOL PENTAMIDINE: THE NEED FOR ADVOCACY

Ryan White, diagnosed with AIDS three years ago at age 13, has become well known to the nation through media coverage of his situation. White, exposed to AIDS through a hemophilia treatment, was banned from the local school and forced by prejudice to move from Kokomo, Indiana to Arcadia, Indiana, where he and his family found acceptance. Three years ago, doctors predicted he had six months to live.

In January 1988 Ryan White was hospitalized for a recurrence of pneumocystis. Michael Callen, co-founder of the People With AIDS Coalition in New York, called White's family to make sure they knew about aerosol pentamidine. It turned out that the family had not been told about that treatment, or any other preventive for pneumocystis.

Callen sent a packet of information for the physician. Ryan White is now using aerosol pentamidine and doing well.

It surprises us that even in so well known a case, the family was not told about the option of pneumocystis prophylaxis. While not formally approved by the FDA—due to research delays like those cited above—prophylaxis by aerosol pentamidine or other treatments has become the standard of care of experienced AIDS physicians. An editorial in the *New England Journal of Medicine* (October 15, 1987) recommended it for those at risk for pneumocystis.

Note: Michael Callen, a well-known singer as well as AIDS activist, was diagnosed six years ago and not expected to live past 1984. He is very much alive and just released his first solo album, *Purple Heart,* a collection of songs about being gay in the age of AIDS. *Purple Heart* is available through Significant Other Records (see Appendix B).

DEXTRAN SULFATE, IMUTHIOL (DTC) AND "ALTERNATIVE" TRIALS: CONVERSATIONS WITH DONALD ABRAMS, M.D.—PART II

Part I of this interview (*AIDS Treatment News,* Issue Number 54) concerned the activities and plans of the County Community Consortium. Part II concerns dextran sulfate, imuthiol, and other clinical trials at San Francisco General Hospital in which Dr. Abrams has been an investigator.

Dextran Sulfate

JJ: How did the dextran sulfate trial get started?

DA: After the II International Conference on AIDS (Paris, June 1986), I went to a conference in Japan to do a presentation, and at that time I was introduced to two people from Ueno Fine Chemical Company in Japan who thought they had something with potential anti-HIV activity in the laboratory. Normally I get mail from people who have the cure for AIDS every day; if I listened to all of them I would spend all my time listening and corresponding with these people.

But the Ueno people showed me a graph of data from Dr. Samuel Broder's lab at NIH, which had some of the preliminary studies on dextran sulfate. And they asked me if I was interested in helping them bring this drug to the U.S. for testing in a carefully-controlled phase I trial. They were a chemical company and had no experience doing clinical research. I said, let's do it.

They wouldn't tell me the name of the compound, they said it was confidential and they wanted to make sure I really was going to collaborate, so they gave me the code name, UA001. I wrote a protocol with an unknown substance, using the model of what a phase I study is. Just because something works in a test tube doesn't mean it's going to work in human beings. So what we do when we take a drug that's new is see what its tolerances and toxicities are.

They said that this substance had been used in Japan for 20 years, but unfortunately there was no real background data. Our FDA has some baseline requirements before they allow people to buy and take a prescribed drug, and I think that's there to protect us. I'm not concerned about our FDA. I think that sometimes they can be a little bit much, but overall they are here to protect the consumer.

So I wrote the protocol. We did have a lot of communication between us and the FDA with regard to eligibility, who should be on it, and how to keep the study absolutely pure and make sure the patients were only taking this substance. We needed a group of patients in whom we could really measure the effects of UA001 on their systems.

In a phase I study you just give increasing dosages to see what the maximum dose is. When you find that, then you can see if the drug has any effectiveness. That's called the phase II study, when you're looking for effectiveness. Sometimes with AIDS these two phases are combined, into a phase I/phase II trial.

Then they told me that UA001 was dextran sulfate, and we began a study. I mentioned it to a few people here, and they said it's a non-specific antiviral that they use in culture media; it prevents viruses from entering cells in the culture media. But it's a large polymer; if you take it by mouth it will be digested and it won't be the same substance that they're using in the test tube that will get to HIV-infected cells, because the body will digest it or won't absorb it, because it's too large a molecule. It could not be pharmaceutically effective, they said, because it has a molecular weight of seven to eight thousand and would not enter cells. People were skeptical, saying this would never work, don't do it. But we had a study. Recruitment was slow, however, because most people were using AZT, and didn't want to give it up.

Since we were testing doses that were higher than people ever take in Japan, the FDA required patients to be on the low doses for two weeks (a month at the higher doses) before we could start the next group on the next higher dose.

After a while, people heard that we were testing dextran sulfate, just as people heard that we were testing DTC and started obtaining DTC by their own means and taking it as well. It seems like every time we try to study something, people think that because it's being studied maybe it's the cure. Or people read the scientific literature about what it does in the test tube.

Here we are doing our dextran sulfate study, and suddenly it's all over the streets. We're told that patients on our lowest dosages might not be taking the dose that we think they're taking.

We have seen some toxic effects of this drug, especially in patients taking the highest dose.

We are conducting an eight-week study, not using a placebo, but using escalating doses instead. And to be fair to patients who participated for the eight weeks, we let them continue their dose after that if they can tolerate it. Studies don't always do that; but we want to be thankful to our people who are participating, and also gain some information as to the longer term safety, tolerance, and efficacy of the drug. Eight weeks is a good time to observe for toxicity, but seeing if something works may take longer.

After the eight weeks, we monitor the patients who choose to continue using the drug just as we did during the eight weeks. But now we learn that some of the people we started to see toxic effects on, at what we thought was the lowest dose, may actually be taking what we're giving them plus some more they're getting on the street. So how can we make any statement now about toxicities or the side effects of this particular dose, when the people that we think are taking it aren't? A bit of a problem.

JJ: It is a problem. But looking at it from another point of view, it's not right to keep thousands of people from taking something so that a few can be forced into a study. The approach, then, would be to find people who don't have a strong feeling one way or another about the drug, they're in it not because it's the only way they can get the drug, but they're in it for the free blood work...

DA: Why would thousands of people want to take something if it doesn't work or if it's toxic? This is the same argument we went through with suramin. People demanded that we make suramin available to everybody, and it killed people. If you don't study it, how are you going to know if it does anything or if it's harmful or helpful?

JJ: What about the controversy over whether the oral drug you are using could get into the bloodstream? Why is there any question when this drug has been used orally for 20 years in Japan?

DA: Our phase I study also drew blood from patients so that we could measure the drug, to demonstrate that it got into the bloodstream. My Japanese collaborators have not been able to demonstrate that this drug has entered into the bloodstream of my patients taking it.

They showed me from healthy people in Japan that they were able to demonstrate that the drug entered the system after being swallowed. But you cannot import HIV-infected blood into Japan. Ueno's researchers took 50 specimens back with them to Japan in January. They tried to get somebody here to do the measuring, but they couldn't find anybody to perform the test satisfactorily.

They had to heat-inactivate the specimens (to legally take them into Japan for testing). By doing that they precipitated the dextran sulfate with the plasma, so they were unable to find it. So there is no evidence that drug is absorbed into anybody's bloodstream, at this point in time, to convince to anybody's satisfaction that there is oral bioavailability.

JJ: I don't understand. People have been using this drug orally for 20 years in Japan. How could it not be absorbed?

DA: The drug isn't licensed in the United States for the same indications.

JJ: You say in Japan they found it got in the bloodstream?

DA: From three healthy volunteers. I've learned to be cautious. I'd like to know what the levels are in my patients.

We've been doing the study now for almost a year and we haven't found any laboratory here (to measure it in the blood). It's a stumbling block.

JJ: What groups of patients enrolled in the dextran sulfate trial? The patients enrolled mostly had lymphadenopathy. The reason that it's weighted toward these patients is that the eligibility criteria said they could be on no other medications, because we want to see the effects of dextran sulfate. And it's hard to find a patient with AIDS who isn't taking something. So there are only four people with AIDS in the entire trial. The FDA wants to see what this drug does by itself.

I looked for patients who had a greater than 20 percent increase in their T-helper number from week zero to week eight, and that was one-third of the low-dose groups. (The high-dose groups have not yet had their blood work done, so they are not included in this result.) Without a placebo we don't know how many would have shown that increase without treatment.

JJ: As you know, there is a rumor that you were responsible for making it hard for Americans to buy dextran sulfate. I have never seen evidence for this rumor. Do you want to say anything to clarify the situation?

DA: It's so upsetting to me. When in the course of my day did I have time to deal with whatever agencies are necessary to block importation of agents into countries? I don't know where this rumor came from. I've heard that it's very widespread, nationwide, that I am some sort of an ogre who set up roadblocks at borders. How am I so powerful?

JJ: People assumed you must have called Ueno, and Ueno had a way with the Japanese companies to get them to stop selling to Americans, in order to support their trial. That's what some people believe.

DA: We're working together, and they (Ueno) realized that the drug was flooding the market. Whatever happened happened, and I don't know how I could have any control over this. I was told that a patient was trying to bring dextran sulfate in, and also DTC, across the border from Mexico and was allowed to bring his DTC but was told he couldn't bring dextran because there's a study being done in San Francisco. I hear about these things second hand.

JJ: What future plans do you have to study dextran sulfate?

DA: I told the AIDS Clinical Trials Group (at NIH) that I wanted to present a phase II study to evaluate the antiretroviral activity of dextran sulfate in patients who are P24 antigen positive. The P24 test is what they want now as a criterion for their studies. I said let's extend this study for six months, no placebo, to get this information.

In the meantime I've asked the Japanese to get me an intravenous preparation of the drug, and I've submitted to the FDA the protocol we wrote.

Robbie Wong and myself wrote a pharmacology study, intravenous vs oral. We'll measure the levels after an IV dose and compare it to an oral dose.

Also I've just written a protocol for a combination of dextran sulfate and AZT, which we're going to do here.

For me it remains a compound that has some interest, especially because it appears to have a different mechanism of action compared to the other antiretroviral agents, in the test tube.

The Imuthiol (DTC) Study: Why No Results Yet?

Note: We reported on the imuthiol study over a year ago (*AIDS Treatment News*, Issue Number 29). The San Francisco General Hospital arm of the study has long been finished. Many people are concerned that the results have not yet been released.

Dr. Abrams discussed this question on several occasions. We summarized the conversations, adding background information to clarify the matter for our readers.

• The imuthiol clinical trial is sponsored and financed by the drug's manufacturer, Institut Merieux, in Lyon, France. Several U.S. medical centers conducted this placebo-controlled trial.

• Some of the centers were unable to recruit their full quota of patients. As a result, San Francisco General Hospital was asked to recruit more patients, and did so.

• When there still weren't enough patients, Merieux added two new centers, at Key West, Florida, and Downstate Medical Center in Brooklyn, NY. It naturally took time to set up the program at these centers. (And we heard from another physician— not Dr. Abrams—that at least one of the new centers had serious delays in recruiting.) Some patients are just now starting the trial, meaning that they will not complete it for six months.

• So far Merieux has chosen not to release preliminary data, but to wait until all patients are finished at all centers, despite repeated pleas from Dr. Abrams. (San Francisco General Hospital does not have the data except from its own patients, and it does not know which of them were on the placebo.)

• To make the best of the situation, Dr. Abrams asked Merieux to supply additional imuthiol so that patients finishing the trial could go on "open label," receiving the drug if they chose—whether or not they had been on placebo originally. Merieux agreed. So these patients are obtaining treatment, and long-term data is being accumulated.

• The larger problem is that physicians and persons with AIDS do not have information they need to make treatment decisions. And other scientists, even the leading researchers at NIH, do not know how to prioritize DTC for future studies. Dr. Abrams has urged the company to do a preliminary analysis, even if it does not choose to unblind the study (by telling which patients got the placebo). We do not know when results may be released.

"We went to a meeting (with Merieux) in San Diego last Tuesday. I used your story (AIDS Treatment News, Issue Number 54) to take up to the scientific directors, and said, this is a problem, you have not lived up to your part of the bargain, we have had patients on this trial for over a year now and there is no cracking of the code, we're dragging our feet, and we are losing the respect of our community that we need to participate in these trials." At that meeting, Merieux also gave Dr. Abrams its view of whether the prescription drug antabuse would be an effective substitute for imuthiol. The company has a strong interest in this question, because if the answer is yes, then the imuthiol they have been developing for several years may have little commercial value.

"The Merieux people are quite adamant that they have all the data they need to demonstrate that antabuse does not break down into DTC (imuthiol). Robert Gorter (a physician at San Francisco General who worked with Dr. Abrams on the imuthiol trial) is going to try to pursue that further, because it differs from his understanding.

"I told you before about my skepticism about drug companies. That skepticism is important."

Meanwhile, what could be said about DTC, before we have the data? Dr. Abrams seems happy with the results. There have been surprisingly few deaths in the study, and the patients seem to be doing well.

"Alternative" Treatment Trials: A Hidden History

We learned recently that Dr. Abrams has designed and often conducted a number of clinical trials largely unknown to the AIDS community. Some of these trials tested "alternative" treatments, that is, those initiated by patients themselves rather than by drug companies or the National Institutes of Health. Dr. Abrams approached these treatments neither as a believer nor disbeliever, but as an investigator who felt that substances people were using deserved scientific study to find out whether they worked or not.

Here is an annotated list of protocols (some for alternative treatments) designed, co-designed or conducted by Dr. Abrams:

Interferon alpha (1984). This trial involved 18 patients, half on placebo. Dr. Abrams presented the results at the II International Conference on AIDS (Paris, June 1986), but did not publish them, because the study did not find much; on the whole, patients on the drug did no better than those on the placebo. One of the treatment patients has been a long-time survivor and is still taking the interferon, however.

"Now the wheel has come full circle almost, and Tony Fauci (at NIH) is treating asymptomatic seropositives with interferon alpha."

Isoprinosine (1985).   Dr. Abrams became one of the investigators in a multi-centered trial of isoprinosine.

"I did it because there was a lot of interest in the community in isoprinosine. I knew people were going to Mexico to get it. I knew it was an antiviral and decided to look at it with a placebo-controlled trial.

"We put 24 patients on the trial very quickly. People knew they might get a placebo, but they were taking it only for one month. Then we followed them for three months.

"I participated, not believing that this was going to be the miracle cure, but to confirm the original data that was coming from New York, data that was getting people excited. We wanted to see if this drug was worth pursuing.

"But while the study was in progress the drug company got itself into some difficulty by making claims about the drug that could not be supported."

Due to the political controversy and confusion, Dr. Abrams (and the patients and the public) never learned the results of that trial—not even today, three years later.

Vitamin C (1985).   "Through personal friends and acquaintances I met some of the early people who felt that vitamin C was part of the answer. These contacts in the community put me in touch with investigators at the Linus Pauling Institute. For a year I informed them about AIDS, and they informed me about their results with vitamin C in cancer patients. We decided what dosage we would try.

"We wrote a protocol and sent it to NIH. We worked for a year and a half trying to get this study funded someplace. The government didn't want it. So we submitted it to the Universitywide Task Force On AIDS, but their reviewers didn't think it was worth investing in, so we didn't do the study.

"In the meantime, unfortunately, most of the people who helped me realize that the community wanted to look at vitamin C had died of the disease. So it became clear to me that it probably wasn't a cure."

Relaxation and Imagery (1986).   "There was a movement a few years ago saying that relaxation and positive thinking, such as the Simonton approach, was the cure. There was a patient written up in the Sunday paper who reportedly was cured of AIDS through positive thinking. Now he has died of the disease, but at that time there was more interest in it.

"I said, okay, nothing I have is the answer, so I'm willing to investigate it. I wrote a study with Inge Corless, who was a postdoctoral nurse with the Robert Woods Johnson program.

"We did a controlled trial. For six weeks half of the patients were just followed by me in the clinic, the other half were seen intensively by Inge Corless. She did a program composed of relaxation, imagery, and therapeutic touch.

"We investigated its effects on platelet counts, helper suppressor ratio, and adrenal function. We found no particular change in these parameters, but patients in the intervention group were less stressed, and had better psychological adjustment scores.

"This study, as most of the studies I've been involved in, was not funded by any granting agency; it's something I did because it's an alternative approach that may have some foundation in reality, but it needs to be tested."

Ribavirin (1985). "I felt we should look at ribavirin as well, because so many people were going to Mexico to get it. For the same reason: if this works, we should know about it; and we're not going to know about it unless we do a controlled study.

"You know the ribavirin mixup?" (Part of this long and controversial story appeared recently in the *Wall Street Journal*—April 13, 1988, "Shop Talk" column, page 31).

"I was only peripherally involved in the ribavirin study."

Chinese medicine (1988). Dr. Abrams is working with Barbara Bernie, president of the American Foundation of Traditional Chinese Medicine. "This study will evaluate certain herbal treatments, breathing exercises, and other traditional Chinese medical interventions. Since it is currently not funded, and staffing is required for monitoring at the AIDS Clinic, the logistics are becoming difficult. Hopefully we can work something out in the near future."

DNCB. Within the last month Dr. Abrams has worked with Elswood, of the grassroots DNCB movement in San Francisco, to write a protocol for a scientific test of this AIDS treatment which has been used by thousands of people through "guerilla clinics." He just sent the protocol to the FDA. Even if the FDA approves the study, funding must still be found. Funding may be a problem because DNCB is not patentable so no drug company has any incentive to investigate it; and NIH has not been interested.

Consortium Studies. Dr. Abrams is also involved with several studies planned by the County Community Consortium in San Francisco. Their aerosol pentamidine study, which is already in operation, was described at length in part I of this interview.

Other studies now in preparation include:

• An alternative treatment registry. Private-practice physicians will work with their patients to monitor whatever they are trying, whether or not prescribed by a physician. If the researchers see any trend in either clinical, virologic, or immunological parameters, the treatments which may be responsible can be studied with more control.

• A zidovudine registry. This will monitor long-term side effects and benefits from AZT (zidovudine).

• A study of prophylaxis against MAI.

• An attempt to alleviate anemia caused by AZT.

Issue Number 57
May 20, 1988

VIRX: NEW AIDS CLINIC OPENS IN SAN FRANCISCO

A new kind of AIDS clinic and treatment research center is seeing its first patients this week in San Francisco. We interviewed its founder, Robert E. Anderson, M.D.

ViRx Medical Group, Inc. aims to bring together patients seeking the latest AIDS research information and access to experimental treatments, with pharmaceutical companies which have promising drugs to test. ViRx differs from government and university research centers in that as a private company it has more flexibility and hopes to move faster in conducting trials. ViRx has also assembled top people in AIDS research, such as Dr. Luc Montagnier of the Pasteur Institute in Paris, who will serve as a consultant to keep ViRx informed on the most interesting treatment developments in Europe and elsewhere.

During its current start-up phase, however, ViRx is not yet conducting clinical trials, so patients will not have access to experimental treatments yet. Meanwhile they can benefit from the company's treatment expertise and its state-of-the-art research facilities. These facilities—the laboratory and an extensive in-house database of treatment information—are paid for by the investor, a major venture-capital company, and not out of patient fees, which are comparable to standard physician and laboratory charges.

Patients may also benefit because ViRx is spending considerable resources to inform itself of interesting treatments being tested anywhere; it will inform persons of such options even if ViRx itself cannot acquire them and must refer its patients elsewhere. Another advantage for patients now is that they can register to be informed immediately if any clinical trials for which they qualify do begin at ViRx.

ViRx will charge customary rates for its patient consulting and monitoring services, which should be covered by insurance. Any additional costs for sponsored clinical trials will usually be paid by the drug company. Later, ViRx may also sponsor its own trials, with the pharmaceutical company providing only the drug; then the cost of additional monitoring required might have to be paid by the patient, since insurance companies do not pay for experimental treatments. For nontoxic drugs, the routine monitoring being done anyway may be sufficient, meaning that the total additional cost to do the trial may be very small.

All this means that patients should usually be able to participate in most experimental trials through ViRx at little or no cost, beyond the cost of routine monitoring which is recommended anyway and covered by insurance.

Patients should be aware, however, that ViRx insists that it "is not a supermarket" for AIDS treatments. It will only use experimental treatments as part of scientific protocols. Therefore new treatments will seldom be available unless the company which owns a drug wants to run trials, and uses ViRx to do so.

Besides counseling and laboratory monitoring, ViRx would prefer not to provide primary care, handle hospitalizations, etc. Its clients will usually have their own physicians, and ViRx will be cooperating rather than competing with community physicians. But ViRx will expand patient services if its patients require them.

ViRx is seeking patients at all stages of HIV infection, from asymptomatic to persons with ARC or AIDS.

Personnel

The founder of ViRx, president Robert E. Anderson, M.D., has been Chief of the AIDS Section of the California Department of Health Services, and was the Public Health Medical Officer for AIDS in California. He also co-founded the San Francisco Men's Health Study. He is a specialist in laboratory testing procedures, and has authored or coauthored over a dozen papers or presentations on AIDS.

Other key consultants and personnel are:

- Dr. Dannie King, who was head of infectious diseases at Burroughs-Wellcome when AZT achieved its rapid licensing. "He knows how to make the FDA work."

- Peter Hutt, former general counsel of the FDA, and an expert on the history of drug regulatory law. He was involved in negotiating the treatment IND regulations.

- Gary Wilcox, a molecular biologist.

- William Lang, M.D., consultant and clinical supervisor.

- Bruce Decker, in business development.

ViRx is currently recruiting a full-time physician for both clinical and research work.

Facilities

ViRx has its own state of the art laboratory and can do T-cell subsets and P24 antigen testing on the premises. ViRx will use several quality-control checks not usually done in commercial labs to assure more accurate counts.

ViRx also has a computer network throughout the facility. Every examining room has a terminal. Patient records are coded with numbers to protect confidentiality; all identifying information is kept separately. The computer will also be used to monitor results of whatever treatments patients are already using.

Comment

ViRx hopes to conduct dozens if not hundreds of drug trials. It hopes to significantly speed FDA approval for the drugs it studies, by more quickly providing the data required by that agency. If it succeeds, the company could make a major contribution to AIDS treatment development.

What does ViRx offer to patients? Eventually it will provide access to experimental treatments which may be unavailable elsewhere. Already it has a top-quality laboratory, as well as an in-house database of treatment information, with staff who are informed about treatment options and have time to discuss them with patients.

ViRx can make an important contribution to AIDS drug development and to patient services. But since it is seeing patients for the first time this week, it is too early to know how successful this company will be in attracting patients and sponsored research.

MM-1: SECRET DRUG TESTED IN EGYPT AND ZAIRE

MM-1 is an antiviral drug developed and tested by a team of physicians in Egypt and Zaire. Several hundred people so far have received the drug, which is given as a series of 20 intramuscular injections over several weeks, and the results from several dozen persons have been reported.

The developers have made impressive claims for efficacy, and widespread news reports have generated much interest. But "MM-1" is only a code name; the developers have not revealed what the substance is. Therefore other physicians and scientists have been unable to evaluate the treatment. Most observers have kept a healthy skepticism, while agreeing that MM-1 is certainly worth a closer look.

The Claims

A one-page report from four physicians (reference below) outlined results of a test with 49 patients. MM-1 was given as one intramuscular injection every other day for 10 injections, followed by one every third day for the remaining 10.

No side effects were reported. Nine of the 49 patients died, mostly from advanced opportunistic diseases which they had before beginning treatment. The other 40 "were considered as cured and are conducting a normal life since completion of the treatment six to 10 months ago. Meanwhile, all of the 40 control patients died during the first six months."

Other Published Information

Wire-service reports published in newspapers last Fall quoted one of the physicians who developed MM-1 as saying the drug is inexpensive, and should cost about $10 per injection.

The developers have not revealed what the code name "MM-1" stands for. Rumors in Zaire were that the abbreviation stood for "Mobutu-Mubarak-1," named after the leaders of Zaire and Egypt.

Unpublished Information

We heard the following from confidential sources which seem credible, but is not well known to us. We have not been able to confirm this information independently.
  We have heard:

- That there is one side effect—a high fever, 102 to 103 degrees, 20 minutes after each injection.

- That the developers are so concerned about secrecy that patients remain in a hospital throughout the treatment, lest someone get their blood analyzed and learn what the chemical is.

- That the "cure" may not be permanent; no one knows how long it will last. Apparently at least one person has received the treatment twice.

Speculation

It is widely believed that MM-1 is a commonly available substance. The reason for secrecy may be that the secret is all the developers have to sell.
  The fact that the one alleged side effect—the fever—was not reported in published material suggests that it might be an important clue. It is even conceivable that the drug works by inducing a fever. Perhaps the fever, or the body's reaction which produced it, had a beneficial effect.
  This speculation is consistent with the "honeymoon" period which often follows a first attack of pneumocystis, which causes high fevers. Fevers induced by drugs could be adjusted and scheduled for optimum benefit, without the antigenic stimulation and other disadvantages of fevers produced by a serious disease. A number of experimental treatments for AIDS do in fact cause fevers; could that be responsible in part for their benefit? This possibility deserves a closer look.

Attempts To Learn More

NIAID (the National Institute of Allergy and Infectious Disease) has committees to seek AIDS drugs for testing. It sent a letter to one of the African physicians, but had not heard back yet.
  The buyers clubs in New York and San Francisco raised the money to send a physician to Africa, if such a trip will be productive. At least one U.S. health-care worker has already traveled to either Egypt or Zaire to learn more about MM-1.
  More information may be released at the Stockholm AIDS conference, June 12–16.

REFERENCE

Lurhuma, Z., A. Shafik, M. Diese, and J. Wane, "Role Of MM-1, an Antiviral Agent in the Treatment of Patients with AIDS." (This one-page summary has the latest information we have seen.) An earlier article with the same authors and title was published in *The Egyptian Medical Journal* 4(3) (October 1987).

STOCKHOLM SCIENTIFIC CONFERENCE, JUNE 12-16

The major scientific AIDS conference of the year will take place June 12–16 in Stockholm, Sweden. The "IV International Conference on AIDS" is the fourth in this international series; last year's was in Washington, D.C. in June 1987. Thousands of scientific papers on all aspects of AIDS will be presented.

AIDS Treatment News will be there; we also plan to interview physicians and other participants on what treatment developments they consider most important. We will probably devote several issues primarily to covering this conference.

AIDS COMPUTER CONFERENCE FROM STOCKHOLM

Those who cannot go to Stockholm may be able to participate in a computer conference arranged by the IV International Conference on AIDS.

At this time we do not know how U.S. computer users will connect directly to the "1st AIDS Computer Conference" (1ACC), which will run on a computer called "QZCOM" in Stockholm. But the messages entered into 1ACC will probably be available on various systems in the U.S.

Those familiar with "Usenet," an electronic message system that runs on university computers using the Unix operating system, can probably receive the messages in "sci.med.aids" on that system. Those using Bitnet (available mostly through academic institutions) should check on "AIDSNEWS." Users of these systems will probably redistribute the messages onto various AIDS-related computer bulletin boards, where anyone with a home computer and modem can read them.

A computer conference could potentially have the great advantage of continuing indefinitely, not just for several days of each year. Researchers, physicians, officials, journalists and others could communicate with each other from wherever they are. But successful computer conferences are difficult to organize, so we don't know how well this one will work.

AIDS/HIV EXPERIMENTAL TREATMENT DIRECTORY

The American Foundation for AIDS Research is publishing the latest edition of its important treatment directory this month. Formerly called the *AmFAR Directory of Experimental Treatments for AIDS and ARC,* it will now be titled *AIDS/HIV Experimental Treatment Directory.* This new edition will include background information for people with AIDS.

A one-year subscription, including the directory and updates, costs $30; a single issue is $10. AmFAR will continue its policy of sending a free copy of the directory to any person with AIDS who cannot afford one.

This directory, like the previous editions, includes only treatments for HIV, not those for opportunistic infections. AmFAR does plan to include treatments for opportunistic infections in future editions.

To order the directory, contact AmFAR (see Appendix B).

BUYERS CLUBS ASSIST ACT NOW, MM-1 RESEARCH

On April 28, The Healing Alternatives Foundation (THAF, formerly named Healing Alternatives Buyers Club, or HABC) gave a $1500 emergency grant to ACT NOW to help in coordinating the Spring AIDS Actions of 1988. ACT NOW is a national network of ACT UP and similar local organizations throughout the country (including the AIDS Action Pledge in San Francisco).

THAF and a similar New York buyers club, the PWA Health Group, also pledged several thousand dollars to send a physician to Africa to learn more about MM-1 (see article above), if and when such a trip would be helpful.

These grants were arranged in days, not the weeks or months most funding sources require. They show the potential of the buyers clubs as a major community resource—able to move quickly at critical times, willing to fund treatment and advocacy work which mainstream AIDS organizations have ignored.

Buyers clubs are nonprofit self-help groups formed by persons with AIDS to make available health products, such as AL 721 substitutes, which are hard to find or much more expensive from other sources such a health-food stores. They have also become important channels for all kinds of treatment information.

To contact The Healing Alternatives Foundation, see Appendix B.

AIDS POLITICAL FUNERALS?

Political funerals occur in many parts of the world, for example South Africa and the Middle East. Now this form of protest is being discussed for AIDS.

We first heard the idea several months ago, as plans to scatter human ashes on the White House lawn as a protest of the Reagan Administration's mismanagement of AIDS education and treatment research. But no such action took place.

More recently people are talking about real funerals—with real bodies in the coffins or ashes in the urns—outside of the Japanese embassy in Washington, or consulates throughout the country, in protest against the boycott by Japanese companies against Americans trying to buy dextran sulfate for AIDS/ARC treatment—after the drug had been sold over the counter to anyone for 20 years. (One U.S. AIDS physician called this boycott "immoral and close to murder.")

At this time negotiations are taking place on the dextran sulfate issue, and the protest against Japan may be unnecessary. The White House, of course, remains an appropriate site. But whatever the immediate situation, political funerals will deserve and require careful thought, planning, and work in advance. Whether such funerals ever do occur or should occur, the community should start discussing the possibility now.

The biggest obstacle preventing political funerals is that they will require much detailed work such as overcoming legal difficulties, notifying the press appropriately, and otherwise making detailed arrangements which persons who are dying, and their families and loved ones, would seldom want to do at that time.

An organization would have to take on these arrangements. Like the Neptune Society, which offers burial at sea, a specialized group could handle the details.

Then persons who wanted a political funeral could write their choice in their will, and be spared the burden of arranging the details.

CONGRESS LOOKS AT AIDS RESEARCH DELAYS

On April 28 and 29, Representatives Ted Weiss (D-NY) and Nancy Pelosi (D-SF) held hearings on AIDS research delays and treatment-access problems. These hearings were held in Washington, D.C. by the Subcommittee on Human Resources of the House Government Operations Committee, chaired by Mr. Weiss. Witnesses included top Federal officials in both NIH and FDA, as well as AIDS physicians and treatment advocates.

AIDS Treatment News has already reported the most spectacular single revelation from these hearings—the admission of Dr. Anthony F. Fauci, who is in charge of the AIDS clinical trials run by the U.S. government, that lack of a single staff person delayed testing and approval of aerosol pentamidine for over a year, while similar delays postponed dextran sulfate and other potential AIDS treatments even after they had been given the highest priority by the government's own scientific advisory committees.

These hearings mark the first time members of Congress were well prepared on AIDS research issues, the first time top Federal AIDS officials had to answer to anyone in authority who would not take "fluff" answers and the most shallow of bureaucratic self-justification as revealed, unquestioned truth.

The *New York Times* reported the hearings on page one (Saturday, April 30), but most of the press ignored them. For example, none of the San Francisco daily papers mentioned the hearings at all—despite over a thousand AIDS deaths already in the city, thousands more inevitable unless the research gets results, and—if that weren't enough local relevance—the fact that Nancy Pelosi's Congressional district includes most of San Francisco. (Even San Francisco's gay newspapers largely ignored the hearings, suggesting that the press default stemmed not from conspiracy or homophobia, but from the great difficulty of the press and public alike in getting a grasp on AIDS treatment research and access issues.) Congress will eventually publish the full text of the hearings, several hundred pages, but few will read the fine print. So to convey the impact of the information we interviewed Dr. Steve Morin, a legislative assistant to Congresswoman Pelosi and one of the staff people involved in the hearings, which were arranged and conducted by the Human Resources Subcommittee chaired by Mr. Weiss.

"The Subcommittee put (top Federal officials) under oath, and subpoenaed their records," Morin explained—meaning that for the first time the officials could not simply deflect or ignore the questions and deliver the Reagan Administration line. Morin told us that the message he most wanted to get out is that there are people who care and are working to overcome the obstacles blocking progress in AIDS treatment research.

We asked Dr. Morin for his overview of the hearings, and his sense of what was most important there. Our own comments are in parentheses.

The Interview

"The first witness was a father of an infant with AIDS. He testified anonymously behind a screen, for fear of identification and discrimination. He told about the lack of access of his infant daughter to AZT, in essence because the FDA did not approve the use of AZT for infants. He described his repeated efforts to try to get the drug for his daughter, how he ran into bureaucratic difficulties at every step, how she was now on a respirator and expected to die.

"The next witness was Iris Davis, M.D., a black woman from Brooklyn. She talked about lack of access to experimental protocols for women, IV drug users and ethnic minorities. In Brooklyn these groups are rarely included in clinical trials. The trials tend to go to academic centers, not to the centers that treat the majority of the people with AIDS infections.

"Then Nan Hunter from the ACLU spoke about access to clinical trials for women and ethnic minorities. The trials are seen as offering hope, and the hope was not being offered equally.

"The second panel started with Tom Merigan, M.D., from Stanford University, where he is Principal Investigator of Stanford's AIDS Clinical Trials Unit. He spoke from the perspective of planning and oversight of drug trials, especially the work at Stanford on DDC. He expressed some optimism about that program.

"Dr. Merigan said the investigators run the program by participating in initial review of candidate drugs, devising the protocols, and setting priorities. He said that a total of $64 million in annual funding would be needed for the original 19 AIDS Treatment Evaluation Units, part of the Federal government's AIDS clinical trials program.

"Ms. Pelosi tried to pin down Merigan on community consultation issues, what kind of input did they have from potential participants in the trials. He tried to sidestep the issue as best he could."

(We commented that as far as we knew, the Stanford program had no community input.)

"They have none. He said that the goal is to work for a better patient-physician relationship. In essence it was beyond his way of thinking to involve the AIDS community in the actual planning (of clinical trials).

"Ms. Pelosi raised the issue of dextran sulfate with Merigan, and that started quite a debate. My memory is that he was very critical of the Japanese for not accepting blood samples to test the pharmacological issue of absorption. Apparently the Japanese government just didn't want the contaminated blood coming in to the country. Various lack of cooperation has delayed researchers' ability to say anything definitive out of Donald Abrams' studies.

"Dr. Mathilde Krim, Chairman of the American Foundation for AIDS Research and a leading advocate for more effective and humane treatment development, presented a series of recommendations. Many would require leadership from the administrative branch of government. NIAID (the National Institute of Allergy and Infectious Diseases, part of the National Institutes of Health) should have independent construction authority, as it did not have the facilities to do the research it was being asked to do.

"Ms. Pelosi posed the question (San Francisco AIDS activist) John Fox has posed in our community meeting. When a drug is past phase I, known to be safe, makes theoretical sense that it could be effective but there's no efficacy data, should people be allowed to have access to it? Krim has historically waffled on this question, but she's coming around to a position where she couldn't come up with any good reasons why they shouldn't. It does give people hope, so perhaps these substances should be made available.

"Dr. Krim also described critical staffing shortages at NIAID and the FDA."

(We commented that there was some cynicism in the AIDS community about the FDA's need for more staff, since it already has enough to move against safe and plausible treatment options, without any reason to believe that they are harmful or ineffective.)

"Mr. Weiss and Ms. Pelosi cross-examined Fauci (on staffing problems at NIAID, not FDA), and the total staff working on AIDS drug development, that includes everybody, amounted to 22. This count includes some who may not actually be working on AIDS.

"It's quite unbelievable that they are expected to coordinate all these trials, make these complex decisions about candidate drugs, staff the meetings, bring in scientists to advise, collect and analyze data, with a staff this small."

(The *New York Times*, April 30, page 1, quoted Congressman Weiss as commenting to Fauci that, "The dimensions of the shortfall is such that you can't possibly meet your needs.")

(Part II of this interview appears in *AIDS Treatment News*, Issue Number 58.)

Issue Number 58
June 3, 1988

FLUCONAZOLE FOR CRYPTOCOCCAL MENINGITIS: ANOTHER SUCCESSFUL REPORT

Last September 25, *AIDS Treatment News* published a full report on fluconazole, an experimental drug which seems to be a major advance in treatment of systemic fungal infections, especially cryptococcal meningitis. Unlike amphotericin B, the conventional treatment, fluconazole is given orally, freeing the patient from long-term dependence on intravenous medication. Also it seems to have few, if any, side effects.

The only drawback is that because of red tape, fluconazole is hard to get in the United States. Pfizer Inc., the manufacturer, does supply it for cryptococcal meningitis and certain other conditions when all approved treatments have failed. But in practice many physicians do not know about fluconazole or how to get it, and many patients—perhaps most—who should get the drug, die instead.

In Europe fluconazole is much more available, and thousands of people have used it, even for much less serious conditions such as skin or vaginal yeast infections. But in the U.S., there is a widespread official belief that compassionate-use drugs should not be widely available to persons with AIDS. Various excuses are used, various obstacles are allowed to block treatment access.

Part of the problem is that little has been published on fluconazole. We only know of two case reports in the medical literature of fluconazole used for AIDS-related cryptococcal meningitis. One, published by physicians at the Pasteur Institute (*Annals of Internal Medicine,* May 1987) was cited in our earlier report (*AIDS Treatment News,* Issue Number 41).

The other, the occasion for this article, appeared in the March 1988 *Annals of Internal Medicine* (Byrne, W.R., and C.P. Wajszczuk, "Cryptococcal Meningitis in the Acquired Immunodeficiency Syndrome (AIDS): Successful Treatment with Fluconazole after Failure of Amphotericin B," Volume 108, Number 3, pages 384–385). Fluconazole was used after amphotericin B and other treatments became ineffective; the amphotericin had been used for 15 months. Two weeks after the change

317

to fluconazole, improvement was "dramatic;" and the cerebrospinal fluid culture became negative for the first time in a year, and stayed negative. The patient has done well at home on fluconazole for a year. There have been no side effects.

For medical information about fluconazole and how to obtain it, physicians only should call Pfizer Central Research (see Appendix B).

Readers can help to make fluconazole and other drugs more available by lobbying AIDS organizations—or gay, medical, or other organizations—to educate themselves and appoint a person or committee to work to overcome the red tape, ignorance, inertia, mismanagement, and commercialism blocking the research which should be done and the drugs which should be accessible to physicians and patients. Waiting for the system to move at its own pace will result in thousands of unnecessary deaths. The major AIDS organizations, fearing controversy and loss of funding, have so thoroughly ignored this issue that even a little effort will go a long way.

HYBRIDONS: MAJOR RESEARCH ADVANCE RUMORED; CALL FOR INFORMATION

A well-informed source recently told us that researchers are excited about a designer drug being developed by major pharmaceutical companies. We have not been able to confirm this report, but chose to publish what we heard, in case any of our readers have more information about this project and can help us assemble a complete picture.

Apparently scientists prepared a mirror image of part of the "tat" gene of HIV—a gene which regulates the activity of the virus. This chemical was then attached to a sulfate group to make it water soluble. In this form, according to the report, it enters every cell, and shuts down HIV, with little toxicity to the cell.

The drug has not yet been tried in humans. But according to our source, the same idea was applied to a form of mouse leukemia caused by a virus, and it did work; when given to mice, the mouse version of the drug arrested the disease.

A paper on this technology, called "hybridons," was published two years ago (Zamecnik *et al.*, 1986). It has not received much attention, perhaps because the idea of a designer drug which enters cells and blocks a specific gene seems futuristic, not something imminent. Yet that early paper reported HIV inhibition up to 95 percent in cells in the laboratory, and suggested that the approach seemed useful for treating patients with AIDS or ARC.

What may be new, according to the report we heard, is that this approach has worked in mice, and is generating much excitement among the professionals who know about it. This technology could apply also to cancer, certain genetic defects, and other retroviral diseases, as well as AIDS.

Apparently the drugs are fairly easy to make, with a specialized machine called a DNA synthesizer. But there are billions of different possible chemicals of this class, and most would be ineffective or harmful.

If you have any other information about hybridons or any related project, please call or write to me here at *AIDS Treatment News* (see Appendix B).

REFERENCES

Goodchild, J., P.C. Zamecnik, R.C. Gallo, and P. Sarin, "Inhibition of Expression of Human T Lymphotropic Virus Type III Proteins in T Cells by Anti-Sense Oligodeoxynucleotides (Hybridons)," *Federation Proceedings* 45(6) (1986), p. 1752 (abstract only).

Zamecnik, P.C., J. Goodchild, Y. Taguchi, and P.S. Sarin, "Inhibition of Replication and Expression of Human T-cell Lymphotropic Virus Type III in Cultured Cells by Exogenous Synthetic Oligonucleotides Complementary to Viral RNA," *Proceedings of the National Academy of Sciences USA* 83(12) (June 1986), pp. 4143–6.

OCTREOTIDE FOR CRYPTOSPORIDIOSIS

Octreotide, a synthetic substitute for the naturally-occurring hormone somatostatin, is a new designer drug with the same general structure as peptide T. (Both are artificially created peptides with eight amino acids.) Octreotide would be expected to provide symptomatic relief for severe diarrhea, such as that caused by cryptosporidiosis, even when nothing else worked.

In a case reported earlier this year, physicians found that octreotide was helpful for a patient with AIDS with severe cryptosporidiosis. Stool volume was reduced from five to ten liters per day to two to three, and the patient could be discharged from the hospital. The patient did well at home for five months, but then deteriorated and died from other AIDS-related causes.

The octreotide (also called Sandostatin) was obtained as an experimental drug. For more information, see the report by Katz, *et al.*, 1988.

REFERENCE

Katz, M.D., B.L. Erstad, and C. Rose, "Treatment of Severe Cryptosporidium-Related Diarrhea with Octreotide in a Patient with AIDS," *Drug Intelligence and Clinical Pharmacy* 22 (February 1988), pp. 134–6. Also see the editorial and the review article in the same issue.

FDA REFORM: MAJOR NEW POSITION PAPER

A short, 12-page report published in April by a conservative think tank and now widely circulating in Washington, D.C. provides perhaps the best call ever written for major reform of the FDA drug-approval process. The AIDS community might consider using this proposal as a rallying point. It suggests a workable, politically possible change which could solve part of the AIDS "drugjam," and remove the need to travel abroad or use underground sources to obtain rational, well-supported treatments.

Red Tape For the Dying: The Food and Drug Administration and AIDS recommends fundamental reform, in clear language anyone can understand:

"Something clearly is wrong when a regulatory program aimed at protecting the health of Americans sends thousands of its supposed beneficiaries into covert action to obtain potentially effective drugs. What is needed is fundamental reform of the FDA. The agency's power to block new drugs should be eliminated. While FDA should continue to certify drugs that it finds safe and effective, licensed physicians should be allowed, with the patient's informed consent, to prescribe drugs that are not so certified."

The report, which applied to all serious diseases not just AIDS, is published by The Heritage Foundation. For a copy, send $2 to The Heritage Foundation (see Appendix B). Be sure to ask for their "Backgrounder Number 644."

Why It's Important

• The report is accessible to anyone who can read a newspaper; no special background is required. Yet it has enough substance that we learned much from it, despite our familiarity with the subject.

• The paper provides an excellent overview of what is wrong with the current FDA system, and how and why the problems developed. It summarizes previous ineffective attempts at reform, such as the "treatment IND" regulations announced last year, and explains why they failed.

• It is full of authoritative references—for example to government reports, the *New York Times, The Wall Street Journal*—which individuals and organizations can use to support their case.

• It arrives at a critical time when interest in drug regulatory reform is stronger than ever.

• It has its own momentum which the AIDS community can build on.

For Example: Explaining Unbalanced Judgment by FDA

Two kinds of error by the FDA—wrongly approving a drug, or wrongly denying or delaying approval—can cost lives. Yet there is so great an institutional bias toward fear of the first kind of error that the second kind is hardly considered at all. The report explained why.

First it quoted a former FDA commissioner: " '. . . in all of FDA's history, I am unable to find a single instance where a Congressional committee investigated the failure of the FDA to approve a new drug. But, the times when hearings have been held to criticize our approval of new drugs have been so frequent that we aren't able to count them. The message to FDA staff could not be clearer. Whenever a controversy over a new drug is resolved by its approval, the Agency and the individuals involved likely will be investigated. Whenever such a drug in disapproved, no inquiry will be made. The Congressional pressure for our negative action on new drug applications is, therefore, intense. And it seems to be increasing. . .' "

Then the report suggested that ". . . in large part this is due to the fact that the victims of a mistakenly approved drug are often highly visible, while the victims of a wrongfully delayed drug rarely even realize that they have been injured."

The report listed some consequences of this imbalance. U.S. drug innovation fell by 50 percent after the FDA obtained its current powers in 1962. England, for example, has four times as many new drugs which are not available in the U.S., as the U.S. has which are not available in England. In cardiovascular, respiratory, and gastrointestinal medicine, U.S. drug development has all but stopped; almost all the new drugs are available in England (and elsewhere) but not to Americans, except those who make periodic trips abroad to pick up personal supplies.

And according to an article in *The Washington Post*, quoted in the report, unjustified FDA delays in approving the heart-attack drug TPA caused three thousand needless deaths in the United States.

An Objection, and Our Reply

Objection: "The proposal would allow unsafe and ineffective drugs to be marketed to desperate people, for profit."

Reply: The proposal would apply only with a prescription, a prominent warning, and informed consent. It would in no way weaken the laws against false or unproven claims, or other forms of fraud.

We should be very careful of the idea that seriously ill persons are "desperate" and therefore unable to decide properly for themselves. Even a decision to try a dubious therapy is often the best, most rational choice among the unattractive options available to that person. The efforts to disempower those seriously ill may stem less from efforts to protect them, than from the fact that persons facing major illness or death may free themselves from the constraints of conventional structures—structures which have evolved to reflect the interests of the most powerful groups (here drug companies, bureaucrats, and professionals) much more than those of the patients, who in the past have not had a seat at the negotiations through which the conventional structures developed.

In other words, persons seriously ill are deprived of the right to make their own decisions, not to protect them, but rather to control them for the benefit and protection of powerful vested interests.

FDA Media Note

You may have noticed the FDA much in the news recently, in its favorite role of hero and protector. The agency has an impressive ability to generate press attention when necessary to divert the thrust of widespread calls for reform.

Don't be misled—no one wants to end the legitimate and necessary consumer protection functions of the FDA. That isn't the issue. Instead, we need reforms to give patients and their physicians final say in an emergency, final say when the agency doesn't know best or has not had the time or resources to get around to making a decision, final say when commercial or bureaucratic empire building would override the best interest of the patient.

Consumer protection has nothing to do with sending thousands of people to their deaths in order to safeguard the FDA's regulatory process, or the market shares and profits of the giant corporations which know best how to work the system and have the contacts and money to do so.

BETA: NEW TREATMENT NEWSLETTER AVAILABLE; FIRST ISSUE, AZT

The first issue of the *Bulletin of Experimental Treatments for AIDS (BETA)*, published by the San Francisco AIDS Foundation, is now in press and will be available soon. Copies can be ordered now (see below).

BETA "is published as an educational resource for people considering experimental treatments for AIDS, ARC and HIV infection." It "reviews available scientific data on AIDS treatments as well as anecdotal information provided by physicians, researchers, people with AIDS and ARC, and individuals infected with HIV." Publication by *BETA* of information about a treatment does not, of course, imply endorsement of that treatment by the San Francisco AIDS Foundation.

The first issue, on AZT, gives a readable, comprehensive overview on the use of the drug—including areas of controversy where physicians disagree. About five thousands words in length, the article includes:

* Dosage, toxicity, and side effects;

* Combining AZT with other drugs;

* AZT use by asymptomatic seropositives—pro and con;

* Experiences of people taking AZT;

* Physicians' comments;

* A glossary; and

* A resource guide to experimental treatment information.

Each issue of *BETA* gets a careful medical review by the Scientific Review Committee of the San Francisco AIDS Foundation.

For a copy of *BETA* contact the San Francisco AIDS Foundation (see Appendix B).

PNEUMOCYSTIS DIAGNOSIS DELAYS— NURSES' STATEMENT

Delays as long as 12 days in diagnosis of pneumocystis have become a major problem. Recently the AIDS/ARC Interest Group of the Golden Gate Nurses Association (Region 12 of the California Nurses Association) published a statement on the problem. Their statement may help AIDS service organizations elsewhere obtain more effective (and incidentally less costly) medical services in their localities.

To obtain the statement, or for more information, contact the Golden Gate Nurses' Association (see Appendix B).

FREE AEROSOLIZED PENTAMIDINE TREATMENT IN SAN FRANCISCO STUDY

Persons who have had pneumocystis in the last six months may be able to receive aerosol pentamidine without charge, in a study by the Institute for HIV Research and Treatment at the Davies Medical Center in San Francisco. Patients may continue using AZT or other antivirals during this study.

No placebo will be used. Instead there will be two doses, 30 mg and 150 mg, every two weeks.

There has been some controversy over whether 30 mg is enough; also, no one knows for sure how large a dose will prove safe for long-term use. We are hearing that when pneumocystis does occur in persons using aerosol pentamidine, it tends to be mild; there have been very few deaths from pneumocystis in such studies, even at the low 30 mg dose. In any case, an independent company will audit the charts of patients in this study, so that the trial can be stopped if the low dose turns out to be too small.

Other Options

Persons at risk for pneumocystis should know that there are other options—such as dapsone, or Septra—if they cannot obtain aerosol pentamidine. These are more likely to cause side effects, but seem to work well if patients can tolerate them. They are much less expensive. What is most important is that those at risk for pneumocystis should use some form of prophylaxis.

AIDS Treatment News has published several warnings about fansidar, another drug sometimes used for pneumocystis prophylaxis; it can cause serious or fatal reactions, and patients using it must get appropriate warnings from their physicians so that they will stop the drug and get medical help immediately if symptoms develop. Recently we have heard that fansidar is much more likely to cause problems if used by patients who are also taking AZT.

DESERT AND MOUNTAIN STATES PWA COALITIONS URGE TREATMENT FOCUS, LOBBYING OF AIDS ORGANIZATIONS

At a meeting on May 14 and 15, People With AIDS Coalitions in six states issued a call for AIDS organizations to work toward a unified approach with more attention to treatment access issues.

The Desert and Mountain States Regional Conferences of People With AIDS Coalitions, representing PWA coalitions in Albuquerque, Denver, Phoenix, Salt Lake City, and Tucson, urged the National Association of People With AIDS (NAPWA), NAPWA board members, and the AIDS community, to:

• Focus and direct political action by AIDS organizations. "We feel that the time has come for a single focus, rather than a thousand voices crying in the wind."

• Work for the release and availability of lifesaving treatments.

- Lobby all AIDS organizations to involve themselves in making treatments more available.

- Urge persons with AIDS and their friends to pressure the FDA and other agencies or organizations to speed the study and release of treatments.

- Ask all PWA groups and leaders to work toward finding appropriate treatments and making them available.

For a listing of PWA Coalitions by state, see Appendix C.

SUNLIGHT HARMFUL TO PERSONS WITH HIV?

The "guerilla clinic" movement, best known for its interest in DNCB as a possible AIDS treatment, has collected and distributed evidence that sunlight or other ultraviolet light might stimulate the growth of HIV and be harmful to persons with HIV infection. Now a new laboratory study, published May 5, 1988 in *Nature,* greatly increased the concern.

- It has long been known that ultraviolet light can damage or suppress the Langerhans cells of the skin. These cells are an important part of the immune system, and have recently become a focus for intensive research on AIDS.

- Researchers at the Centers for Disease Control have found the onset of AIDS, as well as almost all opportunistic infections, peak in the summer, when ultraviolet exposure from sunlight is highest.

- The recent article in *Nature* reported that ultraviolet light increased the activity of HIV genes as much as 150 times in laboratory tests. (An unrelated virus, tested as a control, showed little or no such effect.) Exposure to half an hour of direct sunlight increased the HIV activity 12 times. HIV is known to infect Langerhans cells in the skin, which are exposed to ultraviolet light from the sun or other sources.

We asked two AIDS-knowledgeable physicians what they knew about the dangers of sunlight to persons with AIDS, ARC, or asymptomatic HIV infection. Neither had seen the *Nature* article; both urged normal caution. One warned especially that a number of drugs used by persons with AIDS make the skin much more sensitive to the sun than usual.

For more information, see "A Warning About Sun Exposure From the Guerilla Clinics." This short article has 20 technical references. For a free copy send a self-addressed stamped envelope to: Jim Henry (see Appendix B).

CONGRESS LOOKS AT AIDS TREATMENT DELAYS—
PART II

AIDS Treatment News, Issue Number 57, published part I of our interview with Dr. Steve Morin, legislative assistant to Congresswoman Nancy Pelosi. Part II continues here. Dr. Morin's remarks are in quotation marks; our comments are in parentheses.

(We commented to Dr. Morin that the staffing problem could also explain the inability to investigate the suspicion that the AL 721 now being used in NIH/NIAID trials may be seriously deficient and perhaps ineffective. After hearing the reports, NIH planned to conduct its own quality control through a government or commercial laboratory; we have heard ambiguous reports about whether it did so. And one well-informed source told us that NIH refused to allow physicians running the trials to provide samples of the material to the buyers clubs, which routinely test AL 721 substitutes and wanted to do the same tests on this AL 721 at their own expense.)

"We heard one after another after another of that kind of story (at the hearings). It spoke eloquently of the lack of coordination, the lack of staff to actually monitor the implementation of the studies that the scientific advisory groups were giving high priority. Fauci admitted as much in the Friday hearings.

"The next witness was Jeffrey Beal, a physician from Tulsa, Oklahoma. He's one of the primary caregivers in Tulsa, he has 80 patients who are HIV positive. He told us that the average time from diagnosis to death in Tulsa was five months—compared to about 14 months median in San Francisco.

"Apparently many people (in Tulsa) delay seeking treatment for fear of discrimination. People arrive very sick, they're fearful of losing jobs and insurance, as well as being ostracized by the community.

"There seem to be real problems in Tulsa. The nearest of the original 19 AIDS Treatment Evaluation Units is 500 miles away. They don't have the kind of information that's available on the coasts. A lot of people come home to die there, they have a lot of people who do not seek active treatment, coming from somewhere else.

"The Thursday afternoon panel was mostly activist groups from New York and San Francisco: ACT UP, Community Research Initiative, Project Inform. They told how the Community Research Initiative model had developed. People had been frustrated with FDA and NIAID. They wanted to be involved in the whole process.

"Martin Delaney (co-founder of Project Inform in San Francisco) focused on problems with the treatment INDs, how that was really more of a public-relations effort than an actual option."

(The "treatment IND," a plan purportedly to speed access to drugs to persons with serious or life-threatening diseases, was implemented on paper last May, but has had almost no practical effect since then.)

"Day 2 of the hearings opened with Admiral Watkins, who presented in essence the recommendations of the Presidential Commission on the HIV Epidemic. He was wonderful, the recommendations were wonderful, very critical of the FDA and NIH.

"Then Fauci and others (from NIAID) were questioned for about three hours. As reported in *The New York Times* (cited above), Fauci requested 127 new positions and got only 11 from the Reagan Administration.

"Fauci sounded completely frustrated in being able to get anything done, in a way he hasn't sounded before in interviews.

"Probably the most heat came out of the discussion of aerosol pentamidine, and their 13-month delay on that. Fauci said one of the major reasons was that they didn't have a single staff person they could assign to be on top of it. It became abundantly clear, whatever the cost of that one staff person, if you calculate the cost of Medicaid of all the hospitalizations, even aside from human suffering, how much it was costing the government not to have a person escort that drug and speed it up, it's just ridiculous.

"We also heard from LyphoMed, Inc., the manufacturer of aerosol pentamidine, on the pricing issue. I thought the LyphoMed people had a good explanation for the pricing. They showed the cost of the research that would lead to the eventual licensing of the drug for that use. They paid the cost of supplying the drug through the Community Research Initiative (which is doing a study supported by LyphoMed). Also they have people in the field, staff which drives up prices. It has to do with the hoops they have to jump through for the FDA. LyphoMed didn't have to do any of that (earlier) when pentamidine was only an orphan drug; they weren't trying to license it then.

"LyphoMed outlined exactly what they had to do, and how much it cost, and it all computed. It was a reasonable explanation.

"The corporate drama around aerosol pentamidine is a good sign, because it indicates people really believe it is going to be effective, a long-term hopeful approach.

"Frank Young (the Commissioner of the FDA) was on the entire afternoon, along with Ellen Cooper and some of the others there. That was quite a lengthy question session. A lot focused on the treatment IND issue. They basically maintained that none of the drugs they knew of were good enough to qualify."

(We asked how a lay person could challenge such an argument. The FDA has secret information on the drugs. Do they simply have to say that none of the drugs is good enough to release? Must the rest of the world simply accept such statements with no criticism, no checks and balances, as an ultimate truth from on high?)

"Commissioner Young had just had an operation. Ms. Pelosi asked what he would do if it turned out that he were given contaminated blood and had an HIV infection, would he take any of these alternative treatments that showed theoretical potential but had not been proven effective? He admitted yes he would take them, because they would be the only option he had.

"They tell you one thing in the official capacity, and then they tell you that they would go ahead and take the drugs (if it were for themselves personally). What kind of message is that? It's a message that the bureaucratic stuff is just that."

(We told Morin that we saw the FDA's standard dog-and-pony-show at the Presidential Commission, which did not question the FDA witnesses in any serious way, just patted them on the back. The witness sitting next to me said he had seen the same presentation time and time again, that the FDA's top officials are in the business of making a living giving this show to high-level officials. The slick, well-designed presentation simplifies the whole confusing situation on AIDS drugs—provides clean, strong, simple concepts like phase I, phase II, phase III—it wraps up everything in a nice package for officials. The FDA becomes the focus point, the nerve center, the central gateway of the whole drug development process, so all the complexity now fits into place. The officials—confused, uniformed, at sea in all the complexity—love it.)

"They had all of that, the (same) graphs. It was well packaged. Linguistically it sounded very compassionate."

(We commented that linguistically it also sounded very rational, to appeal also to those who think that way.)

"But they (FDA) do have expedited review, they do have a lot of things that NIAID does not have, that speed things along. But they have so many hoops to go through."

(They'll speed up the paperwork, yes.)

"But the things they say in the paperwork that people have to go through to get to the next step are very time consuming.

"To sum things up, there is a human element to this. Alternative treatments that are safe and have theoretical potential to be effective but haven't been proved effective, do give people hope. And giving people hope is very important in an epidemic like this, where there isn't that much hope in the media. The media doesn't talk much about the people who are long-term survivors.

"What could be done to give people hope, was the focus. The FDA was not being a helpful participant in thinking of it that way."

Morin commended Chairman Weiss for his continuing leadership on AIDS issues. "The hearings gave me new hope."

MAJOR DRAFT REPORT FROM PRESIDENTIAL COMMISSION

Just before going to press we received the recommendations of Retired Admiral James D. Watkins, Chairman of the Presidential Commission on the HIV Epidemic, to be considered by the full Commission before it issues its final report. This important document includes hundreds of specific recommendations for better management of the AIDS epidemic. We cannot review it now; for more information see the story in *The New York Times* (Friday June 3), page one.

Issue Number 59
July 1, 1988

STOCKHOLM AIDS CONFERENCE: THE UNTOLD STORY

The "IV International Conference on AIDS," June 12-16 in Stockholm, Sweden, included over three-thousand scientific presentations—more than twice as many as last years' meeting in Washington, D.C. We covered these conferences to gather information on promising treatment possibilities and related scientific research. This article gives our overview; details will follow in the next several installments, starting below and continuing every other issue.

What's Right?
Despite largely pessimistic press reports, we found more good news than bad from the Stockholm conference:

- Tremendous nuts-and-bolts progress in basic research represents major advance toward an eventual cure or highly effective treatment—for AIDS and many other diseases as well. Little of this progress makes headlines, however.

- The conference reflected a new stage of effective worldwide mobilization in many areas of AIDS. (Unfortunately there are also glaring deficiencies, illustrated below.)

- In civil liberties and related areas (outside our treatment focus) the world's experts have developed strong consensus which recognizes the concerns and dignity of persons with AIDS. For example, balancing the rights of infected persons against those of the uninfected is seen as a false issue; on the contrary, antidiscrimination protection is regarded as absolutely crucial to effective control of the spread of the virus. Far from being opposed, the interests of those with AIDS and the larger society correspond.

The developing consensus easily crosses national borders. For example, telephone hotlines throughout the world are now providing roughly the same information.

328

This writer is too busy covering treatments to give nondiscrimination and related issues the attention they deserve. Those working in these areas should examine the Stockholm results and other forums for ammunition against the political demagoguery still very much with us.

Behind the Bad News: Analysis and Comment

The bad news is the lack of major treatment advances in the last year.

Most commentators have assumed that lack of progress on treatments reflects the difficulty of the disease. But analysis of the Stockholm presentations contradicts this assumption. The evidence suggests another cause for lack of treatments.

If the intractability of the disease were responsible, we would have expected to see a string of treatment failures at Stockholm—many reports of drugs or other therapies which were tried but failed to work. In fact there were very few such reports. Very few new treatments failed in the last year. Very few were tried at all.

The problem is political, not technical. The impressive worldwide mobilization around basic research, prevention, and other areas has glaringly omitted any serious mobilization or commitment to save the lives of those now infected or ill. These people were written off several years ago, and since then there has been no institutional constituency for mobilizing research to save lives.

The major thrust of the scientists at Stockholm has been to find a cure through elegant molecular biology, maybe in five to ten years. There is no urgency or mobilization to test the dozens if not hundreds of treatment possibilities widely agreed to be available now—dozens of which could be tested within the next few months if only there were the will.

Some of the scientists now realize that there is a problem, in that current policies all but guarantee that hundreds of thousands of people will die of AIDS during the next few years. Some have reached the "isn't it a pity" stage. But few have broken through the aura of inevitability to see the problem as resulting from human attitudes and decisions which can and should be changed.

The one common factor behind virtually every treatment attempt receiving serious research attention—AZT, vaccines, interferons, CD4, Ampligen, IMREG-1, and a few others—is hot prospects for commercial gain. No major institution, government as well as private, will seriously consider a treatment solely on its medical and scientific (as opposed to commercial) merit. If it's a plant that anyone could pick, a food in general use, a common industrial chemical, or a health-food product, it won't be considered, no matter what the evidence.

Scientists as well as corporations have vested interests. It has unfortunately always been hard to find financial support for basic biological and medical research—work which doesn't make headlines, but on which future progress depends. AIDS is now driving huge advances in fundamental knowledge of viruses and the immune system, as well as related technology such as improved scientific tests. The research community involved in this effort has never had it so good.

No one is deliberately conspiring to keep AIDS going to feed the multi-billion dollar research and pharmaceutical industries. No one has needed to. For the interests of the powerful are only threatened by doing what needs to be done—creating a mechanism to promptly test the dozens of promising treatments already known and available, regardless of commercial prospects—each with perhaps ten to 20 volunteers. The problem isn't money—this testing wouldn't need to cost much—but pervasive obstructionism throughout the institutions involved.

This problem may seem so big as to be hopeless. But there is a key place to start, where attainable public effort can have critical results: namely the lobbying of AIDS, gay, hemophilia, and physicians' organizations to investigate and address the issues of clinical trials and treatment access for saving the lives of the millions of people already infected with the AIDS virus.

The decision to write off those already ill probably started from homophobia. But now it continues from its own momentum, due to the almost total lack of institutional support to change it. We saw this lack in Stockholm, when scientists didn't even feel the need to address the issue of the "drugjam" in clinical trials.

Like the first candle in a dark room, the first advocacy makes all the difference when there has been none before.

TREATMENTS AT STOCKHOLM

Dozens of treatment possibilities appeared somewhere among the three-thousand presentations at Stockholm. Most were largely ignored, however, with their poster sessions usually empty; the scientists just walked by. Usually no evidence suggested that these treatment prospects were any worse than the ones getting the attention. They lacked political and commercial currency, not necessarily scientific merit.

Nobody could cover all three-thousand presentations in the few days of the conference; scientists naturally focused on what was hot in their fields. In our own coverage, however, we decided to emphasize those treatments most likely to be overlooked. Therefore we de-emphasized those which will get attention, namely AZT, interferons, vaccines, and the very important area of improved medical management. We will cover these subjects mainly by interviewing physicians who were at the conference; we spent our own time gathering as much information as possible about other treatment leads. We may have been the only journalists at the conference whose primary business was to seek out precisely those treatments most likely to be overlooked.

Treatments possibilities not at the conference which we would like to have seen there included BHT, DHEA, DNCB, garlic, and MM1. Apparently nobody submitted papers on these.

Treatments or leads presented in Stockholm which we plan to cover include (in alphabetical order) acyclovir, aerosolized pentamidine, AL 721, ampligen, antabuse, antisense DNA, apurinic acid, AS 101, avarone, carrisyn, castanospermine, CD4, corticosteroids, dapsone, DDC, dextran sulfate, fluconazole, foscarnet, fusidic acid, ganciclovir (DHPG), germanium, ginseng, glycans, glycopeptides, glycyrrhizin, GM-CSF, gonadotropins, heparin, HPA-23, Immunotoxins, interferons, IMREG-1, imuthiol, isoprinosine, itraconazole, ozone, peptide T, pine cone extract, PMEA, prostaglandin inhibitors, ribavirin, rifabutin, selenium, somatostatin, THF, thymostimulin, trimetrexate, tumor necrosis factor, and zinc.

We will also look at new research directions and improved methods, such as new scientific tests.

Covering treatment news at the "IV International Conference On AIDS" presents unusual difficulties—problems which help explain why treatment developments received less press coverage than they deserved.

Reporters faced a huge mass of information with no organizing principle, and no help in deciding what was important other than following the "conventional wisdom" of what was in style among physicians and scientists. No single treatment or small group of them compelled special interest based on actual data presented at Stockholm— although chances are good that a number of treatments discussed may prove very important in the future. But for now, even from the mass of reports taken together, no pattern emerged.

Mainstream reporters complained that you could take any angle you wanted at this conference, and support it. As one commented, you could shoot anywhere and hit something. This excessive freedom makes the reporter's job more difficult, because no guidance emerges from the material itself. Reporters do not want their basic relationship to the story to be arbitrary.

In this situation we owe the reader some explanation of our own biases and approach, as we begin a series of several articles on dozens of specific treatment possibilities about which information was presented in Stockholm.

First, we have not considered treatments unless we saw some thread of possible usefulness in the foreseeable future. But many of the potential treatments we report are not ready for people to use now, and some will never be.

We considered selecting what to report from the point of view of what information is most useful now, but decided against this approach for several reasons. First, hundreds of practicing physicians attended the conference, and they are in the best position to know what is immediately important. We can interview them about this information, and plan to do so.

Second, no one can know at this time which treatment leads presented at Stockholm will turn out to be important. The more suggestive, unproven developments are the ones most likely to be overlooked by the conference attenders; often in the history of science and medicine valuable information is lost for years in this way. We want to make this information available to those who did not happen to attend the conference and read a particular poster.

The remaining question is how to make coherent to our readers a massive body of facts which fits no particular pattern, no particular categories. We expect to organize each article as a guided tour, using particular treatments to illustrate concepts or viewpoints which may help in understanding the overall picture of AIDS research. We cannot organize the articles in advance, however, as it will take us several weeks to go through the material, as we are writing about it; and in any case we have not found useful ways to categorize the treatments. Each article will consist of what emerges at that time from material not covered so far.

HOE/BAY 964 (Poster #3656)

We never heard of this substance before, and conference attenders could easily have missed it, as no mention appeared in the published book of abstracts (abstracts submitted months in advance, therefore lacking the most current information). Instead, HOE/BAY 964 appeared only at the conference itself, at the end of a poster ostensibly about something else. The poster, titled "Development Of HIV-Variants With Higher Resistance Against AZT Under Treatment With AZT," was presented by seven German scientists from two research institutions in West Germany, and one from the Karolinska Institute in Sweden. What caught our attention was the statement that this substance is already in clinical study in Germany; therefore we thought we should know about it.

The poster primarily reports on a study of what may be a reason that the effectiveness of AZT often falls off after long-term use—development of drug resistance by HIV.

Other reports have suggested that evolution of HIV within each patient may be an important part of the natural history of disease. HIV evolves far faster than other viruses or organisms, and the development of drug resistance may occur independently within each person. It is certainly conceivable that due to prevention methods such as safer sex—which patients will probably have adapted well before their diagnosis and treatment with AZT—the resistant virus would be unlikely to spread to others, and therefore the cumulative development of resistant strains may not be a problem. (This possibility reinforces the advice that persons who are HIV positive or who have AIDS must avoid unsafe sex with each other.)

The poster (#3656) included a summary, the first two paragraphs of which were identical to the published abstract (except for updating the number of persons known to have developed AIDS from 64,000 when the poster was submitted to 84,000 when the conference took place). The researchers followed 60 AIDS patients receiving AZT for periods up to one year, and during this time AZT did not reduce the ability to culture virus from the patients' blood.

Three of the 60 patients were studied more intensively by testing the susceptibility of their virus to AZT in the laboratory. The researchers found that the virus from these patients was significantly less sensitive to AZT late during the course of the treatment, meaning that drug resistance had developed.

Then the summary included the following apparently new results, introducing HOE/BAY 946 almost as an afterthought:

"In contrast, HOE/BAY 964 (chemically a xylan/hydrogensulfate disodium salt), an inhibitor of HIV currently under clinical investigation in Germany, did not show significant differences in the inhibition of the RT from sequential virus isolates from these patients."

The poster also included a diagram with the chemical structure of HOE/BAY 964, and clinical results from the three patients whose virus was studied.

We could not be sure from the poster that HOE/BAY 964 had been tested in humans. But as this issue went to press, we heard from a physician who talked to the researchers who presented the poster (#3656). They told him that they are using HOE/BAY 964 with patients, especially those who need to discontinue use of AZT. (Therefore it seems especially important to investigate this new antiviral now, as many people have been using AZT for about a year, and may need to find another treatment soon if the AZT becomes less effective due to development of drug resistance by HIV.)

AmFAR (The American Foundation For AIDS Research) is following up on HOE/BAY 964 for possible inclusion in the new issue of its treatment directory. AmFAR is in an excellent position to collect this kind of information, since it is a well-'nown, respected organization, and it gives several million dollars a year in research ants. We will continue to report on this treatment possibility as more information omes available.

Note On Treatments

More readers have asked us questions about dextran sulfate and AL 721 than about any other experimental treatments. We will cover these later when we have time to assemble the information. Briefly, both dextran sulfate and AL 721 had some new information presented at Stockholm, but nothing spectacular. Perhaps the biggest news was the great interest in dextran sulfate among physicians and scientists at the conference. Only a little new human data was available, however.

NOTES AND ANNOUNCEMENTS

Stockholm Conference Abstracts Available

In San Francisco: A copy of the abstracts of all three-thousand presentations at the Stockholm conference is kept at the library of The Healing Alternatives Foundation (formerly the Healing Alternatives Buyers' Club) (see Appendix B). There is a keyword subject index and an author index, so you can find the abstracts on the above treatments, or on other subjects. Individual abstracts can be photocopied at the library for five cents each.

Long-Term Survivor Study

The AIDS Healing Alliance (a San Francisco organization not to be confused with The Healing Alternatives Foundation) is conducting a long-term survivor study. It needs participants for its pilot study within the next week. It is seeking persons who have had

- An AIDS diagnosis for at least two years, or
- An ARC diagnosis for at least seven years, or
- A seropositive status for at least seven years.

Participants will fill out a medical and lifestyle survey questionnaire.

Major New York Fundraiser July 10

A little-known group which organized a very successful fundraiser last year hopes to do even better this July 10. This effort can also be a model for fundraising elsewhere. People Taking Action Against AIDS (PTAAA) last year raised more than $120,000 at a single event, with less than $5000 in expenses. The key was an auction of donated work by well-known artists, some world famous, at an event at a home in Bellport, Long Island. PTAAA gave $50,000 to the Community Research Initiative to fund a lipid study, and the remainder to a local AIDS service organization, LIAAC, the Long Island Association for AIDS Care.

This year PTAAA will not only help the same beneficiaries, it will also reserve money for small seed grants to help other communities organize their own events. It is particularly interested in supporting organizing outside of major metropolitan centers, in areas where there is currently not much AIDS activity or information access.

For information about the community grants, or how similar events might be organized in San Francisco or elsewhere, contact People Taking Action Against AIDS (PTAAA) (see Appendix B).

California: Help Needed Against Dannemeyer Initiative

An "AIDS Initiative" which would close California's anonymous testing sites and force physicians to report anyone they know or "suspect" to be antibody positive will be on the November ballot in California. It would also allow insurance companies to use the HIV antibody test to deny coverage, and require anyone who has tested antibody positive to report themselves to authorities within seven days.

While the voters just rejected the similar LaRouche Initiative by a large margin, the Dannemeyer "AIDS Initiative" is much stronger politically. It has important Republican Party support and is not associated with La Rouche. Also, it may have insurance industry support because it would repeal the current law against using the HIV antibody test for insurance.

This initiative threatens the movement to get people to be tested earlier and treated earlier. It gives everybody strong reasons to delay getting tested as long as possible, delaying medical intervention and AIDS-prevention counseling. It is likely to exacerbate the AIDS disaster.

Comment on HIV Testing and Insurance

Legislation which passed the California Assembly this week would let insurance companies use the HIV antibody test to deny health insurance to persons with HIV (a provision also included in the Dannemeyer "AIDS Initiative," above). This issue illustrates a long-term problem for the whole U.S. health-care system, not just AIDS. For the HIV antibody test is only the first of an expected wave of high-tech tests to detect persons at higher risk for cancer, heart diseases, arthritis, and other expensive illnesses, as well as AIDS.

In the past the whole point of insurance has been to share the risk. But in the future the industry will inexorably drive to use the new tests to cut costs, by excluding those at risk and betting only on a sure thing—clients screened to exclude any detectable risks. Others will be dumped onto the increasingly overburdened public sector. They may also face employment discrimination, as they cannot qualify for the often-mandatory "benefit" of group health insurance—or would raise the employer's premium if they were hired.

FDA Backs Off on AL 721

ast week the FDA moved against two suppliers of AL 721 or related products: Ethigen ᵓoration, the patent and trademark holder on AL 721, and Nutricology Inc., in

San Leandro, California. Protests began immediately and the FDA rescinded both actions in the same week. It appears that the central FDA office near Washington, D.C. did not even know about the actions of the regional offices until the protests began.

The four people central to the negotiation for the AIDS community were attorneys Jay Lipner and David Barr with Lambda Legal Defense in New York, Martin Delaney with Project Inform, and Curtis Ponzi, attorney for The Healing Alternatives Foundation in San Francisco. We spoke to both Lipner and Ponzi; they saw the outcome as a message of community empowerment, but Lipner commented that the ultimate results are unknown and warned that we must keep watching the FDA in the future.

The New York Times ran a page-one story on these events on Sunday, June 26, 1988.

Issue Number 60
July 15, 1988

AFFORDABLE TREATMENT OPTIONS: YOU CAN HELP

The Stockholm AIDS conference will continue to be a major theme for the next several issues of this newsletter. But due to reader requests we are also starting a theme of affordable treatment options—whether they were discussed in Stockholm or not.

The list below shows some of the treatments we plan to investigate; we don't yet know about safety, rationality, or availability/affordability of some of them. You could help by bringing others to our attention, especially any which have worked well for you or persons you know.

We have no exact cut-off for affordability, but are aiming for treatments costing less than a dollar a day; some cost only pennies a day. Because of this cost criterion, many treatments which patients should consider, such as AZT, acyclovir, and dextran sulfate, do not appear on this list. The big question, of course, is what role the substances listed should have in AIDS/HIV treatment, if any. The list so far, in alphabetical order:

- acidophilus
- aloe vera
- antabuse (as DTC substitute)
- aspirin (or indocin, as prostaglandin inhibitor)
- BHT
- Chinese herbs
- chlorophyll (including wheat grass, algae, chlorella, etc.)
- coenzyme Q
- dapsone
- DHEA
- DMG, TMG (dimethylglycine, trimethylglycine)
- DNCB
- DTC (imuthiol)
- fatty acids
- ganoderma
- garlic
- germanium
- homeopathy
- hydrogen peroxide
- lecithin

- linaza seeds (used in Central America for nausea)
- lysine
- macrobiotics
- monolaurin
- naltrexone

- propolis
- selenium
- septra
- shiitake
- vitamins: C, B12, others
- zinc

We may also look at attitudinal approaches, lifestyle changes, and self care.

What distinguishes the "affordable" list from more mainstream lists of experimental treatments, such as found in the *AIDS/HIV Experimental Treatment Directory* (compiled and published by the American Foundation for AIDS Research), is not that the "affordable" ones are necessarily inferior, but that less is known about them. Neither industry nor government has had any serious interest in treatment possibilities which do not have commercial potential. Yet the treatments which develop a grassroots following without promotion, like most of those above, would be excellent candidates for small, well-managed, scientific clinical trials. For one thing, the grassroots treatment possibilities are generally safer than the high-tech options which generate commercial, government, and professional interest. And they are available now, not after several years of bureaucratic delay and frequently ill-designed, unethical, and unworkable trials.

The U.S. needs public policy which recognizes that people must and will make treatment decisions, and then supports them in that process.

We at *AIDS Treatment News* are becoming increasingly unhappy about reporting on treatments which have only fragmentary, anecdotal, or theoretical evidence of effectiveness—such as many of those listed above. At this stage in the epidemic, there should be direct scientific evidence that treatments actually benefit certain groups of patients. But until we have a public commitment to do the research needed to help people stay alive, we see no choice but to continue to report what evidence there is.

PCR TEST NOW AVAILABLE

Update: Readers please note the article "PCR Test Cautions," which appears later in this volume, in Issue Number 62, page 352.

A new HIV test far more sensitive than any other is now available commercially to physicians.

The new test, called PCR (polymerase chain reaction), often detects HIV infection months before the antibody test; in one case reported at the AIDS conference in Stockholm, it detected HIV three-and-a-half years before seroconversion. Some persons who are negative on the antibody test, P24 antigen, viral culture, and all other tests have been found to be positive on the PCR. PCR will prove especially useful for testing infants, because only about 40 percent of the infants who test antibody positive for HIV are really infected; the others are only carrying their mother's antibodies temporarily, and the usual antibody tests cannot tell the difference.

No one knows how many people will be found to be positive on the PCR even though they are negative on the antibody and all other tests. And no one knows whether everyone who is PCR positive will become antibody positive eventually, or whether some people who are positive only on the PCR might have controlled the virus successfully.

The PCR detects very small amounts of a particular sequence of DNA, which contains the hereditary information of cells. For HIV diagnosis, the PCR test is used to detect genetic information inserted into the DNA of human cells by HIV.

Unfortunately the current version of the PCR only tells whether or not the DNA created by HIV was detected—it does not give any indication of how much. Therefore the test now available cannot be used to monitor how well patients are responding to treatment—or as an indicator of how well experimental drugs are working—because once a person is positive on the PCR, he or she will presumably remain positive, short of being completely cured. Later improvements in PCR technology may enable the test to give quantitative results, so that it could be used to monitor therapy and drug trials.

How It Works

The PCR (polymerase chain reaction) is a major scientific advance which will be an important tool for many kinds of basic research, and for diagnosis of other diseases as well as AIDS.

The PCR test works by taking advantage of the fact that DNA can make a copy of itself, as it does during normal cell division. The sample being tested is treated in such a way that each piece of the DNA being tested for will double into two pieces. The treatment is repeated, and the two pieces become four, then eight, then 16, etc. After 20 or more repetitions, the DNA (if any) will have multiplied more than a million times, and then it can be detected by ordinary biochemical tests.

The PCR can detect HIV infection even if it is completely latent, in the DNA of macrophages or other cells, not causing the replication of virus or the production of antibodies.

Persons who are antibody positive would presumably always test positive with the PCR. Those who are antibody negative despite high risk of exposure to HIV could use the PCR for reassurance if they are negative, or to start early infection control, periodic blood work, or early treatment if they test positive.

For more background on the PCR, see "Multiplying Genes by Leaps and Bounds," *Science* (June 10, 1988).

Where To Get the PCR

The PCR is now available with a physician's prescription everywhere except New York State, which requires special licensing the companies have not yet obtained. The cost for the test itself is $145, and it takes about five days to get the results.

Cetus Corporation, a biotechnology company in Emeryville, California, developed the PCR. Last week Cetus licensed two companies to provide the test commercially. Physicians who want to order the test should call customer service at either (1) Pathology

Institute, Berkeley, California (see Appendix B), or (2) Specialty Laboratories, Inc., Santa Monica, California (see Appendix B). The PCR might also be available through whatever laboratory the physician uses already, by subcontract with one of these two companies.

SURAMIN DISASTER: THE STORY IS TOLD

An article in the July/August issue of *San Francisco: The Magazine* traces the history of the suramin drug trial in 1985—the first multicenter test of an antiviral AIDS drug in the United States. This disastrous trial killed some of the participants and became a major setback for AIDS research, delaying the progress of clinical trials for perhaps as much as two years or more. It has provided the foundation for justifying the slow pace of trials, restrictions on access to experimental treatments, the movement to accept and romanticize death in the gay community, and the corresponding attitude in government, business, medicine, and the media to write off those already ill or infected, and not bother with the practical clinical research or other public policy commitments designed to save their lives.

Yet for the last several years word-of-mouth reports circulating among those in the AIDS community close to the suramin trials said that major mistakes in the conduct of the trials had contributed to a disaster that was at least in part avoidable. The current article in *San Francisco,* by *San Francisco Sentinel* reporter Charles Linebarger, brings some of this history into public view for the first time.

We learn, for example, that the National Institutes of Health didn't tell the investigators running the trial that adrenal damage was a possible side effect of suramin because "any doctor can make a clinical diagnosis of adrenal insufficiency." But the symptoms of that condition can mimic AIDS symptoms, so they were not recognized until too late. If the physicians running the trials had been warned, they would have included a simple test for adrenal damage.

The *San Francisco* article may help to shake the fatalism which resulted in part from the suramin trials—a fatalism which has allowed U.S. public policy to accept projections of hundreds of thousands of AIDS deaths with remarkably little effort to avert them.

DALLAS AIDS GROUP SUES COUNTY HOSPITAL ON AIDS CARE

A major lawsuit over substandard care of persons with AIDS in Dallas may establish national precedents on whether indigent patients have a right to health care.

Parkland Memorial Hospital, the large county hospital comparable to San Francisco General here, treats over 1,000 patients with AIDS, ARC, or who are HIV positive. Only one full-time and one half-time physician have to handle this patient load, with 700 patient visits per month. Typical AIDS patients are persons who lost their jobs as the disease progressed, and exhausted their savings, thus becoming indigent.

The lawsuit, brought by the Dallas Gay Alliance and the American Civil Liberties Union AIDS Project, seeks to end these practices:

- A waiting list for AZT. The cost of the drug is not the issue, because the AZT is provided by a State program with Federal funds. But the hospital does not assign enough physicians to monitor patients using the drug.

The lawsuit also names the University of Texas Southwestern Medical Center, which provides medical personnel—students, residents, fellows, and professors—to the hospital. This medical school rotates its personnel through all 132 of the clinics at Parkland Memorial, except for one—the AIDS clinic. This discrimination exacerbates the shortage of physicians in the AIDS clinic.

The hospital admitted that in the one-month period from April 7 to May 6, 1988, seven people on the AZT waiting list died. These were patients for whom AZT was medically prescribed but not available due to the hospital policy.

- Arbitrary denial of aerosol pentamidine prophylaxis and treatment. The hospital's full-time AIDS physician, after his recent resignation, pointed out that pentamidine costs the hospital about $100 per month per patient, while each hospitalization for pneumocystis costs the hospital $10,000 for the average stay of seven days.

- Rationing of AIDS beds. Persons with AIDS have been forced to wait for a rationed AIDS bed until another patient is discharged or dies, even though other beds are empty. Patients ill enough to need hospitalization have had to wait 12 hours or more for a bed.

Legal Results So Far

The lawsuit was first filed in a state court. Judges in Dallas are assigned at random, and a conservative judge was assigned to the case. But even he ruled against the hospital, forcing it to end the AZT waiting list, deliver aerosol pentamidine, and end the AIDS bed control. He gave the hospital 30 days to comply.

Then the hospital moved the case to the Federal court system. This time a moderate-liberal judge, with a reputation for being very thorough and fair, has been assigned.

Recently the Dallas Gay Alliance has asked the court for permission to change their pleading to a class-action lawsuit, which would include 28,000 people and have a wider impact. The ruling on this motion is pending.

This article cannot do justice to the excellent organizing and action around the Parkland hospital case by the Dallas Gay Alliance and other organizations. This work is a model for organizations elsewhere and may set important legal precedents concerning health care for AIDS and other conditions as well.

SAN FRANCISCO: VOLUNTEERS NEEDED

The Healing Alternatives Foundation needs volunteers for several projects:

- Improving its AIDS library;

- Implementing a "doctor report card" and "treatment case history" file;
- Facilitating small treatment study groups;
- Helping out in selling nutritional products such as egg lecithin lipids.

Volunteers can work evenings or weekends, as well as weekdays, on many projects. For more information call The Healing Alternatives Foundation (see Appendix B).

The Healing Alternatives Foundation is a nonprofit organization based on the philosophy that AIDS is a treatable disease.

WASHINGTON, D.C.: WELLNESS WORKSHOP SERIES

The Whitman-Walker AIDS Program in Washington, D.C. will offer a "Wellness Workshop Series" of nine weekly meetings Thursday evenings starting July 28. Topics include AZT, experimental drugs in clinical trials, acupuncture, Chinese and American herbs, nutrition, guided imagery, and spiritual issues.

AIDS TREATMENT RESEARCH POLICY: WHAT MUST BE DONE TO SAVE LIVES?

(Statement distributed at the Lesbian and Gay Health Conference and AIDS Forum, Boston, July 1988)

For over two years we have published biweekly articles on experimental and "alternative" AIDS treatments and research, in the *San Francisco Sentinel* and as *AIDS Treatment News*. We could not come to Boston this July, so we prepared this statement to contact health organizers about what is needed in AIDS research policy, how we can help, and how you can help.

Barring a miracle, hundreds of thousands of people in the United States alone are expected to die of AIDS over the next several years—and the Federally-controlled research establishment as it is currently operating will have little impact on this catastrophe. No one disputes the projections of what will happen without better treatments. And just last week FDA Commissioner Dr. Frank Young told Senator Kennedy's Senate Committee on Labor and Human Resources that he expected little to come out of the official drug development process in the next three years. In other words, hundreds of thousands of deaths are virtually inevitable under current policies.

Everyone agrees that these predictions are horrifying. The question is, are they inevitable?

Few now dispute that U.S. public policy has written off almost everyone who is now ill or HIV positive. National policy has consigned these people to death with remarkable equanimity, with no serious debate, and no serious effort to develop alternative strategies for a different outcome.

In over two years of researching these matters and publishing over 60 articles on AIDS treatments, we have never found any compelling *scientific* or *medical* support for believing these deaths are inevitable. Instead we have found that *commercial* and *political* reasons account for the continuation of policies which will allow hundreds of thousands of deaths.

For example, no HIV treatment has been approved since AZT, and no new approvals are now in sight. But meanwhile, dozens of unapproved, "underground" AIDS treatments have acquired a grassroots following, most with little or no commercial promotion. Solid evidence that these treatments work is admittedly scanty. But the evidence that they *don't* work is far scantier, often nonexistent. The research establishment simply assumed these treatments do not work, without evidence, because the ideas did not come from the mainstream of corporations, agencies, and professionals—a network which does not pursue leads unless they have commercial potential, or relevance to elegant, commercially desirable science such as biotechnology.

Besides the basic research in fields such as virology, which is already being done well, we need a mechanism to test dozens or even hundreds of attractive treatment leads which are available now, in small, fast (but well designed and well managed) scientific clinical trials. Any treatment known to be safe, and which acquires either a significant grassroots or scientific following, should be tested.

We may not find a cure this way. But we probably will find therapies to restore health and slow the disease process, perhaps indefinitely, for most people. Then when basic research does find a cure, perhaps in five or ten years, these people will be alive to benefit from it. And billions of dollars in medical costs for hospitalization and care of the dying might well be avoided.

Money isn't the problem; the cost of what amounts to an assembly line for mass production of small clinical trials would be modest. Most of the potential treatments themselves cost little. The problem, rather, is that the kinds of trials needed to save lives in this emergency do not fit into the conventional way U.S. drug development is done. The small trials suggested above, for example, might not count toward FDA drug approval—especially if there is no sponsor to pay the $80 million to $120 million generally recognized as the cost to develop *each* new drug through final U.S. approval. (These trials could contribute indirectly, however, by focusing attention on anything found to work dramatically well.) And releasing drugs without full approval would threaten the investors who have put millions of dollars into the conventional drug development and approval process, threaten regulators who have built their careers on it, and even threaten consumer protection advocates who have made a religion of keeping drugs off the market and away from people before full proof of efficacy—though everyone knows that even when the drugs do work such proof takes years, and is so cumbersome that it may never happen at all. These are the commercial and political obstacles which delay research for years when it could otherwise take weeks or months.

Instead of perfect proof of efficacy, we need practical trials which support patients and physicians in the treatment decisions that they are already making anyway.

Such trials have already begun on a very small scale through organizations like the Community Research Initiative in New York and the County Community Consortium in San Francisco, and through the practical experiences of individual physicians. Therefore we do not need to lobby for something totally new, but rather we need to expand a process already taking place, and to focus some of the central energies of this nation on it.

The first and most important step your organization can take to contribute to this effort is to develop in-house expertise in some aspect of AIDS treatment research policy, somewhere within your organization. Without such knowledge, you will be forced to accept at face value views and analysis by experts dependent on the existing system, analysis loaded with the institutional interests of the most powerful players in the $550 billion dollar per year medical industry. No serious advocacy can operate without its own centers of expertise. The AIDS service community ignored treatment advocacy for the first six years of the epidemic. Fortunately the tide has begun to turn.

We need not overthrow the system, only make room at the negotiating table for one more party. The fortunes, the empires, the turf wars, the games, the maneuvers, the coups, all will continue. But the lives of hundreds of thousands of people must also count when the real decisions are made.

To discuss how we can work together to promote national treatment strategies for saving lives instead of writing people off, call us at *AIDS Treatment News*.

Issue Number 61
July 29, 1988

FDA RELAXES DRUG ACCESS POLICY

In a surprise announcement on July 23 to the Lesbian and Gay Health Conference and AIDS Forum in Boston, U.S. Food and Drug Administration Commissioner Frank Young told an audience of several hundred people that the FDA would allow patients to import small quantities of unapproved medicines for personal use. The policy applies to AIDS and other diseases as well.

For some time the FDA has quietly not objected to patients bringing small quantities of medicines from abroad, if they brought them in personally when returning from a trip. However, most patients cannot afford to fly periodically to Europe, Japan, or elsewhere if they need medicines unavailable in the United States. The controversy about dextran sulfate as a possible AIDS treatment led to negotiations between the FDA and AIDS treatment organizations, leading to a compromise allowing patients to receive dextran sulfate by mail, under certain conditions which both sides could live with. This compromise has now become formalized as a written "pilot guidelines for release of mail importations"—to the surprise and approval of AIDS treatment activists, who had expected the agency to implement the compromise quietly, and only for dextran sulfate or for other drugs for which great pressure developed. (News of the policy announcement appeared on page 1 of the West Coast edition of Monday's *New York Times;* it may have appeared in late Sunday editions elsewhere.)

The last element of the compromise concerned what happens in the minority of cases where packages get stopped by customs. In those cases the patient will have to sign a form to receive the package, acknowledging that he or she knows that the drug has not been proved safe and effective. The FDA wanted a physician's prescription or at least a physician's signature on a letter stating that the patient was being monitored. The AIDS organizations said that such an arrangement was unworkable, as physicians would not sign due to fear of potential lawsuits, and reluctance to put their names on an FDA list. The compromise was that the patient would have to name his or her physician to receive the package, if it was stopped.

The FDA had been reluctant to allow individuals to receive the drugs by mail at all, because it feared the development of offshore businesses set up to sell unapproved drugs to Americans. The agency has made it clear that it will not tolerate commercialization of unproven drugs under its new policy.

Analysis and Comment

The new policy reflects the spirit of the "third moral appeal" of the ARC/AIDS Vigil in San Francisco: "We appeal to the FDA to immediately allow American physicians to prescribe medicines and treatments for ARC and AIDS that are available to their colleagues in other countries." (The ARC/AIDS Vigil has held a continuous vigil and AIDS information center outside the Old Federal Building in San Francisco, with people there 24 hours a day every day for over two years.)

The recent FDA announcement could mark a major improvement. On the other hand, it might prove unworkable or ineffectual; or it might be abused, leading to pressures for its cancellation. At the time of this writing—two days after the announcement—we believe that the FDA deserves credit for a good-faith effort to develop cooperation with the AIDS community.

This policy does not address all of the research and access problems, however. For example, it will probably do nothing to make drugs like ampligen more quickly available.

Potential Benefits

• If it proves workable, the new policy could let us move attention away from the underground mindset and operation, in order to focus on the more important issue of what drugs do work, and how should the drug trials be organized. While the question of a person's freedom to use a treatment whether or not it works is indeed an important issue—for empowerment and for other reasons—the more important question is what treatments do in fact work, and how can the evidence be collected, evaluated, and applied quickly and effectively. If the FDA's new announcement proves effective in practice, it will let everyone focus less on fights over access, and more on how we can work together to get treatments tested and made available.

• Second, the new policy could remove major red-tape obstacles hindering community-based trials of some of the drugs most interesting to scientists and physicians. We have heard that some of the most highly regarded physicians are delighted that now they can set up community-based clinical trials for the benefit of their patients, using the most appropriate experimental treatments that otherwise were in practice prohibitively difficult to get. If the patient can order a personal supply of the drug from France, Japan, or elsewhere, certain well-justified trials which otherwise would not happen can now take place, leading to faster AIDS research for everyone's benefit.

• Researchers hope that the new policy will reduce the incidence of patients in drug trials secretly violating the trial conditions by using other treatments and not telling the investigators. Such secret treatment while one is in a trial degrades the data and harms everyone, by casting a pall over any trial results. But as long as patients are put in "lie or die" situations by poorly designed clinical trials, which compare medically unjustified treatment options such as one drug alone vs. a placebo, without proper management of opportunistic infections in either study arm, no amount of preaching will be effective.

The new FDA announcement moves away from the policy of forcing patients into trials by denying other means of access to treatments. If those who only want dextran sulfate, for example, can get it on their own and not only through a trial, then the motives for volunteering for a trial can shift more toward altruism, rather than drug access.

Much work remains to be done in reconciling the needs of researchers with those of patients and their physicians. For example, many trials cannot recruit volunteers, often because the studies have imposed conditions so much against the volunteers' interests that physicians will not recommend that their patients participate. We are seeing some hopeful signs that researchers are moving away from forcing patients into trials, toward making the trials more attractive—for example, by using blood-test "markers" such as poor blood counts as study endpoints, instead of severe illness or death.

*   And legal access to drugs not yet approved in this country could end the festering scandal of drugs used by thousands of people in Europe, Japan, or elsewhere being unavailable to Americans, even when they are unquestionably the only appropriate treatment for the patient. In the past these drugs have been accessible only to those Americans who could afford to travel to pick them up—a loophole for the rich and influential which allowed the system to continue, because if enforcement had been tightly applied to everyone, political opposition would long ago have forced reform. Allowing patients to receive the drugs by mail will help to end this shameful situation of one medicine for the rich and another for everyone else.

It takes six to eight years to get a drug approved in the United States—and the clock starts only after the physicians, scientists, and investors most knowledgeable about the drug have good reason to be interested in it. The process costs so much that companies often don't bother with U.S. approval, even for drugs which unquestionably do work, meaning that Americans will never have regular access to drugs in common use elsewhere. The system must be reformed, but reform takes time; allowing Americans to order drugs not approved here is a stopgap which can save lives in the meantime.

Potential Risks

*   The new policy might prove unworkable in practice—as happened with the "treatment IND," announced by the FDA over a year ago to speed access to experimental drugs for serious or life-threatening conditions, which has had almost no practical effect since then.

We believe that today's situation is different, however. With the treatment IND, all the initiative had to come from the top. Nothing happened unless both the FDA and a drug company agreed—and neither one had incentive to act. But allowing patients to order personal-use quantities of unapproved drugs decentralizes the initiative to patients and physicians. No central approval or other action is needed.

And if patients and physicians are frustrated in their attempts to obtain appropriate treatments, the public will know of the problem right away. With the treatment IND, it took a year of hoping that something was happening behind the scenes for the public to realize that the system wasn't working.

• Another danger is that fast-buck artists will abuse and discredit the system. They could, for example, use their First Amendment rights to promote dubious treatments in the U.S., while secretly benefitting from businesses they set up abroad.

There is no quick fix for this problem. The AIDS community will have to put more effort into warning itself about frauds, and urging people to talk with their doctors before they part with their money. In the past we have had to work first and foremost for access. Now, if the FDA's new policy proves workable, patients can focus less on how to get a drug, and more on whether or not they should do so.

CHINESE HERBS SCREENED
FOR ANTI-HIV ACTIVITY

Two researchers, one at the University of California at Davis and the other at the Chinese University of Hong Kong, have screened 27 herbs used in traditional Chinese medicine for treating infections. Five of the herbs almost completely stopped HIV in laboratory cells; six others also showed significant activity (see lists below). The scientists published this work in the journal *Antiviral Research* earlier this year.

The first step in the study was to select the herbs. The researchers used a computerized database of traditional Chinese medicinal herbs, compiled at the Chinese University of Hong Kong, to select the 27 herbs to test. Many others would also be appropriate for the same screening.

Then crude extracts were prepared by boiling "under reflux," meaning that special apparatus was used to condense and recirculate vapors. After further purification steps, the researchers ran tests to find the greatest concentration of each extract which was not toxic to the cells and did not inhibit their growth.

Then each of the 27 herbs was assayed by adding HIV to the cell cultures in the presence of the largest nontoxic concentration of the extract. Every assay was repeated three times. To be considered as showing anti-HIV activity, every one of the three assays had to reduce the percent of infected cells by at least three standard deviations from the average value in control assays (which were done in quadruplicate).

For example, the herb which did best, Viola yedoensis, reduced the percentage of infected cells from 12.8 to zero in the first assay, from 3.8 to .4 in the second, and from 21.5 to .4 in the third—using the maximum concentration of herbal extract not toxic to the cells.

The five best herbs were Arctium lappa L., Viola yedoensis, Andrographis paniculata, Lithospermum erythrorhizon, and Alternanthera philoxeroides. The other six which also passed the test in all three assays were Epimedium grandiflorum, Lonicera japonica, Woodwardia unigemmata, Senecio scandens, Coptis chinensis, and Prunella vulgaris.

The researchers studied one herb, Viola yedoensis, in greater depth. They found that it did *not* kill or inactivate HIV on direct exposure, did not induce interferon production by the cells, and did not inhibit herpes or other viruses against which it was tested. The mechanism of action against HIV is unknown.

Comments

The fact that a drug stops HIV infection in the laboratory does not mean that it will work in people. And in this experiment, the concentrations of herbal extracts tested—the maximum concentration which did not harm the cells which the HIV was infecting—was probably much higher than could be achieved in the body. Presumably blood levels were not measured because of the many obvious difficulties of conducting any human experimentation. If the researchers had set out to run human trials, their project would not have happened at all.

Yet despite this caution in interpreting the results, it seems clear that a medicine long used in humans and which almost completely stops infection of cells by HIV at a concentration harmless to the cells deserves a closer look. How will this research be carried out?

The authors stated in their paper that they do not have the expertise or facilities to isolate and identify the anti-HIV compounds. Drug companies could do this work. But even if one took an interest—and few of even the largest pharmaceutical companies have any antiviral program—it would take years to isolate the chemicals, learn how to manufacture and use them, and get them approved as drugs.

The alternative, of course, is to test the herbs themselves, with the help of herbalists familiar with them. Such a trial might be done through a community-based research organization such as New York's Community Research Initiative. That way the trial would meet all legal standards for protection of patients, and also meet scientific standards of good study design and data collection and analysis, so that the results would be credible.

In practice it will take a long time to get any such study going, because there are so few organizations now doing community-based trials, and so many candidate drugs to test. Meanwhile people are likely to try some of the herbs on their own; most if not all of those mentioned above are widely available. Anyone trying herbs should at least check with herbalists, physicians, or other experts about dosage, precautions, and any other information on how to use them safely. Even though herbs are "natural," they are medicines and must be used appropriately.

For More Information

For more information on screening the herbs for anti-HIV activity, see R. Shihman Chang and H.W. Yeung, "Inhibition Of Growth of Human Immunodeficiency Virus By Crude Extracts Of Chinese Medicinal Herbs," *Antiviral Research* 9 (1988), pp. 163–76.

Note that we have only reviewed the article here. We have not interviewed the authors, or herbalists or other experts. We hope that others, perhaps an organization of herbalists or of persons interested in AIDS treatments, will look further into these potential treatments.

We do not know of anyone following up these leads at this time.

AUTOVACCINATION REPORT

An autovaccination treatment developed at the University of Dusseldorf in West Germany has shown impressive results in the 14 AIDS/ARC patients treated so far, according to a letter published last month in *The Lancet*. Forty-two additional patients have now entered the study.

The 14 patients started the treatment in 1985 and 1986. Twelve have shown clear and often major clinical improvement—including those who had had pneumocystis once or more before beginning. (Of the other two, one left the study in 1986 and died a year later; the second, an IV drug user who also has hepatitis B, is still alive although his condition has worsened since he started the trial in June of 1986.)

Comment

The treatment consists of a heat-treated, killed-virus vaccine prepared from each patient's own blood. This approach overcomes the usual vaccine problem of the great variation among different strains of HIV. A vaccine prepared for one strain usually will not work for others; but here the patient's own strain is used.

Autovaccination also eliminates the worry of reinfection with a different strain in case some of the virus should survive the heat treatment.

But how could it help to inoculate the patient with antigens which he or she already has? The answer may be that the AIDS virus subverts the process by which the body normally produces antibodies, causing it to produce more virus instead. But the killed virus cannot infect the T-helper cells, so it might allow the body's normal defenses to work, even when they could not work against the live virus.

For More Information

For more information about autovaccination as an AIDS/ARC treatment, see the letter by H. Bruster *et al.*, *The Lancet* (June 4, 1988), pp. 1284–5. Most of the other information now available—referenced in that letter—has been published only in German.

AMFAR SUPPORTS COMMUNITY TRIALS

The American Foundation for AIDS Research awarded $30,000 to New York's Community Research Initiative, and $50,427 to San Francisco's County Community Consortium, for testing AIDS treatments through patient volunteers in physicians' private practices. Such community-based trials can be set up much faster than the usual trials at university or government medical centers.

AmFAR has also earmarked up to one million dollars—to be raised at a Carnegie Hall concert organized by Leonard Bernstein—for additional community trials. The benefit concert is scheduled for World AIDS Day, December 1, 1988.

Since 1985, AmFAR has awarded $11 million in seed or start-up grants to more than 170 research teams. These grants have usually been for AIDS laboratory studies. Support for community-based clinical trials represents a new direction for the organization.

DEXTRAN SULFATE AVAILABLE FASTER

Positive Action HealthCare in San Francisco (see *AIDS Treatment News*, Issue Number 47) has arranged for a supplier in Japan to ship small quantities of dextran sulfate for personal use. Delivery should take 10 to 14 days—compared with four to six weeks usually required in the past, when people had to collect orders and fly to Japan to fill them. Anyone using dextran sulfate should be monitored by a physician; and U.S. Customs will occasionally hold a package and ask the addressee to name his or her physician before the drug is released.

SAN FRANCISCO: ORGANIZE AIDS BENEFIT

SoMARTS AGAINST AIDS, a group of South of Market galleries and businesses, has organized a series of benefits in August, including:

• Gran Fury representative Tom Kalin speaks on August 6; admission is free to this event. Gran Fury, a collective of artists in all fields, has done outstanding work with ACT UP in New York. Kalin will discuss options for organizing similar projects here.

• Other events include photographic exhibitions on kissing (Bruce Velick Gallery), on monuments and memorials (New Langton Arts), and on women with AIDS (The San Francisco Arts Commission Gallery). Performances include a work in progress by Ellen Sebastian (August 20), a reading "Eros and Writing" (August 5), and a wrap-up party on a ship at Fort Mason (September 4).

Beneficiaries include *AIDS Treatment News*, the San Francisco Suicide Prevention Hotline, the AIDS Emergency Fund, and the San Francisco AIDS Foundation Food Bank.

SAN FRANCISCO: PROJECT INFORM NEEDS VOLUNTEERS

Project Inform, which provides information about new and experimental AIDS and HIV treatments, urgently needs volunteers for hotline and other work. Due to increasing publicity, its hotlines now handle 4,000 calls a month, a major increase in just the last two months.

Volunteers benefit by helping a larger cause, working one on one with people in need, and staying current on AIDS treatment information.

Those who can work during the day can help on the hotline. In the evening there is other work in the office.

Hotline training consists of one day of classroom instruction, followed by three weeks of supervised work. On the last week trainees answer calls while a more experienced volunteer listens in.

If you might be able to volunteer, call Project Inform (see Appendix B) and ask for a volunteer application.

SAN FRANCISCO: DR. LEVIN SPEAKS, AUGUST 9

As we went to press, we learned that Dr. Alan Levin of Positive Action HealthCare will speak at the weekly meeting of The Healing Alternatives Foundation, Tuesday, August 9, 1988 at 7:30 PM, at the Metropolitan Community Church, 150 Eureka Street, San Francisco. John S. James of *AIDS Treatment News* will also be on the panel.

Issue Number 62
AUGUST 12, 1988

FDA DRUG APPROVAL: MAJOR REFORMS CONSIDERED

A behind-the-scenes effort to reform the Federal drug-approval process has recently become public through an editorial in *The Wall Street Journal* (August 2, 1988), and a major article in *The New York Times* (August 7, 1988).

The effort, spearheaded by Vice President George Bush and his Presidential Task Force on Regulatory Relief, apparently seeks the following changes:

• Regulatory hurdles could vary with the severity of the disease. For example, a treatment for AIDS, cancer, or Alzheimer's disease could be approved more quickly than a new cold remedy or sleeping pill.

• For life-threatening diseases, the current "phase III" testing (large-scale efficacy trials) could be eliminated. This phase takes the longest, yet it contributes the least, since the great majority of drugs which begin phase III are eventually approved (after several more years) for marketing. These drugs have already been proved safe in phase I, and probably effective in phase II.

• The FDA would be allowed to require a "phase IV," or post-marketing monitoring of the drug. This step is important because one of the current obstacles to earlier approval is that once approval is given, the FDA loses control of the drug and the company has no further incentive to complete its research. Instituting phase IV could allow the FDA to let patients get the drug while the research continued.

(The importance of finishing the research is illustrated by the problems in surgery, where new procedures do not need to prove efficacy. Some experts believe that a large fraction of operations are unnecessary, and that some accepted procedures may not be effective or do more harm than good. The issue isn't whether drugs should prove efficacy, but whether drugs that probably work should be denied to patients in an emergency, pending lengthy, final proof.)

• The FDA would also work more closely with companies during phase I and phase II, to design trials which could lead quickly to approval, and avoid the need to redo trials because of ambiguities in the results.

Comment

These reforms could be very important—or they could fail, in many ways. The AIDS community must be vigilant to see that the needs of persons with life-threatening ill-nesses are addressed.

The forces which wrecked previous reform attempts like the "treatment IND" could sabotage this one too. A process as complex and delicate as drug approval inevita-bly leaves room for obstructionism. Could the proposed reforms deal with the depth of problems which have occurred?

Time and again the AIDS drugs closest to approval have had extraordinary bad luck:

• Going into the recent Stockholm conference, the only drug close to approval was Imreg-1. Four days later it was so vilified by exaggerated criticism that the researchers were terrified of loss of their professional reputations. Criticism of the research design was legitimate. But the crowd lost the perspective to ask whether, even if all the criti-cism were true, the drug still should be available to patients.

• A year and a half ago, ribavirin was closest to approval. Early release of ques-tionable data led not only to justified criticism, but to extraordinary vilification of leading researchers who were completely innocent of wrongdoing.

• Imuthiol (DTC) looks good in every way. But the U.S. trial results on which U.S. approval depends are being kept secret, for about a year, pending the completion of the last straggling arms of the multicentered trial. Apparently the developers feared that what happened to ribavirin could happen to them if they did not wait for full com-pletion. What they are doing makes sense if the existence of an emergency is ignored.

• DHPG (ganciclovir), the only accessible treatment for AIDS-related blind-ness, got caught in regulatory limbo long ago because after compassionate use in thou-sands of cases everybody knew that it worked—and that scientific trials to "prove" it worked would require deliberately letting people go blind. When the FDA acted against this drug, apparently to punish the company for not doing the scientific trials, other compassionate-use treatments such as fluconazole for cryptococcal meningitis suddenly became less available. It is well known that the FDA does not like compas-sionate use for AIDS drugs.

The common factor in each of the cases above is that the drugs were close to approval. All were threats to AZT, which takes in more money than anything else in AIDS, and therefore has more clout.

The corporations victimized by these abuses seldom dare to speak out, for fear of retribution not only against the drug in question, but against their non-AIDS drugs as well. Government agencies will not speak out. Researchers dare not, for doing so would damage their career prospects with almost any potential employer, public or private. Funded AIDS organizations have feared loss of funding if they speak about treatments not already approved by the FDA. In short, no major institutions nor any of their employees can tell the public what is wrong—which is why these problems were not recognized, addressed, and corrected long ago.

For these reasons we are only cautiously optimistic about the proposed reforms. The AIDS community must be cautious about fine print which could destroy the goal of faster approval—such as the rumored proposal to start the reform by moving all AIDS drugs back to phase I, requiring that all the trials be redone.

In particular we should note whether the new policy has written standards specifying the conditions under which a drug can be released. The "treatment IND" system had no such standards, meaning that drug companies set their course depending on their reading of internal FDA politics. The real decisions were made privately, with public scrutiny excluded.

The U.S. drug-approval process was deliberately designed to be impervious to outside pressures and influences. Clearly a case can be made for setting up the system that way; for otherwise, powerful companies could buy or pressure their way to approvals not medically justified. But this system has also resisted scrutiny and challenge of the ill-concealed, de facto public policy decision to write off those already ill or infected with HIV.

The FDA is not the whole problem. The NIH, and private drug companies, have done no better. Few major drug companies even have an antiviral program. Almost all of the ballyhooed business interest in AIDS research concerns only new tests or other non-treatment products—and much of the rest is stock manipulation.

The fundamental problem has been a pervasive lack of political will to save the lives of people with AIDS. During the last year we have seen the beginning development of this political will. But still it must overcome the legacy of previous years—the inertia of legions of officials and professionals less inclined to do the job than to argue why it can't be done.

Ultimately this battle will be won; this country will not sit still while hundreds of thousands die from public neglect. The question is how long victory will take, and that depends on the effort we bring to the struggle.

THE EMPEROR HAS NO CLOTHES: NOTES ON AIDS DRUG TESTING AND ACCESS
by Nathaniel Pier, M.D.

The following comments were edited from an August 5 telephone conversation with Nathaniel Pier, M.D., a New York physician treating several hundred patients with AIDS and related conditions:

"We have lost something in the struggle to find therapies for AIDS. The individual patient with the counsel and guidance of his or her physician must have the right to make choices, to have options. People with AIDS and at risk for AIDS have abdicated their responsibility far too much to the medical establishment and the research establishment to make this decision for them.

"The primary role of a clinician such as myself is to synthesize a course of action with a patient that makes sense. That means every patient is offered the opportunity of choosing from the options that are available, under the careful guidance of their clinician. This should not be a major issue.

"The current system of doing drug studies has failed. It has bureaucratized to the point where it takes two to three years to test a drug that should be tested in two to four months. There is no proof that this system works. So let's go back to the old system where individual clinicians are given the opportunity of synthesizing a course of action.

"Under supervised protocols from a national group, we should get access to drugs that are in phase II trials, including drugs that have not had efficacy demonstrated, and clinicians should be allowed to authorize the option of trying these drugs if patients want to. (Editor's note: drugs in "phase II" testing have already passed the "phase I" test for dosage, toxicity, and safety.) It should be up to the patient with the clinician's guidance to make such decisions. The fact that we have to wait two to four years for a drug like lentinan or dideoxycytidine to come down as a potentially useful drug is not fair to the patients who have no other options, who are simply going to die.

"The system is essentially telling patients with immune deficiency disease, 'We don't care about you, go home and die. We will cure this disease in our own time with our designer drugs.' Every patient should demand that anybody with HIV disease should have access to a number of experimental options through their clinician, and these options should be offered to them as supervised protocols.

"A good example is the multi-drug protocols for cancer. If you're diagnosed with colo-rectal cancer, for example, your oncologist ties in to a national computer where your statistics are kept confidentially; out the other end comes a protocol. Not only are you allowed to participate in a potentially lifesaving drug regimen, but the data that's collected from you goes back to a center that very quickly will collect information as to whether this particular combinations of drugs works.

"We should be doing this in AIDS. There is no reason that after 18 months of AZT, we shouldn't be allowed to combine other drugs for both antiviral and immunomodulatory effect. We could do this on thousands of patients overnight if there were a national registry and a system for doing it.

"We wouldn't need to do complex virological or immunological tests. The studies requiring such tests should be done in smaller protocols at major medical centers. Otherwise, once a month the physician would do the blood work specified in the protocol, and send the data to the NIH, and the physician will fill in clinical data. Probably within three or four months we could find out which treatment combinations are best. People with AIDS should be demanding that the system be reformed to allow anybody at risk access to these drugs under supervised protocols.

"It seems that groups advocating for people with AIDS have lost this primary goal, that it should be the *patient's* option, to use experimental drugs under guidance, supervision, and monitoring.

"The system now in place for developing and testing and distributing AIDS drugs is not working, it is not producing new therapeutic options. In the last two years all we've had is AZT. AIDS advocates need to start saying that the emperor has no clothes. So let's start a system that is going to work—one where people with AIDS-related problems get rapid access to experimental drugs in protocol, on a routine basis through their clinicians, whether private physicians or at a clinic.

"Let's stop wasting time. I have done my rounds of researchers, and there is nothing, there are no new drugs close to approval. It's a scandal that our system with its funding still isn't producing.

"The system claims to be working, but isn't. Why aren't more people demanding access to these drugs which are potentially effective and are safe to use? We must stop this idea that testing drugs on a small number of patients, then on a slightly larger number of patients is a reasonable approach when people are dying. We want to make experimental therapies available to people as a matter of course, as a matter of therapy, so that clinicians caring for AIDS patients can get access to these drugs under supervised protocols. Not only would patients have more options, we also would learn quickly what works.

"It is completely unreasonable that two years after AZT there is no new drug, and combination therapies using antivirals and immunomodulators are not available. It is unreasonable that Frank Young of the FDA says that very few drugs are likely to be approved between now and 1991, when we're losing 48 people a day to this disease.

"It's not working, so let's come up with a new system. Let's use experimental treatments as potential therapy for ailing patients, and do it in a manner that's going to provide useful information. Set up a national registry, check out protocols of combination therapies, and let people use them. Similar systems have been used for cancer and heart disease.

"For example:

"At the recent Stockholm conference, information from NIH demonstrated that an AZT and dideoxycytidine on alternating weeks may be an effective alternative for people who can no longer take AZT continuously. Why isn't this drug combination available to these people, who have few other choices?

"NIH made dextran sulfate a top priority drug in January 1988. It has taken eight months since then to get ready to start its first study, a multicenter trial with all of 60 patients. When thousands of people have no other choice, it's inhuman not to make such a safe drug available to patients through their doctors, as part of a study.

"Where are new antivirals such as DDA or DDI? NIH has been recruiting for clinical trials for about six months.

"My problem with the treatment underground is that for the last two and a half years we have tried naltrexone, AL 721, antabuse, dextran sulfate. Something has come along every few months that has offered people hope, and access to therapy that they couldn't get other places. That's very important. But I as a clinician am tired of my patients not knowing which of these therapies is the best to choose, tired of patients being bamboozled by people into taking this or that or the other thing, tired of not being able to assess whether or not an approach or combination is really benefitting the patients. We need a system so that when a therapy comes along, we can evaluate the efficacy very quickly.

"What I'm proposing is very clear. We need a national registry, and if a patient has an AIDS-related problem at any stage of the illness, and if that patient elects to try to intervene, there should be protocols available to that patient's clinician. There should be multiple protocols for every stage of the disease, so that we can quickly assess which intervention might in fact make a difference.

"These protocols should be available not just through a few selected centers, not just to the lucky few who can afford to go to doctors who can get them into these studies. They should be available to every physician who treats AIDS patients, not just in the major cities. We know enough about this disease to develop a logical approach involving antiviral, immunomodulatory, prophylactic, and anti-inflammatory therapies.

"There are enough drugs to be tried so that we could develop these protocols in a few weeks and make them available to clinicians through a national computer. The data from these combination trials could start pouring in, and we would know within a few months which of the available combinations are working best, rather than the years and years that it's currently taking.

"This approach will give patients hope, and access to humane, well-supervised medical treatments, instead of allowing them to live in fear or desperation, or search for the few trials available. At the same time it will allow them to participate in a larger effort, to find what therapies work best for everybody, making their situation meaningful not only for themselves but for the world.

"We want to participate, to know what is happening with the research and what the future plans are. We want to reduce the secrecy, the sense that scientific data is proprietary or exclusive in the face of this epidemic.

"The current system simply has not produced the goods. And if Dr. Frank Young's prediction (of few new drugs approved by 1991) is any indication, it will not produce the goods for a long time to come. This consigns large numbers of people to death without giving them a dignified chance to fight back. This is not an acceptable human or reasonable approach to doing research in this epidemic.

"After five years of being on the front lines, my heartfelt feeling is that the top priority for people with AIDS and people who care about AIDS is to demand access to experimental therapies to try to save their lives.

"I appeal to people to organize this effort immediately, to bring it forward in their local groups, then present the case to their political people, and to the people who are running the present medical system of testing drugs. It's time we told them that the emperor has no clothes, that the current system is not working. It's time to insist on wider access to promising therapies, and rapid testing of existing drugs to develop better treatment options."

CD4 TREATMENT TEST NEAR?

An article in the August 9 *San Francisco Chronicle* first reported that Genentech, a biotechnology company in South San Francisco, had been granted permission for human tests of CD4, its genetically-engineered AIDS treatment. The company applied for permission in January.

In the week before the article, two people who were considering volunteering had asked us what we knew about the treatment.

CD4 is the protein found in the CD4 receptor site on T-helper and certain other cells. In the laboratory, manufactured CD4 provides an alternate target for HIV, preventing it from infecting new cells.

There will be a risk for the first person or first few persons who try this treatment, however. Some experts fear that injecting CD4 could cause the body to develop antibodies against its own T-helper cells, making AIDS symptoms worse. Animal and laboratory tests have been successful, but because this drug is so specific for the human immune system, these tests cannot rule out the possible danger.

Despite the risk, CD4 represents an important potential treatment for many people. It should be tested quickly. San Francisco General Hospital and other medical centers are now preparing to run initial trials.

PCR TEST CAUTIONS

Issue Number 60 of *AIDS Treatment News* described the new PCR test, a very sensitive biochemical test for HIV. After reading the article, Joseph Sonnabend, M.D. called to alert us to the controversy over whether this research test is ready for clinical diagnostic use, because of the unknown risk that it could produce false positives or false negatives. Dr. Sonnabend and others, some speaking off the record, alerted us to the following information and concerns:

- The PCR test is so sensitive that sometimes it can detect a single molecule of the DNA being looked for. Therefore it is also extremely sensitive to even the tiniest contamination of laboratory glassware, reagents, etc.

- Even small variations in the chemicals used in the test can cause large differences in the result. And no one has yet made sure that the test works in a standard way when performed in different laboratories.

- Although about 200 people at least have already been tested with the PCR, this number is too small to provide very accurate data on the risk of false positives or false negatives.

- It is too early to be sure of the clinical meaning of a PCR test.

Most experts seem to agree (1) that the PCR should not be used by itself for diagnosing patients, and that (2) this very important research test may also be useful for diagnosis after more is known about it. Whether the PCR should be used at all at this time for diagnosing patients remains controversial.

ROADS TO RECOVERY: RESOURCE BOOK FOR PERSONS WITH AIDS

Roads to Recovery, an 860-page loose-leaf compendium of AIDS information from a PWA perspective, has been compiled by Jeremy Bell and published by Face to Face, an AIDS service organization in Sonoma County, California.

The articles selected represent many points of view—including mainstream medicine, minority medical views such as some of the syphilis theories, and spiritual approaches. Most of the material concerns treatment options, especially non-approved or alternative treatments. Chapters on "AIDS 101" (basic background information), coping, doctor-patient relationships, legal issues, a glossary, and resource lists also are included.

The high price, mainly to pay for photocopying over 800 pages, and the mass of material and mixture of different viewpoints will deter some from using this book.

We think that *Roads to Recovery* will be most useful as a reference. Libraries, service organizations, support and study groups, and individuals who want in-depth information or who have limited information available in their localities may want a copy.

Roads to Recovery, provided in loose-leaf form to allow future updating, is available for $50 donation ($65 for hospitals, institutions, or physicians) from

Face to Face (see appendix B). Please include $6 for shipping and handling. This project is a fundraiser for the PWA Emergency Fund.

AMFAR GUIDE TO AIDS EDUCATIONAL MATERIAL

The American Foundation for AIDS Research has published the *AIDS Information Resource Directory*. It includes descriptions of over 1,000 AIDS brochures and pamphlets, videotapes and films, curricula and instructional programs, posters, public service campaigns, manuals, and periodicals.

A panel of 34 experts reviewed the material for medical accuracy, appropriateness to the target audience, and production quality. The directory divides material by target audience, for example, "Gay and Bisexual Men," "Black Community," and "Health Care Professionals and Service Providers."

The *AIDS Information resource Directory* costs $10, and can be ordered by calling AmFAR (see Appendix B).

Issue Number 63
August 26, 1988

HYPERICUM: COMMON HERB SHOWS
ANTIRETROVIRAL ACTIVITY

A chemical in a common plant used in herbal medicine (St. John's wort), and previously tested in humans as an antidepressant, has been found to strongly inhibit retroviral infections in animal and laboratory tests. Researchers writing in the July 1988 *Proceedings of the National Academy of Sciences* (abbreviated *PNAS*) suggested that hypericin, an active ingredient found in plants of the *Hypericum* family, commonly known as St. John's wort, might become a useful AIDS therapy.

The fact that the drug can be given by mouth, has already been used in humans, and is found in a widely available plant customarily used as a medicinal herb and sold at little cost, suggests that this treatment possibility might also be developed through the herbal and alternative-treatment traditions, avoiding the years of delay built into mainstream pharmaceutical development. But the herb must be used carefully, because large doses have poisoned grazing animals when they fed on it, and because many questions about its possible use as an AIDS treatment remain unanswered.

No human trials for HIV have yet been conducted. We have heard through guerilla clinic sources that several persons have started using the herb for this purpose, but they started only a few days ago, so it is too early to see any results.

Antiviral Tests of Hypericin

The July *PNAS* article (Meruelo *et al.*, 1988) gave a detailed account of tests of hypericin against two retroviral diseases of mice. (A closely related variant, "pseudohypericin," is also found in the herbs and has similar antiviral effects; this article will use "hypericin" to refer to both chemicals.) Most of their research did not use HIV, presumably because this virus does not cause diseases in animals, preventing direct animal tests of HIV treatments. Also, there is a serious shortage of laboratory facilities set up to work with HIV. But researchers are increasingly interested in testing possible

360

AIDS treatments in the "animal models" which are available—animal diseases caused by retroviruses, such as feline leukemia in cats, or the mouse retroviral diseases used here.

Meruelo and colleagues did mention that preliminary laboratory work showed that pseudohypericin could reduce the spread of HIV.

Most of the testing reported in the July *PNAS* article used the Friend leukemia virus (FV) in mice. A single small dose of hypericin, given up to one day after the injection of the virus, completely prevented the rapid development of disease and death. Long-term survival, for at least the 150-day period of the experiment, was 44 percent for the treated animals, while all the untreated animals died before the 25th day.

No virus could be found in the infected but treated mice. Also, there was no enlargement of the spleen in treated mice ten days after infection, while the spleen was several times the normal size in untreated mice at that time.

The researchers found no toxicity or side effects from the small treatment dose—even though they ran a panel of 25 blood tests to look for toxicity.

In this study, the hypericin was given by injection—a more precise way to administer a drug than orally, and more convenient in animal tests. But oral administration also proved effective.

Hypericin and AZT

The exact mechanism of antiviral action of hypericin is unknown. But Meruelo and colleagues found that it had no effect against reverse transcriptase, meaning that it works by a different mechanism than AZT. This finding suggests that hypericin might work well in combination with AZT.

An earlier published study, cited by Meruelo and colleagues, showed that AZT alone protected mice from FV infection. But the AZT had to be given repeatedly, at doses highly toxic to the animals. Hypericin suppressed the virus with a single small dose, without toxicity.

What about treatment after disease has already developed? Meruelo and colleagues administered the drug early—up to one day after exposure to the virus. But their paper mentioned unpublished, apparently preliminary work in which "combinations of hypericin/pseudohypericin with (AZT) have been found remarkably effective in curing mice from FV-induced leukemia at concentrations and frequencies of administration in which each of the two drugs separately was ineffective."

Human Therapeutic Experience: Medical and Scientific Papers

No human study of antiviral effects of hypericin has been published. But there is safety information from at least four decades of testing *Hypericum* extracts in humans, as an antidepressant and antibiotic. Some of this research suggests that there may be antibiotics or antivirals other than hypericin in the plant.

Meruelo and others cited a 1949 article on antidepressant use in humans. Several more recent articles have been published, mostly in German and Russian; see references below for a partial list. Medical *Hypericum* extracts may be available in Germany, the Soviet Union, or other countries, but we do not have details at this time. (West Germany has nearly twice as many approved drugs as the United States.)

Herbal Use

We examined several herb books with information about *Hypericum*. The books were: John Lust, *The Herb Book* (New York: Bantam, 1974); Mrs. M. Grieve, *A Modern Herbal* (New York: Hafner Publishing, 1967); Michael Weiner, *Weiner's Herbal: Guide to Herbal Medicine* (New York: Stein and Day, 1980); and Paul Schauenberg and Ferdinand Paris, *Guide to Medicinal Plants* (New Canaan, CT: Keats Publishing, Inc., 1977).

Different plant species have been studied. All the herb books, and most of the scientific papers on hypericin which we found by a computer search, used *Hypericum* perforatum. But Meruelo and colleagues extracted hypericin from *Hypericum triquetrifolium* Turra—a different species in the same family. The readily available *Hypericum perforatum* is also known to contain hypericin.

It is hard to summarize the traditional medical uses of this herb (commonly called St. John's wort), because different herb books list different uses. Antidepressant and related applications predominate.

Most but not all of the herb books warn readers about the potential toxicity of the plant.

Toxicity

All sources we have seen referred to only one form of toxicity of St. John's wort: that excessive doses makes the skin abnormally sensitive to light. Such "photosensitizing" is a side effect of various drugs.

Meruelo and colleagues cited reports that in livestock exposed to very high doses and intense light, the reaction can be severe or even fatal. But in their test of hypericin with over 800 mice, they found no serious toxicity. And toxicity has not prevented human use of herbal extracts as an antidepressant.

Weiner's Herbal recommends against internal use because the plant contains hypericin, and light-skinned persons can suffer dermatitis, burning, and blistering of the skin if exposed to sunlight after using the herb—depending on the amount ingested and the amount of sunlight.

John Lust's *The Herb Book* warns that St. John's wort has poisoned livestock and can make the skin sensitive to light. But it does include the herb in a number of combinations for medicinal teas.

It would seem prudent for anyone trying St. John's wort to stay out of the sun. Sunscreens have been prescribed for patients taking other photosensitizing drugs.

One well-regarded herbalist, reached shortly before press time, told us that despite earlier concerns about St. John's wort, the toxicity seen in grazing animals has not been a problem in humans. He believed that the difference was due to the very different stomachs of ruminants. We have been unable to find any published reports of cases of human toxicity; however we have not obtained a number of papers on the herb, so such reports might exist.

Our main concern is that herbal preparations can vary greatly in the amount of active ingredients they contain. Standardized preparations and careful medical monitoring will be needed to determine safe and effective doses (if any) for persons with HIV infection. Fortunately the chemical properties of hypericin suggest that herbal extracts should be easy to prepare, test, and standardize.

Chemical Properties of Hypericin

The *Merck Index* gives the following information:

- Hypericin decomposes at 320 degrees C. (Therefore it will not be harmed by the heat of boiling water if prepared as a tea.)

- It dissolves in water, providing the water is alkaline.

- Hypericin solutions in water are red below pH 11.5; above pH 11.5 they are green with red fluorescence. These properties should make it easy to test whether an extract contains hypericin, and how much. The *Merck Index* cites articles which published absorption and fluorescence spectra, which laboratories might use for precise tests.

- The *Merck Index* also noted that "very small quantities appear to have a tonic and tranquilizing action on the human organism."

Interview with Dr. Meruelo

We called Daniel Meruelo, Ph.D., the principal author of the *PNAS* article. He is concerned that people have started using St. John's wort or commercial extracts, and hopes they will wait for more scientific evidence. He added that it is unfair to people to develop this potential treatment in an improper way; that people could be made hopeful or desperate to get the substance before it is clear that it could be helpful. The result could be hype, distress, profiteering, and potentially great harm.

We expressed our concern that even if hypericin does work, it would take years to become available as a pharmaceutical; why not try the herb in the meantime? Dr. Meruelo replied that his team had found only minute amounts of hypericin in the commercial preparations they have tested. He doubted that it would be possible to get enough of the chemical from the herb. We asked how that could be a problem, if it is possible to get a toxic dose by taking too much of the herb; no one would want to use more than that. He answered that the hypericin did not seem to be responsible for the toxicity, as his mice showed little or no evidence of toxicity when given the purified chemical.

St. John's wort contains at least 50 chemicals, not only hypericin. Dr. Meruelo commented that earlier published studies which reported no toxicity from medical herbal preparations had not published blood tests to confirm the lack of toxicity.

Dr. Meruelo also said that the work was proceeding very rapidly; more would be learned in the next several months, and if all went well clinical trials might start within a year. Right now his team cannot obtain enough purified hypericin to do toxicity tests in dogs or higher animals; they get relatively little by extraction from St. John's wort, or by known means of chemical synthesis. They are now working on a better method for producing the chemical synthetically; that work is just beginning, however.

Dr. Meruelo also emphasized that everybody involved, at NIH or elsewhere, has been very cooperative with this project; everyone recognizes its urgency. The team, so far financed only by the researchers' institutions (New York University, and the Weizmann Institute of Science in Israel), has been working very hard for almost two years. Now that they have data they hope to get more funding, and to interest a pharmaceutical company.

We asked Dr. Meruelo why he and his colleagues decided to try hypericin in the first place. He replied that there was no reason to believe that there would be an anti-retroviral effect. But earlier papers had reported possible effectiveness of St. John's wort extracts against other viruses, such as herpes simplex and influenza (see references below); since retroviruses are a more urgent problem than herpes, and since one of the team members is a professor of organic chemistry at the Weizmann Institute and had an interest in the plant, they decided to try it.

Comment

Many questions remain. But despite Dr. Meruelo's understandable caution, we do believe it is important to investigate whether a useful treatment based on a simple herbal extract could be developed.

Until now the scientific community has believed that hypericin was largely responsible for the toxicity of excessive amounts of St. John's wort. The lack of side effects in Dr. Meruelo's mice casts doubt on this hypothesis, but does not conclusively disprove it. The question is crucial, because if hypericin does cause the toxicity, then it should be possible to get all of it one could use through herbal teas or other preparations, avoiding the need to wait for chemical synthesis and official drug approval.

The fact that the researchers are just beginning to learn how to synthesize hypericin efficiently, and will then start toxicity tests on dogs, and do not yet have a pharmaceutical company involved, suggests that it will take some time before hypericin arrives in the drugstores. Human testing alone usually takes seven to ten years for U.S. drug approval.

Hopefully standardized herbal extracts can be tested in community-based trials, with good medical supervision and scientific control so that we can quickly learn whether or not the treatment is helpful. Any such efforts using the herbs must be distinguished from efforts to develop the purified chemical. We hope both projects will move quickly.

Meanwhile several people have just started using a St. John's wort tea for HIV, outside of a formal trial. While their reports will be anecdotal and not the equivalent of a scientific trial, they will be the first information we will have on human use of the herb for AIDS/HIV.

Anyone considering using St. John's wort for AIDS/HIV should realize that there is no human experience yet with such use, serious questions remain on whether enough hypericin could be obtained this way, and there might be toxicity if one is exposed to sunlight or other strong light. For these reasons, we believe that this herb should not yet be considered a routine alternative treatment. Those who try it at this time are pioneers; they should educate themselves thoroughly, work with others, and take all appropriate precautions.

We have so far heard from two people who made a tea from dried St. John's wort; the tea did not have the characteristic red color of hypericin, suggesting that little of the chemical was present. One person reported nausea after drinking a dose of the tea much larger than suggested in the herb books.

Kolesnikova (1986) reports that extracts from St. John's wort leaves and flowers work better as antibacterials than decoctions (teas prepared by boiling)—and also allow better control of the dosage. We have seen only an abstract of the article and do not know how the extracts were made.

Various tinctures and other extracts of St. John's wort are routinely sold in health-food stores; some do have the expected red color. But companies can legally call a product *Hypericum* (or St. John's wort) extract even if it contains only infinitesimal quantities of the herb. Clearly we need chemical testing to answer serious doubts about whether various preparations contain enough hypericin to be worth trying. Independent non-profit groups such as HIV-positive buyers clubs could easily standardize doses by testing each lot of commercially available extracts and publishing the results—avoiding the complications of re-mixing and re-bottling a standard product of their own.

Alternatively, physicians may be able to obtain standardized medical extracts from abroad.

In the United States, St. John's wort is usually harvested in July and August. If more of the herb is needed, it will not be necessary to wait another year, because the same plant species is common in Australia, which has its summer during our winter. The old plants, incidentally, contain the most hypericin, while the young plants seem most toxic to livestock (Horseley, 1934).

AIDS Treatment News will continue to cover hypericin and St. John's wort, publishing updates as new information becomes available.

REFERENCES

Derbentseva, N.A., *et al.*, "Action of Tannins from Hypericum Perforatum L. on the Influenza Virus," Language: Russian. *Mikrobiol ZH* 311(6), (1972), pp. 768–72.

Hoffmann, J., and E.D. Kuhl, "Therapy of Depressive States with Hypericin," Language: German. *ZFA* (Stuttgart) 55(12) (April 30, 1979), pp. 776–82.

Horseley, C.H., "Investigation into the Action of St. John's Wort," *Journal of Pharmacol. Exp. Ther.* 50 (1934), pp. 310–18.

Kiriliuk, ZhI., "Treatment of Suppurative Infection with St. John's Wort and Kalanchoe Preparations," Language: Russian. *Vestn Khir* 119(9) (September 1977), pp. 112–16.

Kolesnikova, A.S., "Bactericidal and Immunocorrective Properties of Plant Extracts," Language: Russian. *Zh Mikrobiol Epidemiol Immunobiol* 3 (March 1986), pp. 75–8.

Meruelo, D., G. Lavie, and D. Lavie, "Therapeutic Agents with Dramatic Antiretroviral Activity and Little Toxicity at Effective Doses: Aromatic Polycyclic Diones Hypericin and Pseudohypericin," *Proceedings of the National Academy of Sciences, USA* 85 (July 1988), pp. 5230–4.

Muldner, H., and M. Zoller, "Antidepressive Effect of a Hypericum Extract Standardized to an Active Hypericine Complex: Biochemical and Clinical Studies," Language: German. *Arzneimittelforschung* 34(8), pp. 918–20.

Nozaki, J., *et al.*, "New Antiviral Agent Isolated from *Hypericum erectum* with Activity Against Herpes Simplex, Influenza, Rabies, Hepatitis B Virus, etc.," Abstract #C84-129876; we do not have the complete reference.

MEDICAL VIROLOGY CONFERENCE, SAN FRANCISCO, SEPTEMBER 22–24

The 1988 International Symposium on Medical Virology, sponsored by the Department of Pathology, University of California, Irvine Medical Center, will be at the Ramada Renaissance Hotel in San Francisco, Sept. 22–24.

Scientists will provide "a comprehensive overview of the diagnosis, clinical manifestations, and treatment of human viral diseases. In addition, poster sessions will provide an opportunity to discuss specific research and developmental work in new areas of medical virology. The symposium is directed to all individuals involved in the diagnosis and management of patients with viral infections, including microbiologists, internists, pathologists, infectious disease specialists, and medical technologists."

The conference is coordinated by Luis M. de la Maza, M.D., Ph.D.

STANFORD: NUTRITION AND AIDS CONFERENCE, SEPTEMBER 10

A one-day conference on nutrition and AIDS, organized by the ARIS Project (an AIDS service organization) and the Stanford AIDS Education Project, will take place at the Dinkelspiel Auditorium on the Stanford campus, Saturday, September 10. Registration at the door is 7:30 to 8:30 AM; a talk by Donald Kotler, M.D., gastrointestinal AIDS specialist at St. Luke's / Roosevelt Hospital Center in New York, starts at 9:00.

Cost is no more than $35.; credit is available for pharmacists, registered nurses, and registered dietitians. PWAs can register in advance for free admission.

DEXTRAN SULFATE SIDE EFFECTS

Alan Levin, M.D., of Positive Action HealthCare in San Francisco, asked us to warn people about possible gastrointestinal side effects of large doses of dextran sulfate.

In recent weeks he has seen at least six people with explosive bloody diarrhea after taking 3000 mg or more of dextran sulfate per day. Two of them had colonoscopies, and showed evidence of what looked like ulcerative colitis.

When these patients discontinued dextran sulfate, their symptoms resolved and stools became normal. One had a repeat colonoscopy, and the lesions seen earlier had resolved.

Dr. Levin is suggesting that the dose be lowered from 3000 to between 1800 and 2400 mg per day. He has three hundred patients who are using dextran sulfate; most had been taking about 3000 mg per day.

Donald Abrams, M.D., who is running a dextran sulfate study at San Francisco General Hospital, has also reported gastrointestinal symptoms as a side effect of the drug. The diarrhea has also led to questions about whether dextran sulfate is well absorbed.

In Japan, dextran sulfate has been used without a prescription for over 20 years. But the doses have been lower, commonly 900 mg per day.

SAN FRANCISCO: CHINESE MEDICINE PROGRAMS FOR SEROPOSITIVES

(1) Quan Yin Acupuncture and Herb Center in San Francisco will sponsor a new herbal program and study for 100 persons who are HIV positive. The 12-week program, which is partially subsidized and offered in conjunction with the Institute of Traditional Medicine in Portland, Oregon, and the Oriental Healing Arts Institute in Long Beach, California, still has 35 places open. Participants must call immediately to avoid missing the starting date of the program.

The cost of the herbs is $55 a month. A monthly consultation with an herbalist is included at no extra charge. Other costs are for two acupuncture sessions per month with any acupuncturist at Quan Yin (required as part of the program—sliding scale $20 to $75 per session), and a CBC blood test once per month (cost about $10). Quan Yin does accept insurance, does accept MediCal for acupuncture, and will help people with their insurance and financial planning.

(2) Separate, comprehensive HIV-positive (and AIDS/ARC) programs run by the San Francisco AIDS Alternative Healing Project (AAHP) will start in early September. These programs include acupuncture, herbal consulting, nutritional counseling, nutrition groups with Tom O'Connor, massage, individual counseling, hypnotherapy, chiropractic as needed, donated nutritional supplements, a support group run by a counselor, and additional consulting with Misha Cohen, clinical director of the HIV programs.

The programs require a 26-week commitment, and costs $140 per week for the HIV-positive program, and $170 for the AIDS/ARC, which is more intensive. AAHP does accept insurance, and does help people plan for financing, but it is a non-profit organization with no outside funding, so it must support itself through fees.

AAHP is just completing a six-month herbal treatment study with 22 persons with HIV infection and six with chronic fatigue syndrome.

The new programs will start in mid September.

(3) Other programs: Both Quan Yin and AAHP have or are developing other HIV programs. Some can be started at any time; but the advantage of the ones which begin at set times is that they are group programs, meaning that participants regularly meet each other and can more easily compare experiences. For more information about any of these programs, call the organizations at the numbers given in Appendix B.

TOM O'CONNOR ON NATIONAL TOUR

Tom O'Connor, author of *Living with AIDS: Reaching Out* (see review in *AIDS Treatment News,* Issue Number 38) may be able to speak to your group this Fall or Winter. He will be in the Carolinas to Toronto area in October, Hawaii in November, the Midwest and then Southern California in December, and the Gulf Coast (Texas to Florida) in January.

WASHINGTON, D.C. DEMONSTRATIONS, CONFERENCE, OCTOBER 5~13

A week of meetings, cultural events, and demonstrations, including a National AIDS Activism Conference (October 8), an activists meeting (October 9), and demonstrations at the Department of Health and Human Services (October 10) and the Food and Drug Administration (October 11), will mark the anniversary of last year's March on Washington for Lesbian and Gay Rights. Those who want to go should make travel plans now to get the low rates.

ACT NOW (AIDS Coalition to Network, Organize, and Win), a national coordinating group of various local ACT UP organizations, is sponsoring the treatment meetings and demonstrations. The Names Project, the National Gay and Lesbian Task Force, and other organizations, are sponsoring other events during the week.

United Airlines is offering group discounts, plus a donation to the Names Project for each ticket sold. Nicholas Sempeti of FOG Travel Service in San Francisco gave us pointers on buying tickets. For those who might be arrested at the FDA demonstration, where nonviolent civil disobedience is planned, he suggested a "refundable" rather than "nonrefundable" round-trip ticket. The refundable one, which costs a little more, allows changes with a 25 percent penalty for any leg of the trip changed. The nonrefundable ticket is lost if not used at the reserved time, requiring an expensive one-way trip back for those who spend time in jail. And of course it's important to buy tickets early; even if airline rules set a deadline for low fares such as two weeks before the flight, only a certain number of tickets are set aside for those fares, and often they sell out before the official deadline.

SAN FRANCISCO: CRI PROJECT NEEDS ADMINISTRATOR

The PWA Coalition of San Francisco is looking for an administrator to help it organize a community research initiative (CRI) to facilitate community-based trials. A medical/clinical research background is preferred. Applicants should have organizational and interpersonal skills, knowledge of HIV treatment options, word processing and writing skills, fundraising experience, and commitment to the project. Volunteers are also needed.

AIDS TREATMENT SURVEY: YOU CAN HELP

AIDS Treatment News is conducting a survey asking its 5,500 subscribers what AIDS/ARC/HIV treatments they believe worked best for them, and which ones seemed worst. The results will be published in *AIDS Treatment News*. You can help people everywhere by sharing your experience of what worked or didn't work for you. The following partial list of treatments may be helpful. But please feel free to include treatments whether they are on this list or not. Sometimes there is more than one name for a treatment, e.g. AZT, Retrovir, and Zidovudine. You can use any name; we will combine totals when appropriate.

- Acidophilus • Acyclovir • Acupuncture • Aerosol pentamidine • AL-721 (or workalikes—please specify) • Aloe vera • Alpha interferon • Amphotericin B • Amino acids (please specify) • Ampligen • Ansamycin • Antabuse • AS 101 • AZT • Bactrim • Bee propolis • BHT • Carrisyn • Castanospermine • Chemotherapy • Chinese medicine (please specify) • Coenzyme Q • Dapsone • DDC • Dextran sulfate • DHEA • Dideoxycytidine • DNCB • D-penicillamine • DTC • Echinacea • Egg lecithin lipids • Erythropoietin • Fansidar • Fluconazole • Foscarnet • Fusidic acid • Gamma globulin • Garlic • Germanium • Glandular extracts (please specify) • GM-CSF • Ganciclovir • Ginseng • Glycyrrhizin • Herbs (please specify) • Homeopathic treatments (please specify) • HPA-23 • Hydrocortisone • Hydrogen peroxide • Hyperimmune globulin • Imreg-1 • Imuthiol • Interferon (please specify) • Interleukin-2 • Iscador • Isoprinosine • Ketoconazole • Lecithin • Lentinan • Lysine • Methionine enkephalin (MEK) • Milk from hyperimmune cows • MM1 • Monolaurin • Mycelex • Naltrexone • Nutrition (please specify) • Nystatin • Ozone • Penicillin (megadose) • Peptide T • Plasmapheresis • Prosorba column • Proteolytic enzymes (Wobenzym, etc.) • Radiation therapy • Retrovir • Ribavirin • Rifabutin • St. John's wort • Salk polio vaccine • Salk HIV vaccine • Selenium • Septra • Shiitake mushrooms • Spiramycin • Spiritual approaches (please specify) • Stress reduction techniques • Thymic humoral factor • Thymopentin (TP5) • Thymostimulin • Transfer factor • Trimetrexate with leucovorin • Tumor necrosis factor • Typhoid vaccine • Visualization • Vitamins (please specify) • Wheat grass juice • Zidovudine • Zinc

Editor's Note (1989): This is not a current survey.

Issue Number 64
September 9, 1988

COMMUNITY-INITIATED AIDS DRUG TRIALS: INTERVIEW WITH LELAND TRAIMAN

Leland Traiman, a nurse practitioner now working as clinical research manager for Marcus Conant, M.D. and managing Dr. Conant's trial of the experimental treatment TP-5 (thymopentin), discussed what makes the difference between a good or poor clinical trial, at the weekly public meeting of The Healing Alternatives Foundation on August 23. Mr. Traiman stressed that he was speaking for himself only, not representing Dr. Conant.

Due to audience interest in actually organizing and conducting community-based clinical trials in San Francisco—following or changing the model created by the Community Research Initiative in New York, which was organized within the People With AIDS Coalition there and is now conducting several AIDS drug trials—discussion at the meeting shifted to how such an effort might work here. For continuity and easier reading, we selected the most important information and arranged it under the headings or questions below.

JJ: What are the most important differences between good vs. poor clinical trials?

LT: "The researchers must define very clearly at the beginning of a study whom they will admit, what medical entry criteria will be required.

"Also, a trial needs a clear definition of success; not an amorphous goal like 'we want people to get better,' but a clear clinical definition of success or failure: symptoms, blood work, skin immune assays, and activity of the virus in the blood.

"Unfortunately, we still do not have very good tests to measure viral activity. The more we use the P24 test (a test for a viral protein), the less reliable it seems to be. The beta-2-microglobulin test might be a good one, but it's still too early to tell. Until we get a better test, much of this research is going to be iffy."

JJ: Meanwhile, people are making treatment decisions.

LT: "While it's empowering to take treatments such as AL 721 substitutes or what-ever, the buyer should beware. People are basing large investments on anecdotes and sketchy science. Unfortunately, there is little more than sketchy science, so we should encourage people to do as much of their own research as possible, and keep asking questions."

JJ: Explain some of the problems with anecdotes.

LT: "Here is an example. A person I know, a friend of a physician, had a T-helper count of 800 a few years ago. He decided to adopt a healthier lifestyle. So he stopped smoking, drinking, and hard drugs—he had used a lot of drugs. He lost weight, went to the gym, etc.

"But after a year his count was 600. So he figured why bother, and he started drinking, taking drugs, abandoning his healthy lifestyle. A year later his count was 1300, and has stayed that way for the next several years.

"You can find an anecdote for everything. Helper cells can improve, spontaneous remissions can happen, regardless. If a person had started taking substance X before it happened, then people say it must be working.

"Until we get better information, more well-designed studies, I encourage people to keep questioning about every treatment or study, and question those answers."

JJ: How can we support people in making better decisions?

LT: "Since so many people are using treatments, I wish we could set up our own entry criteria and run our own community study, on AL 721, or dextran sulfate, or whatever. We could organize 15 to 20 people in each group and follow them for three, six, eight months and see what happens. Chart them on a number of medical parameters.

"There are so many people doing many things, and many doing just one thing, and people starting all the time, that we could surely find 15 to 20 people to study the treatments which are already popular in the community. I wish this could happen, but it needs somebody to organize it.

"If people are going to be using treatments, then it would be very helpful if there were some way of organizing 15 or 20 people using the same treatment, and monitoring them—whether they are using dextran sulfate, ozone, hydrogen peroxide, or whatever."

From a member of the audience: "I'm doing dextran sulfate, and acyclovir, and just three pills a day of AZT; I tried higher doses of AZT but couldn't tolerate that much. I feel a need for people who are using the same treatments to get together to talk about our experiences, to learn from each other."

From the audience: "Stay up on the research, write letters to the researchers. We can pool our brain power."

From the audience: "Keep a diary."

LT: "If we can find 15 to 20 people interested in the same treatment, who decide exactly what they are going to do and do it for three months—the same dosage, etc.—and if we follow up everybody and get consistent data, from the same laboratory, then we can take that data to any reputable physician who's a sentinel physician in this town, and he or she will take notice. Physicians will start saying that maybe they should look into this. That's the only way to convince physicians about the value of a treatment."

From the audience: "If everybody is doing combinations, you are never going to find enough people who are just doing AL 721, or just doing dextran sulfate."

LT: "I disagree. I talked with over a thousand people, to recruit them for the TP-5 study. I put an ad in the newspaper.

"As of tomorrow, we will have 32 people in the study. Over 150 people have come in to be screened. One-hundred ten of them couldn't be in that study because their viral cultures didn't grow. (A positive viral culture is one of the entry criteria for the TP-5 study.) These people want to be in a study.

"Many people don't believe in doing anything by themselves, but they do want to be part of research—thousands of people."

JJ: Meaning that it's not true that it's impossible to study anything because people are using so many treatments on their own already.

LT: "You could put an ad in the newspaper for people who are not doing anything and say we are going to start on whatever. And take baseline tests. You'll get 15 to 20 people, I guarantee you.

"If there was a person running these studies, a physician or nurse practitioner, to do clinical evaluations on these people to go along with all their blood work, it can happen. I've spoken to a thousand people."

From the audience: "We're a tremendous resource amongst ourselves. We might have a lot of pieces of the puzzle, we have to respect that, although we don't have the titles, we don't have the M.D. or Ph.D.

"We're ready to go to the next level, because we have thousands of us now. It's fascinating that we're not able to get into the regular research projects. When you can desire to be studied, contribute to humanity.

"We can get, say, ten people, and it's up to each individual to do his or her own treatment. We don't have to wait for the FDA."

From the audience: "Set up your own research trials, put an ad in the paper, say, 'I'm on dextran sulfate, I'm here because I want to go on something. . .'

"You set up a group, and each person in the trial, through their own individual doctor, says 'I'm on dextran sulfate.' "

JJ: One way to handle the drug-combination issue is to organize trials to test the combinations that people want to do anyway.

From the audience: "It needs a leader, some group to hire the nurse practitioner. The same thing has come up for months. I don't have the time; everybody is busy with what they are doing already. The project doesn't get off the ground."

Terry Beswick, Healing Alternatives: "I'm pulling together a meeting, getting the ball rolling. This is an idea we can plug into a CRI (Community Research Initiative) model."

From the audience: "If the gay dating services can organize to bring people together, then we can, to save lives."

From the audience: "Agree with your doctor that for six months you're going to take dextran sulfate, acyclovir and AZT—or whatever—then put an ad in the paper."

From the audience: "A lot of it is each individual's initiative. Each person does it on their own, through their own doctor."

From the audience: "Everyone participating instead of waiting for someone else to do it."

LT: "The only caveat: along with the other criteria, one of the defining things is to agree to use lab X for the study, so that the data from different people is compatible. And if your doctor doesn't use that lab, just say send it there. They'll take the business."

Note: The PWA Coalition of San Francisco is looking for an administrator to help organize community-based trials. For more information see the announcement in *AIDS Treatment News,* Issue Number 63. Volunteers are also needed.

PRESCRIPTION DRUG PRICE COMPARISON
by Denny Smith and John S. James

Are you getting the best prices for prescription drugs? Could you save money by using a mail-order pharmacy? *AIDS Treatment News* called pharmacies in seven cities, and also two mail-order pharmacies, to see how much prices varied. We found some great variations—in one extreme case, a ten-fold variation in price for equivalent products; it is a good idea to compare.

Usually mail-order pharmacies are close to each other in price—as would be expected, since geography doesn't matter and customers can easily call and compare. They consistently have good prices, but not always the lowest.

At community pharmacies (not mail order), prices can vary greatly. We found that cities like New York and San Francisco usually had the highest prices, while smaller cities like Nashville had the lowest. This variation suggests that persons in big cities may save the most by filling their prescriptions by mail.

But individual pharmacies often have surprisingly low or high prices for a particular drug. (And an earlier survey of five pharmacies in San Francisco, reported to *AIDS Treatment News,* found some price variations as much as 50 percent or more for the same drugs in the same city.)

Generic drugs—chemical equivalents of brand-name products for which patents have expired—can offer the biggest savings; prices are often a fraction of those charged for the name brand.

The most extreme price differences we found were for Septra DS. You could pay $154.65 at one pharmacy. Or you could buy a generic equivalent by mail for $11.19.

Are the less expensive drugs as good? Few doctors insist on the more expensive brand-name drugs. Ask your doctor if he or she knows any reason not to use a generic equivalent.

Mail-order pharmacies are poorly regulated at this time, and some critics have claimed that they may be more likely than others to make errors in filling prescriptions. Since errors are possible in any case, you might check when refilling a prescription to make sure that the pills look the same. If you want to check the first time you receive a medication, the *Physician's Desk Reference,* available in most public libraries, includes color pictures of prescription drugs.

Some legal requirements can vary by state. In some states, if the patient wants a generic drug the physician may have to specify that on the prescription. In others (including California), a pharmacist may substitute a generic equivalent (with the patient's consent), unless the physician writes "do not substitute" on the prescription; these days few physicians do. In these states you can get the generic (if one is available) by asking the pharmacist for it, even if you did not bring up the matter with your physician.

Another legal technicality to note is that California and some other states prohibit refilling an out-of-state prescription. Therefore if you are using an out-of-state pharmacy, you will probably have to send a new prescription each time, even if you could otherwise just ask for a refill. Watch your drug supply to avoid running out; most physicians will mail you a new prescription when necessary, and then you can mail it to the pharmacy.

The great price differences suggest that it would be wise to check prices at several pharmacies, including at least one mail-order pharmacy, before spending much money for prescription drugs.

Price Ranges (September 1988)

We agreed not to publish the prices of specific pharmacies; these change frequently in any case, so published prices would quickly become obsolete. Instead we show the range of prices—the lowest and highest for traditional pharmacies (not mail order), and the lowest and highest for prescriptions filled by mail.

	NOT MAIL ORDER		MAIL ORDER	
	LOW	HIGH	LOW	HIGH
AZT (100 mg, 100 caps)	$159.97	$195.39	$155.60	$169.75
Acyclovir (200 mg, 100 caps)	56.97	75.35	56.77	60.35
Mycelex (10 mg, 100 tabs)	49.99	79.55	49.30	51.65
Septra DS (160 tabs)	75.00	154.65	92.00	98.08
Septra generic equivalent	25.19	49.60	11.19	19.40
Nizoral (200 mg, 50 tabs)	75.99	118.55	75.02	92.75
Dapsone (25 mg, 80 tabs)	14.50	18.75	12.75	14.45
Ativan (1 mg, 50 tb)	21.69	25.95	20.84	23.85
Ativan generic equivalent	9.39	17.34	9.49	10.55

Note: Stores sometimes sold the same medicines in different quantities, complicating comparisons. In these cases we asked the stores to prorate the prices they reported to us.

The Pharmacies

We did not select the pharmacies in this survey systematically; we either picked ones we knew about, or we asked PWA organizations to suggest one in their city. While the pharmacies selected this way are probably better than average, there are many others which we did not consider. All those we did call were helpful and cooperative.

The two pharmacies selling by mail were Family Pharmaceuticals of America (see Appendix B), and Huntington Plaza Pharmacy (see Appendix B). The seven others were The Apothecary (Bethesda, MD, near Washington, DC), Bigelow (New York), Corsons (Philadelphia), Ike's (Nashville), Kaiser (San Francisco), Pay'n Save (Seattle), and Walgreen's (Minneapolis).

HYPERICUM UPDATE

The major article in the last issue of *AIDS Treatment News* concerned *Hypericum* (St. John's wort), a medicinal herb containing an ingredient which showed strong anti-retroviral activity in animal tests.

Hypericum, considered moderately safe but not totally safe by herbalists, has long been used for other medicinal purposes, and various preparations are available in some health-food stores. But there are doubts whether they contain enough hypericin, the active ingredient, to be useful. And so far we do not have even anecdotal reports of human use for AIDS or HIV; no one has yet said that they think the herb did (or did not) help them, because no one has used it long enough. For these reasons, we do not think this potential treatment is ready for widespread use, until there is more experience with it.

A few people are trying different extracts at this time. Also we have learned that chemical testing to compare the extracts should be inexpensive, around $30 for each sample analyzed. However we have not yet obtained a "standard," a sample of the pure chemical to calibrate the testing equipment; without the standard, the laboratory can compare the concentrations of hypericin in different extracts, but cannot accurately measure absolute amounts.

NEW AMFAR DIRECTORY OUT

The August edition of the *AIDS/HIV Experimental Treatment Directory* is now available from the American Foundation for AIDS Research. Besides new and updated listings, this edition has improved maps and other aids for locating clinical trials, a new article on testing potential AIDS drugs in macrophages, and, for the first time, some information on experimental treatments for opportunistic infections.

A one-year subscription, including the directory and updates, costs $30; a single issue is $10. AmFAR will continue its policy of sending a free copy of the directory to any person with AIDS who cannot afford one.

To order the directory, contact AmFAR (see Appendix B).

MAJOR AIDS BILL IN CONGRESS

The most important AIDS bill yet, HR 5142, will be considered by the House of Representatives in late September. This comprehensive bill includes many different research, prevention, and treatment programs. Congresswoman Nancy Pelosi, a friend of persons with AIDS, has asked for help in supporting the bill.

You can help by asking your Representatives to vote for HR 5142, for Pelosi's amendments on early-treatment research and on mental health treatment programs, for Congressman Henry Waxman's amendment to provide compassionate access to drugs shown to be potentially effective, and against all amendments which would eliminate the confidentiality and consent provisions of HR 5142.

SAN FRANCISCO:
AIDS PUBLIC-ADMINISTRATION CONFERENCE

The 2nd annual National AIDS Conference, sponsored by the San Francisco Department of Public Health and co-sponsored by the U.S. Conference of Mayors and over 20 other organizations, will be held September 28 through October 1 in San Francisco's Civic Auditorium.

The conference will "examine how systems of AIDS education, prevention and care are designed, implemented and evaluated. Administrative issues and policies related to AIDS programs will be addressed. The role of the local health department and its interaction with community-based organizations will be emphasized." Registration is $175 regular, $50 for staff of non-profit community-based agencies, and complimentary for persons with AIDS or ARC. Continuing-education credit is available.

SAN FRANCISCO:
STRESS AND HAIRY LEUKOPLAKIA STUDY

Persons in the San Francisco area who have had hairy leukoplakia and are not currently taking antivirals are wanted for a one-month study at the University of California, San Francisco. The study, conducted by Doctors Tom Coates, Marcus Conant, and Susan Folkman, is non-invasive; participants will fill out questionnaires daily for 28 days.

IN MEMORIAM: JOHN FOX, 1948-1988

John Alan Fox, one of the founders of the Healing Alternatives Buyers Club, died in Glenwood Springs, Colorado on August 26, 1988. He had had AIDS since October 1986. The immediate cause of death was never diagnosed.

John was a leading organizer and president of the board of directors of the buyers club (now The Healing Alternatives Foundation) until three months ago when he became too ill to be active. He had become a leading expert on AIDS treatments, spending much of his time on the phone with physicians, scientists, and persons with AIDS throughout the United States and beyond. People in San Francisco will remember his talks on treatments almost every Tuesday night, at meetings of Healing Alternatives. He also answered questions on treatment options from hundreds of persons around the country, especially on new therapies for KS. John worked with his oncologist and other physicians to devise a successful low-dose triple chemotherapy.

John tried many experimental treatments. He obtained lentinan through Japanese connections in 1987—one of the first Americans to do so. He had his own ozone machine, which he believed was helpful. Occasionally, however, he suffered serious side effects from some of the treatments he tried.

John had access to the best medical care, but during his final illness was unhappy with what was available for AIDS. In our last conversation he commented that physicians "don't think;" that even the better doctors simply ordered the obvious diagnostic tests and then gave up when they all came back negative. No one could diagnose his repeated fevers, weakness, and shortness of breath.

On August 6, accompanied by his brother and an attendant, John went to Glenwood for a last treatment attempt, with an unorthodox therapy there. Before leaving, he had made plans for his memorial service.

Friends of John Fox are looking for a permanent memorial to him and his contribution—perhaps through Healing Alternatives. John's courage, enthusiasm, and willingness to help others will never be forgotten by those who knew him.

Issue Number 65
September 23, 1988

CHINESE HERBS SHOW EARLY RESULT; MODEL FOR COMMUNITY-BASED TRIALS?

Keith Barton, M.D., C.A., a Berkeley, California physician who is also a certified acupuncturist trained in Chinese herbal medicine, has prepared a combination of six traditional Chinese herbs, all of which have shown antiHIV activity in laboratory tests. (See "Chinese Herbs Screened for Anti-HIV Activity," *AIDS Treatment News,* Issue Number 61, which reports on the laboratory testing.) The only patient so far to use the combination went from P-24 antigen positive to zero in three weeks; he was using no other treatment during this time.

One other patient started the herbs but had to stop after a potentially dangerous drop in white blood count which might have been caused by the herbs. His count recovered in three weeks.

What's limiting further research now is lack of patients who are antigen positive and not using any other antiviral treatments—for example, persons who could not tolerate AZT. Such patients or their physicians could contact Dr. Barton.

No conclusions can be drawn from one patient, of course. But the fact that P-24 antigen became zero (unlikely with no treatment), that this therapy has good laboratory rationale as well as thousands of years of human experience with the component herbs, that the treatment if it works could be readily obtained and applied, and that further testing would be easy, rapid, and inexpensive, suggest that this approach is worth pursuing.

Protocol Details

The six herbs are Lonicera japonica, Lithospermum erythrorhizon, Prunella vulgaris, Viola yedoensis, Epimedium grandiflorum, and licorice root. The first five were from the eleven found to have antiviral activity (by R. Shihman Chang and H.W. Yeung,

378

published in *Antiviral Research* 9 (1988), pages 163–176). Licorice root has shown anti-HIV activity in other research, in Japan.

The herb mixture was provided in bags to be prepared as a tea according to written directions. Patients used one bag per day for the first two weeks, two bags a day on the third week, and four bags daily in the fourth week. After the fourth week, patients are taken off herbs for two weeks, while laboratory tests continue.

Neither the patient who used the herbs successfully nor the one who had to stop had any obvious symptoms of side effects, except for some fatigue. But for safety, as well as good monitoring of the results, extensive laboratory testing was done, including baseline (before treatment began) and weekly complete blood count (CBC), chem 16 blood chemistry panel, urinalysis, PT, PTT, platelet count, P-24 antigen, and beta-2 microglobulin. In addition, HIV cultures were done at baseline and every two weeks thereafter, and T-cell subsets at baseline and monthly.

For more information send a self-addressed stamped envelope to: Keith Barton, M.D. (see Appendix B).

A Model for Community-Based Trials

This test of certain Chinese herbs suggests a model for community-based trials in several important respects:

- The treatment has a rationale. The herbs all showed anti-HIV activity in the laboratory; and all had been in human use for other purposes for many years.

- The treatment is available, legal, easy to use in a physician's practice, and safe under medical supervision.

- The trial has clear entry criteria (P-24 antigen positive, overall health stable, not using other antivirals within the last month).

- The trial has clear success criteria (P-24 antigen becoming negative within six weeks).

An organization to support community-based trials will not have to start from scratch, but instead can develop and refine existing work. Such an organization could contribute in several ways:

- A scientific review committee will select the best options to test, and the best ways to organize the trial—how many subjects, what success criteria should be used, etc.

- Many physicians will be involved, so it will be possible to recruit eligible patients more quickly.

- The consensus of a scientific review committee, an institutional review board, a number of participating physicians, and perhaps representatives of Federal agencies, will give each study more impact. Successful results will be disseminated, accepted, and used more rapidly than if only one physician were involved.

SCIENTIFIC JUSTIFICATION
FOR COMMUNITY-BASED TRIALS

The kinds of studies which we believe are appropriate for community-based trials (such as the antiviral herb study above, or the kinds of trials proposed by Leland Traiman, interviewed in *AIDS Treatment News,* Issue Number 64) have sometimes been dismissed by establishment scientists, who have argued that only the much more elaborate studies such as those run by NIH can produce valid data. Some AIDS organizers have been led to believe that there was no scientific support for the kind of research the AIDS community is coming to believe is needed. Those of us working to develop community-based trials have so far heard from only one side of an ongoing debate.

An important book which reviews both sides is *Ethics and Regulation of Clinical Research,* by Robert J. Levine, M.D., published by Yale University Press, New Haven, Connecticut, 1988. Dr. Levine is Professor of Medicine at Yale, and a well-known ethicist.

A chapter on randomized clinical trials (RCTs) includes a four-page section titled "Excessive Reliance on RCTs," which reviews papers by scientists proposing other study designs. These scientists see randomized trials as a valuable tool—but imposed excessively on U.S. medical research by the FDA and the National Cancer Institute of the NIH, "agencies which control the entry of new therapies into the practice of medicine...through their refusal to accept data developed with other methods." Others have shown through statistical studies that randomized trials have often failed to prove what they claimed to have proved.

One analyst described the conflict between "pragmatic" researchers (including most clinicians), and "fastidious" ones (including biostatisticians), with the fastidious school dominating clinical trials. The result is "clean" study designs which do not reflect actual medical practice. And a larger problem, though barely hinted at in Dr. Levine's book, is that the practical difficulties of meeting "fastidious" study requirements often cause grave delays, or even prevent important research from being done at all.

The arguments we have heard against more practical designs are:

• That each separate drug must first be tested by itself to show efficacy; it is not okay to test a treatment consisting of a combination of drugs not already tested and approved separately. (This argument supports the commercial needs of pharmaceutical companies, which want each of their products tested and approved by itself, not in combination with competitors' products.)

• That new antivirals cannot be tested in doctors' offices. Instead, such "phase I" trials often hospitalize patients in medical centers for the first weeks, for elaborate testing. (We agree with this procedure for new, high-tech drugs such as CD4 or DDI—but not for herbs, foods, common chemicals already in human use, or prescription drugs—which already have long records of human use, with toxicities either unimportant or known.)

• The only good way to prove efficacy is with a randomized clinical trial, meaning that patients who volunteer do not know which of two or more treatments they are going to get (one may be a placebo). (We agree that such trials have a major place—but they involve great practical difficulties which have often delayed results for years.

Most of the delays and difficulties can be avoided by tight, scientifically designed trials built around the kinds of medical intervention which patients would be receiving anyway.) The mainstream drug trials commonly take a year or much more before they even begin, to get approvals and funding. Many have such impractical entry criteria that it takes months to recruit even a single patient; these studies are doomed before they start, but they go through the motions anyway, giving the impression that something is being done. Other trials do collect potentially useful data, but keep it secret for a year or more until the slowest trial centers complete their last patients. Then results can take months to analyze, sometimes because the only people important enough to make decisions are too busy to find mutually acceptable times to meet. Finally the results must be kept quiet and unavailable to most physicians and patients for the months or more until publication. And even after publication there is no organized way to get the results to the attention of most of the physicians who could use them.

This system usually takes years to test each interesting possibility—if it ever does. This slow "turn-around time" has a disastrous effect on research results and productivity, because years are required for each full cycle of idea, test, and evaluation, and many such cycles may be needed to get practical results.

These problems represent poor management, not good science. The research establishment is now coming to accept the concept of community-based trials—a concept endorsed by the Presidential Commission on the HIV Epidemic. But we fear that this establishment wants to keep community-based trials in the same straightjacket as conventional studies.

If community trials are required to repeat the unfeasible designs and procedures common in mainstream trials, they will be just a pale, underfunded imitation of the ineffectual system we already have.

Dr. Levine's section on excessive reliance on randomized trials mentions an alternative design, called observational case control studies, which is practically identical to the drug-trial proposals developing in the AIDS community:

"This design entails systematic observation of patients as they are treated by practicing physicians. Inclusion and exclusion criteria exactly like those used for RCTs are used to determine who will be observed. After the outcome has been established, patients are sorted by outcome, e.g., fatalities and survivors. Causes of the outcome are evaluated as in case-control studies."

Anyone organizing community-based trials should scan *Ethics and Regulation of Clinical Trials* and the literature it cites (the book has over 700 references). The AIDS community does have authoritative scientific support for the kinds of studies which need to be done.

DRUG-TRIAL CONSTIPATION

One of our subscribers wrote to his Representative, Congresswoman Patricia Saiki of Hawaii, about delays in AIDS drug trials. Congresswoman Saiki forwarded the letter to NIH, and received a reply dated July 18, 1988 from James C. Hill, Ph.D., Deputy

Director, National Institute of Allergy and Infectious Diseases. In the process of defending the system, Dr. Hill also illuminated what is wrong with it. We quote two paragraphs from his letter:

> To help decide which drugs are the most promising, the NIAID established an AIDS Clinical Drug Development Committee (ACDDC), composed of Government and non-Government experts, to evaluate candidate drugs for entry into NIAID-sponsored clinical trials. The goal of this effort is to ensure that any drug showing scientific promise and receiving a high priority rating by the Committee will be evaluated in a clinical trial. Some concern has been expressed that there may have been undue delays from the point at which the ACDDC designates a drug as "high priority" to its being entered into a clinical trial and patient accrual begun. However, it is important to point out that the initiation of clinical trials with investigational new drugs is often complicated and requires extraordinary coordination among Government, research institutions, and pharmaceutical manufacturers. There are many issues that limit our ability to go rapidly from the designation of a drug as "high priority" to patient accrual into a clinical trial.

> At either the stage of ACDDC review of a drug or the drug's subsequent referral to the AIDS Clinical Trials Group committee, there are often a variety of issues that still may need to be resolved: recommendation for additional safety and efficacy studies in animals; extensive negotiations with the manufacturer are often needed to ensure the production of sufficient quantities of clinical grade material prior to the further development of the protocol(s); all supporting preclinical information, manufacturing processes, and intended trial design must be approved by the Food and Drug Administration; the pharmaceutical manufacturer must agree to supply the drug required to conduct the study as well as agree to the design of the protocol; Institutional Review Boards at the individual medical centers must also review and approve the proposed protocol; case report forms must be designed and reviewed with statistical input to assure that the measurements taken throughout the study are being collected in a manner that will provide the necessary data to meet the predetermined objectives; and finally, patients must be screened in order to select the population that meets the intended protocol entrance criteria. The failure of any one or more of these elements to be accomplished in a timely fashion can cause unforeseen delays in the initiation of the clinical trial.

AUTOPSY STUDY PINPOINTS DIAGNOSIS FAILURES

A study of autopsy records at two major New York hospitals found that half of the persons who died of AIDS had cytomegalovirus (CMV) infections not suspected while they were alive. Several other opportunistic conditions were also undiagnosed; three quarters of the patients who died were found to have unsuspected AIDS-related complications.

This study, published July 9 in *The Lancet* by researchers at the New York University School of Medicine, New York City Department of Public Health, and New York Hospital-Cornell Medical Center, can help physicians by letting them know which complications are most often missed, so that they can check carefully for these, especially in patients with undiagnosed problems.

Of all AIDS death records between May 1981 and May 1987 at two large teaching hospitals, one public and one private, 101 adult patients had autopsy and all other records available. The major unsuspected AIDS-related conditions were: • CMV infection, 49 percent (of all 101 cases); • Systemic fungal infection, 20 percent; • Systemic KS, 14 percent; • MAI infection, 11 percent; • Systemic herpes infection, 9 percent.

Other problem diagnoses were fungal pneumonias (undiagnosed despite bronchoscopy and even biopsy), tuberculosis, and central nervous system lymphomas (sometimes treated unsuccessfully as toxoplasmosis).

Bacterial pneumonias—presumably treatable—were important contributors to death in 30 percent of the patients.

Successful diagnosis was found for pneumocystis (over 90 percent of cases), and cryptococcal infection and CMV retinitis (diagnosed correctly in all cases).

Previous autopsy studies (when the cause of death was not AIDS related) have also found that many infectious diseases are missed.

For more information, see Wilkes, M.S. *et al.*, "Value of Necropsy in Acquired Immunodeficiency Syndrome," *The Lancet* (July 9, 1988), pp. 85-8.

LABORATORY TESTING: SAVING MONEY WITH PACKAGE PRICES

AIDS Treatment News talked with two physicians who negotiated large price reductions with testing laboratories by setting a price for panels of dozens of different tests. These examples may help other physicians make similar money-saving arrangements.

(1) Positive Action HealthCare in San Francisco obtained a price of $168.40 from Roche Biomedical Laboratories for a panel including T- and B-cells with subsets (including T-helper cells of course), beta 2 microglobulin, P-24 antigen, sedimentation rate, CBC (complete blood count), a SMAC chemistry panel with about 20 different measurements, the RPR syphilis serology, and urinalysis.

(2) Keith Barton, M.D., in Berkeley (see article on Chinese herbs above) obtained a similar package which in addition included an HIV culture, from another company for under $200. (Most laboratories may not offer so low a price for an HIV culture; this company is developing its own tests, and may have subsidized the price to obtain blood samples in order to compare its tests with the standard ones.)

Prices can be kept even lower by minimizing expensive tests. Even some of the research trials funded by major corporations use only two or three T-cell subset tests, and avoid HIV cultures entirely. The other tests are much less expensive.

Low prices on testing will facilitate community-based trials. Such trials can be integrated into the medical care the patient is receiving anyway, so they can cost very little in addition, and the cost of the tests can usually be paid by insurance. (The drugs likely to be tested in this way are seldom very expensive.) In other words, much community-based AIDS treatment research can be done with no external funding—largely eliminating the institutional delays which have made most existing research ineffectual. Community organizing, bringing together the knowledge and talents of persons with AIDS, physicians, and scientists, is the only limiting factor in how much can be accomplished.

CALIFORNIA: "NO ON 102" EFFORT NEEDS FUNDS

A right-wing AIDS initiative on California's November ballot would close anonymous testing centers, require doctors and researchers to report the names of anyone they believe to be HIV positive, and allow employers and insurance companies access to HIV test results. The legislative analyst's official estimate of the cost of implementing this initiative is tens to hundreds of millions of dollars. This destructive initiative, called Proposition 102, even has a provision prohibiting the California Legislature from amending it without resubmission to the voters—a time-consuming process which would prevent the State from adjusting public-health policy to changing conditions.

While directly affecting only California, this initiative would impact public health everywhere by greatly impeding AIDS treatment research in California, since it would forbid researchers from keeping the names of their subjects confidential. It would also end the anonymous testing and counseling programs which have proven successful in greatly reducing the spread of the virus.

Two economics professors at the University of California at Berkeley recently estimated that other effects of this initiative, such as forcing the firing of over 30,000 teachers and food handlers found to be HIV positive, would cost California over three billion dollars a year in direct and indirect expenses.

The normally conservative California Medical Association (CMA) went to court in an unsuccessful attempt to keep Proposition 102 off the ballot. Many other groups such as the California Nurses Association, California Association of Hospitals and Health Systems, and Health Officers Association of California officially oppose the initiative. An unusual development is that major corporations such as Levi Strauss, AT&T, and Apple Computer, which usually would not take a position on such an issue, are also opposing it. Others opposed include the California Chamber of Commerce, League of Women Voters, California Taxpayers Association, California Federation of Labor, and both California Senators.

But polls show that the initiative would pass if the election were held today, because people do not understand its provisions. The measure was designed to sound reasonable to the uninformed, and the California ballot is loaded with measures. Polls show that voters reject the initiative if they know that it would ban anonymous testing, and allow employers to require HIV tests and fire or refuse to hire anyone testing positive. It will cost hundreds of thousands of dollars for the media time needed to get this information to the voters before November.

If you can help in any way, with money, volunteer time, contacts, publicity, etc., contact Californians Against Proposition 102.

WOMEN'S AIDS SERVICE PROGRAM BEGINS
by Denny Smith

The San Francisco AIDS Foundation has received special funding to serve women with AIDS and ARC, and their partners and children. This program, possibly the first of its kind in the nation, is already serving 80 women.

Women with AIDS have faced unique, severe problems. For example, only five of the 80 clients in this program are now on AZT, and only five are on aerosol pentamidine. Only two of the 80 are now using an experimental treatment, such as dextran sulfate or AL 721.

Seventy of the 80 are low income; food and rent bills must compete with treatment costs. Many women are uninsured or underinsured. Women are often excluded from trials of experimental drugs. Long waits in public clinics are often impractical for women with young children and no childcare. Women with AIDS seldom have the community support and institutions available to gay men. Because of these and other obstacles, women with HIV-related symptoms are often late to receive treatment.

The new program runs ongoing discussion groups for sharing treatment and other resource information. With the help of Catholic Social Services and the Shanti Project, it hopes to open two houses for women with AIDS or ARC.

For more information about this program, contact the San Francisco AIDS Foundation (see Appendix B).

Issue Number 66
October 7, 1988

TREATMENT RESEARCH IDEAS FOR
COMMUNITY-BASED TRIALS

The U.S. system of testing new treatments against AIDS or other diseases has become so cumbersome that many promising possibilities never even start the testing process. A new system called community-based research, pioneered by the Community Research Initiative in New York and the County Community Consortium in San Francisco, organizes scientifically sound drug trials through the practices of private physicians, whose patients can volunteer for the studies.

By integrating scientific trials with normal medical practice, community-based trials allow credible testing of treatment options with far less administrative delay than usually involved, and at far less cost; often the main expense is laboratory tests which the patients should be receiving anyway. These trials differ from everyday medical practice in being designed in advance by a research professional, and being approved by scientific and by ethical review boards. Criteria for patient selection and for evaluating the success of the therapy are as rigorous as in any other trials. And patient compliance can be better in community-based than in other trials, because of the closer physician-patient relationship, and because community-based trials often test treatments which are already available, meaning that no one is forced into the studies to get treatment, so there is no incentive to cheat; volunteers come forward only for altruistic reasons. The greatly reduced cost of community-based trials encourages research by pharmaceutical companies, and also allows testing of medically attractive treatment options which lack commercial or scientific glamor, and thus would not be studied otherwise.

Community-based trials are most suitable for testing potential therapies which already have known safety records in human use—including most of the treatments which have developed a grassroots following among patients or scientists without commercial prompting. Drugs which are unusually dangerous, difficult to use, or untried in humans usually need to be studied in major medical centers, not through private physicians' offices in community trials.

Grassroots Treatment List; What the Community Wants To Test

Most treatments already being studied in community-based trials are products being developed by pharmaceutical companies. The immediate reason for this focus is of course financial; it has been hard to fund trials of substances which are medically promising—or used by thousands of people—but which are unpatentable or otherwise lack commercial potential. Certainly the commercial treatments must be studied; "second generation" HIV drugs can be the most promising possibilities. But we also need trials of the "grassroots" treatments which the public is using, for at least two reasons: (1) to give patients objective assessments of risks and benefits of different options; and (2) because treatments attractive enough to have developed a following among patients, physicians, or scientists, with little commercial or organized promotion, may well have objective benefits which academic research and medicine should consider.

While community-based trials clearly should study both the industrial and grassroots treatment possibilities, in our list below we focused on those with a popular interest or following (some also have commercial sponsors). We chose this focus for the practical reason that *AIDS Treatment News* has better information about treatments with grassroots support, which usually come to our attention, than about treatments being developed by pharmaceutical companies, which are often kept secret.

We selected the treatments listed below because there is public interest in them, they have some medical or scientific rationale, and they appear suitable for community-based research. This list is not nearly complete, and we welcome suggestions for additions.

Readers should note that the rationales we present below are necessarily sketchy; we could not research every treatment thoroughly by press time. We published this list to emphasize the wide range of treatment possibilities suitable for testing in community-based research.

Potential Treatment List (Alphabetical)

Acidophilus. Acidophilus preparations, available in health-food stores, contain live beneficial bacteria, intended to help crowd out harmful micro-organisms in the gastrointestinal tract. (For more background information, see *AIDS Treatment News*, Issue Number 32).

A community-based study of acidophilus could begin by asking clinicians experienced with it to specify (a) how to select the patients believed most likely to benefit, and (b) what benefits should occur, and when.

While community-based trials would seldom use a placebo, a randomized double-blind placebo trial might be appropriate in this case because:

• The placebo would be strictly voluntary, as anyone who wanted could obtain acidophilus outside the study. The only reason for volunteering would be to contribute to the advancement of knowledge, not to obtain treatment.

- Benefits of acidophilus (if any) are likely to be noticed very rapidly. The placebo phase of the trial would probably need to last for only a few days.

- Evaluating the success of this treatment might necessarily be subjective, through patients' reports that they were feeling better. Lack of laboratory measurements of success increases the danger of a false positive outcome of the trial due to "placebo effect," making a double-blind design more necessary.

Incidentally, it should be easy to make a placebo which looks and tastes like acidophilus, simply by heat treating the capsules or otherwise making sure the organisms were dead.

AL 721 or substitutes.   The Community Research Initiative in New York is already conducting a community-based trial of egg-lecithin lipids. The study is fully enrolled, and preliminary results should be available in a few weeks.

Aloe vera.   Aloe vera preparations are used for medicinal purposes in many cultures. For AIDS/HIV, the most systematic studies are being done by advocates of carrisyn, a chemical found in aloe vera and now being moved through the FDA approval process by Carrington Laboratories in Dallas, Texas.

Carrisyn may take months before showing improvement (usually measured in T-cell numbers). It would be difficult to ask patients to stay off other treatments during this time. Therefore the study could be designed not as a test of carrisyn (or other aloe preparation) by itself, but rather of whatever combination therapy patients are most likely to want to try anyway. Such patient-led design should make it easier to recruit patients, reduce any incentive to cheat, and also take advantage of any practical knowledge in the community of patients and front-line physicians on how best to use carrisyn (or other aloe preparations).

Amino acids.   A number of people are using lysine, readily available in health-food stores, as an antiviral for herpes and/or HIV. Some are convinced that at least two other amino acids should be avoided—not supplemented or used in large amounts—as they are believed to encourage the growth of viruses. We have heard of this use of lysine from at least three well-informed sources; however one nutritionist who is familiar with the literature on amino acids had never heard of using them in antiviral treatment.

The scientific review committee would need to research whether there is credible justification for this therapy, and if so, what patients should be selected and what measurable endpoints used to look for beneficial results.

Antabuse.   Thousands of people are using this prescription drug as a substitute for imuthiol (DTC), an immune modulator developed in France but not easily available in the United States. Much of the antabuse taken becomes imuthiol in the body. The Community Research Initiative in New York is now conducting a monitoring study of antabuse.

Anti-inflammatory therapy.   Various published and unpublished information suggests that certain anti-inflammatory drugs such as indocin or even aspirin may be helpful to some patients. Others might not be helped or might be harmed by the drugs.

By reviewing the literature and interviewing clinicians, some of whom have been using this treatment for years, the scientific committee could determine which patients are likely to benefit, what measurable results could be expected, how long it should take to see them, and what is known about risks of long-term use of the drugs by persons with AIDS or ARC (less relevant to the safety of this short-term study than to the usefulness of a positive result).

If benefits could be expected very quickly (perhaps within days) it might be feasible to use a placebo and double-blind design for only the first week or two of the test, after which everyone would go on the drug. Only volunteers would risk the placebo; the rest would start open label immediately. This protocol not only eliminates the unethical extortion of withholding treatment to force participation in a placebo study, it also removes any incentive to cheat. Only those who volunteer to help research may get the placebo—and only for a short time.

AZT for cryptosporidiosis. At the June Stockholm conference, six researchers at a Paris hospital presented results from 16 patients (poster 3672). Marked improvement was found in 14 of the 16 in the first month; diarrhea disappeared in 10 of the 15 patients who were treated for at least three months. Half and full doses of AZT seemed to work equally well. Unfortunately this poster session received less attention than it deserved, because it was not indexed under cryptosporidium in the abstract book.

Other scattered reports have suggested such an effect—not as surprising as it may seem, since AZT is an antibiotic as well as an antiviral, effective against a number of micro-organisms including at least one intestinal parasite, giardia. An anticryptosporidiosis effect of AZT may explain why this disease has been less common than had been feared.

It might be hard to find patients for the trial, as most of those ill enough to have cryptosporidiosis would already be using AZT, unless they could not tolerate it.

BHT. This food preservative is very effective against most lipid-coated viruses in the test tube, and has prevented viral infections in animals. One published human trial found it effective for treating herpes. One laboratory test found particular activity against CMV. (See *AIDS Treatment News,* Issue Number 10.)

For several years hundreds of people have been using large doses of BHT, about one gram a day, to help control herpes. Few have tried it for AIDS-related conditions. Laboratory results with HIV are mixed, with NIH finding no efficacy.

In recent months public interest has greatly increased, perhaps due to widespread publicity about encouraging laboratory results mentioned by R.C. Aloia *et al.* in the *Proceedings of the National Academy of Sciences USA* (February 1988), pages 900–904. This public interest in a readily available chemical makes it even more important to have a trial with medical monitoring to learn more about safety as well as efficacy of this potential treatment.

Other Possibilities

We had not written annotations for the following by press time. These and others may appear in future issues.

- Bile salts
- Chinese medicine
- Chlorophyll
- Coenzyme Q
- Dapsone
- DDI
- Deficiency testing and supplementation
- Dextran sulfate
- DHEA
- DNCB
- Fatty acids
- Ganoderma
- Garlic
- Germanium
- Ginseng
- Homeopathy
- Hydrogen peroxide (or chlorine dioxide)
- Imuthiol (DTC) from France
- Iscador
- Japanese herbs (over 100 paid for by national health system)
- Lentinan
- Macrobiotic diet (investigate status of earlier study)
- Milk antibodies (or colostrum, or veterinary antibodies from whey)
- Naltrexone
- Nutrition improvement
- Ozone
- Peptide T
- Plasmapheresis (and related, e.g. Prosorba column, packed washed red cells)
- Polio killed-virus vaccine
- Propolis
- Selenium
- Typhoid immunization
- Vitamins: A, C, E, others
- Zinc

DECISIONS FOR COMMUNITY-BASED TRIALS

Recent conversations with leaders of the Community Research Initiative (CRI) in New York suggested several issues that a community-research organization should consider. We prepared this report, drawn from our phone notes, to help others develop similar research elsewhere.

- Is the goal to do monitoring studies, prospective trials, or both?

Monitoring studies—for example, collecting records from physicians' offices of patients who have used a particular treatment—are much easier and less expensive. In New York, volunteers have done much of the legwork. Such studies can show trends; but the research community considers them only suggestive that further research should be done, if a treatment looks good.

Prospective trials, which are more definitive, ask patients to follow protocols designed in advance by research professionals, instead of simply recording what the patients are doing anyway.

The New York CRI has both kinds of trials under way.

- There is a major shortage of principal investigators to design and manage AIDS treatment trials. NIH and pharmaceutical companies have a big problem finding qualified people, the CRI has had major problems, and for a new organization it could be even more difficult.

The principal investigator (PI) does not need to be an M.D.; many are Ph.D., although the combination of both degrees is strongest for getting published. The PI does need to know about AIDS, know how to design clinical trials, and have the time; it often takes about 20 hours a week to manage a study: write the protocol, get it approved by committees, negotiate among all the parties, recruit subjects, manage the data collection, analysis, writing and publication, etc.

Often the PI trusts someone with less training, such as a research nurse, to draft the protocol and change it as required, make phone calls when possible, etc. The PI must sign off on the result, of course. Perhaps the ten to 20 hours a week could be reduced to two or three this way, making it much easier for top people to serve as the PI.

• Pharmaceutical companies are very unhappy with the NIH clinical research system, because it is too slow and for other reasons, so they are looking for alternative ways to test their drugs. The New York CRI has had a number of requests from both large and small companies to run trials for them. If a community-based research organization is credible, and is an attractive site for testing pharmaceutical-industry drugs, it will probably be able to do this work. On the down side, such organizations might be seen as a bread-and-butter threat by other researchers, making it harder to get the effort off the ground.

• Promoters with money have also approached the New York CRI, trying to get favorable publicity for dubious products. Any research organization must be careful.

• New York had much difficulty getting funding to study non-commercial treatment options (like most of those listed below). Therefore it had to focus on what pharmaceutical companies wanted to test. CRI had to live for a long time on its $5,000 seed money from the PWA Coalition. But now it should be possible to raise money much more quickly, because the community-research concept has become well known and established.

• If such funding is available, an organization could build a reputation for doing quality research on grassroots treatments. Clearly this work should be done—we need to study what people are in fact using—but because of lack of funding, this research is now largely neglected.

• A typical community-based prospective study with 10 to 20 people lasting several months might cost $30,000 to $70,000. Much of the expense is for laboratory testing. Also, someone needs to be hired for "keeping the books" on the data. There is also the cost of physician examinations. And of course there is overhead—rent, staff, telephone, etc., for the organization.

• What about minimizing expenses by building the study around laboratory tests which patients will be doing anyway? CRI considered this approach. Two potential difficulties are (1) community objection that only those insured or who can pay for their care could participate, and (2) concern that insurance companies should not be billed for research (against which others say that if the blood tests are going to be done anyway for treatment, there is no ethical imperative to waste the data). These issues were discussed in the CRI, but not resolved.

It may be possible to conduct scientifically sound, credible research ultra-cheap—by carefully designing studies which organize elements of patient care which already exist and are paid for. But if funding is available, it should be used to assure faster results by following more conventional, better tested procedures.

• The CRI obtained space for a clinic—to facilitate administering aerosol pentamidine, drawing blood to be sent to the same lab, and data collection. Physical examinations, however, are still done at the offices of individual physicians, who then send a form to the CRI.

• Community-research organizations need to involve many professional people besides physicians in support of their effort—for example, fundraisers, statisticians, and attorneys. The clergy can be helpful in making connections. Many people in the business community would be ready to help but have not yet been asked.

• In New York, the CRI has developed many procedures and documents that others can use. For example, its IRB (institutional review board) recently approved a set of documents providing a flow sheet of what the IRB must do for a trial. New efforts for community-based research can benefit from the experience of the CRI, and of other organizations that want to help.

CHINESE MEDICINE SYMPOSIUM OCTOBER 23 IN LONG BEACH, CALIFORNIA

A one-day symposium, "AIDS, Immunity, and Chinese Medicine," will be presented by the Oriental Healing Arts Institute, on Sunday, October 23 from 9 AM to 5 PM, at the Marriott Hotel, near the Long Beach airport. Speakers include well-known herbalist Subhuti Dharmananda, orthopedist and traditional Chinese doctor Qing-Cai Zhang, M.D., Dr. Misha Cohen, clinical director of the Quan Yin Acupuncture and Herbal Center of San Francisco, Keith Barton, M.D., a Berkeley, California physician who is also a certified acupuncturist, and H.W. Yeung, Ph.D., Director of the Department of Microbiology and Biochemistry, Chinese University of Hong Kong, and co-author of "Inhibition of Growth of Human Immunodeficiency Virus by Crude Extracts of Chinese Medicinal Herbs," published in *Antiviral Research,* and reviewed in *AIDS Treatment News,* Issue Number 61. Continuing education credit is available.

AVOIDING THE 20 PERCENT COPAYMENT ON INSURED PRESCRIPTION DRUGS

Since running our earlier article on the prices of prescription drugs, the following information was brought to our attention by Ron English, whom we know through his work as a major fundraiser for the Community Research Initiative in New York. Mr. English is also working for Preferred Rx, of Independence, Ohio, the company discussed here.

Most patients who have insurance coverage for the cost of prescription drugs still have to pay 20 percent of the price; the insurance pays 80 percent (after any deductible has been met). Preferred Rx offers a plan which allows patients to avoid this 20 percent. It fills the prescription through its arrangement with a mail-order supplier, and accepts an insurance payment of 80 percent or more as payment in full.

The plan works by taking advantage of the difference between common retail prices of prescription drugs, and the lower prices available through mail-order pharmacies. Insurance companies cannot force patients to use the cheapest way to fill their prescriptions, as long as the price is reasonable. Preferred Rx bills the prescription at a reasonable price, receives 80 percent of that, and profits by filling the prescription for less.

There is an annual $25 dues for using this system—waived in certain cases such as for Medicare patients. If you do not have insurance coverage of prescription drugs, Preferred Rx is comparable to other mail-order pharmacies.

For more information, contact Preferred Rx (see Appendix B).

Issue Number 67
October 21, 1988

PASSIVE IMMUNOTHERAPY: EFFECTIVE TREATMENT FOR ADVANCED AIDS?

In a study described last June at the Stockholm AIDS conference and published last month in *The Lancet,* researchers treated six persons with advanced AIDS by transfusing blood plasma from donors who were healthy seropositives selected for having a high level of the antibody against the p24 protein of the AIDS virus. The patients had no detectable antibody to p24 before the treatment. But after a single treatment, these patients had the antibody for several weeks—the length of time depending on how much plasma they were given—and showed impressive clinical as well as laboratory improvements. For example, there were ten opportunistic infections among the six patients in the two-month period before treatment, but only one in the two months the treatment was in effect.

This treatment possibility, which is still unproven and not yet in use, is important because it might save lives which could not be saved by any other known means. And technically it would be easy to set up; the only possible obstacle is red tape. Community organizing and support for such an effort may be necessary.

The study is also important because it strongly indicates that persons with even advanced AIDS can recover, if the disease process can be stopped.

How the Study Was Done

We will only outline the procedure used because those who need more information can obtain the paper (Jackson *et al.,* 1988).

First the researchers selected two donors who were HIV positive and had very high levels of antibodies to p24 (see "Background" section, below). Then they used plasmapheresis, a routine procedure in blood banks, which separates plasma from cells in the blood, allowing the cells to be returned to the donor. (Plasmapheresis is used in blood banking because donors can replace plasma much more rapidly than cells, allowing more frequent donation, and the plasma itself is often all that is needed for transfusions or for making blood products. Also, plasma usually does not need to be separated by blood type, as whole blood does.)

Then the plasma was frozen and thawed, to rupture any remaining cells, and heat treated to kill any virus. Varying amounts of this treated plasma were infused intravenously into the recipients.

These six patients were severely ill. For example, in the two months before the treatment, five of the six had pneumocystis, and altogether there were ten opportunistic infections. During two months after treatment, there was only one new infection—a fatal case of pneumonia in one patient who had liver disfunction and other complications before the infusion was given, and who did not benefit from the treatment. But after the treatment was discontinued (as part of the experimental design) and after the infused antibodies had disappeared there were nine opportunistic infections among the patients in a two-month period. Other improvements during treatment included weight gain, improved Karnofsky score (a rating of overall health), increased T-helper cells as well as T-8 and T-11 cells, and an immediate disappearance of P24 antigen after infusion of the anti-P24 antibodies. The one test which did not improve was skin sensitivity to antigens.

Before the treatment, viral cultures from the plasma of four of the six patients had been positive. While the treatment was in effect, only one of 36 plasma cultures done was positive. After the treatment period, when the infused antibodies had disappeared, all of nine plasma cultures which were done were positive again. This difference is statistically significant—as was the reduction in opportunistic infections.

Since according to the study design the treatment was not repeated, even if successful, no long-term data was obtained. The treatment proved harmless, however, and there was no indication of viral resistance developing, suggesting that long-term use should be possible.

Background

Previous studies had shown that patients with a high level of antibodies against p24 or p17, which are core proteins of the AIDS virus, usually remained healthy. These and other observations suggested a model of AIDS progression which has become widely known and accepted.

In this model, antibodies to *surface* proteins of HIV, such as gp120, remain high in patients regardless of whether they do well or not. These antibodies do not tend to neutralize or inhibit the virus.

But antibodies to *core* proteins of HIV, such as p24, are important indicators. These develop a short time after infection. While they remain high, the person remains a healthy seropositive.

But eventually, for unknown reasons, most patients lose their ability to produce these antibodies, and the level falls to zero, or at least so low that it is undetectable. Then over the next several months, the patient is likely to develop p24 antigenemia, meaning that the p24 viral protein can be detected in the blood. This is what the p24 antigen test measures. (Do not confuse the p24 antigen test, which measures a protein produced by the AIDS virus, with the test for the *antibody against* the p24 antigen.

You want the antigen to be negative, and the antibody against the antigen to be high. The test for the anti-p24 antibody is not widely available, however.) Patients with high levels of p24 antigen are more likely to progress to ARC or AIDS during the following months or years. However, some patients with AIDS do not show the p24 antigen.

One study of 57 patients suggested that lack of anti-p24 antibody might be an earlier indicator of risk of progressing to AIDS than the p24 antigen itself, or tests in common use such as T-helper count (Forster *et al.*, 1988). Loss of anti-p24 antibody could precede AIDS by as much as 40 months. We have not yet obtained this paper, only an abstract, so we do not know if any of the 57 patients progressed to AIDS despite having the antibody, or if any remained healthy for a long time without it.

Yet despite the clear fact that lack of anti-p24 antibody was associated with a greater risk of AIDS, it was still not clear that providing this antibody to patients who had lost the ability to make it would be helpful. In fact, during the questioning session after the Stockholm talk by Dr. Jackson, a talk attended by leading AIDS researchers from such institutions as Johns Hopkins, Harvard, and the University of California, San Francisco Medical Center, questioners were impressed but also surprised by the clinical improvement. Questioners expected the immediate disappearance of p24 after infusion of the antibody—which was observed—but did not expect antiviral activity. In most studies, antibodies to HIV had failed to neutralize (inhibit) it. Dr. Jackson pointed out that some posters being presented at the Stockholm conference had shown that there was at least one site on p24 where an antibody would be neutralizing, although there were other sites where it would not be. In other words, antibody to p24 could have an antiviral effect, although until recently many experts would not have expected it.

Technical Issues

We asked Lisa Bero, Ph.D., a pharmacologist now with the Institute for Health Policy Studies who has several years experience in drug development and has worked extensively with antibodies, to comment on possible technical problems with this treatment. She was concerned that the freezing and heating required to kill the virus might damage the antibodies. While the process seemed to work in the experiment reported, it might not work consistently. Other ways might work better to kill any virus in the plasma. There are standard methods (used in preparing gamma globulin) which can separate antibodies in blood without danger of the product transmitting HIV.

Some tests for the antibody level in the patients treated with the plasma could detect antibodies even if their structure had been damaged by the heat. The particular test (EIA) used by Dr. Jackson's team was a good choice, because it is less likely than others to make this error.

Another possible problem is that patients might develop antibodies against the injected antibodies. This could cause "serum sickness," as well as making injected antibodies ineffective. No sign of such a problem has been observed, however.

Practical Considerations

How long does each treatment with the plasma containing anti-p24 antibodies last? In the study by Dr. Jackson and others, the protective antibodies stayed in the blood from 30 to 70 days, depending on the amount given. With 50 ml of the plasma, antibodies of the recipient would last for about 30 days; with 500 ml, they would last about 70. The data suggested that as little as 5 ml might be effective.

These numbers suggest that one healthy seropositive donor could provide antibodies to maintain at least several people with AIDS, or people at high risk of developing AIDS due to loss of their anti-p24 antibodies.

The treatment did not harm any of the recipients. But precautions were taken, such as observing the patients in the blood bank for one to two hours after the plasma infusion, and then releasing them with an accompanying person.

Would donating protective antibodies be harmful to the donor? It seems unlikely. Six weeks after plasma donation, both donors had antibody levels twice as high as when they donated. In fact, there is substantial evidence that plasmapheresis (the plasma donation) itself can be beneficial to some persons with AIDS, apparently by lowering the level of harmful substances which otherwise accumulate in the blood.

The Next Steps

We do not know of anyone who is using this passive immunotherapy treatment now. Nor could we find anyone by press time who understood how this treatment could fit into the regulatory process and be made available quickly to patients. One activist described what was needed at this time as "breaking the ice"; that is, persons and organizations will have to pioneer and explore options for how the treatment might be made available.

Technically, it would be easy to do. However, private-practice physicians would probably need the cooperation of a blood bank or clinic to do the plasmapheresis and heat treatment of the plasma. They would also need to consult with medical specialists who were up to date on the research. And someone would need to find plasma donors who had high levels of appropriate antibodies.

Two things should be done. We need more research to confirm that the treatment really does work—and to help physicians know how to use it most effectively. Pharmaceutical companies, or community-based research organizations such as the Community Research Initiative, or the U.S. National Institutes of Health, could conduct this research.

But research can go on for years, during which time few people will have access through the trials, so we also need whatever organizing is required to support patients and physicians who want to try passive immunotherapy before all the research is complete. Since plasmapheresis and transfusion of plasma are already standard medical procedures, already regulated to assure good medical practice and patient safety, the same procedures already in use should be available in this case. Physicians clearly have the right to use a standard drug or procedure for a new treatment purpose. Patients who need this treatment, especially those who have no other options, should have access to it without waiting the many years required for approval of new drugs. Results of the treatment should be closely monitored, so that others can benefit from the experience as it becomes available.

Unfortunately the FDA seems unlikely to allow their "treatment IND"—the rules announced over a year ago to make early treatments more available for serious or life-threatening diseases—to be used for passive immunotherapy. (See

"Beyond an Unreasonable Doubt: Comments on Drug-Approval Delays," below.) All options will need to be explored.

REFERENCES

American Foundation for AIDS Research, *AIDS/HIV Experimental Treatment Directory*, passive immunotherapy section (August 1988 and later).

Forster, S.M. *et al.*, "Decline of Anti-p24 Antibody Precedes Antigenemia as Correlate of Prognosis in HIV-1 Infection," *AIDS* (England) 1(4) (December 1987), pp. 235–40.

Jackson, G.G. *et al.*, "Passive Immunoneutralization of Human Immunodeficiency Virus in Patients with Advanced AIDS," *The Lancet* (September 17, 1988), pp. 647–52.

AMPLIGEN: STUDY STOPPED AFTER POOR RESULTS

An article in *The New York Times* (October 14, 1988) confirmed rumors that had been circulating for weeks—that ampligen was not proving effective in the current double-blind trials.

After 20 patients in that study progressed to AIDS, the code was broken for those 20. Twelve of them were taking ampligen, compared to eight who were taking the placebo—indicating that ampligen was not stopping the progression to AIDS.

According to a phone call from one patient in the study, a higher-dose arm of the trial might still be continued.

Ampligen had been considered a very promising treatment after an earlier study, published in June 1987, reported good results in 10 patients with AIDS, ARC, or lymphadenopathy—especially reductions in viral cultures or other measures of viral activity. That study did not have enough patients to look for prevention of progression to AIDS.

Apparently no one knows why the two studies of the same drug produced such different results. Finding out why might help prevent similar errors in the future.

FDA ISSUES RULES TO SPEED DRUG TESTING

On October 19, the U.S. Food and Drug Administration announced new regulations to speed the development and commercial release of some drugs. Initial reaction by AIDS organizations has been mostly negative (see *The New York Times,* October 20, page 1). Project Inform expressed limited support.

The rules essentially codify what was already done with AZT. They ask drug companies to work more closely with the FDA to design an expanded phase II (efficacy study), after which drugs could be released without going through a phase III (larger efficacy study). But there are no commitments to use the new procedures in any particular situations; and some have questioned whether the FDA has enough money or staff to handle accelerated approvals.

These rules were adopted after months of bitter infighting behind the scenes. Powerful FDA officials who never wanted this reform may try to sabotage it.

The previous "treatment IND" (now called "treatment protocol") remains as before. In theory those rules permit the early release of treatment for life-threatening or severely debilitating illness; in practice they have almost never been used since they were announced over a year ago.

The current new rules do not change the real intentions and operations of the agency concerning early release of drugs before full commercial approval. The FDA still adamantly refuses to allow early release through the treatment protocol (treatment IND) *unless it believes that the data supports approval for full commercial marketing* and only paperwork remains. The treatment protocol can be used only to get the drug to patients during the time of this considerable paperwork; it is only a steppingstone toward commercial release. The FDA sees no drug as eligible for commercial release (and therefore none eligible for a treatment protocol) at this time.

For reasons outlined in "Beyond an Unreasonable Doubt," below, we believe that this new FDA ruling will do nothing for AIDS in the foreseeable future, probably nothing for at least two years. Yet it may be an important long-range step toward improving U.S. drug regulation.

Martin Delaney, co-founder of Project Inform, called the rules "only a small step, not the whole solution to the problems we have been addressing for the last three years. . . . Nevertheless, they stake out new philosophical ground for the agency, acknowledging for the first time that drugs must be evaluated flexibly, that the rules should be different when a life-threatening illness is involved, and that approval should be based on a risk-benefit analysis rather than rigid, standard rules."

The new rule will appear in the Code of Federal Regulations, 21 CFR 312 as a new Subpart E, "Drugs Intended to Treat Life-Threatening and Severely-Debilitating Illnesses."

BEYOND AN UNREASONABLE DOUBT: COMMENTS ON DRUG-APPROVAL DELAYS

The new FDA rules are unlikely to make any practical difference for two years or more, because they concern procedures for expanded "phase II" trials which have not yet even been designed, let alone recruited for, conducted, and analyzed. The new document fails to address the most important FDA issue for AIDS: allowing access to treatments which have been proved safe (or which have known and acceptable risks), and which do show good, credible evidence that they may be effective, but which *do not have enough scientific data yet* to justify full release for commercialization. (Such commercialization includes glossy ads in medical journals, sales forces and promotional campaigns targeting doctors who do not have time to read the literature and make their own evaluations, doctors using the new drug for non-approved and non-emergency purposes as well as approved or emergency ones, etc. It is understandable that the FDA insists on very thorough proof first.)

Why does the FDA refuse to allow a separate standard and procedure for early, less commercial, conditional release in an emergency? The agency purported to do this with its "treatment IND" announced over a year ago. But the treatment IND has almost never been used; and FDA officials do not conceal the fact that they never intended to let the treatment IND employ any lesser standard of proof than required for full commercialization. The treatment IND (called "treatment protocol" in the new regulations) was never intended to allow early release until the FDA already knows, based on its access to proprietary data concealed from the public, that the drug will qualify for full commercial release, and only paperwork remains to complete the approval.

Why does the FDA ask patients to wait years for treatments for life-threatening illnesses when it is known the treatments are safe, and that they probably do work (though none yet is a cure for AIDS)? Why not let patients and their physicians make their own decisions based on the specifics of each case—specifics the FDA cannot possibly respond to, as it cannot know them in advance? Why does the FDA refuse to do in reality what it pretended to do when it announced the treatment IND, over a year ago?

We can only guess at the motives of the agency. But one particular guess clarifies mountains of confusion about FDA policy. This explanation also reveals why the treatment IND failed (why it never represented the real intent of the staff), and why the FDA strongly discourages compassionate use and punishes companies which make their drugs widely available that way (such as Syntex with ganciclovir, also called DHPG).

For if early emergency release required any less data than full commercialization, then some drugs allowed into emergency use would later fail to meet the criteria for general marketing. Then what would happen to the hundreds, maybe thousands of people who were using the drug and were convinced, wrongly or rightly, that it was helping them stay alive? (Even drugs rejected for commercial marketing can in fact save the lives of some people, even if not enough people for statistical proof.) If the FDA or the manufacturer were to cut these people off, there would be tremendous protests—much more than if the drug had been denied in the first place, before the patients had any personal experience with it. In politics there is a saying that people don't fight to get, they fight to keep. Those who have used a drug and found that it helped them will protest much more forcefully if it is taken away, than if they had only read about the drug in a newspaper—or not heard about it at all.

But if the FDA or the manufacturer did not cut the patients off, then the drug companies would need to maintain manufacturing (and the FDA to maintain regulation of good manufacturing practices, etc.) indefinitely for a dead-end drug never expected to be approved. For how long—until the last person no longer wanted it? The drug would stay in limbo—in use, but going nowhere.

By simply holding up emergency release under the treatment protocol (treatment IND) until it is clear that a drug will eventually get full commercial approval and awaits only the paperwork, the FDA prevents in advance the awkward dilemma of ever having to take a drug back—or to allow the creation of a new class of drugs never to be approved but officially released and permanently in use anyway.

Thousands of lives *are* being lost and will be lost to this policy of refusing to allow early treatment release in emergencies, without the full proof required for commercialization. This policy gravely delays the drugs which are good enough to eventually be approved, and it impedes research by preventing physicians from developing practical knowledge early.

Treatments affected include the passive immunotherapy discussed above, imuthiol, fluconazole (which might get a treatment IND as it may already meet standards for marketing), trimetrexate (which has a treatment IND, the only one for an AIDS drug, but is highly restricted and cannot be tried for other infections such as cryptosporidiosis), aerosol pentamidine (available anyway without official sanction), dextran sulfate (available anyway), and colony stimulating factor (not usually available, and a serious problem for patients and physicians who cannot obtain it). Other treatments which might soon be ready for early release, but which probably will not be allowed due to the FDA policy discussed above, include CD4, ddC, and ddI.

This policy grossly mis-serves the public but still will be hard to change. For a triple alliance composed of drug companies, the FDA, and good-government, consumer-protection advocates, who usually have different interests which roughly balance each other, are on the same side of this issue:

• Drug companies want full commercial approval. They do not want the profitless bother and liability of early release, which may lead to dead-end drugs which will never be approved, but which they cannot discontinue without serious public-relations cost.

And companies big enough to afford the $80 million to $120 million bill for each new drug approval do not want to make openings for smaller competitors. (The code words for this corporate wing of the triple alliance are that small "fly by night" companies could profit by "quack" remedies, if allowed earlier, easier emergency release of their products.)

• The FDA fears bad publicity, and greatly fears any independent public movement for a drug, beyond its control. Early release invites just such a movement, if the FDA later rejects the drug. In other words, the agency could lose control if allowed early release before it was clear that the drug would eventually be approved for marketing. So it blocks emergency access, often secretly by pressure behind the scenes, with catastrophic consequences for patients—not for their benefit but for its own. (The code words are "greatest good for the greatest number," to justify policies clearly against patients' interests.)

• Consumer-protection advocates have fought step by step for decades to control dangerous and unscrupulous drug-company practices. The fight over early emergency release exposes a basic flaw in our whole system of drug development and regulation. Regulation advocates fear a weakening of the walls they have so laboriously built up. (The code words are that "standards" of "science" should not be "weakened" because of the AIDS emergency.) Also, the problem will be hard to fix because it is hard to imagine any graceful solution. Any emergency release based on a standard of evidence short of that for full marketing approval will by definition either create awkward take-backs, or create an indefinite limbo for dead-end drugs. But thousands die unnecessarily because patients are denied access to safe and effective treatments pending full justification for commercialization, and because this system greatly delays research by requiring years of red tape to finance, set up, and run elaborate studies to get academic answers when physicians could otherwise get practical answers in weeks.

The standard now in use could be called proof beyond unreasonable doubt. Any possibility, no matter how farfetched, of erroneously approving a drug which does not work must be ruled out.

Society may well want this meticulous standard for routine medical improvements. But it is deadly in an emergency. If AIDS had affected all people equally and not been concentrated in unpopular groups, it is hard to believe that no accommodation would yet have been made. The current policy of withholding emergency treatments until they meet standards for full-scale commercial release amounts to genocide by business as usual.

The new FDA rules try to reduce the pressure for emergency release by promising to speed final commercial release for life-threatening or seriously disabling illnesses. But these rules apply to studies yet to be devised, so they will not help anyone with AIDS in the foreseeable future.

The problem today is the same as it has always been. Agencies, corporations, and professionals have been in business for decades and have negotiated arrangements in their own interests. Patients, unwilling newcomers to the world of medical policy, have had vastly less influence. That is why U.S. drug-approval policy sacrifices thousands of lives for regulatory and corporate convenience.

The public usually avoids the complex and rarified world of regulation. But AIDS is different from other regulatory issues because at least a million U.S. citizens have a life-or-death interest in FDA decisions. Along with the giant corporations, the bureaucrats, and the good-government advocates who were formed in an earlier era, these citizens must and will be heard.

Issue Number 68
November 4, 1988

CHINESE MEDICINE AND AIDS: WHAT HAS BEEN LEARNED? INTERVIEW WITH MISHA COHEN

Misha Cohen, O.M.D., C.A., founder and clinical director of the Quan Yin Acupuncture and Herb Center in San Francisco, has worked extensively with persons with AIDS and HIV infection for five years. We asked Dr. Cohen to outline the most important lessons from this work—and also to suggest practical treatment options available now, even for persons living in areas which have no access to Chinese doctors or practitioners.

AIDS Treatment News (ATN): What basic themes or messages are most important to give to our readers?

Dr. Cohen (MC): "We believe that a combination, integration of Eastern and Western concepts is necessary to fully benefit in treating AIDS/HIV. Traditional Chinese medicine is a system in itself, with concepts very different from those of Western medicine.

"Some Chinese doctors have examined persons with AIDS, recognized various syndromes they commonly treated with herbs, and said, 'We can treat those.' But when they tried, often it didn't work. They were masters with herbs, but they had no experience with AIDS.

"For over five years we have been working with AIDS and ARC. It has taken that long to get to where we are now, learning to use Chinese concepts, and also to look at Western concepts, such as viruses, opportunistic infections, and the pathogenesis of the disease as seen by Western medicine. We had to combine Chinese principles in use of herbs, etc., with Western ideas. Others should not start from the beginning all over again.

"Chinese medicine, and natural therapies in general, are very strong on immune enhancement. But by itself that's not enough. With AIDS the major problem has been antiviral.

"Chinese medicine has hundreds of potentially antiviral herbs. But only recently has it been possible to discover which ones have anti-HIV properties, by modern research. (See "Chinese Herbs Screened for Anti-HIV Activity" in *AIDS Treatment News,* Issue Number 61.)

"We are working with the well-known herbalist Subhuti Dharmananda, of the Institute for Traditional Medicine in Portland, Oregon on antiviral and immune enhancing combinations.

"The antiviral work is the leading edge of herbal medicine for AIDS today. The hope is to find strongly antiviral herbal combinations without serious side effects.

"We need to caution readers, don't just take the antiviral herbs. In Chinese medicine, these are known as anti-infection herbs, which 'clear heat, clear toxin.' But also they are, in Chinese medical terms, 'very cold.' You want a balance of cold, hot, warm, cool. To take only these herbs together is unbalanced, and people will not feel well, just from the herbs. They may feel drained, colder, and find it hard to digest the herbs. It's much better to use combinations designed according to Chinese medicinal principles, including both antiviral and immune enhancing herbs."

Practical Options

ATN: We know that Chinese medicine is highly individual, so it is better if people can see a practitioner to tailor any treatment to their own situation. How can people start (1) if they are near San Francisco or in another area where experienced practitioners are available, and (2) if they cannot get to a practitioner but are living in an area where all they can do is obtain herbal formulas by mail? First tell us what options you have available or know about for persons within commuting distance of San Francisco. Also, our readers should know the approximate costs of the various options, and your policies on accepting insurance.

MC: "In the San Francisco area, and also in Chicago and New York, there is an herbal treatment and research program sponsored by three organizations: Quan Yin in San Francisco (mentioned above), the Institute for Traditional Medicine in Portland (mentioned above), and the Oriental Healing Arts Institute in Long Beach, California. At Quan Yin, 105 people are currently participating in this program, and that number will increase by 50 every 12 weeks. In addition, 40 to 50 are in the program in Chicago, and about 60 in New York.

"This particular program has a reduced cost because it is partly subsidized by the companies which supply the herbs. The exact cost depends on what subsidies are available at the time. At this time, the entire 12-week program costs about $150. If the same herbal formulas were bought at retail, they would cost about $150 per month.

"In addition, since this is a research program, anyone participating will have to have blood work done, which is a good idea anyway. The tests currently required for the study, such as the complete blood count or CBC, are not expensive.

"In San Francisco, this program will have 50 new places available on December 15, and 50 more every 12 weeks thereafter. That's for people who want to reduce the cost by participating in the research. You can start similar treatment programs any time.

"Anyone who wants more information about our treatment/research program can contact us at Quan Yin (see Appendix B). Arrangements are being made so that persons outside of the San Francisco area can participate in this research through their physician or practitioner wherever they are, receiving the formulas by mail, provided they agree to share the results with us by returning the data forms we provide.

"Incidentally the results of our last study were presented by Qing-Cai Zhang, M.D., at a symposium in Long Beach on October 23. The proceedings will be published by the Oriental Healing Arts Institute; they should be ready in December or January. For more information, contact the Oriental Healing Arts Institute" (see Appendix B).

ATN: What was the most important finding in that study?

MC: "The formulas we used at that time generally made people feel better, and be able to fight certain infections better, and seemed to raise red blood levels. But we also know that those formulas had very little if any effect on T-cell counts, white blood counts, and viral levels in the blood.

"That is why we encourage people to consider other antivirals, including AZT for some people, when used correctly. We hope that there are anti-HIV antiviral herbs which work well with little toxicity, but that hasn't been established yet.

"We have changed the formulas since last time, especially by using the laboratory anti-HIV results to develop a stronger antiviral formula, called 'Isatis 6.' It has that name because it contains Isatis and five other herbs, a total of six in the combination.

"Yet even with the previous formulas, at the beginning of our study, 8 of 23 persons with AIDS, ARC, or HIV could not work because of illness. One of them died in the first month of the study. But by the end of the study, all of the other seven were able to go back to work."

(Note: Two of the seven were temporarily hospitalized at the end of the study for complications unrelated to herbal treatment. One had an infection from a central line used for DHPG, the other had pneumothoraxes. Both are able to work now.

And to complete the account of everybody with HIV who entered this study, one person with ARC dropped out for financial reasons. He was healthy enough to work both at entry to and exit from the study.)

ATN: Besides the research program, what other options do you offer?

MC: "At Quan Yin, we also offer a general Chinese medicine and herbal healing clinic—not just for AIDS/HIV. Besides herbs, we have acupuncture, massage, hypnotherapy, nutritional counseling, psychic counseling, and other therapies. We also have a full Chinese herbal pharmacy. And we refer clients to medical doctors, chiropractors, and others.

"Quan Yin does accept MediCal, private insurance, Workman's Compensation, personal injury (through insurance companies), and of course Catholic Charities and the AIDS Emergency Fund."

ATN: What other programs are you involved with in San Francisco?

MC: "The San Francisco AIDS Alternative Healing Project (AAHP) has comprehensive programs for persons with AIDS or ARC or who are HIV positive—including acupuncture, herbs, and weekly sessions for counseling, hypnotherapy/visualization, massage, and support groups. These are group programs which run for six months, so people have to join when a new group is starting. The programs are intensive, with six to eight hours per week in appointments. For more information, people can call AAHP (see Appendix B)."

ATN: And what options can you suggest for people outside of San Francisco? What about those who cannot find any experienced Chinese practitioner where they live?

MC: "In some cities they can find a practitioner. The AAHP also runs a referral and information phone service, at the same number (see Appendix B). We mentioned that there are related programs in Chicago and New York. AAHP can also refer people in some other cities; for example, Austin, Texas has a group doing similar work."

ATN: What if they cannot find a Chinese practitioner? What is the best in that situation?

MC: "They should be working with a physician or someone who is following them. Then I could suggest the following four-part program of herbal formulas. Sometimes these formulas can be bought in a local health-food store; if not they can be obtained by mail. These specific recommendations will change over time as we gain more experience from the research treatment programs.

"For people locally, these formulas are available from Quan Yin. But we do not sell mail order, so those who cannot find them in a local health-food store can order directly from the suppliers listed below.

"**(1)** The 'Astragalus 10+' formula for immune enhancement (from Institute for Traditional Medicine, in Portland, Oregon; see Appendix B; or Cascade Mushrooms, also in Portland; see Appendix B. Cascade sells by the case only).

"**(2)** The 'Isatis 6' formula is the one we are now trying for antiviral effect. It contains some of the Chinese herbs found to have anti-HIV properties."

(Note: Isatis 6, developed by Subhuti Dharmananda of the Institute for Traditional Medicine, is distributed through practitioners and not sold in stores. Dr. Dharmananda discourages people from ordering it directly and recommends obtaining it through a practitioner, but the Institute will sell it, especially for people following a protocol, such as the one from Quan Yin. The Institute cannot provide any consumer literature about how to use this product. Persons interested should obtain the protocol, from Quan Yin's Chinese Herbal Treatment Program for HIV Infection, at the phone number or address given in Appendix B.

The six herbs in this formula are Isatis leaf and root, Lonicera, Andrographis, Dandelion, Viola, and Prunella.)

"**(3)** Some form of ganoderma mushroom for a general tonic. Satisfactory formulas include 'Power Mushrooms' (from Health Concerns, Alameda, California; see Appendix B; and 'BIOHERB Instant Reishi' from BIOHERB, Inc., Schaumberg, Illinois; see Appendix B).

"(4) The fourth element is more difficult to get at this time. In the research study, we are using 'Antler 8,' a formula containing deer antler, which is highly valued in Chinese medicine. It is hoped that this formula will help the bone marrow and increase white blood cells, red cells, and T-helper counts. However, the Institute for Traditional Medicine has not released this formula commercially until it gains more experience with it and learns that it does work as expected for people with HIV.

"In the meantime, people may be able to get deer horn slices, or 'Pantocrin' (a liquid herbal formula with deer horn), from a Chinese herb company, which can usually be found in Chinatown in various cities. Deer horn is expensive, commonly over $100 per pound." (The Institute told us that it expects to have 'Antler 8' in about three weeks. It recommends obtaining this formula through a practitioner.)

ATN: What about dosage? Do the formulas usually have adequate suggested doses on the bottle? What about the deer horn? Can people call the phone referral service at AAHP to ask these questions?

MC: "For information on dosage, call or write to the Chinese Herbal Treatment Program for HIV Infection at Quan Yin (see Appendix B)."

ATN: For general background, could you recommend a beginning book on the principles of Chinese medicine?

MC: "For theoretical background, people could start with *The Web That Has No Weaver: Understanding Chinese Medicine,* by Ted J. Kaptchuk, published by Condon & Weed. It is available in bookstores and is now in paperback. This book covers basic Chinese medical theory, including syndromes and diagnosis, such as pulse and tongue diagnosis. It is used by acupuncture students, as well as lay people, as their first contact with Chinese medicine. The book has no treatment information.

"A recent and important book is Subhuti Dharmananda's *Chinese Herbal Therapies for Immune Disorders,* published by the Institute for Traditional Medicine. To obtain this book, contact the Institute" (see Appendix B).

ATN: One final question. I know it is very difficult to raise money for research on Chinese or any kind of herbal medicine. The U.S. research establishment has little interest, it wants to test single chemicals, because those fit with our system of pharmaceutical companies and drug regulation.

If you could find a good fundraiser or a private donor who could help you find money for this work, what could you do with more resources? How could you speed the research on Chinese-medicine options for AIDS, and also what could be done on making these options available to people who cannot now afford them?

MC: "If we had funding, we could subsidize people who cannot afford even the reduced rate for the herbal treatment/research program. We would do full laboratory testing on every person. Today we cannot afford to do T-cell counts.

"We would also greatly expand the program, and test different groups of herbal formulas at the same time. We do have the organizing ability; what limits us now is the money.

"Also we would have quicker turnaround as we could tabulate the data, do the statistics, and get papers published more quickly. We could move faster and have more opportunity to find what formulas worked the best."

ATN: Anything else you would like to add?

MC: "We are happy and gratified to have maintained good relations with the medical doctors who are treating persons with AIDS. We refer patients to them, and they to us. This cooperation is basic to the comprehensive approach of combining Eastern and Western medical ideas. No one has the whole answer. Everyone benefits by communication and cooperation among the different disciplines."

CALIFORNIA: PROPOSITION 102

This issue is going to press before the election, so we do not know whether Proposition 102, the AIDS reporting initiative, will pass. (For background on Proposition 102, see *AIDS Treatment News,* Issue Number 65). In case the measure does pass, we are including this section to address the immediate fear and confusion, and will later report on what people are doing to minimize the damage.

The information here comes from our notes of a meeting of representatives of AIDS agencies and organizations to address the legal and other consequences of Proposition 102. However, we did not have time to get back to the attorneys and other speakers to check the correctness of this report. It is correct as far as we know.

The most important points to know now are:

• Organizations and agencies (including *AIDS Treatment News)* are not legally required to turn over your name. Only doctors, blood banks and plasma centers, and people who run alternative test sites would be required to report names of clients they know or believe are HIV positive.

It is conceivable but unlikely that local health departments would sue organizations for the names of their clients—guaranteeing lengthy litigation for which the proposition appropriates no money.

AIDS Treatment News will never divulge names of subscribers under any circumstances. And we have taken other precautions, such as not keeping track who subscribed at the reduced rate for persons with AIDS or ARC—which is why our bills always have both options. It is encouraging to know that we will not have to take drastic measures to protect our subscribers, such as moving out of state.

• The measure requires persons who know they are HIV positive to report everyone from whom they might have been infected, or whom they might have infected, within seven days. But it does not require them to report themselves.

This section is probably unenforceable, since it would be hard to prove that someone did not report as required—since no record could be found if they reported anonymously or under a false name, as they could legally do.

In any case, the measure will only apply to unsafe sexual contacts; safe sex need not be reported.

Do *not* report obviously false sexual contacts—e.g., with public figures such as Ronald Reagan—as doing so would raise a red flag to officials and invite prosecution.

When will the law go into effect? There is confusion, but most experts we talked to think that it will go into effect immediately after the election (not January 1). However, county health departments may choose to wait for administrative guidance from the State before implementing some of its provisions.

A court challenge has already been prepared and will be filed within the first week after the election, if the measure passes.

• Physicians are only required to report those with whom they currently have a doctor-patient relationship. This relationship can be terminated by a letter from either party—suggesting one way to resolve a doctor-patient impasse over reporting, in some cases.

If Proposition 102 passes, we will have more reports on what people are doing and what the real options are.

NEW YORK: COLUMBIA CONFERENCE ON AIDS/HIV TREATMENT, NOVEMBER 19

The second annual conference, "AIDS: Improving the Odds," will take place on Saturday, November 19, from 9:00 AM to 6:00 PM, at Columbia University, Kathryn Bache Miller Theater, 116th Street and Broadway, New York, NY. Press registration begins at 8:30. The panelists are: Donald Armstrong, M.D., Charles A. Barber, Michael Callen, Martin Delaney, Barry Gingell, Michael H. Grieco, M.D., Ronald Grossman, M.D., John S. James, Richard Keeling, M.D., Donald Kotler, M.D., Michael Lange, M.D., Craig Metroka, M.D., Ph.D., Richard Price, M.D., Joseph Sonnabend, M.D., and Daniel William, M.D. The conference will be moderated by Laura Pinsky and Paul H. Douglas, Columbia Gay Health Advocacy Project.

Admission is free, but tickets will be required due to limited space.

CMV RETINITIS STUDY SEEKS VOLUNTEERS

The National Eye Institute of the National Institutes of Health (NIH) is recruiting patients with CMV retinitis for a study of treatment with foscarnet. Previous uncontrolled studies have shown a 70–85 percent favorable response for treatment of CMV retinitis with this drug, which also has activity against HIV.

This randomized trial includes three arms: foscarnet alone, AZT alone, and foscarnet plus AZT. To avoid eye damage to persons in the control group receiving AZT alone, the study's entry criteria specify that the CMV lesion is located where it does not threaten sight, and the study will be stopped before vision is endangered. After the study, all patients will be eligible to continue foscarnet on compassionate use.

The study will take place at the National Institutes of Health in Bethesda, Maryland, near Washington, D.C. All expenses are paid, including travel and lodging for patients from outside the area.

Patients will need to spend three to four weeks at the National Eye Institute in Bethesda, followed by weekly visits. The number of visits depends on the course of the disease. During this phase of the study, patients may return home or remain in Bethesda, and NIH will pay all travel or lodging expenses, either way. Afterwards, patients can be treated with foscarnet through their home physician, making further visits to Bethesda unnecessary.

So that patients and their ophthalmologists can quickly determine whether they are eligible, we quote the inclusion and exclusion criteria.

Inclusion criteria: "Patients with AIDS (age 18–60) and cytomegalovirus retinitis located more than 3000 microns from the fovea and more than 1500 microns from the optic disc unless the vision is less than 20/400 in that eye in which case any location is eligible. One or both eyes may be involved by the retinitis.

"Serum creatine less than 2.0 mg/dl; total neutrophil count greater than 1000/mm^3; total hemoglobin greater than 8 gm/dl; platelets greater than 25,000/mm^3."

Exclusion criteria: "Previous therapy with ganciclovir or foscarnet. Concomitant therapy with marrow toxic or nephrotoxic agents excluding AZT. Concomitant therapy with oral or intravenous acyclovir. A history of intolerance to AZT."

Issue Number 69
November 18, 1989

AIDS TREATMENT NEWS SURVEY: PRELIMINARY REPORT

Last August, *AIDS Treatment News* sent a survey questionnaire to its subscribers, asking for their overall evaluation of any treatments they had used for AIDS, HIV, or any related condition. We asked subscribers to name up to three treatments that had worked best for them or for others they knew personally. We also asked them to name the three worst treatments from their experience—meaning those which either didn't work or seemed harmful. The survey included several questions, and left space for open-ended explanations.

Of the 5725 questionnaires sent, 391 were returned by the deadline (October 1, later extended to October 10). This preliminary article reports the number of times each treatment was listed as one of the three best, vs. one of the three worst, in all 391 questionnaires.

Many of the results were as expected, but others were surprising. Some unorthodox and conventional treatments alike did worse than we had expected.

Some of the tabulations below could be misleading; the obvious interpretation may not reflect what is really happening. We will explain some of these potential errors, to warn the reader about the limitations of this survey. It can indicate which treatments seem to be working for people, but must not be taken as gospel.

	BEST	WORST		BEST	WORST
Acidophilus	4	1	*Amitriptyline*	1	1
Acupressure	2	0	*Amphotericin B*	3	5
Acupuncture	21	0	*Ampligen*	2	4
Acyclovir	114	10	*Antabuse*	8	16
AL 721	85	46	*Antibiotics*	0	5
Aloe vera	8	7	*Aspirin*	2	1

	BEST	WORST		BEST	WORST
Attitudinal healing	3	0	Hydrocortisone	0	2
AZT	204	87	Hydrogen peroxide	6	6
Bactrim (Septra)	19	46	Interferon alpha	4	7
BHT	2	4	Interferon beta	1	1
Chanting	2	0	Iscador	2	0
Chemotherapy	8	4	Isoprinosine	5	5
Chiropractic	2	1	Leucovorin	2	0
Coenzyme Q	8	4	Lecithin	2	0
Cortisone	0	2	Love	3	0
D-penicillamine	1	2	Massage	2	0
Dapsone	5	9	Meditation	7	0
ddC	2	1	Minerals	3	0
De Veras beverage	3	1	Monolaurin	4	4
Dextran sulfate	61	15	Mycelex	10	8
DHEA	2	1	Naltrexone	13	6
DHPG	13	0	Nizoral	11	6
Diet	40	3	Nystatin	5	6
DNCB	3	9	Ozone	2	1
Doctor	2	5	Pau d'arco	2	1
Doxycycline	2	0	Penicillin	2	4
DTC	8	6	Pentamidine (?)	12	2
Echinacea	2	3	Pentamidine aerosol	105	1
Erythromycin	0	2	Pentamidine iv	4	11
Exercise	13	0	Positive attitude	11	0
Fansidar	5	16	Prayer	2	0
Fluconazole	3	0	Prednisone	3	1
Folic acid	2	1	Propolis	1	3
Fusidic acid	0	2	Protein powder	2	0
Garlic	8	1	Psychotherapy	5	0
German enzymes	1	0	Radiation	6	5
Germanium	6	2	Relaxation	4	0
Gamma globulin	2	1	Rest	4	0
Ginseng	2	1	Revici method	2	2
Group	2	0	Ribavirin	6	18
Herbs	22	6	Salk polio vaccine	4	3
Homeopathic	5	1	Selenium	3	0
Hospitalization	0	2	Shiitake Mushrooms	1	3
HPA 23	0	3			

	BEST	WORST		BEST	WORST
Sleep	3	0	*Trimethoprim*	2	4
Spiritual	25	3	*Trimetrexate*	1	1
Steps program	2	0	*Typhoid vaccine*	2	1
Steroids	0	3	*Visualization*	16	0
Stress reduction	19	1	*Vitamins*	47	12
Sulfa drugs	0	2	*Work*	2	1
Supplements	2	0	*Zantac*	2	0
Thymus	2	0	*Zinc*	4	1
Transfer factor	8	3			
			TOTALS	**1117**	**489**

How We Conducted the Survey

We had intended to enter all the information from the returned questionnaires into a computer database, then select various groups of survey respondents (such as those who did well with one particular treatment but poorly with another), and compare these different groups. But many people gave us several pages of comments, or medical information such as lab reports. Often the information they provided was so diverse that there was no straightforward way to process it by computer. So we computerized only the best and worst treatments, miscellaneous questions like medical degree if any and ZIP code, and brief comments. We arranged the forms for easy access by sequence number, so that we can select interesting groups by computer, then collect and examine the corresponding physical questionnaires, in the hope of finding insights into why certain treatments do or do not work for certain people.

Only the "best" and "worst" tabulations are available for this preliminary article, however.

Treatment Categories and Names

The following decisions affected the results reported below:

Treatment Combinations.   We asked respondents to list combinations as if they were single treatments. For example, an AZT/acyclovir combination should be listed as one of the best (or worst) treatments, not as two different treatments.

But often there was no clear dividing line between what was and what was not considered a combination. For example, AZT and aerosol pentamidine might be listed together by one respondent, even though they have separate purposes, and listed separately by others.

Another problem is that there are so many different possible combinations of drugs that it is difficult to categorize them meaningfully.

Because of this confusion around treatment combinations, we decided to break combinations apart, and count each drug or treatment individually in the tabulations below—noting the important combinations here in the text.

Fortunately for the analysis of this survey, only two combination occurred often enough to greatly affect the results:

- AZT and acyclovir was listed 28 times as one of the best treatments, and only twice as one of the worst.

- Persons using food supplements often listed the entire treatment regimen as a combination. We could not analyze this information for this preliminary article, so usually we grouped them as "vitamins" or "herbs" in the tabulation.

Combining Related Treatments in the Tabulations. For this preliminary report, we grouped all "herbs" together, also all "vitamins," and all "spiritual" approaches. Later we will try to report more detail, but this information is difficult to categorize, as each person's combination is often unique.

We did notice that astragalus was named in 6 of the 22 "best" herb entries, none of the 6 "worst." And in the vitamin group, vitamin C appeared 15 times in "best" and 5 in "worst." These results may change when we go back to the survey forms for more detail. Other herbs and vitamins were much less prominent in the computerized information we have examined, and we could not get meaningful numbers, at least without scrutinizing the survey forms.

Using Uniform Names. We combined "nutrition" with "diet," "septra" with "bactrim," "disulfiram" with "antabuse," "ketoconazole" with "nizoral," "ganciclovir" with "DHPG," and "imuthiol" with "DTC." We usually chose the names most frequently used by respondents.

We combined "carrisyn" with "De Veras beverage," but kept them separate from "aloe."

In *AIDS Treatment News,* Issue Number 63, with which we sent the survey, we included an extensive list of treatment names. Treatments not on that list may have been under-represented in the survey results, relative to their actual use in the community.

Interpreting the Numbers: Comments and Cautions

Respondents listed more than twice as many treatments under "best" than under "worst." Apparently they tended to believe that treatments they had used were helpful. A rule of thumb for reading the table printed above could be that unless a treatment has a two-to-one favorable rating in this survey, it was rated worse than the average.

But a low rating does not necessarily mean that a treatment should be avoided. A drug may have a low rating because of side effects, but still be medically advisable.

Some comments on particular therapies:

AZT: is the most common single drug, with 204 of the 391 respondents listing it as one of their three best treatments, and 87 of the 391 as one of their worst. (A person could list a treatment as both best and worst, but we did not let any respondent count the same treatment as "best" or "worst" more than once.)

AL 721: looks slightly below the average treatment in this survey, with 85 "best" listings and 46 "worst." The large total for AL 721 among subscribers to *AIDS Treatment News* may reflect this newsletter's early coverage of that treatment, and not accurately represent its prevalence in the community.

Pentamidine, Aerosol: with 105 "best" and only 1 "worst," may look like the top treatment of all. While it may well be one of the most valuable drugs, we expect that this survey may have unduly favored it. For most patients use pentamidine aerosol as a preventive, so they do not feel its benefit directly; what doesn't happen counts. Therefore few respondents would have listed this drug on the basis of personal experience; they must have been guided by its reputation instead. For this reason we believe that the lopsidedly good result of 105 to 1 is too extreme.

Visualization: rated 16 "best" to zero "worst;" meditation 7 to zero, and spiritual approaches 25 to 3. Clearly some people are finding these methods valuable. But the lack of negative ratings should not be assumed to mean that these approaches work all the time. Visualization and meditation, for example, seem unlikely to be listed as treatment failures, if only because of the dynamics of how we talk and think about them.

Antibiotics: rated zero "best" to 5 "worst," shows the opposite bias. Successful treatment would seldom be attributed to "antibiotics" in general; more likely the specific drug or drugs would be named. Therefore the successes would not show up under "antibiotics," and only the failures would remain—as seems to have happened here. Clearly it would be wrong to conclude that antibiotics are worthless. This example, like some of the others above, shows that the survey must be interpreted carefully.

Bactrim (septra): also looks bad, with 19 "best" and 46 "worst," probably because it is often used as a preventive, meaning that patients do not notice the good that it does, while they do notice any side effects.

Dextran sulfate: looks good, with responses four to one in its favor. This result may reflect real benefits. Or it could reflect the drug's reputation and publicity, plus the struggle people had to go through to get it.

A number of seemingly popular treatments look worse in this survey than we would have predicted. (When reading these numbers, remember that an "average" treatment will have about twice as many "best" responses as "worst," as explained above.) For example (in alphabetical order):

- Aloe vera (8 "best," 7 "worst");
- Ampligen (2 "best," 4 "worst;" the clinical trial also showed lack of result);
- Antabuse (8 "best," 16 "worst," probably reflecting side effects);
- BHT (2 "best," 4 "worst," too few responses to give a reliable picture, although these numbers suggest that the treatment is not widely used);
- DNCB (3 "best," 9 "worst," probably due to side effects, but showing disappointingly few reports of good results);
- Hydrogen peroxide (6 "best," 6 "worst," hardly the much-touted miracle cure);

- Propolis (1 "best," 3 "worst," too few to tell anything for sure, but much worse than from the anecdotal reports we had heard);

- Ribavirin (6 "best," 18 "worst");

- Shiitake mushrooms (1 "best," 3 "worst;" this result may change when we analyze the herbs more completely).

Other treatments which look good or at least passable in this survey, in addition to the attitudinal and spiritual approaches mentioned above, include:

- Diet (40 "best," 3 "worst;" clearly a major success);

- Exercise (13 "best," zero "worst;"

- Stress reduction (19 "best," 1 "worst");

- Garlic (8 "best," 1 "worst");

- Coenzyme Q (8 "best," 4 "worst," probably reflecting the fact that it only helps those who have a deficiency);

- Germanium (6 "best," 2 "worst," although this result should be taken cautiously, because the drug can make people feel speedy and might improve its "best" rating for that reason alone);

- Homeopathic treatments (5 "best," 1 "worst");

- Naltrexone (13 "best," 6 "worst," and low-cost and harmless);

- Rest and relaxation (each 4 "best," zero "worst");

- Transfer factor (8 "best," 3 "worst," but expensive, given by injection, and not widely available);

- Zinc (4 "best," 1 "worst"); and

- Selenium (3 "best," 0 "worst," but beware of overdose).

Herbs and vitamins also look good. But as mentioned above, this preliminary report did not count them completely.

SAN FRANCISCO: AIDS FOUNDATION NEWSLETTER ON 14 ANTIVIRALS

Last week the San Francisco AIDS Foundation published issue #2 of *BETA (Bulletin of Experimental Treatments for AIDS)*. This issue reviews 14 different antivirals, and also includes an update on AZT, the focus of the first issue of *BETA* (#1).

BETA is exceptional because it combines openness to treatment options, extensive and careful research and references, and a presentation easy for non-medical people to understand.

The antivirals covered in issue #2 are: AZT, Dextran sulfate, Iscador, AL 721, Ribavirin, Carrisyn, BHT, and (available only to people in clinical trials) CD4, CD4-pseudomonas exotoxin, Foscarnet, ddC, Alpha interferon, Beta interferon, and Gamma interferon.

The San Francisco AIDS Foundation distributes *BETA* free within San Francisco. It will also send free copies (of issue #2 only) to persons elsewhere; later, it plans to accept subscriptions, free from within San Francisco and paid from elsewhere.

To get a subscription to *BETA*, contact the San Francisco AIDS Foundation (see Appendix B).

SAN FRANCISCO: CHANGES AT *SENTINEL* NEWSPAPER

For over two and a half years part of the material published in *AIDS Treatment News* has also appeared biweekly in the *San Francisco Sentinel,* a gay newspaper distributed free in San Francisco. Last week a dispute between members of the staff and the newspaper's new owner resulted in the resignation of the entire editorial and production departments, nine persons in all, including the people we worked with at the paper. This week's *Sentinel,* in which the survey results published here would ordinarily have appeared, was not published.

The *Sentinel* situation does not affect *AIDS Treatment News,* which is independent. We do want to continue to appear in a newspaper in San Francisco. We are exploring all the options.

WASHINGTON, D.C.: NEW HIV-POSITIVE ORGANIZATION; ACUPUNCTURE TALK

A new HIV-positive organization called Options +, sponsored by Lifelink and the Whitman Walker Clinic, has organized a talk by Dr. Wu and associates from the Green Cross Acupuncture Clinic. The talk will be at St. John's Lafayette Square Church, at 7:30 PM on December 15. For more information about Options +, call them (see Appendix B).

Issue Number 70
December 1, 1988

COMMUNITY RESEARCH ALLIANCE: NEW SAN FRANCISCO EFFORT FOR COMMUNITY-BASED TRIALS

Update 1989: The Community Research Alliance began its first clinical trial, a hypericin monitoring study, in June, 1989.

For over two months this writer has been a founding board member of the Community Research Alliance (CRA), a San Francisco organization modeled after the Community Research Initiative in New York. *AIDS Treatment News* has not reported on the CRA, because the board asked its members not to publicize the organization until it had better defined its identity. Earlier this week the board ended the request to avoid publicity. This article is the first published description of the CRA.

Like New York's CRI, San Francisco's CRA began under the fiscal sponsorship of the PWA Coalition. Initial funding came from pledges of $1000 from each of five organizations: *AIDS Treatment News,* The Healing Alternatives Foundation, Project Inform, PWA Coalition, and the San Francisco AIDS Foundation. Other donations, including office space, use of computers, and especially the work of a volunteer administrator, allowed the CRA to begin swiftly, without waiting for major funding.

Background on Community-Based Trials

Community-based trials is a concept pioneered in different ways by two organizations: the County Community Consortium in San Francisco, and the Community Research Initiative in New York. Within the last year this concept has won widespread recognition and support, from groups including the Presidential Commission on the HIV Epidemic which commended New York's CRI, from Congress which appropriated over $5,000,000 for community-based trials, and from the National Institute of Allergy and Infectious Diseases (NIAID), which is administering these Congressional funds. (See

"NIH Announces Program for Community-Based Trials," in this issue, page 428.) What are community-based trials?

Traditionally, clinical trials of experimental drugs or other treatments were done in major medical centers, usually connected with leading universities. Everyone agrees that some trials must be carried out in such specialized institutions—for example, tests of dangerous treatments, or of chemicals never before taken by humans. But other trials do not need such special facilities.

Anything that happens in major medical centers is expensive and time-consuming. So in New York the Community Research Initiative, started as a project of New York's PWA Coalition with $5,000 from that organization, set up all the arrangements legally required to conduct human trials with patient volunteers in the practices of private physicians. The CRI, which is now running five trials, is believed to be the first organization in history set up by patients to conduct fully sanctioned, professional scientific research for testing new treatments. (The current CRI trials are aerosol pentamidine, egg lecithin lipids, antabuse monitoring study, erythropoietin, and bovine milk immune globulin. Four more trials are in advanced planning: DHEA, lentinan, dextran sulfate, and pyrimethamine prophylaxis for toxoplasmosis. The aerosol pentamidine trial, originally financed by LyphoMed for one year, was recently extended for six months. The trials of lipids and of DHEA are financed by fundraising events organized by People Taking Action Against AIDS, a Long Island group which raises money for AIDS work.) For more background on community-based trials and the CRI, see *The New York Times*, March 15, 1988. Also see our articles about the CRI in *AIDS Treatment News*, Issues Number 38 and 45.

Two Models of Community-Based Trials

The phrase "community-based trials" means scientific tests of experimental drugs or other treatments conducted through the practices of private physicians. But two different approaches to such trials have developed. Much confusion and sometimes debate stem from the failure to understand the differences.

The two approaches are illustrated by the two different organizations, the Community Research Initiative described above, and the County Community Consortium.

In San Francisco, the County Community Consortium (CCC), organized primarily by researchers at the University of California, San Francisco Medical Center, conducted the first community-based trials anywhere. At this time, the CCC is conducting seven trials; its meetings are attended by almost every physician with an AIDS practice in San Francisco. This organization works closely with the AIDS Clinical Trials Group sponsored by the U.S. National Institutes of Health and located in San Francisco General Hospital, which has developed an efficient system of running clinical trials. (The seven trials currently open are two with aerosol pentamidine for pneumocystis prophylaxis, two monitoring studies (an AZT database, and an alternative treatments database), clofazimine for MAI prophylaxis, AZT with vitamin B12, and megace. None of these trials is sponsored by pharmaceutical companies.) Both the Consortium in San Francisco and the Community Research Initiative in New York conduct trials through the practices of front-line AIDS physicians. Both run trials designed by leading researchers, approved for scientific merit by a Scientific Advisory Committee, and approved for ethical treatment of patients by an Institutional Review Board (IRB).

The difference is in the degree of PWA participation in the organization of the research.

In both cases, the *scientific and medical* issues are decided by qualified professionals. But the Community Research Initiative, operating under New York's PWA Coalition, includes much participation by PWAs in policy decisions concerning the research.

In San Francisco, community-based trials developed differently. The County Community Consortium was started so that university researchers could inform community physicians about the latest AIDS medical information, and improve coordination between private-practice physicians and San Francisco General Hospital, which is closely affiliated with the University of California, San Francisco Medical Center. Later, some of the physicians wanted to participate in trials of experimental drugs; as a result, community-based trials began. But patients had nothing to do with the development of the trials; their involvement began when they signed up for a study. Until a year ago, most persons with AIDS in San Francisco probably did not know that the Consortium existed. Recently, however, the Consortium has set up a Community Advisory Board, to improve communication and allow input from persons with AIDS/HIV and treatment advocates. (For more background on the Consortium, see "Conversations with Donald Abrams, M.D.," *AIDS Treatment News,* Issues Number 54 and 56.)

New York's Community Research Initiative, started by a PWA Coalition, has much patient involvement in research policy. The PWA community has funded at least two trials through fundraising events, has set its own policies on placebo use, and has insisted that trials under its sponsorship be effectively open to women and minorities, not only to gay men. Such prior community involvement in policy issues around the selection and conduct of trials makes recruitment easier and increases patient-experimenter cooperation, for example by greatly reducing any need to "cheat" in the study by taking other drugs without telling the researchers.

Why the CRA?

Why should there now be a second organization (the CRA) to conduct community-based trials in San Francisco, when the Consortium is already doing so? The CRA has not officially answered this question, but the answers we suggest below seem representative of views found in the organization.

(1) The Consortium can only conduct a handful of trials at one time. More needs to be done. The CRA will not duplicate work of the Consortium. Instead it will do additional studies which otherwise would not have been conducted.

(2) PWAs want to be involved in the policy making, organization and administration of the research. Otherwise, the PWA community would remain only a passive recipient of research efforts conducted in its behalf by others.

(3) The Consortium does not have its own Institutional Review Board (IRB); the CRA plans to establish one. There is concern that existing IRBs may be too conservative to respond appropriately to the AIDS emergency. PWAs fear—rightly or wrongly—that many physicians will not be able to get approval for formal scientific tests of well-supported treatment options which they may in fact already be using in

their practice. (Physicians do not need IRB approval to use non-approved "treatments" for their patients; they do need approval, however, if the same treatments are called "research." This system, intended to protect patients against exploitation and unconscionable risks at the hands of scientists or pharmaceutical companies using them to get data, has also had the unfortunate side effect of creating a physician underground, forcing legitimate, legal treatments out of the public arena, preventing proper research and open communication of results. An IRB created by PWA organizations would allow physicians to submit these treatments they are using without fear of automatic rejection.)

Research Policy Issues: The Need for Patient Involvement

There is a common assumption that since everyone is on the same side, doing their best to find treatments for AIDS, we can leave the whole matter to professionals, since the only decisions are scientific and medical ones which must be made by specialists, not policy decisions in which affected citizens need a voice. Some simple examples will show how this assumption is wrong:

(A) Drugs approved under the current system will be expensive, because pharmaceutical companies are only likely to support products which will provide them with the highest return. And because trials are expensive, scientists and physicians can only conduct research that someone will pay for. It is no coincidence that AZT, one of the most expensive drugs in history, has become most intensively studied— while readily available treatments are hardly studied at all.

Persons with AIDS or HIV, by contrast, want affordable treatments. U.S. insurance companies, hospitals, employers, and public agencies are increasingly dumping patients who cannot pay the extreme costs of U.S. medicine. Patients want studies of treatments which could be made available to all, not only those with money or insurance.

(B) A number of antibiotics which may be essential for saving lives of persons with AIDS are in common use in Europe but not available in the U.S., because their manufacturers do not want to spend the years and tens of millions of dollars required for U.S. approval.

Here again the interests of patients and professionals differ. Patients want the drugs tested, and want their physicians to have the option of recommending them. If red tape gets in the way, they are willing to rock the boat.

But for scientists, the professional incentives are to stay away from drugs without commercial sponsorship in the U.S. Here again, the interests of patients and professionals differ.

(C) When preliminary studies of a new treatment show very good results, research professionals not surprisingly want to do more studies, which will take years. No one objects to the studies; the issue is access by patients who need the treatment now. There is no institutional incentive to provide this access until double-blind studies have been designed, cranked up, run, analyzed, and published, and then delayed several more years for FDA approval.

The interests of the research community, the pharmaceutical industry, and regulators have all been well represented. None of these have put the patients' needs first.

And unless the PWA community is involved in the many difficult details of organizing actual trials, it will not have the depth of knowledge needed to effectively articulate and realize its interests. The PWA community must have organizations which understand the administration of AIDS research as well as any university, corporation, or government agency.

The Community Research Alliance is committed to always having effective PWA representation on all decision-making bodies: the Institutional Review Board (IRB), the Scientific Advisory Committee, and the board of directors. As far as we know, it is one of only two clinical-research organizations in the country to do so; the other is New York's Community Research Initiative.

The CRA Today

At this time the CRA board of directors includes people listed below. The board is seeking new members to broaden its base in all parts of the AIDS community. Because it is hard for a large group to conduct routine business, a smaller executive committee makes recommendations to the full board, which makes the final decisions.

To date (December 1, 1988) the Scientific Advisory Committee has not met. But 16 physicians and scientists have so far expressed interest in working with this group. And 19 physicians with private practices in the Bay Area have expressed interest in participating in the trials. (Nine are on both groups). Several physicians have already proposed research studies.

The Institutional Review Board has not yet been formed.

The CRA has an office and a full-time administrator, Tom Wilcox, who recently moved to San Francisco from New York, where he was manager of the PWA Health Group, and worked closely with the Community Research Initiative.

We list the current CRA board members below. Note that some of the organizations with which these people are affiliated have not taken any position on the CRA; therefore this listing does not imply organizational endorsement.

Ron Baker	Editor and co-author, *Bulletin of Experimental Treatment for AIDS,* San Francisco AIDS Foundation.
Keith Barton, M.D., C.A.	Private practice in Berkeley, California.
Terry Beswick	Director, The Healing Alternatives Foundation, San Francisco.
Misha Cohen, O.M.D.	Founder and Clinical Director, Quan Yin Acupuncture and Herb Center, San Francisco.
Martin Delaney	Co-director, Project Inform.
Rick Graham	PWA Coalition (alternate for Hank Wilson).
John S. James	Editor and publisher, *AIDS Treatment News.*

Tom O'Connor	Author of *Living with AIDS: Reaching Out.*
Jim Palazzolo	Co-author, *Bulletin of Experimental Treatments for AIDS,* San Francisco AIDS Foundation (alternate for Ron Baker).
Curtis Ponzi	Attorney.
Pat Sanders, M.S.N., C.A.	Unit Manager, NIH HIV Research, Kaiser Permanente, San Francisco, and licensed acupuncturist in private practice, San Francisco (alternate for Tom O'Connor).
Hank Wilson	PWA Coalition, San Francisco.
Tim Wilson	National Task Force on AIDS Prevention, of the National Association of Black and White Men Together.

Funding

Because of donations of office facilities, and of the time of volunteer administrator Mike Lipson who was invaluable in starting the organization, little money has been spent. With pledges and a matching grant totaling $8,000 so far, about $4,000 additional will carry the organization through the next three months, which should be enough to complete the development of the Scientific Advisory Committee and IRB, and start evaluating research proposals from physicians and scientists.

Later, the organization will need major funding for the trials themselves. Trials can cost $2,000 or more per patient, mostly for laboratory tests, which are usually paid for by the study. There may also be additional physical examinations. Usually the drugs are donated by the manufacturer, so they would not be an expense for the CRA.

In New York, most of the studies now being conducted by the Community Research Initiative are financed by pharmaceutical companies, which were eager to participate because of their frustrations in getting their drugs tested through other channels. The CRA may also do such studies. But it hopes to raise money from foundations, corporations, individuals, and other contributors, so that it can focus research attention on what may be the fastest, most cost-effective way to get results—including the study of medically promising treatment possibilities which have been overlooked so far because for various reasons they are not commercially attractive.

CRA does not yet have this funding and will need community help in getting it.

How You Can Help

CRA is building a skills list of friends who can help this project in any way—fundraising, organizational skills, helping us contact people we should be working with, technical skills such as computers, graphics, or printing, medical and scientific experience of course, etc. If you want to help, contact them by calling or writing (see Appendix B).

The CRA greatly needs volunteers. It plans to follow the CRI model of having one person be volunteer coordinator, with most of the work done by volunteers. This approach not only controls expenses; it also allows for participation by PWAs who are on disability and not permitted to earn money without risking their benefits.

Contributions to CRA are tax deductible. Make checks payable to "PWA Coalition," and send them to the CRA at the address given in Appendix B.

The organization would like to form a "Friends of the CRA" auxiliary, to be a social organization which would also raise money, find volunteers, develop contacts and community coalitions, and otherwise promote the work of the CRA.

ALPHA INTERFERON APPROVED FOR KS; OFFICIAL DOSE TOO HIGH?

On November 21, the FDA approved use of alpha interferon to treat KS. The drug, already available by prescription since June 1986 and previously approved to treat hairy cell leukemia and genital warts, is being marketed under two brand names, Intron-A (Schering Corp.) and Roferon (Hoffman-La Roche). The two versions have slightly different molecular structures.

After the FDA approval, *AIDS Treatment News* talked with Mathilde Krim, Ph.D., founding chairperson of the American Foundation for AIDS Research. While best known for her work with AmFAR, Dr. Krim is also a leading expert on interferon. In 1975 she became co-director and then director of an interferon laboratory at Memorial Sloan-Kettering Cancer Center in New York, a position she held until 1985 when she left to do AIDS work.

Dr. Krim is concerned that the doses on which the FDA based its approval may be much too high. Two weeks ago, at an international meeting on interferon research in Japan, Dr. Ernest Borden showed that as long as the dose was enough to produce the desired effect, a higher dose made little difference; this result was based on human as well as test-tube work. Other researchers, including Dr. Clifford Lane and colleagues, who used high dose interferon and published an article in *The Lancet* (November 26, 1988), showed that those who responded well usually started with over 150 T-helper cells, while those who did not respond had fewer. The important factor seemed to be the state of the immune system, not the dose.

Also, clinical studies with the high doses, 20 million units a day or more, caused such unpleasant flu-like side effects that in order to keep the patients in the study, physicians had to reduce the dose to half or a quarter. Yet the beneficial effects continued.

Dr. Krim also noted that much smaller doses have been found effective in treating hairy cell leukemia, in some cases as little as one and a half million units given twice a week.

But the early studies of alpha interferon for KS had used large doses, because the dominant thinking, derived from chemotherapy, was that the dose should be as high as the patient could tolerate. The FDA had to use the data available, much of it from early studies, as the basis for the approval. This may give patients and physicians the impression that they need high doses. But these doses cause unpleasant side effects, and also are very expensive, conceivably costing as much as $50,000 in a year.

Dr. Krim believes that alpha interferon would probably be effective at much lower doses, and would be well worth trying.

PASSIVE IMMUNOTHERAPY: MAJOR NEW ARTICLE— AND PATIENT SUPPORT GROUP IN SAN FRANCISCO

In October, *AIDS Treatment News* (Issue Number 67) reported on passive immunotherapy, a treatment which consists of taking plasma from healthy HIV-positive donors who have high levels of antibodies against the core proteins of the AIDS virus, and infusing the plasma into persons who have lost the ability to produce those protective antibodies. That work, by researchers at the London Hospital Medical College, the University of Illinois College of Medicine, and Abbott Laboratories, had been presented at the Stockholm AIDS conference in June, 1988, and also published in *The Lancet* (September 17, 1988).

Now other researchers at Cambridge University in England have published a report of their study of ten patients with AIDS or ARC who received monthly passive immunotherapy treatments in the December issue of *Proceedings of the National Academy of Sciences USA*. We have not seen this article before going to press. But news reports quoted the researchers as saying that the virus disappeared from the blood of all ten, nine of whom are still alive and reasonably healthy nine months later.

A principal developer of the treatment, Dr. Abraham Karpas, assistant director for research for the Department of Hematological Medicine at Cambridge University in England, described passive immunotherapy as completely nontoxic, and said that while more studies are needed, he saw no reason it could not be made available now.

A year ago August, Dr. Karpas noted that in a small test with four patients, "there was considerable subjective improvement in the patients noted by both the medical and nursing staff."

The October/November issue of *Positive Directions News,* a publication of Positive Directions, an association of HIV-positive persons in Boston, Massachusetts, interviewed AIDS researcher Dr. Clyde Crumpacker of Harvard Medical School about the Stockholm AIDS conference (June 1988). Most of the published interview concerned passive immunotherapy, which Dr. Crumpacker called one of the most interesting findings presented at that conference.

Since our earlier article, we have heard the following from physicians:

(1) Precautions must be taken to minimize any risk of transmitting different strains of HIV, or any other viruses, to the recipient. Viral cultures may be used to make sure the donor's HIV has been killed by the heat treatment of the plasma.

(2) The plasmapheresis step might be avoided, simply by centrifuging tubes of blood to obtain the plasma, and not returning cells to the donor. Avoiding plasmapheresis, which requires complex equipment, could make the treatment less expensive and easier to administer. (The drawback is that the donor could not donate as often.)

(3) There is concern that red tape could delay the availability of this treatment.

HOW TO OBTAIN MEDICAL ARTICLES

AIDS Treatment News often cites articles in medical journals. How can you get copies of these articles if you do not have access to a medical library?

A number of commercial document-retrieval services can take orders by telephone and copy and mail the articles within a few days, usually for less than $10. They can obtain hard-to-find published articles on any subject.

The service we are using is Dynamic Information Corporation in Redwood City, California (see Appendix B). Prices for most articles are $4.80 plus 20 cents a page plus copyright (usually $1 to $1.50) plus shipping; copies can usually be mailed within two days if the article is available on the library shelf. Articles not found at major university libraries cost somewhat more. Rush service, overnight delivery, fax, etc., are available. Credit card or prepayment is required on orders from individuals.

ANTABUSE/DTC: CONTROLLING GASTROINTESTINAL SIDE EFFECTS

Many people using antabuse (or using DTC, also called imuthiol) as an immune modulator experience cramps and diarrhea the day after taking the medication. Bernard Bihari, M.D. asked a nutritionist about possible diet supplements to control these effects. The method suggested completely controlled the problem in seven of eight persons using antabuse who have tried it so far; the eighth was much improved. (It has also worked for two people who obtained imuthiol from Paris.)

The diet is simply:

(1)   Include a bowl of high-fiber cereal (4 to 5 grams per serving) with breakfast every day; and

(2)   On the days the antabuse or DTC is used, take two tablespoons of olive oil an hour before lunch; then take the medicine with lunch.

The recommended dose of antabuse, which is a prescription drug, is 500 mg twice per week. Precautions are to avoid alcohol, of course, and also to watch out for cough syrups and other liquid medicines, which may contain alcohol. Alcohol-free formulas are available.

SAN FRANCISCO: FREE MEDICAL CARE IN TWO STUDIES: ERYTHROPOIETIN (EPO) FOR ANEMIA; AZT IN EARLY ARC (FOR VETERANS)

Administrators of two clinical trials in San Francisco told *AIDS Treatment News* about their need for volunteers. While both these studies do use placebos, they were designed with more concern for the patients' welfare than most placebo studies in the past. Both monitor blood work, and take patients off the study if they show disease progression, and offer open-label treatment (without placebo) instead.

(1)   Positive Action HealthCare is doing a trial of EPO, a substance which causes the body to produce more red blood cells, and therefore can substitute for transfusion in cases of anemia. All expenses are paid; you do not need to be a patient of Positive

Action. Patients must have anemia (hematocrit under 30), and cannot have taken AZT or certain other drugs during the last 30 days.

The placebo study will run 12 weeks, then all patients will be eligible for EPO for six months. But patients will be monitored monthly, and if they show signs of disease progression, they will receive free outpatient treatment (including EPO if needed). Positive Action has also negotiated to cover free outpatient care for a year for participants, including transfer factor and dextran sulfate as appropriate; however, the clinic cannot cover the cost of AZT.

(2) The second study, AZT for early ARC, is for veterans, and is being conducted at the Veterans Administration Medical Center at 4150 Clement St., San Francisco. Patients must have 200–500 T-helper cells, and be mostly well, but with one ARC symptom. Patients for this study cannot have AIDS, nor presently be taking AZT; certain other antivirals such as ribavirin or isoprinosine are also exclusions. AL 721 is okay.

A placebo is used, but if patients go under 200 T-helper cells they are taken off the study and given open-label AZT.

This trial is being conducted by the Cooperative Studies Project (CSP), the same group that did the study with doctors taking aspirin to see if it prevented heart attacks. This AZT study is identified as CSP #298.

SCIENTISTS: JOBS AVAILABLE IN AIDS RESEARCH

Scientists (Ph.D., M.S., B.S., bench or administrative experience) interested in AIDS work can contact Kalvert Personnel Services, Deer Park, Long Island, New York (see Appendix B). They represent several biotechnology companies looking for persons with expertise in one of the following areas: immunoassay development, or molecular biology, or protein chemistry, or virology, or clinical microbiology. Jobs are on both the East and West coasts. All fees are paid by the employer.

AL 721™—TRADEMARK CONFUSION

Ethigen Corporation of Los Angeles, California called to remind us that the name "AL 721" is their registered trademark, and should not be used to refer generically to egg lecithin products. We had used it that way in recent articles.

In the future we will use "egg lecithin lipids" to refer generically to egg lecithin products (including AL 721) in which the 7:2:1 ratio of NL, PC, and PE is present or intended, and "AL 721" to refer to the Ethigen product.

There is more confusion. Ethigen Corp. will also introduce the same product under a new trademark name, "Altrigen," for over-the-counter sales in the U.S. It will continue to be called "AL 721" in clinical trials, and in Europe, where it is now available by prescription in England, although it cannot be promoted there until trials are complete.

The "Altrigen" name apparently resulted from a compromise with the FDA, which objects to products being sold as food supplements if they are also in clinical trials for approval as a drug. Ethigen will be allowed to sell its remaining stocks which are already labeled as "AL 721." Until recently, Ethigen was unable to speak publicly about this situation, due to its negotiations with the FDA.

You can order AL 721 (which will soon be called Altrigen) from Ethigen by calling them (see Appendix B). You can obtain generic products through buyers' clubs (see list in Appendix C), or from some health-food stores.

Editorial Note: The current situation with egg lecithin lipids is complex, ambiguous, and controversial. There is much speculation (but no compelling proof from scientific human trials) about whether this treatment works at all, or whether any particular version works best.

Our impression from talking with persons using this treatment, plus what little scientific clinical information is available, is that egg lecithin lipids are a significant help to some people. But we have also heard several reports of growing skepticism among physicians and others in New York, where more people are using the lipids than anywhere else. We will provide more information as it becomes available.

AIDS TREATMENT NEWS, PROJECT INFORM RECEIVE BAPHR PUBLIC-SERVICE AWARDS

The Bay Area Physicians for Human Rights (BAPHR), an organization of gay physicians in the San Francisco Bay Area, presented community service awards to organizations, to both *AIDS Treatment News* and Project Inform, at its annual awards meeting on November 18.

Other award recipients included Donald Abrams, M.D., organizer of the County Community Consortium.

AIDS Treatment News thanks BAPHR for this recognition. To us it marks the theme—reinforced by observances of World AIDS Day on December 1—of an end to an era of isolation which began for *AIDS Treatment News* in our early days, when very few AIDS organizations would touch treatment issues. Today there is a growing interest in consensus building, cooperation, and involvement by AIDS organizations in treatment issues.

NIH ANNOUNCES PROGRAM FOR COMMUNITY-BASED TRIALS

On November 22, the National Institute of Allergy and Infectious Diseases, a branch of the National Institutes of Health, announced a new program to involve community physicians in AIDS research. Contracts for this research "are targeted to individual or group providers, public and private clinics, community organizations, or hospitals that may have no prior experience in conducting clinical trials." The program is coordinated by Lawrence Deyton, M.S.P.H., M.D., who will serve as NIAID Assistant

Director for Community Research, advising NIAID Director Anthony S. Fauci, M.D. Dr. Deyton and staff will assist organizations and individuals in preparing contract bids.

Note: On the week of this announcement, NIAID invited representatives from a number of AIDS organizations to Washington to discuss this program. We talked with Martin Delaney of Project Inform, who attended the Washington meeting and thought that the program was beginning well. He was impressed by the openness of NIAID officials to communication with AIDS organizations and physicians. Everyone acknowledged that clinical trials cannot by themselves meet the need for access to health care; this problem must be dealt with directly. And many specific problems remain, for example in the ganciclovir and foscarnet trials for CMV retinitis. But the improvement in communication between NIH and community groups is an important step forward.

Issue Number 71
December 16, 1988

CMV RETINITIS—GANCICLOVIR, FOSCARNET, AND OTHER TREATMENTS: BACKGROUND, HISTORY, AND EMERGING CONTROVERSY

In the last two weeks we heard from two persons with CMV retinitis in immediate danger of going permanently blind because they have fallen between cracks in the red tape surrounding drug development and treatment access. Both had failed using ganciclovir (also called DHPG), one of the two experimental but recognized treatments for CMV retinitis. But because they had used that drug, they are ineligible at this time for trials of the other recognized treatment, foscarnet. They were excluded not because of medical incompatibility, but because the researchers want clean data, unaffected by prior use of a different drug. (A "salvage" trial of foscarnet, for persons who cannot use ganciclovir, will hopefully start by March, 1989.)

For other serious diseases such as cancer, a system called compassionate use has filled such gaps. But for reasons discussed below, a Federal consensus has recently developed that compassionate use of non-approved drugs should not be allowed except as part of scientific studies to determine whether or not the drugs work. While plausible in theory, this policy may cause severe problems in practice, problems which threaten not only the lives and health of patients, but continued progress in scientific drug research as well.

We have heard that the manufacturer of foscarnet is getting five to six calls a day from physicians and patients seeking that drug because for medical reasons they cannot use the only other available treatment, ganciclovir. Because of the recent movement against compassionate use, these patients can seldom get foscarnet, either—but for bureaucratic reasons, not medical. As a result, many of these people are now going blind.

Behind this situation is a bizarre and complex history—and it includes good news as well as bad. This history touches on some of the most central issues in U.S. drug development—not only on what is wrong, but also on steps now being taken to improve the process.

430

Exclusion from treatment for CMV retinitis could become a major, bitter, and confusing dispute. The people affected need to know what their options are. And they may need political support; therefore the larger community must be informed.

CMV Retinitis

CMV retinitis is an infection of the retina of the eye by cytomegalovirus (CMV). The opportunistic infection causes blindness if left untreated. Because damage can occur very rapidly, persons with AIDS should see a physician immediately if they notice blind spots, blurred vision, or loss of peripheral vision. Sometimes there are no symptoms, and the disease is discovered during a routine eye examination.

While it has not yet been documented, experts strongly suspect that the risk is much greater for persons with fewer than 50 T-helper cells. Since 15 to 45 percent of persons with AIDS will eventually develop CMV retinitis (according to a press release from Syntex Corporation, which has the most experience in treating this condition), such persons would probably benefit from a screening for the disease, or from routine eye check-ups from a private physician. Apparently CMV retinitis is becoming a larger problem because persons with AIDS are living longer.

CMV can also affect other organs besides the retina of the eye, such as the intestines or the lungs. It may also be a cofactor causing HIV itself to progress further. One study of autopsy reports found that half of the persons with AIDS who died had active CMV infections unsuspected while they were alive (see *AIDS Treatment News,* Issue Number 65).

The same treatments used for retinitis may also be effective for treating CMV infections elsewhere. A program for distribution of the drug ganciclovir (see below) intends to allow anyone with life-threatening CMV to obtain the drug, even if they do not have retinitis. For more information, call the Ganciclovir Study Center (see Appendix B).

Ganciclovir (DHPG)

During the past three years, over three thousand persons with CMV retinitis have been treated with ganciclovir, which stops the progression of the disease and usually saves the person's remaining eyesight. Unfortunately ganciclovir has side effects, especially bone-marrow toxicity; therefore it usually cannot be combined with AZT, which has similar toxicity. Patients have often had to give up AZT in order to use ganciclovir to save their sight. Also, ganciclovir must be given intravenously.

Ganciclovir has not been approved by the FDA. But its developer, Syntex Corporation of Palo Alto, California, has made the drug available for several years through compassionate use at no charge to the patient, at a cost to the company of over 25 million dollars, mostly in research and development expenses.

Unfortunately the widespread availability of ganciclovir for compassionate use led to a bureaucratic nightmare involving the manufacturer and the FDA. Everybody knew that the drug worked, but the only way to "prove" under the regulations that it did work would involve a trial in which patients were deliberately allowed to go blind, which everyone agreed was unethical. FDA rules insist that a drug must be shown to work through formal scientific trials. But Syntex could not ethically run such a study.

It would be bad enough if a drug could not be approved in spite of the fact that it was known to work. But this situation was even worse. Ganciclovir could not be tested and approved because it was known to work. This knowledge itself meant that complying with the regulations necessary for approval would be universally recognized as unethical.

In an attempt to end this impasse, Syntex presented published articles and reports of thousands of cases to the FDA, asking for an exception in this case because it was so obvious that the drug was effective. But over a year ago, on October 26, 1987, an FDA advisory committee shocked the medical community by recommending against approval (see "DHPG Blindness Drug Threatened," *AIDS Treatment News*, Issue Number 44).

Despite fears that the company might then abandon the drug, it continued to make it available for compassionate use, while working with the FDA and the National Institutes of Health (NIH) on what to do next. But meanwhile, all other compassionate access to AIDS drugs became much more difficult, if not impossible. Companies were determined that what happened to Syntex would not happen to them. It is clear that many deaths have resulted from this side effect of the ganciclovir rejection; but it is difficult to address this fact politically because it would be difficult to prove which ones. Physicians seldom ask for access to a drug if they know they will not get it. So in most cases no record of the rejection, and no audit trail of the public policy behind it, is ever made.

It is clear that the FDA feared that approving the drug without the scientific trials normally required would set a precedent of allowing companies to do an end run around the regular process of drug approval, by means of widespread compassionate use and the resulting political pressure. The FDA was determined that Syntex would not get away with this, would not receive approval without doing a trial. (The thousands of cases recorded under compassionate use did not constitute a formal trial, because these cases occurred as physicians treated patients, not according to a randomized protocol designed in advance by scientists to exclude potential errors such as biases in patient selection, or poor record keeping.) So the impasse remained.

In jurisprudence there is a saying that hard cases make bad law. In the case of ganciclovir, a public-policy stampede against compassionate use was triggered by an unusual situation. Scientifically designed trials are not only the right way to prove drug efficacy, they are usually the cheapest way, too, because uncontrolled use requires far more patients to get convincing information. There should be no need to abolish compassionate use in order to force companies to do proper trials, because they have an economic incentive to proceed that way anyway.

But when ganciclovir was first discovered, Syntex and Burroughs-Wellcome were engaged in litigation over rights to the drug; Syntex eventually won. It appears that the companies were unwilling to invest in trials because they did not know whether or not they would have the rights to the drug.

But Syntex made ganciclovir available by compassionate use, to a few patients at first. Once it was clear that the drug did work, the company was stuck. The FDA refused to accept the drug without scientific clinical trials, and the company was ethically barred from conducting the trials required.

Oral Ganciclovir

Ganciclovir is always given by intravenous infusion, usually requiring daily visits to a medical center. An oral form has been created, however, and a successful but very preliminary human test was published over a year ago (Jacobson *et al.*, "Human Pharmacokinetics and Tolerance of Oral Ganciclovir," *Antimicrobial Agents and Chemotherapy* 31(8), August 1987, pages 1251–1254.) As far as we know, no further testing has been done.

Syntex has applied to the FDA for an IND for permission to test oral ganciclovir. That IND is pending. Syntex will not make public when it first applied, but many months ago we had heard that a proposed trial of oral ganciclovir could not get an IND and therefore would not take place.

An aerosol form of ganciclovir has also been tested, and found effective against CMV lung infection in an experiment in animals. (Debs *et al.*, "Aerosol Administration of Antiviral Agents To Treat Lung Infection Due to Murine Cytomegalovirus," *The Journal of Infectious Diseases* 157(2), February 1988, pages 327–331).

The New Treatment IND and Clinical Trial

Recently a new attempt to resolve the problem was announced by the National Institute of Allergy and Infectious Diseases, a branch of the NIH, the FDA, and Syntex Corporation.

Under the plan, which will replace the compassionate use system in effect until now, everybody who has already been using ganciclovir will be allowed to continue receiving it. New patients will be examined by an ophthalmologist to determine whether the CMV lesions are near the center of the field of vision and therefore immediately sight threatening. Those with immediately sight-threatening disease will be allowed to receive ganciclovir under a system called the "treatment IND," new rules for earlier access to experimental drugs approved in mid-1987 but seldom put into effect since then ("IND" stands for "investigational new drug").

Those with CMV retinitis which is not sight threatening will instead be directed to a controlled clinical trial. No placebo will be used, but patients will be randomly assigned either to receive immediate treatment, or to receive later treatment if there are signs of deterioration (allowing them to remain on AZT longer if appropriate).

Among persons with AIDS and physicians we have heard from, this plan has been greeted with mixed feelings. On the negative side, it reduces treatment options for those with less serious disease. We have also heard medical questioning of specifics of the study design.

The overall plan (the treatment IND combined with the clinical trial) may be a brilliant and partly successful effort to find a medical reason for a study really being done for regulatory-political purposes. The ostensible question is whether it is better to start ganciclovir immediately or wait in cases of non-sight-threatening disease; but what the study is really trying to prove is that Syntex and other manufacturers cannot get away with substituting compassionate use for clinical trials.

Yet despite these negatives, we see the new ganciclovir plan as possibly a watershed advance, moving toward a new compromise and consensus on how to reconcile the scientific requirements of good studies with the needs of patients and their physicians.

(1) In the past, clinical trials usually required eligible patients to stop other treatments and then risk getting a placebo. And persons who did not meet the scientific entry criteria for the study were simply abandoned. By contrast, this plan for ganciclovir serves everyone who needs the drug—and takes patients' needs into account.

(2) In the past, trials of AIDS treatments typically used death, pneumocystis, or other severe deterioration as "endpoints" of the study. Patients have often been subjected to bad medical management—such as being required to stop aerosol pentamidine—in order to make these endpoints more likely for the placebo arm, increasing the power of the trial to tell whether the drug worked better than no drug. But here, the patients not given ganciclovir will receive "very close monitoring for clinical deterioration," according to an FDA press release announcing the new ganciclovir treatment IND and clinical trial—presumably to take them out of the study and give them the drug before serious damage is done.

(3) The ganciclovir plan sheds light on what we believe is a hidden but awesomely important impediment to the overall success of clinical trials, as well as to compassionate treatment access by patients. We call this problem the "mandate for ignorance" which follows from certain ethical requirements on placebo-controlled or other randomized trials, as they are now designed. (See "Drug Trials: A Mandate for Ignorance," below.)

For More Information on Ganciclovir

For information about entering the ganciclovir program, physicians and patients can call the Ganciclovir Study Center (see Appendix B). There is no charge to patients, as costs are paid by Syntex Corporation.

Foscarnet

Foscarnet, often used in Europe as a first choice for treating CMV retinitis because it does not require that the patient stop using AZT, may also have some effectiveness against HIV. Its manufacturer, the Swedish company Astra, had intended to test the drug as an AIDS treatment in the U.S. But according to an editorial in *The Wall Street Journal* (April 21, 1987), Astra left those trials due to frustration with bureaucratic obstacles to AIDS research in the U.S.

Foscarnet, like ganciclovir, must be given intravenously. It does not cause bone-marrow toxicity like ganciclovir. But it can cause kidney toxicity, which may be reduced by giving the patients enough water, sometimes by intravenous infusion.

Published reports of European experience in using foscarnet for CMV retinitis are mixed. It seems clear that the drug does stop the disease during a high-dose "induction" phase of the treatment. But patients are then put on a lower "maintenance" dose, and relapses during this maintenance phase have often been reported. According to information from the National Eye Institute, a branch of NIH, a 70–85 percent rate of favorable response has been reported.

NIH is now running two different studies of foscarnet. One, by the National Eye Institute, was reported in *AIDS Treatment News*, Issue Number 68. This study requires trips to Bethesda, Maryland, near Washington, D.C., but all expenses are paid.

The other NIH study is a multi-centered trial taking place in San Francisco, New York, and Los Angeles. In San Francisco (and probably the other locations also), these studies are recruiting patients now who have not been treated with ganciclovir or foscarnet before. The main advantage of foscarnet over ganciclovir is that patients can continue using AZT; foscarnet is also believed to have some anti-HIV activity.

Both these trials are excluding patients who have previously used ganciclovir. NIH does plan to start a multi-center "salvage" protocol for such patients, hopefully early next year. Meanwhile, for patients who have failed ganciclovir the only access to foscarnet at this time is in Houston, Texas; patients must pay their own travel, lodging, and hospitalization expenses, unless their insurance will cover part of the cost.

One other group of patients may also be left out—those who are using ganciclovir successfully, but should be on foscarnet instead so that they could use AZT. We brought this potential problem to the attention of the group designing the protocol.

For those who fall between the cracks, compassionate use of foscarnet should be available. But the FDA recently led the charge against such access. NIAID is trying to devise plans which can include everyone. When all goes well, these plans may do their job. But when things go wrong and studies are delayed, the current policy against compassionate use makes the patients pay.

It seems clear that foscarnet is not a miracle drug, although it will probably have an important role in treatment. European physicians are using it to treat CMV retinitis, often as first choice over ganciclovir. When nothing else works, U.S. patients and physicians should have the option of using it.

Other Treatment Possibilities

Besides ganciclovir and foscarnet, other possible treatments have been suggested. We have not been able to research these fully by press time.

Acyclovir. This drug may have some effect. NIH plans to study a combination of acyclovir and AZT to treat CMV retinitis.

Anti-CMV Antibodies. Passive immunotherapy using donors with high CMV antibody levels was described as producing conflicting results for CMV disease (Reed, H.C., and Meyers, J.D., "Treatment of Cytomegalovirus Infection, *Clin. Lab. Med.*, USA 7(4), 1987, pages 831–852). But several European articles describe the use of "Cytotect" from Biotest Pharma, a product containing CMV-specific hyperimmune globulin, for prevention or treatment of CMV. The option of using this treatment should be available to U.S. physicians.

(S)-HPMPA or (S)-HPMPC. These new drugs are highly active against CMV in the test tube. We do not know of any human use. For background, see De Clercq *et al.*, "A Novel Selective Broad-spectrum Anti-DNA Virus Agent," *Nature* 323(2) (October 1986), pages 464–469. Or see De Clercq *et al.*, "Antiviral Activity of Phosphonylmethoxyalkyl Derivatives of Purine and Pyrimidines," *Antiviral Research* 8 (1987), pages 261–272.

BHT.   Over two years ago, *AIDS Treatment News* reported interest in BHT as a possible anti-AIDS treatment (Issue Number 10). BHT, used in small amounts as a food preservative, has been an underground herpes treatment used by hundreds of people during the last several years; one clinical trial found some effectiveness in treating herpes in humans. One laboratory report found that BHT was highly effective against CMV in the laboratory (Kim *et al.*, "Inactivation of Cytomegalovirus and Semliki Forest Virus by Butylated Hydroxytoluene," *The Journal of Infectious Diseases* 138(1), July 1978, pages 91–94).

BHT must be used carefully, because large doses are toxic. Even lower doses involve some risk. Letters in medical journals have reported several cases of toxicity, especially gastrointestinal problems, from doses commonly used to treat herpes.

We have not systematically researched BHT since writing the August 1986 article. But recently we talked to a person with AIDS in San Francisco, who has used BHT as his only treatment for CMV retinitis, and is convinced that it did slow although not stop the progression of the disease.

This patient started using BHT in 1986 or early 1987. In January 1988 he stopped temporarily, for about six weeks, following a doctor's advice; during this period without BHT he developed CMV retinitis, which "started galloping;" he saw new blind spots daily. He went back on BHT, using a very large dose for about six weeks, four grams per day dissolved in oil and taken rectally; he reported an instant "high" from the mental effect of this dose. After six weeks, he went back to smaller doses, about two grams per day used orally (still a large dose). In the eight months since, there has been slow deterioration of vision; he can still read, but with difficulty. While this person is convinced that BHT has worked partially for him, and would not dare discontinue it again, he also emphasizes that there is no proof that it has helped.

Toward a Way Out

Recently a top FDA official suggested an idea for reconciling the need for scientific, rigorous studies with the need of patients for access to treatments.

The approach is to have a small, tightly controlled scientific trials with rigorous entry criteria. But in addition, as a condition for approval to conduct a study, the company would also make the drug available on a compassionate basis or "treatment IND" to other patients who needed it—with careful monitoring and reporting, both to enhance patients' safety and also to collect more information about the drug.

What we like about this proposal, which is similar to what is already being started with ganciclovir, is that everyone receives treatment, no one is abandoned. (Placebo studies are now becoming less common, with controlled trials usually comparing one treatment option against another, not against no treatment. It is true that controlled studies reduce the patient's power to choose, since for scientific reasons patients must be assigned at random to the different treatment groups. If there are not enough volunteers, a lottery might be necessary to decide who goes into the controlled trial, and who receives treatment through the compassionate-access, monitoring study.)

This approach will not solve all the problems. But it may allow researchers to conduct tightly controlled studies without sacrificing vital interests of any patients, whether in the study or not. It would certainly improve on the present system, in which treatment is denied in order to force patients into ill-designed trials, with those who don't qualify being abandoned.

DRUG TRIAL SNAFU: THE MANDATE FOR IGNORANCE

We use the term "mandate for ignorance" to refer to a hidden but, we believe, enormously important problem in the effective management of clinical trials.

It is widely agreed that a placebo trial (or any other drug trial in which patients are assigned at random to two or more treatment possibilities) is unethical unless the researchers can state an honest "null hypothesis"—that is, unless they really do not know which of the treatment arms is better. For example, a placebo trial is unethical *if the researchers know that* the drug works better than no treatment. But if they *do not know,* then the study is okay, and they are free to proceed with it.

This ethical standard is obviously intended to safeguard the welfare of patients who become subjects in experimental trials. The idea is that subjects should not have to risk a placebo unless nobody knows whether the drug or placebo is better. But the ganciclovir history shows that this well-meaning ethical standard also has monstrous consequences, because it puts a premium on ignorance.

Why have drug companies become so adamant about refusing compassionate access to AIDS treatments, access commonly available for cancer or other diseases? One reason is to force patients into placebo trials—trials often so poorly designed and poorly publicized that few would enter them voluntarily. But another reason is that drug companies must remain ignorant of how well their own products work, lest that knowledge ethically bar them from conducting the very trials which the FDA requires for approval!

This catch-22 is exactly what happened to Syntex with ganciclovir. And it has terrified other companies into denying compassionate use, and thereby refusing to learn how to use their new drugs effectively except as the result of cumbersome, years-long formal trials.

What should Syntex have done with ganciclovir? Everyone seems to agree that the company should have run placebo trials early—in what is being called "the window of opportunity" to conduct clinical trials—before the public or even the researchers know whether the drug works or not. In other words, the trial must be run before compassionate use—lest the knowledge that the drug does work make it impossible to run the trials. But in practice, trials have usually taken years to set up and conduct. Therefore, compassionate use must be denied for those years.

This mandate for ignorance not only denies compassionate access to patients; it also saps the vitality of the entire clinical-research enterprise. It requires that companies not know that their drug works until after they run formal trials—not before. But companies have little motivation to invest money in trials unless they believe that the drug does work—the same belief that would make those trials unethical. So nothing happens.

One consequence is that drug companies refuse to cooperate when physicians want to test new uses for products in development. Besides other problems such as fear of liability if things go wrong, the company could lose its window of opportunity if things go right.

Therefore the mandate for ignorance not only destroys the commercial incentive to run trials, it also forbids the normal exploratory phase of science—which here would be physicians trying experimental drugs in compassionate, well-supported attempts to treat patients. As a result, clinical trials must be designed in a vacuum—based on whatever theories are fashionable, rather than on exploratory experience of what actually does work in practice. The result is irrelevant, indecisive, and ultimately ineffectual clinical trials, when they happen at all.

In a recent editorial in the *Journal of the American Medical Association*, a former head of the FDA urged a re-examination of "all of the assumptions on which the scientific requirements of the present system (of drug approvals) are based" (November 25, 1988; see also *The New York Times*, Medical Science section, December 6, 1988.) We hope that this mandate for ignorance will be among the issues addressed.

SAN FRANCISCO: CHINESE MEDICINE RESOURCES

In *AIDS Treatment News*, Issue Number 68, we described work at the Quan Yin Acupuncture and Herb Center, and the San Francisco AIDS Alternative Healing Project. Another important San Francisco resource on Chinese medicine is the American Foundation of Traditional Chinese Medicine (AFTCM), a non-profit foundation.

AFTCM founder Barbara Bernie, C.A., has worked with Chinese medicine since 1972. She contributed to the successful effort to pass California legislation which since 1975 has allowed acupuncturists to be licensed and practice openly in the state. She has made many trips to Asia and Europe to meet experts in the field of traditional Chinese medicine.

AIDS Projects

• Herb study with San Francisco General Hospital: AFTCM introduced a highly experienced Chinese physician, Dr. George Zhao, to Donald Abrams, M.D., Assistant Director of the AIDS Division at San Francisco General Hospital, to design a scientific study of Chinese herbal medicine for persons with moderately severe AIDS. Forty patients will be enrolled, 20 using herbs and 20 being controls, with evaluation and crossover at 12 weeks. Unfortunately this study will cost over $200,000 and only $30,000 has been raised so far. If you can help with fundraising, contact Barbara Bernie at the phone number below.

• Qi Gong classes starting in January: Qi Gong is an ancient system of breathing exercises—over one thousand exercises in all. It is the root of tai chi, and of many martial arts. AFTCM will teach classes in medical Qi Gong starting in January; morning and evening sessions will be available. For information, call AFTCM at the number below.

• Other services: AFTCM publishes a newsletter, distributed on a donation basis. It is translating Chinese medical books not previously available in English; two have been translated and published already. It sponsors lectures and other public programs, announced through its mailing list.

AFTCM is bringing together traditional Chinese physicians practicing in the United States with experience in treating AIDS. It plans to offer an AIDS treatment program, and also advanced classes for practitioners, but these are not ready yet.

AFTCM maintains extensive contacts with experts in China, Taiwan, Korea, Japan, and other countries. It hopes to become an international center for medical practitioners, and for persons interested in improving health care around the world.

For more information, contact Barbara Bernie at the American Foundation of Traditional Chinese Medicine (see Appendix B).

NEW YORK: PASSIVE IMMUNOTHERAPY NEEDS DONORS

Nathaniel Pier, M.D., a New York physician who has been interviewed in *AIDS Treatment News,* called to tell us about a study of passive immunotherapy in New York. This important study needs to collect 2,000 liters of plasma—enough to treat 100 persons for a year—and will use the plasma for treatment. Volunteers must be HIV positive, but should be generally healthy. They will be screened by a health questionnaire and by blood tests.

Plasma donors will not be paid, but will have high priority to receive the treatment, if they should later need it. Also, it is widely believed that the process of donating plasma is itself beneficial to some persons with HIV.

If you are a potential donor in the New York area and want to help with this study, call Medicorp (see Appendix B).

TYPHOID SHOTS: PROJECT INFORM URGES CAUTION

The use of typhoid injections as an AIDS treatment is being aggressively promoted in the media. Many physicians are concerned that general immune stimulation might also stimulate the growth of HIV and cause AIDS to progress faster; but many of the typhoid-shot advocates believe that AIDS is really syphilis and HIV doesn't matter.

Most of the information available about the typhoid treatment has come from its advocates. Many people are using or considering using the treatment; they should be able to hear from different perspectives, not only from the advocates.

Recently Project Inform, a San Francisco organization which for several years has provided information about non-approved treatments, wrote to Spin, a music magazine which had carried a highly favorable article about the typhoid-shot treatment. Project Inform's three-page letter included detailed criticisms of the AIDS-is-syphilis theories and of the claims for the typhoid injections.

The letter also noted that Project Inform had heard from many patients treated with typhoid shots, and that most of them had reported negatively, saying that their bloodwork continued to decline.

You can obtain more information from Project Inform (see Appendix B).

A stronger negative comment about typhoid-vaccine shots recommended by researchers who think that syphilis not HIV causes AIDS—"I think (they're) quacks—and don't know the first thing about AIDS"—came from Barry Gingell, M.D., a physician who has AIDS and who edits *Treatment Issues,* an AIDS treatment newsletter distributed without charge by the Gay Men's Health Crisis in New York. Dr. Gingell was quoted in an article published in *7 Days,* November 23, 1988.

We believe that the best way to resolve the issue is to find out how people are doing who started the typhoid injections a year or more ago. There was a flurry of interest at that time, especially on Long Island. A telephone survey could find out how these people are doing—how many are still alive, whether they have continued the treatment, and what they think about it a year after starting. Such a study could determine long-term results quickly, with little expense.

PIGEON HEALTH HAZARD— AND AN EFFECTIVE REPELLENT

Bird droppings, a breeding ground for disease-causing fungi and other organisms, can be a health hazard especially to persons with immune deficiencies. In San Francisco, pigeon droppings have become a growing public concern. Many people do not know that there is a simple, effective repellent to keep pigeons from lighting on window sills, etc.

The Healing Alternatives Foundation in San Francisco had a problem with pigeon droppings, and learned from a contractor about a product called "Bird Tanglefoot," a sticky substance which birds avoid. For the Healing Alternatives building it has been close to 100 percent effective. The product costs a few dollars in hardware stores, and an application should last for about a year. If you cannot find this bird repellent locally, you could call The Tanglefoot Co., in Grand Rapids, Michigan.

WASTING SYNDROME: GOOD RESULTS WITH PRESCRIPTION DRUG

Megace (megestrol acetate), a readily available drug usually used to treat advanced breast cancer in women, showed good results in treating wasting syndrome (cachexia) in every one of 14 persons with HIV (13 of whom had AIDS) reported in an article published last month (Von Roenn *et al.,* "Megestrol Acetate for Treatment of Cachexia Associated with Human Immunodeficiency Virus (HIV) Infection," *Annals of Internal Medicine* (November 15, 1988), pages 840–841). The patients selected for the study were all HIV positive, and had all lost at least 10 percent of their body weight and were losing weight when they began the treatment. All patients gained weight on the treatment, at an average rate of .5 kg per week. All reported improved appetite, and seven also reported a marked improvement in sense of well-being. No side effects were noted. However, four patients have died from recurrent opportunistic infections.

In San Francisco, the County Community Consortium plans to begin a trial of megace in January. Any physician in the San Francisco area can participate in this trial. Physicians can of course also prescribe the drug on their own.

Issue Number 72
January 13, 1989

JANUARY 1989: AIDS TREATMENT STATUS

What do we see happening with AIDS treatments in the coming year?

While no cure is yet in sight, some very promising new treatment possibilities are now in view. Any one of them might lead to major improvement in AIDS therapy this year, even for those seriously ill. While more research is needed to make sure that these treatments do work, the big question in 1989 will be access. Will the research be done? Will treatments get to patients when clearly appropriate, despite formidable bureaucratic, commercial, and political obstacles in the way? Existing institutions will not automatically provide access. Much will depend on grassroots efforts and organizations.

Here are some of the developments and treatments we see as most important in 1989:

Early Treatment.   Some physicians believe that early treatment can reliably halt disease progression, perhaps indefinitely. Others disagree. Because of the slow development of AIDS/HIV disease, it will take time before we know for sure. But systematic, unbiased followup of cases, both successes and failures, could quickly sharpen the available answers and improve decision-making guidance for patients and physicians.

Practical Clinical Trials.   While comprehensive lists are not available, it is clear that much more useful testing of treatments is being done now than a year ago.

Unfortunately, most of the current management of clinical trials still does not reflect a sense of emergency; needless delays of weeks or months, caused by dysfunctional rules, are still easily tolerated. But many more trials, and more important trials, are happening now than a year ago.

And during 1988 the relevant establishment—the medical, political, and media leadership—became far more willing than ever before to acknowledge major shortcomings in drug development management, to openly discuss the issues and consider the possibilities for improvement.

442

New Drugs. Many promising antiviral and other treatments are now in view (see our list in the article below).

While not cures, these treatments might be better than any now available. They could also provide options when existing treatments do not work, as well as new possibilities for combination therapies.

Unfortunately, the treatments themselves and the research needed to make them useful are still usually out of reach. Existing government and corporate structures will not bring them to patients in 1989. But community activism could do so, through community-based research, through political advocacy, and through ongoing nuts and bolts work by self-help organizations.

Community-Based Research. The recognition and momentum achieved by New York's Community Research Initiative (CRI) is now allowing other organizations, such as San Francisco's Community Research Alliance (CRA) to develop much faster than otherwise possible.

Community-based research not only empowers patients and organizes additional trials. It also builds a knowledge base to support expert public advocacy, sometimes for the first time ever, for correcting deficiencies in the medical-research system. (Advocacy-only organizations are also essential, but by themselves they are unlikely to develop as much depth of knowledge about what does and does not work in the research process as groups which routinely work with the FDA or state authorities, pharmaceutical companies, principal investigators, scientific and ethical review boards, etc.)

Other Advocacy and Self-Help Organizations. ACT UP continues to focus attention on lost opportunities to save lives. Some of the groups now have ongoing research arms to investigate behind the scenes and discover the causes of research bottlenecks and access obstacles.

And a new kind of self-help group—exemplified by the passive immunotherapy support group in the San Francisco area, which is doing the organizing necessary to provide access to this treatment option for its members and others—may have long-range importance in providing a serious patient role in all fields of medicine and medical research, for AIDS and other diseases as well.

The New U.S. Administration. At this time, a week before the inauguration of President-elect George Bush, initial signs look good. Transition-team staff members are well-informed. President-elect Bush must know that AIDS will not go away and will be a disaster for his administration unless handled properly.

On the other hand, the new President must focus on economic and foreign problems. The AIDS response will depend on officials whose attitudes are unknown at this time.

Economic Access Issues. Here the prospects look poor, because of the prohibitive cost of medical care and the national budget deficit. AIDS is one disease among others in a nation which is increasingly choosing to control medical costs by simply abandoning those who cannot pay for care they need—not only the poor but also part of the middle class, even some who are well insured.

While the United States does not yet have the political will to seriously address the growing lack of access to care, we believe that some issues can be successfully pursued:

• The AIDS community must resist attempts to pit different disease constituencies against each other. Affordable health care is an issue for everybody.

• All industrialized contries except the United States and South Africa have some form of national health insurance. The AIDS community can build needed contacts with other health groups by contributing to the effort to end the nightmare of unmanageable costs for catastrophic illness, a nightmare which will increasingly affect all but the richest or luckiest Americans, as insurance companies, employers, and government agencies find more sophisticated ways to renege on their clients and the public.

• Localities greatly impacted by AIDS or any other disease—like those impacted by hurricanes or other disasters—need Federal help when the strain on local institutions becomes unmanageable.

• Community-based research organizations can contribute directly to cost containment and access to care by making sure that low-cost treatments are studied. In the United States, the existing research system—including public agencies as well as private companies—only develops the most expensive treatment possibilities. Treatments which may cost a thousand times less, and have unique medical value as well, are usually ignored.

In summary, the elements for major improvements in 1989 are already in place. But no existing institution will bring these benefits to patients automatically. Community activism will determine how much of the existing potential is developed and made available this year.

NEW TREATMENTS TO WATCH, 1989

Here are the potential AIDS therapies that we believe are most likely to become important in 1989.

This particular list only includes treatments for AIDS/HIV itself; therefore it omits other important new developments; for example, better antibiotics for opportunistic infections or treatments for anemia. All the AIDS therapies we selected as most promising turned out to be antivirals—although we did not start out with that criterion.

We included only "new" treatments, meaning ones which were seldom or never available before, but might become accessible for the first time in 1989. Therefore we did not consider existing treatments such as AZT or dextran sulfate.

We based this selection mainly on "quality rumors," choosing those treatments which are generating enthusiasm among medical professionals familiar with them. A few were too new to have rumors; we included them because of the reputations of those involved in their development.

The best source for additional information about most of these treatments is the new *AIDS/HIV Experimental Treatment Directory* (December 1988, Volume 2,

Number 3), published by the American Foundation for AIDS Research. The directory can be obtained from them (see Appendix B for address and phone number).

ddI (dideoxyinosine). ddI is a nucleoside analog (a drug in the same class as AZT), but appears much less toxic.

The first human trial, with 15 early AIDS/ARC patients who have now taken the drug for at least 14 weeks, started last summer at the U.S. National Cancer Institute. Another phase I (dosage and toxicity) trial is taking place at the New York University Medical Center in New York City, and the University of Rochester Medical Center in Rochester, New York; a separate phase I trial is taking place in Boston. No human results have been published, although there are reports of patient improvements.

More importantly from our perspective, we have repeatedly heard rumors that the researchers working with ddI are very enthusiastic about it.

These rumors were indirectly supported by a dispute between top officials of the U.S. National Cancer Institute (NCI) and the FDA. Dr. Samuel Broder, recently appointed head of the NCI, and Dr. Bruce Chabner, director of the cancer treatment division at NCI, strongly criticized the FDA for not allowing NCI to begin tests of ddI in children under two with AIDS, before adult trials were finished. Dr. Broder himself had run the early NCI trial, the first human use of ddI; he must know as much as anyone about how to use the drug. He would hardly have made an issue of the FDA's refusal to allow immediate testing in children if problems had been encountered.

The new AmFAR directory (referenced above) reports that ddI is believed to be ten times less toxic than AZT. "No substantial toxicity or bone marrow suppression have been noted in the NCI study; some patients have complained of mild headaches and lightheadedness. Because ddI is acid unstable, ingestion of an antacid is required prior to oral administration." The phase I clinical trial excludes persons with a history of heart disease or seizure disorder.

ddI appears to be effective in macrophages, and to be able to cross the blood-brain barrier to some extent.

What will happen next? At this writing, the phase I trial in New York City and Rochester has only recruited 9 of 42 subjects. The problem is not lack of interest by patients; New York University at least has a long waiting list. The bottleneck is in the study design. Each dosage level, starting with the lowest, must be tested for several weeks before the next higher dose can be tried (in different patients); this process must continue until the maximum tolerated dose is reached. It is also rumored that limited hospital space has caused delay (each patient is hospitalized for the first two weeks of treatment, as is commonly done in phase I studies). It is possible that Bristol Meyers, which has rights to the drug, will begin a phase II trial without waiting to complete phase I, providing the FDA does not object.

ddI is easy to manufacture. If it is bogged down in red tape and institutional inertia, an underground will be inevitable.

For more information, see the latest AmFAR directory (referenced above) and the information cited there. For the best published report on the dispute between the NIH and the FDA, see the *Chicago Tribune* (January 5, 1989), page 4.

Passive Immunotherapy. This treatment consists of transfusions of plasma from healthy HIV-positive donors, selected to have high levels of effective anti-HIV antibodies, to recipients who lack those antibodies because they have reached a stage in the disease where they can no longer produce them. The plasma infusions, commonly given about once a month, can be dramatically helpful even to some persons with advanced AIDS. Only about 20 people have received this treatment so far, but there is great interest among both professionals and patients.

AIDS Treatment News has already covered passive immunotherapy, so we will not repeat the details here (see *AIDS Treatment News*, Issues Number 67 and 70). You can also call the Passive Immunotherapy Project, a patient support group organized to obtain access to this therapy (see Appendix B for phone number).

At this time the two major concerns about passive immunotherapy are (1) that FDA restrictions may delay access for as long as a year or more, and (2) that some physicians may offer the treatment but not do it properly, endangering their patients. These concerns may seem to be opposites, but in fact they are two sides of the same problem. For the FDA could seriously hamper the organized, professional effort to do passive immunotherapy right—driving this treatment into the separate practices of individual physicians, where the FDA does not have jurisdiction. Excessive restriction could stymie the high-quality, organized efforts, pushing the treatment into settings where there is less quality control.

Antiviral Herbs and Extracts. This category consists of traditional medicinal herbs which have shown antiviral activity in laboratory tests. We listed the following three:

Hypericin. This chemical, found in the St. John's Wort plant, appeared to be an excellent anti-retroviral when tested in animals (against retroviruses other than HIV). It also shows anti-HIV activity in the laboratory. (Since few animals can be infected with HIV, the obvious animal test against HIV infection could not be done.) For background information on hypericin, see *AIDS Treatment News*, Issues Number 63 and 64.

So far we have received only one report of human use for AIDS/HIV, from a physician who has five patients who are using "Hyperforat" (a high-strength, standardized St. John's Wort extract available in Germany), with good to excellent results. It is generally believed that most of the St. John's Wort preparations available in the U.S. in health-food stores are worthless, because they do not contain enough hypericin, the active ingredient. Laboratory testing is now going on to see if any of the U.S. preparations appear likely to be useful.

Compound Q. This experimental treatment (also called GLQ223, and not to be confused with coenzyme Q), is a protein derived from Chinese herbs. It worked very well in stopping HIV in laboratory tests, but no human trials have yet been done. Apparently the drug must be given intravenously, so human experience with the herbs does not prove safety; toxicity tests are now being done in animals. The developer has applied to the FDA for permission to begin human testing.

Compound Q was developed by Genelabs in Redwood City, California, with consultants from the University of California, San Francisco, and the Chinese University of Hong Kong. The project is funded by the Swiss pharmaceutical company Sandoz Ltd., which will have exclusive rights to the product. Genelabs has previously worked with Stanford University in screening chemicals for possible use in AIDS treatment.

For more information about compound Q, see the AmFAR directory (referenced above). Or see the article on new patents in *The New York Times* (January 7, 1989), or U.S. patent number 4,795,739, which was issued to the researchers early this month.

Chinese Anti-Infection Herbs. A screening program conducted by researchers at the Chinese University of Hong Kong and the University of California at Davis tested 27 herbs and found that 11 of them showed anti-HIV activity; five of these almost completely stopped the virus in the test tube. For more information, see *AIDS Treatment News,* Issues Number 61 and 68. We do not have any new results at this time. Anecdotal results seem good.

FLT (fluorodeoxythymidine). In recent Swedish tests, FLT was found several times as effective as AZT both against HIV in laboratory cultures, and against SIV, a related retrovirus, in monkeys. The drug has previously been tried in humans, as it was tested and rejected as a cancer therapy 20 years ago in East Germany.

The recent Swedish results were announced by Professor Bo Oberg, a virologist at Sweden's Karolinska Institute. FLT is being developed by the Medivir research company, which wants to sell the patent rights to a large pharmaceutical company, probably one in the United States. Dr. Oberg previously headed an AIDS research team at Astra, the Swedish pharmaceutical company which also developed foscarnet, an anti-HIV treatment now also being used for CMV retinitis. The team screened almost 2,000 chemicals for anti-HIV activity.

FLT causes bone-marrow suppression like AZT, but it appears to have much less toxicity at an effective dose.

Dr. Oberg was quoted as saying that two years of laboratory and human testing would be required before the drug could be marketed. We suspect that this time-frame reflects the fact that FLT will probably be developed in the United States (Sweden does not have enough AIDS/HIV patients to run trials). In the past, Astra has had major problems trying to conduct AIDS research in the U.S.; see *The Wall Street Journal* editorial of April 21, 1987 concerning Astra's frustration and withdrawal from U.S. trials of foscarnet two years ago.

Many people would be willing to take the risk of trying FLT now, with doses based on what worked in monkeys and on human toxicity data from the earlier cancer studies. We could know in weeks or months whether or not this drug could make a substantial contribution to AIDS treatment. Red tape alone—or rather the empires and vested interests which benefit from it— will extend that time to years, unless the public insists that AIDS be treated as an emergency instead of business as usual.

Azidouridine (AzdU). Formerly called CS-87, azidouridine showed no toxicity when given orally to animals in high doses. In laboratory tests, it is effective against HIV in macrophages as well as in blood cells. The first human trial is planned for early 1989. For more information, see the AmFAR directory.

D4T. Animal and laboratory studies have found this nucleoside analog considerably less toxic than AZT, and about as effective in stopping HIV. Human trials are planned for early 1989. For more information, see the AmFAR directory.

CD4. Despite the publicity about CD4, we put it last in this list of best treatments because so far we have not heard much enthusiasm from those with direct experience with the drug. However, the current trials were not designed to test for efficacy, and they started with very small doses. CD4 may prove effective in further testing.

ABOUT *AIDS TREATMENT NEWS:* PAST, PRESENT, AND FUTURE

(Editor's Note: This article, which appeared originally in Issue Number 72, may be found in the front of this book, as the "Preface.")

IN MEMORIAM: JOHN SCAFUTI, 1949–1989

John Scafuti, who died of AIDS-related lymphoma, was well known in Florida as a pioneering PWA who fought hard to make new treatments available to the community. He worked to make aerosol pentamidine and chemotherapy for KS available to any Orange County, Florida resident, free of charge to those who cannot afford it. John's life inspired countless friends to carry on the fight to survive.

Issue Number 73
January 27, 1989

HYPERICIN/ST. JOHN'S WORT: CALL FOR INFORMATION

Several different research groups are developing protocols for clinical trials of hypericin, which is found in the St. John's Wort plant, as an antiretroviral. Any information about human experience with St. John's Wort extracts, by persons with AIDS or HIV, would help these efforts.

AIDS Treatment News is collecting information about hypericin in order to publish an update, perhaps as early as the next issue. We want to find out what preparations have been used, what doses were used and for how long, and what effects, either good or bad, might have been due to the herb. We also want to hear how people feel about their overall health and well being since starting the treatment, and also about any changes in blood work. We want to know about diagnoses and severity of the disease, and about other treatments being used simultaneously. Consistent with confidentiality, we will share all information with anyone who is developing a clinical trial, as well as publishing our update.

For background information on hypericin, see *AIDS Treatment News*, Issue Number 63. If you have any experience with St. John's Wort or know anyone who does, please call us here at *AIDS Treatment News*.

NUTRITION AND AIDS:
NEW TASK FORCE RECOMMENDATIONS

A task force of top AIDS physicians and dietitians has published recommendations for patients and for physicians on nutritional support for persons with AIDS or any HIV infection. Anyone can obtain free copies of a brochure for patients, and an article written for physicians; the article was also published in *Nutrition* (Volume 5,

449

Number 1, January/February 1989). Organizations can obtain bulk copies by writing to the Task Force on Nutrition Support in AIDS (see Appendix B).

The brochure includes specific recommendations for dealing with mouth pain or sores (which may make eating difficult, resulting in malnutrition), difficulty swallowing, diarrhea, anorexia (loss of appetite), and nausea or vomiting. It also discusses nutritional supplements, and the use of various forms of tube feeding if they become necessary. It includes basic precautions for avoiding bacterial infection from raw foods.

The physician's article gives much more detailed recommendations for optimizing the nutritional status of patients at any stage of illness. For example, it points out that some apparently "neurological" complications are actually caused by malnutrition and are reversible.

The recommendations focus on maintaining adequate intake and absorption of proteins, calories, and all other required nutrients. They do not cover the use of high doses of particular food components as possible therapies to treat specific conditions.

The task force also commissioned its own survey, which found that "although more than 90 percent of caregivers at the major AIDS treatment centers in the United States consider nutrition important, fewer than 20 percent of the institutions have a standard nutrition protocol for people with AIDS."

The eleven-member task force which prepared the recommendations includes Donald Kotler, M.D., gastroenterologist at St. Luke's-Roosevelt Hospital Center in New York and a leading expert on gastrointestinal complications of AIDS; Donald Armstrong, M.D., chief of infectious diseases at Memorial Sloan-Kettering Cancer Center, New York, principal investigator of the National Institutes of Health (NIH) AIDS Clinical Treatment Unit there, and member of the Scientific Advisory Committee of the Community Research Initiative; and Ranuit K. Chandra, M.D., of the Memorial University of Newfoundland, an authority on nutrition and the immune system. It was chaired by Myron Winick, M.D., professor of pediatrics and nutrition at Columbia University. The effort was funded by a grant from Norwich Eaton Pharmaceuticals.

KAPOSI'S SARCOMA:
A WIDE TREATMENT SPECTRUM EMERGING
by Denny Smith

Kaposi's sarcoma occurs in about 35 percent of all AIDS patients. The lesions of Kaposi's usually appear on the skin and must be biopsied to confirm a diagnosis. Recently, the frequency of new KS cases has decreased. More new treatments have become available, and older standard therapies for pre-epidemic KS have been adapted to deal with certain problems of AIDS-related KS.

The treatments reviewed here are fresh applications of conventional therapy. No single agent, new or newly-adapted, has yet worked conclusively. But there are combinations which appear effective in specific stages of lesion growth. Several important factors help determine when and how to proceed against KS: the location of individual lesions, their rate of progression, the advantages of treatments weighed against their drawbacks, and the compatibility of a KS treatment choice with HIV drugs or treatments which one may require for another opportunistic infection.

Where do the lesions appear? They may be localized, especially around the face or lower legs, or widely dispersed, and may involve internal organs. Treatment is definitely warranted if the lesions cause functional impairment, as with awallowing difficulties due to oral lesions, or pain from walking on a foot swollen from lymphatic involvement. Some lesions are treated for cosmetic reasons. For either cosmetic or functional improvement, small cutaneous (skin) lesions can be directly injected with a dilution of vinblastine (Velban), a chemotherapeutic agent. Administered weekly or biweekly for several treatments, these intralesional injections may cause temporary inflammation but can stop or even reverse the growth of some lesions.

Lesions which are coalescent (merging together), or are too large for injection, or located in areas which are difficult to inject such as the eyelids or the bottom of the feet, should be treated with local radiation. We spoke with Dennis Hill, M.D., of Davies Medical Center in San Francisco regarding his application of radiotherapy for treatment of KS. He has used radiation effectively with careful dose volume and frequency for localized treatment of cutaneous lesions, and for edema, or swelling, due to internal obstruction of the lymphatics. He cautions that large volume radiation which may aggravate the underlying immune deficiency is not justified. In addition, too much irradiation of oral lesions can cause a serious inflammatory reaction in mucous tissue. But applied carefully, radiotherapy can obtain good palliative results (relief of symptoms) in many situations. Dr. Hill published his approach in *Seminars in Oncology* (Volume 14, Number 2, 1987). Reprints of the article can be requested from the Department of Radiation Oncology, Davies Medical Center, Castro and Duboce Streets, San Francisco, California 94114.

How aggressive are the lesions? If there are very few lesions and they appear stable, they may not warrant the risk of various unwanted treatment side effects. But if new lesions appear to be progressing rapidly in size or number, they should be treated before they become a functional or cosmetic problem. To inhibit rapid progression, or to deal with slower lesions for which Velban injections or radiotherapy are not useful, a systemic approach with chemotherapy might be considered.

The most commonly used agents against AIDS-related KS are vincristine, vinblastine, etoposide, doxorubicin (Adriamycin), and bleomycin. There is evidence and general agreement that a combination of some of these drugs is more successful than any one used singly, but there is no consensus for which combination, dosage or frequency. The best combination would obtain an effective cytotoxic strength (able to kill KS cells) without corresponding damage to healthy tissue. For example, in addition to their anti-KS activity, vinblastine, etoposide, and doxorubicin can each suppress bone marrow production (myelosuppression), etoposide and doxorubicin are associated with alopecia (hair loss), and vincristine can cause neuropathy. One solution is to alternate the administration of different agents to avoid cumulative toxicity while maintaining anti-tumor effect. Another approach is to balance the dose and frequency such that multiple agents can be used simultaneously.

We interviewed Ivan Silverberg, M.D., also of Davies Medical Center in San Francisco. Dr. Silverberg has obtained good responses with a combination of 1 mg vincristine, 3 mg vinblastine, and 5 units bleomycin, given intravenously once a week. The side effects may include a fever after the infusion, and some minimal hair loss. He has not seen any serious toxicity with this ratio. One friend of ours adapted this combination to one-half mg of vincristine and 2 mg of vinblastine with 5 units bleomycin and after three months decreased the injections to once every two weeks. He felt that his lesions were completely stabilized.

In recent months, two different AIDS newsletters published their own thorough coverage of KS treatment options with a large focus on chemotherapy. Allen Maniker, M.D., wrote for the October 20th, 1988 *Treatment Issues* (published by the Gay Men's Health Crisis; see Appendix B for address). And Lawrence Kaplan, M.D., was the author of an article in the January 1989 *AIDS Medical Report* (published by American Health Consultants; see Appendix B for phone number). Both articles provide a detailed background for people making treatment choices for KS.

How can these choices be integrated into a workable program of AIDS treatments? With any HIV-related illness, the root of the problem is an immune deficiency, so treatment choices must aim carefully to avoid further damage to the immune system. The optimum treatment program would include anti-HIV treatments and possibly an immunomodulator if blood counts call for them and if they are chosen for compatibility with the appropriate KS therapy. Sometimes there is a conflict of treatment strategy between an HIV drug such as AZT and an anti-KS agent like doxorubicin, because they both suppress bone marrow production. But AZT can be administered safely with radiotherapy or non-myelosuppressive drugs such as vincristine.

We have heard reports of people with Kaposi's sarcoma being refused treatment on the assumption that it progresses too slowly to be of concern, or that there are no effective treatments anyway. But many physicians and patients have successfully stabilized lesion growth with flexible combinations of intralesional injections, radiation or chemotherapy. In a future article we will compare new and investigational KS treatments, including interferon, laser therapy, and the prosorba column.

MONTREAL AIDS CONFERENCE—PWA PARTICIPATION

Last week we spoke with Don DeGagne, who is representing persons with AIDS on the program committee of the V International Conference on AIDS—the major scientific conference of 1989, to be held in Montreal, Quebec, in June. After extensive criticism of lack of PWA participation at the previous international AIDS conference in Stockholm, the Canadian AIDS Society and PWA groups lobbied for representatives of community-based groups and PWAs to be involved at Montreal. The organizers of the conference have responded:

• "AIDS, Society, and Behavior," one of the nine modules of the conference, is expected to have persons with AIDS in all of the 20 themes within that module;

• PWAs will be part of the opening ceremony, at least one plenary session, and many panels, discussion groups, and forums. For example, Mr. DeGagne himself is putting together a workshop, "Living with AIDS," in which persons with AIDS from five different regions of the world will talk about their experiences. There will also be a workshop on how to organize coalitions, a concept unfamiliar in some parts of the world.

We asked about PWA involvement in the San Francisco Conference next year. Mr. DeGagne "would strongly urge the organizers of the VI International Conference on AIDS, which will be held in San Francisco at the end of June in 1990, to follow the path of the Montreal Conference by including persons with AIDS in all aspects of the event itself, as well as its planning stages. Collaboration between the groups, consumers as well as doctors and researchers, is a primordial thing. PWAs should be involved from the beginning—for San Francisco, that means now—or it will be hard to catch up later."

SURVIVING AND THRIVING WITH AIDS, VOLUME TWO—COLLECTED WISDOM

People With AIDS Coalition in New York has published volume two of *Surviving and Thriving with AIDS*, edited by Michael Callen—a 368-page book written by persons with AIDS. (The first volume, subtitled "Hints for the Newly Diagnosed," is being reprinted; 20,000 copies have been distributed.) The volume is subtitled "Collected Wisdom."

"The two books are meant to be read together, and in order," according to Michael Callen. "*Hints* is still essential reading for the newly diagnosed. *Collected Wisdom* expands upon the information and ideas contained in *Hints*. It's an anthology of our attempts to cope with AIDS. It's a slice of life which captures what it is like to live with AIDS in America in the late 1980s.

Volume two contains a large section on treatment options, including AZT, aerosol pentamidine, DHPG, TPN, AL 721, and holistic approaches. These treatments are described first hand by people who have used them. The personal accounts include practical perspectives on the decision to use or not use certain treatments. They also give practical hints discovered from personal experience, such as treating thrush and leukoplakia by opening an acyclovir capsule and spreading the contents on one's tongue before going to bed.

Other sections include emotional responses to diagnosis, long-term survivors, love and sex and AIDS, family and friends, women and AIDS, people of color and AIDS, AIDS in prison, political responses, dealing with disability, social security and Medicaide, resource lists, and an index. Throughout the book the first-hand accounts, and pictures, tell much of the history of the development of the PWA advocacy and treatment movements.

Both volumes are offered free to persons with AIDS or ARC; prices for the general public are $10 for volume one and $20 for volume two. We urge those who can afford to contribute more to do so. To obtain either or both volumes of *Surviving and Thriving with AIDS*, send a check to the PWA Coalition in New York (see Appendix B).

SAN FRANCISCO: LENTINAN STUDY RECRUITING

Persons who are HIV positive, have T-cell counts between 200 and 500, and are not using other antiviral or immune modulator treatments, are needed for a three-month study of lentinan at the AIDS Clinic at San Francisco General Hospital. To be eligible, volunteers can be either asymptomatic or mildly to moderately ill, but cannot have AIDS.

Lentinan, an extract of the shiitake mushroom which is given intravenously in 10-minute infusions once per week, has been used in Japan to treat thousands of cancer patients, with very little toxicity. It has immune potentiating effects, and may also be antiviral against HIV. The San Francisco study will look for both effects by blood tests. (For earlier background on lentinan, see *AIDS Treatment News*, Issue Number 19.)

Persons entering the trial will be randomly assigned to one of four groups: 2 mg per week, 5 mg, 10 mg, or placebo. There is one chance in four of getting placebo. However, the placebo is given for only eight weeks (followed by four weeks off treatment, to see what happens when the lentinan is stopped); and the study will be ended early if any dose is found to be clearly effective. And if the lentinan proves effective, all volunteers who complete the study will probably have access to it "open label" (without placebo) without charge; however, this access is not guaranteed.

Aerosol pentamidine and some other treatments are okay during the trial. AZT is probably not.

The study is being conducted by Donald Abrams, M.D., Eric Goosby, M.D., and Roberta Wong, Pharm. D. Financing is from Ajinomoto Co., Inc., Yokohama, Japan, through Lenti-Chemico Pharmaceutical Laboratory, Inc., Teaneck, New Jersey.

Forty patients are being recruited (10 for each arm of the study).

Comment

This study is important for the community. Lentinan might be an effective therapy for delaying or preventing the development of AIDS in persons at early stages of illness. A trial should have been done four years ago, but there was no money then for a U.S. trial, and there were not enough patients in Japan.

Dr. Abrams originally designed the San Francisco study without a placebo. The FDA asked that the placebo arm be added, because if the drug does seem to work it will never again be possible to test it against a placebo, and researchers will be less confident that improvement seen in trials is really due to the drug.

We believe that the placebo is justified in this case. The randomized treatment lasts only eight weeks; the trial is designed to look for blood changes, not serious illness or death. Ten people (not hundreds) will get the placebo. And if the study shows that the drug does work, it will have more credibility and more quickly become available to thousands of people.

This study design is workable and can answer important questions about the drug. We hope that people will volunteer in order to help the AIDS community, despite the personal sacrifice of giving up other treatments temporarily.

AIDS TREATMENT RESEARCH DELAYS: MAJOR INVESTIGATIVE REPORT

A four-part series on delays in AIDS treatment development is appearing Monday, January 30 through Thursday, February 2 (1989) in the *San Francisco Chronicle*. We have seen only the first part by press time, but already this series looks like the most comprehensive report of AIDS drug delays ever published in a major newspaper. Experts and officials who have long been afraid to tell the public what is wrong in AIDS research have spoken more openly in this series than ever before.

The reporter, *Chronicle* correspondent Randy Shilts, also wrote *And the Band Played On,* a history of earlier Federal mismanagement of AIDS prevention, education, and research.

To obtain the *San Francisco Chronicle* articles, you can contact a document delivery service, such as Dynamic Information in Redwood City, California (see Appendix B).

SAN FRANCISCO: COMMUNITY RESEARCH ALLIANCE SEEKS MEDICAL DIRECTOR

The Community Research Alliance (see "Community Research Alliance: New San Francisco Effort for Community-Based Trials," in *AIDS Treatment News,* Issue Number 70) is hiring a medical director, seeking a physician with experience in clinical research and with AIDS. This person will evaluate ideas for clinical trials, help physicians or others write formal protocols for submission to the organization's Scientific Advisory Committee, supervise data management and quality control of research, assist principal investigators with analysis of results, and coordinate with physicians, community groups, pharmaceutical companies, hospitals, clinics, and research organizations.

The position is half time for now and may become full time later. It pays competitive salary commensurate with clinical and research experience.

Issue Number 74
February 24, 1989

HYPERICIN/ST. JOHN'S WORT: EXPERIENCE SO FAR

Issue Number 63 of *AIDS Treatment News* published a report on hypericin, a chemical found in St. John's wort *(Hypericum perforatum)* and related plant species—plants which are common around the world and have long been used as medicinal herbs. A team of researchers at New York University found that hypericin worked as an antiretroviral in animals, in tests with two retroviruses which affect mice; it also inactivated HIV in laboratory tests, and prevented infection of new cells. Hypericin is believed to cross the blood-brain barrier (Meruelo *et al.*, 1988).

Extracts of St. John's wort with chemically standardized hypericin content have been sold over the counter for several years as an antidepressant in Germany, Australia, and Switzerland.

But at the time of our earlier report, there was no information on human use of the herbal extracts for treating AIDS or HIV. This article reports the human experience so far.

A note of caution: The information presented here shows hypericin as a promising treatment possibility. However, this information rests only on reports from eleven persons, all we could find who have used concentrated St. John's wort extracts for treating AIDS or HIV. They have used the treatment only for three months, sometimes less. Many treatments have looked good at first, and later turn out to be useless or harmful.

We were concerned about publishing this article too early, but decided it was better to go ahead than to wait. It is unclear what we would be waiting for. Clinical trials of chemically synthesized hypericin are being planned, but may take a year to even start. Since herbal extracts already available *might* contribute to AIDS treatment, it is urgent that they be given more attention.

Hypericin may be important as a treatment possibility for those who have no other option—who cannot use standard treatments and do not have access to experimental ones. They might want to discuss hypericin with their health care providers, and consider using it with medical monitoring to minimize any risk.

456

But those who have other options and can afford to wait should consider doing so. In a few weeks or months, much more will be known about hypericin, whether it is safe and effective, and how best to use it.

Results with AIDS/HIV

To research this article, we tried to find every case we could locate of anyone who had used any form of St. John's wort or hypericin for AIDS or HIV infection. We interviewed either the persons themselves or their physicians.

We found 19 people overall. The cases divided themselves into two groups. Eleven had used concentrated extracts of St. John's wort, with known concentrations of hypericin; several of them had used the same preparation and same dose, for the same length of time. The other eight had only used herbal teas, or miscellaneous or unknown preparations; in all these cases, the amount of hypericin taken could not be determined. (No one used chemically purified or synthesized hypericin, probably because it was not available.)

Using Known Hypericin Preparations

This is the information collected so far about human use of St. John's wort extracts containing known, significant concentrations of hypericin.

Of the eleven who used known concentrations of hypericin, nine reported successful, often dramatic results. The only failure was a patient near death, who was given the treatment as a desperation measure; it was too late and he died within several days. (One other patient was asymptomatic and had no after-treatment blood work, so there was no indicator of whether the treatment had been helpful or not.)

None of these persons reported any adverse effects from the treatment—except for one who experienced drowsiness when taking very large doses. All ten patients are still using it.

Four of them are patients of one physician, David Payne, D.O., an osteopathic physician in Mesa, Arizona.

Dr. Payne's patients used a standardized German tincture, "Hyperforat" (see "Available Extracts Containing Hypericin," below), which is sold over the counter in Germany for use as an antidepressant. They are taking 40 drops three times a day—120 drops per day total. (The recommended antidepressant dose is 20 to 30 drops three times a day; Dr. Payne increased this amount after discussion with the New York University researchers who had conducted antiviral tests in animals.)

We interviewed Dr. Payne about his experience with hypericin in treating these patients. The following is from the transcript of our phone interview of February 9, 1989:

Dr. Payne: "The clinical experience I've had so far has been very, very good. Every one of the people benefitted—except as I said, one patient who only started the treatment for a few days before he died; he was too far gone to help. But I have had other people who were almost that sick make dramatic recoveries. I called all the patients yesterday, to see how they were doing and make sure there were no side effects. None of them report any side effects from the medication. They say it is very easy to take, causes no distress, no problems. And since starting the therapy around mid-November, they all reported major improvements in symptoms: increase in energy, and so forth."

(Dr. Payne noted that all of these patients had a T-4 (T-helper) count less than 10 when they started, and there have been no major increases. But with counts starting that low, any increase would take time.)

ATN: That's understandable. But what about P24 levels?

Dr. Payne: "We haven't received the P24 back except for one patient. His P24 went from 47 picograms down to 7 (positive to negative)."

ATN: That's good. How much time was there between the tests?

Dr. Payne: "About six weeks."

ATN: (We asked about the individual patients.)

Dr. Payne: "The four patients are Andy, Dan, Chris, and John (the names have been changed). Every one of them is doing very well. Every one of them reports increases in energy. None of them has any symptoms right now. One, Andy, the last T-4 cell count we did on him was nine. He has nine T-4 cells in a white count of one thousand. But he has absolutely no symptoms. He has gone skiing, he is doing everything. So symptomatically, it seems to work very quickly. Their symptoms improve within a matter of weeks. The (T-cell) numbers, however, do not seem to improve as rapidly. Their symptoms, in almost every case, within two weeks had improved."

(Just before we went to press, Dr. Payne reported that Andy's white count is now 2300. It had not been above 1100 for six months.)

"Dan, for instance, was bedfast. He was getting almost all of his nutrition through a catheter. He had to be wheeled into my office in a wheelchair; he was very sick, could not keep anything in his stomach. He was wasting away, fatigued, had no strength or energy in his legs at all. He had mild peripheral neuropathy, not bad. I started him on the hypericin. Two weeks later, he came with his wife, but he walked into the office without any help. He was down to only thirty percent of his nutrition administered through the catheter.

"And two weeks after that, his wife was working, so he drove himself down (a two and a half hour trip), hopped into the office looking like a perfectly normal human being, like there was nothing ever wrong with him, which is astounding. He said he'd been hiking a little bit. He was eating a full diet. His nausea and vomiting had gone away. His energy level was coming up.

"When I saw him a month after that, he was fine, perfectly fine. He had energy, he was happy. He looked like he'd never had anything wrong with him. Really strange. As sick as he was, I thought eight weeks to change from that bad, being bedfast and wheeled in in a wheelchair, to driving himself and walking into the office by himself feeling good—that was dramatic. And I don't know if it is coincidental, but he was not using much else. He could not tolerate AZT, he could not tolerate dextran sulfate. Hypericin is about all he was doing.

"And John had pneumocystis when we started him on the hypericin. So he was not feeling good at the time; we started him on it anyway. We treated him for pneumocystis and continued him on the hypericin. I talked to him yesterday to get an update on it, and he said that he had a little bit of a cold now, but that was it. He said before he got his cold, he had just been in San Diego, and had tons of energy, and was walking all around San Diego. John had also been very sick. He had had pneumocystis over and over again. He was very weak, losing weight. He's gained eight pounds recently.

"Those are the kinds of stories. What is doing it I'm not sure. But I have to attribute some of the improvement to the hypericin. That is the only thing different they are using."

The rest of the interview concerned technical matters such as the possibility of testing for blood levels of hypericin.

Of the other six persons known to *AIDS Treatment News* who used known extracts of hypericin for HIV:

• One had less than ten T-helper cells, and severe diarrhea for several months; the diarrhea could not be diagnosed or controlled. Two days after starting the hypericin (Psychotonin M tincture), the diarrhea stopped. Later, as a test, the patient stopped taking the hypericin, and the diarrhea returned. We do not have other details of this case.

• Another person used very large doses of St. John's wort tinctures (first Psychotonin M, then Jarrow Formulas), several times the recommended dose, in order to test for side effects before suggesting the treatment to friends. He had had severe hairy leukoplakia for a year; it went away completely with the treatment, but later it returned, despite continuing use of hypericin.

Drowsiness was his only consistent side effect. This patient was also using Ativan, which may have contributed to the drowsiness.

• One person used low doses of two different extracts available in the U.S., for two and a half weeks. He reported that swelling in lymph glands was completely gone, after he had had the problem for a year. Also, HIV-related arthritis symptoms in his feet were greatly relieved. (He had used 40 drops per day of a tincture—Jarrow Formulas—for one week, followed by one tablet per day of standardized St. John's wort extract—Yerba Prima Botanicals—for 10 days. For more information on these preparations, see "Available Extracts Containing Hypericin," below.) This person was also taking dextran sulfate (which he had been using for ten months) and a German treatment called "adaptogen," but the improvements mentioned above occurred after he started using the St. John's wort extracts.

This person also reported one side effect of the hypericin—an increase in sun sensitivity, resulting in a mild but unexpected sunburn after being in the sun for about half an hour.

• That person's lover, who has AIDS, took the same preparations and reported significant reduction in peripheral neuropathy (numbness in feet). He also commented that the St. John's wort was the easiest AIDS treatment he had ever taken. He often had stomach problems, but had none whatever resulting from the St. John's wort. The only other HIV treatment he was using was adaptogen.

The following two reports give little information, but we included them for completeness:

• One person took a small amount of a tincture (Jarrow Formulas), together with St. John's wort herbal tea. He was using several other treatments at the same time: acyclovir, ciprofloxicin, isoprinosine, and aloe vera juice (de Veras beverage). He reported increased energy, and also clearing of mucus, making it easier to breathe. He also has KS, and reported that the treatment did not seem to help.

• The final report is from a person who is asymptomatic but who recently became P24 antigen positive. He has been using St. John's wort tinctures for three weeks, and has not yet been retested for P24 antigen. There have been no side effects. But because the patient has no symptoms, and has not yet had blood work after the treatment began, there is no way to tell if there has been any benefit.

No other side effects were reported by any of these patients—only the drowsiness and the increased sensitivity to sunlight, each mentioned by one person as noted above.

Comment

These reports, obtained from informal interviews, omit many details. We did not try to take medical histories; instead we asked people to tell us what seemed important to them. Taken together, we find the reports striking for three reasons:

Consistency.   Except for the patient near death who was given hypericin as a desperation measure, in almost every case there was major, unexpected improvement in symptoms, leading at least to improved quality of life. These people are in different parts of the country, often with different physicians, generally not knowing each other, and using different hypericin products from unrelated manufacturers.

Working for patients who are seriously ill.   Most treatments work best for those who are healthy to begin with. But here, patients benefitted greatly despite being seriously ill to start (needing a wheelchair and tube feeding, pneumocystis again and again, T-helper counts less than 10, etc.).

Speed of improvement.   Clear improvements in symptoms were usually seen within two to three weeks.

In blood work, no significant improvement in T-cells was found in about three months—the longest time anyone has used the treatment so far. Only one person's P24 antigen result is available, and it went from positive to negative (47 to 7 picograms) during the treatment—a good sign, but little can be concluded from a single case.

Using Unknown Hypericin Preparations

The rest of our information on human use of St. John's wort extracts concerns those who only used herbal teas (or, in one case, a homemade extract in brandy, and in another a medicine in France with no labeling for hypericin content and which we could not obtain for analysis). In these cases there was no way to estimate the amount of hypericin taken.

Among the eight persons who used only these preparations, there were no reports of benefits as dramatic as those above. Most believed or suspected it was helping. Most of these people were healthy to begin with, and did not have any before-and-after blood work—meaning that usually there was no indicator to show whether the treatment was helping or not.

Until recently, it was difficult to obtain any St. John's wort extract with a known hypericin concentration in the United States. Most of the patients discussed above obtained theirs by having somebody bring it from Germany; the other two started the treatment in February 1989, when it was possible to obtain apparently comparable preparations in the U.S. But dried hypericin herb (which can differ greatly in quality from one batch to another), as well as a number of tincture and oil extracts, have long been sold in the U.S. in health-food stores. Some of them have only tiny amounts of hypericin—ten times as little as some of the German preparations, or even less. (Some European preparations have very little hypericin, too.)

The eight cases of persons using herbal teas or unknown preparations include two or three treatment failures. In one case the treatment was discontinued because of a drug reaction, a severe rash probably caused by use of St. John's wort; we do not know what kind of preparation was used (herbal tea, tincture, etc.). The rash started about two weeks after the treatment was begun, and went away a week after it was discontinued.

In another case, a person prepared a homemade extract by gathering St. John's wort from nearby fields, and soaking it in brandy. There were no side effects, but after several months of using the preparation, his helper T-cell count had declined from about 400 to 252. He decided that the treatment was unsuccessful, and discontinued it.

In the third case, an older patient developed kidney problems a week and a half after starting using St. John's wort tea; his first symptom was severe swelling in the legs. His infectious disease physician doubted that the herb had anything to do with the problem, because he had seen similar cases where no herb had been used. The patient stopped all medicines he was taking, was treated by kidney specialists, and has largely recovered.

The apparent lack of benefit from herbal teas or other unknown preparations may have resulted from low levels of hypericin in the treatment. On the other hand, they may have resulted from self-selection of *healthier* patients in the herbal-tea group—healthy enough that they had no symptoms to serve as indicators of improvement. Those motivated enough to obtain an extract from Germany were those who had symptoms in which improvement could be seen.

Still, the great difference in the results between those who used concentrated, standardized extracts and those who used the herbal teas suggests that at least until more is known, it would be better to stay with extracts which are standardized for hypericin content, or else have been chemically tested and found to contain significant amounts of the chemical.

Available Extracts Containing Hypericin

Editor's Note: Please see page 475 of Issue Number 75, article entitled "Hypericin: New Dosage Information" for an explanation of corrected information about the dosage. The amounts cited below have been revised accordingly as well.

So far there is more clinical experience for HIV with the Hyperforat product (the one used by Dr. Payne) than with any other; ideally, therefore, that would be the kind to use. Hyperforat has a chemically standardized hypericin content, so every batch of the preparation should be equivalent. But at this time there is no organized way to obtain the tincture from Germany.

To test alternatives which are more readily available, *AIDS Treatment News* bought several U.S. preparations and sent them to a chemist for analysis of the hypericin content. Three may be roughly comparable to Hyperforat; two others failed the test. We suspect that most of the St. John's wort extracts sold in health-food stores are worthless against HIV, as there is no testing or regulation of hypericin content. One of the samples we tested had less than a tenth of the hypericin expected.

Unfortunately, there are several inconsistencies in the chemical test results we have seen. Therefore we cannot reliably estimate how much of the tinctures which are more readily available in the U.S. would be needed to be equivalent to the 120 drops per day used by Dr. Payne. All we can say is that the preparations listed below do appear to contain significant amounts of hypericin. We hope to get more precise chemical measurements in the future—and also results for other preparations which we have not tested. Perhaps buyers clubs could work together to organize such a testing program.

The two German products mentioned favorably by the people we interviewed for this article were Hyperforat, used by Dr. Payne's patients, and Psychotonin M, used by some of the others. Hyperforat is standardized at 0.2 mg (200 micrograms) per ml. We do not know the concentration of Psychotonin M.

If it becomes possible to purchase these products in the U.S., they will probably cost twice as much as in Germany because of shipping expense. It may cost about a dollar and fifty cents per day for the dose Dr. Payne's patients used.

Not all German St. John's wort extracts are satisfactory. Some have only tiny amounts of hypericin.

In the U.S., a St. John's wort tablet from Yerba Prima Botanicals contains a standardized herbal extract obtained from Germany. According to the product label, each tablet contains 250 mg of St. John's wort extract, standardized at 0.14 percent hypericin. Using these specifications, we calculated that two tablets contain about the same amount of hypericin 1.225 mg) as 120 drops of Hyperforat (1.2 mg, assuming 20 drops per ml). *(Editor's Note: this dosage calculation has been corrected since originally published in the newsletter; the amount cited here, in this volume and on this page, is the corrected calculation, as explained in Issue Number 75, page 475.)* The tablets cost about $7 for 60 (retail price), so the total cost of this daily dose is about 40 cents. (The suggested adult dose on the label is less, one tablet twice a day.)

The St. John's wort tinctures from Jarrow Formulas, and from Herb Pharm, were found in our testing to contain significant amounts of hypericin. However, our test results had unexplained inconsistencies, so we do not trust them for computing doses. We do not know at this time what dose would be equivalent to 120 drops of Hyperforat.

Those who have used the tinctures but who cannot take alcohol have been putting the tincture into boiling water and letting it stand for at least two minutes to allow the alcohol to evaporate (instructions on Jarrow Formulas bottle). The heat cannot hurt the hypericin.

How To Order

As explained above, we do not yet know how to order Hyperforat (or Psychotonin M) St. John's wort extracts. The PWA Health Group in New York hopes to carry them. Meanwhile, the herbal extracts listed below are readily available.

When ordering any of these preparations, ask for St. John's wort extract, not hypericin. The people taking the orders seldom know what hypericin is.

Yerba Prima tablets are available in health-food stores nationally, or you can call them (see Appendix B for phone number); ask for "St. John's wort standardized extract" tablets.

For Herb Pharm tincture, call Herb Pharm (see Appendix B) and ask for "St. John's wort tincture."

For Jarrow Formulas product: To find locations of health-food stores which carry the product, or to ask other questions about it, call Jarrow Formulas (see Appendix B). To order by mail, call Vitamin Trader (see Appendix B). Ask for "St. John's wort herbal tincture extract."

Note: You can also purchase St. John's wort extracts through buyers' clubs. We suggest keeping in touch with these groups and seeing what they recommend. The ones we know which are already selling St. John's wort extracts, or will be very soon, are the PWA Health Group in New York; the Healing Alternatives Foundation in San Francisco; the Nutritional Buyers' Club in Los Angeles; and Alliance 7 in San Diego. (See Appendix B or Appendix C for these contact numbers.)

Precautions

The following precautions for using St. John's wort extracts were suggested by one or more of the people we interviewed for this article:

• Let your doctor know what you are doing. At this time, few physicians know anything about this treatment. But if side effects develop, or if the medical community learns other information about St. John's wort which you should know, your physician can pass on the information if he or she knows that you need it.

• People can become abnormally sensitive to sunlight while using St. John's wort. Persons using the treatment should minimize exposure to sunlight or other ultraviolet light.

• We reported some side effects above—especially one case of a severe skin rash apparently caused by using St. John's wort.

• Dr. Meruelo (whose team conducted the animal antiviral experiments mentioned above) suggested using a blood-chemistry panel, such as SMA 25, as an additional precaution. His group found slight, temporary changes in transaminases, LDH, and platelets in some rhesus monkeys, possibly caused by the pure hypericin used. All values returned to normal within 48 hours.

• One paper suggested the theory that hypericin works as a kind of antidepressant called an MAO inhibitor. Certain prescription antidepressants which are MAO inhibitors require avoidance of certain drugs and even certain foods, to avoid dangerous interactions. No one we talked to thought that any foods needed to be avoided with St. John's wort. While this problem seems remote, we thought we should mention the possibility.

• Dr. Rollow Hebert, a naturopathic physician in Seattle, Washington who is familiar with St. John's wort, cautioned that the antidepressant effect might give a false sense of well being, causing people to undertake tasks which are too stressful for them.

• No one knows the effects of long-term use of high doses of hypericin. It is known that the chemical can stay in the body for two weeks or more; therefore, harmful concentrations might build up. Two people we talked to speculated that it might be better to take hypericin intermittently, not every day. There is no data yet either to support or to contradict this possibility.

Clinical Trial Plans

Researchers at New York University, and at the Weizmann Institute in Israel, together applied for worldwide patent rights for antiviral use of hypericin. With the rights secured, they have been able to find funding for animal studies using chemically synthesized pure hypericin, and later clinical trials. A small Phase I trial may start later this year.

Meanwhile, Dr. Payne has written a protocol and already begun a formal trial of hypericin herbal extracts with and without half-dose AZT. He recruited 20 patients in the first few days, and expects to have 100 in as little as two weeks. Even though he is located in Arizona, where there are fewer persons with AIDS or HIV, recruiting has been no problem because the four patients he has already treated have many friends.

The trial with and without AZT is important, because hypericin appeared to be synergistic with AZT in an animal study—meaning that both together might work better than either one by itself.

For more information, researchers and physicians can contact Dr. Payne in Mesa, Arizona.

Doctors Rollo Hebert and Don Brown, both naturopathic physicians in Seattle, Washington, are developing a protocol to test the effect of hypericin on P24 antigen levels and other measures of viral activity.

Keith Barton, M.D., in private practice in Berkeley, California, is interested in monitoring P24 antigen levels. Persons must be located close enough to visit the office, and be P24 positive. Dr. Barton is currently monitoring P24 levels of patients using certain Chinese herbs.

There may also be trials through community-based research organizations such as New York's Community Research Initiative, or San Francisco's County Community Consortium, or Community Research Alliance. There are no detailed plans at the time of this writing, however, because the first human results (reported in this article) are so new.

Call for Information

If you use hypericin, even for a short time, *AIDS Treatment News* would like to hear about your experience. We are especially interested in laboratory test results, including P24 antigen, standard tests including T-helper count and white count, and (if possible) HIV cultures. Call or write John James or Denny Smith at *AIDS Treatment News* (see Appendix B).

Conclusion

At this time hypericin looks promising as a possible AIDS/HIV treatment. It deserves prompt attention.

But many treatments have looked good at first, then proved disappointing later. With only three months' experience and anecdotal reports from a handful of patients, it is too early to know whether hypericin will prove valuable, or how much risk is involved.

People should be cautious, especially until more is known.

REFERENCE

Meruelo, D., G. Lavie, and D. Lavie, "Therapeutic Agents with Dramatic Antiretroviral Activity and Little Toxicity at Effective Doses: Aromatic Polycyclic Diones Hypericen and Pseudohypericin," *Proceedings of the National Academy of Sciences USA* 85 (July 1988), pp. 5230–4.

AEROSOL PENTAMIDINE GETS "TREATMENT IND" APPROVAL

On February 6, the FDA gave tentative approval to use of aerosol pentamidine for prevention of pneumocystis, under the "treatment IND" rules for providing early access to new treatments for life-threatening conditions. The approval was based on data from a San Francisco study started by the County Community Consortium and completed by San Francisco General Hospital.

Aerosol pentamidine was already in widespread use before this treatment IND. Several different doses had been used. The new approval specifies a recommended dose (300 milligrams every four weeks), and nebulizer (Respirgard II). It recommends aerosol pentamidine for "primary" prophylaxis (i.e., for those who have never had pneumocystis) for patients who have a T-helper count under 200—as well as for anyone who has had pneumocystis already. This criterion for primary prophylaxis is based on a yet-unpublished epidemiologic study supported by NIAID.

The treatment IND allows the developer to charge for the drug to recover costs; this is the first time there has been such a charge. LyphoMed is charging the same price as for intravenous use of pentamidine, $99.45 per 300 mg dose. As a result, physicians have been slow to sign up for the program, as there is some paperwork required and no price break. Also, some have chosen to stay with the doses they have been using, at least until they see the full justification of the 300 mg recommendation, data which may not be published for several months.

The new official recognition for aerosol pentamidine should make it easier to get insurance companies to pay for the treatment. (One reason for physicians to sign up for the program, instead of continuing to prescribe aerosol pentamidine as they have done before, is that Medicaid is "likely" to decide to reimburse for treatment administered under it, and if so, reimbursement will be retroactive.) Another benefit of the treatment IND is that research protocols will probably be changed to allow patients to use aerosol pentamidine, if they do not already do so. And the U.S. approval may contribute to efforts to make aerosol pentamidine available in Canada, where lack of access has been a major problem.

LyphoMed has agreed to continue trials of aerosol pentamidine for 24 months, even after full FDA approval, so some patients will receive free treatment through this study.

Physicians and patients can obtain prescription and enrollment information by calling LyphoMed's hotline, Monday through Friday 9 AM through 9 PM EST (see Appendix B). Physicians can request an enrollment packet with forms and instructions.

PROPOSED FEDERAL RULE WOULD BAR REIMBURSEMENT FOR "TREATMENT IND"

A new rule proposed by the U.S. Health Care Financing Administration (HCFA) would effectively sabotage the "treatment IND" (the progam used to make aerosol pentamidine available) by forbidding Medicare to pay for any drug approved under that system. (Medicare itself pays for few AIDS expenses, but Medicaid/Medi-Cal and private insurance companies will probably follow its lead and also refuse to pay, placing the entire burden on the individual.) And even when a drug company provides a drug free under a treatment IND, this proposed rule would probably bar payment for hospitalization and other routine, normally-covered expenses, if a treatment IND is used (see "Insurance/Medicaid Reimbursement Problems," below). The effect will be to deny the treatment IND option to patients and physicians, and delay medical progress for everyone.

The HCFA has asked for public comments on the new rule. Comments must be received no later than March 31, 1989.

The main point of the proposed new rule, called "BERC-432-P," is to codify existing procedure for determining Medicare reimbursement. A single sentence on the treatment IND (which is new and therefore still unresolved, not part of existing procedure), was slipped into 16 pages of fine print, perhaps in the hope that no one would notice in time.

BERC-432-P (the initials stand for Bureau of Eligibility, Reimbursement and Coverage, an office within HCFA) has other problems, too. For example, any drug which has not been approved by the FDA for marketing is not covered—regardless of medical practice in the community. The only exception is certain cancer drugs. All payment for such treatment for all other diseases would be barred. This rule would probably prevent the system which now allows cancer patients to have access to experimental drugs from being applied to AIDS or any other disease. (For background information on the cancer system, see interview with Nathaniel Pier, M.D., in *AIDS Treatment News*, Issue Number 62).

We just obtained the text of BERC-432-P before press time and have not been able to analyze it fully. The complete text is published in the Federal Register (January 30, 1989), pages 4302–4318.

The most damaging section is the sentence, "Treatment Investigational New Drugs (INDs) are approved by the FDA but are still considered experimental and not covered by Medicare." The whole point of the treatment IND is treatment, not research—making drugs available sooner for serious or life-threatening conditions when there is no alternative. Because the procedure is new, reimbursement precendents have not yet been set. The above sentence in BERC-432-P goes beyond the ostensible purpose of BERC-432-P—to codify existing procedures—by trying to slip in a new policy, without consideration, discussion, or debate.

INSURANCE/MEDICAID REIMBURSEMENT PROBLEMS: MOBILIZATION AGAINST AIDS COLLECTING INFORMATION

Mobilization Against AIDS (MAA) is working to get legislation drafted to correct problems with health insurance reimbursement—either private insurance or Medicaid (Medi-Cal in California). The immediate focus of interest is California. MAA needs the help of anyone who has recently been denied treatment because of insurance-reimbursement problems—or their physicians, or any health-care worker who knows of specific examples.

Any such person should send a brief note to Paul Boneberg at Mobilization Against AIDS or call (see Appendix B). These references will be shown to lawmakers to help them in drafting corrective legislation.

Comment

Medical reimbursement problems go beyond AIDS to affect every man, woman, and child in the country, except those so rich that they do not need health insurance. The rising costs of medicine are increasingly prompting public and private insurers to find excuses to avoid covering care.

For example, cancer chemotherapies are often approved officially only for certain specific tumors, when in practice oncologists use the treatments for other tumors, too. But if a tumor does not appear on the FDA's list of approved uses for the drug, insurance companies can refuse to pay, even if the treatment used is in fact the standard of care.

An example in San Francisco shows how such excuses can increase costs and block important research, as well as denying quality care. Physicians at San Francisco General Hospital, one of the world's leading centers for AIDS care, want to try dapsone in the treatment of some cases of pneumocystis. Dapsone costs pennies; lack of reimbursement for it would be no problem. But if dapsone is used, the California office which administers Medi-Cal rules that the physicians used an "experimental" treatment—and refuses to cover the *hospitalization* also, when it would otherwise be reimbursed. (Dapsone is not "labeled" by the FDA for treatment of pneumocystis—and it never will be, because it is one of the cheapest drugs, so there is no commercial incentive to pay for the clinical trials required to obtain such labeling.)

One of the excuses used in such cases is that Medi-Cal is protecting patients from unscrupulous scientists who would use them as guinea pigs. But the real point is to save money by avoiding payment whenever possible—even if it means paying for more expensive drugs, and more hospitalization if the expensive drugs are not as good.

Documenting reimbursement abuses may be difficult, because physicians seldom tell patients that they are using a second-rate treatment for financial reasons; it is easier to give a medical rationale. That is why Mobilization Against AIDS needs support from physicians as well as from patients in its efforts for reform.

It is understandable that insurance companies and public agencies do not want to be billed for some drug company's private research, which they never agreed to pay for. But it is very different to use the FDA lag (typically five to eight years, and often forever) to refuse to pay for appropriate, well-supported treatment. AIDS is especially impacted, because most of the treatments are new; but anyone who becomes seriously ill for any reason could be affected.

Unless these problems can be resolved through legislation, there could be ballot initiatives in California or other states, with the voters deciding directly what Medi-Cal and private health insurance must cover. People may decide to pay a percentage more for insurance that will not run away from them when they need it most. Today you cannot buy that peace of mind at any price.

Issue Number 75
March 10, 1989

ROXITHROMYCIN AND AZITHROMYCIN: TOXOPLASMOSIS, CRYPTOSPORIDIOSIS EXPERIMENTAL TREATMENTS (NOT IN USA)

Update 1989: *Results presented at the "V International Conference on AIDS," (June 1989) in Montreal, showed that roxithromycin was not effective for treating advanced toxoplasmosis.*

Roxithromycin is an antibiotic approved as a prescription drug in France; azithromycin, a similar drug, has been approved in Yugoslavia. They *might* be useful in treating toxoplasmosis, cryptosporidiosis, isospora (an infection which, like cryptosporidiosis, causes severe diarrhea), and possibly MAI.

Despite the need for better treatments for these conditions, we could find nothing being done or planned in the United States to learn whether these drugs might be useful. (We have heard that a trial for toxoplasmosis may start soon in France.) We publish this article to bring attention to these treatment possibilities, so that others can investigate further and organize clinical trials to determine whether these drugs are valuable for treating AIDS-related infections.

Background: Toxoplasmosis

Toxoplasmosis is typically a brain infection caused by the protozoan *Toxoplasma gondii* (which can also affect the eye and other organs). Many healthy people are infected with the parasite, which is commonly present in cats, but usually the immune system keeps the organism controlled. At present, toxoplasmosis is becoming an increasing problem because of AIDS, and also because of wider use of immunosuppressive drugs, for example by organ-transplant patients. Toxoplasmosis is also a threat to the fetus and newborn infant, even in healthy persons without immune suppression.

Toxoplasmosis is usually treated with a combination of pyrimethamine and sulfadiazine (leucovorin must be given with the pyrimethamine). While the drugs are effective, they do not kill cysts of the parasite, so the treatment must be continued as a maintenance dose; often toxicity forces discontinuation of the drug, and relapses result. The statistics are not good, with reported death rates of about 70 percent and median survival of four months, although some people remain alive and healthy for many years after diagnosis. If pyrimethamine and sulfadiazine cannot be used, other drugs such as clindamycin or spiramycin may be used instead. It is important to start treatment early.

One recent study found that one-year survival rates were greatly improved (58 percent vs. 12.5 percent) in patients who were given AZT after starting the maintenance dose (Clumeck *et al.*, 1988). But another paper presented at the same conference reported that AZT interfered with the action of pyrimethamine and greatly *reduced* survival from toxoplasmosis in mice (Israelski *et al.*, 1988). Possibly the important difference is that in the human study, the AZT was not used until after the acute therapy for toxoplasmosis had been successfully completed.

A year ago (January 28, 1988) *AIDS Treatment News* mentioned the case of one person diagnosed with toxoplasmosis who rejected conventional treatments and used large amounts of garlic instead—despite a physician's warning that failure to use the drugs would almost certainly result in death. This patient is still alive today. While rejecting the conventional drugs would seem to be extremely dangerous, this case suggests that there might be some value in using garlic in addition to the treatments recommended by physicians.

It is clear that better treatments are needed.

Note: due to publication deadlines we were unable to review all relevant articles before writing the background summary above.

Roxithromycin and Azithromycin:
Animal and Laboratory Studies

At first glance, roxithromycin looks mediocre in animal studies of toxoplasmosis (see discussion below). This appearance, which may be deceptive, may have discouraged wider interest in the drug. Several published studies have suggested that these drugs are worth trying for treating toxoplasmosis. Our review of these studies is in order by publication date, starting with the most recent.

"Azithromycin, a Macrolide Antibiotic with Potent Activity against *Toxoplasma Gondii*" (Araujo *et al.*, 1988) reported an experiment in which 10 days of treatment with azithromycin protected mice after their brains were infected with *Toxoplasma gondii*. Eight of ten of the treated mice were alive and well on day 30 after infection, while nine of the ten untreated mice were dead by the 14th day and the survivor remained ill. The researchers pointed out that compared to roxithromycin, azithromycin seemed effective in smaller doses. The authors concluded that azithromycin should be studied as an alternative treatment for toxoplasmosis.

"Effect of Roxithromycin on Acute Toxoplasmosis in Mice" (Chang and Pechere, 1987) studied roxithromycin and other drugs, including the conventional treatments for toxoplasmosis, in mice given 500 times the 100 percent fatal dose of *Toxoplasma gondii*. The conventional treatment (pyrimethamine-sulfadiazine) worked well, protecting upt to 100 percent of the mice, depending on the number of doses given. Roxithromycin worked less well, but it also protected up to 100 percent of the mice, depending on the dose. For spiramycin, however, only a 50 percent dose could be determined, because the mice died from toxicity of the drug before a 100 percent protective dose was reached. The authors concluded that roxithromycin might be useful for treating toxoplasmosis, but that clinical studies would be necessary to see how it compared with other drugs.

"Activity of Roxithromycin (RU28965), a Macrolide, against *Toxoplasma gondii* Infection in Mice" (Chan and Luft, 1986) found that roxithromycin was effective in mice, but less so than the standard treatment, pyrimethamine and sulfadiazine. The authors suggested that roxithromycin might be a safe and effective alternative treatment for toxoplasmosis—presumably for use when the standard treatments fail or cannot be used because of toxicity.

"In Vitro Effects of Four Macrolides (Roxithromycin, Spiramycin, Azithromycin/CP-62,993, and A-56268) on *Toxoplasma gondii*" (Chang and Pechere, 1988) tested the drugs in cell cultures in the laboratory. Roxithromycin was the most powerful, spiramycin the least. The authors suggested clinical studies of roxithromycin and other drugs.

Human Experience with Roxithromycin (Not AIDS-Related)

Recently, the *British Journal of Clinical Practice* published a special issue on roxithromycin (Volume 42, Supplement 55, 1988). This issue included several short reports of clinical trials or experience, mostly for lower respiratory tract infections. These reports, from France, Austria, and Argentina, all found the drug effective.

Roxithromycin is a "macrolide"—an antibiotic in the same class as erythromycin, a prescription drug widely used in the U.S. and elsewhere for atypical pneumonias and certain other infections. Roxithromycin is believed to have about the same antimicrobial activity as erythromycin, but better bioavailability—correcting an important shortcoming of other macrolides. Macrolides are considered one of the safest classes of antibiotics (Neu, 1988).

Human Experience Relevant to AIDS

In a study presented at the October 1988 Interscience Conference on Antimicrobial Agents and Chemotherapy (ICAAC), roxithromycin was found to reach very high concentrations in the human brain (Manuel *et al.*, 1988). Researchers in France and Switzerland, noting that roxithromycin had been effective in treating toxoplasmosis in mice, gave the antibiotic to volunteers who were scheduled to undergo brain surgery, so that levels in brain tissue could be determined. (These volunteers did not have toxoplasmosis or AIDS.) The four patients for whom concentrations were measured had much higher roxithromycin concentrations in brain tissue than in blood plasma; two had brain concentrations seven times as high, the other two had fifty times or more roxithromycin in brain tissue than in blood. These measurements were taken 12 hours after the last roxithromycin dose; since blood levels are known to remain high for 12 hours or more, the comparison is a fair one.

This study suggests that roxithromycin is extremely effective in crossing the blood-brain barrier. No other macrolides are known to behave similarly.

In comparable tests in rats, roxithromycin was found *not* to penetrate well into brain tissue—suggesting that the drug may be even more effective in humans than it was in the mouse studies cited above. The potential value for humans might have been missed.

Another human study presented at the same conference (Kazmierczak *et al.*, 1988) found that roxithromycin had much better blood concentrations, 12 and 24 hours after a single dose, than the two other drugs which were compared (spiramycin and trolandomycin).

Taken together, these studies show that roxithromycin, a drug known to be effective against toxoplasmosis in mice, reaches a high concentration in human blood, and a much higher concentration yet in the human brain, where it is needed for treating the disease.

The obvious next step would be to test roxithromycin as a treatment for toxoplasmosis. We have only heard of one case where it has been tried. The physician thought that the drug (brand name "Rulid" in France) had been beneficial, but was not sure, pending study of before and after brain images.

We have heard that a clinical trial of roxithromycin or azithromycin for toxoplasmosis is about to start in France, but we do not have any further information at this time.

Other Opportunistic Infections

A letter in the Journal of Infectious Diseases (Musey *et al.*, 1988) reported that roxithromycin cured one case of *Isospora belli* infection, after several other treatments had failed. This infection causes severe diarrhea; the patient had had chronic diarrhea for two years.

Isospora belli is closely related to *Toxoplasma gondii*, the organism that causes toxoplasmosis. Both are also related to the organism that causes cryptosporidiosis. *Isospora* is easier to treat, however, and often bactrim is effective.

We heard two anecdotal reports of treatment of cryptosporidiosis with azithromycin, a drug approved in Yugoslavia which is closely related to roxithromycin. In one, we talked to a U.S. physician who was convinced that the treatment had worked very well. In the other, we heard from a Project Inform hotline volunteer that a patient had called and said that azithromycin seemed to make his cryptosporidiosis worse; this patient did not leave his name or any way to contact him, so Project Inform cannot investigate further.

It is possible that roxithromycin or azithromycin may also be useful for treating MAI, in combination with other drugs. Physicians are interested because these new macrolide antibiotics penetrate well into monocytes; MAI is often found inside these cells.

FDA Roxithromycin Controversy

On December 15, 1988, *The Alternative,* a Baltimore gay paper which often publishes important, original investigative stories on AIDS treatment research and public policy, reported that a major drug company had applied to the FDA for an IND (Investigation New Drug approval) to study roxithromycin and azithromycin in clinical trials, but that the FDA had rejected the application due to lack of adequate animal studies—even though roxithromycin was already approved and in human use in France. (Roxithromycin was later mentioned in *U.S. News and World Report,* February 13, 1989, page 82.)

We called the FDA and the drug company (Roussel, a French company which also has offices in New Jersey), and found that the agency and the company had different understandings of the facts of this case. The misunderstanding, which came to light by accident, may have helped cause the proposed research to be cancelled.

Both agree that the company did apply for an IND, and the the FDA asked for animal studies. The IND application was to study roxithromycin for AIDS-related cryptosporidiosis and isospora—not toxoplasmosis. The animal studies were to answer certain questions concerning the rationale of the treatment—not to test roxithromycin as if it were a new chemical which had never before been given to humans.

The question at issue is whether the drug was rejected because animal tests showed it was unpromising for cryptosporidiosis and isospora—or whether it was dropped without any tests because of the expense or impossibility of obtaining the information requested.

The FDA spokesperson we talked to believed that the company did do the studies, and based on the results decided it was unlikely that the drug would be effective, and therefore decided not to pursue human trials. He suggested a person at Roussel whom we could call for further information.

We called that person, who needed to check further, as we had called asking about toxoplasmosis, but he had been prepared to reply about cryptosporidiosis and isospora. Our concern was that people were starting to use the drug, and if animal studies had suggested that it would be ineffective, it was urgent that the information be known.

After checking with other people in the company, the Roussel spokesperson called us back and told us that no such animal studies had been done. Instead, after the FDA asked for those studies to confirm the activity of the drug, the researchers at Roussel found no good animal models to answer the questions asked, so the company decided not to pursue the project. The spokesperson also confirmed that the IND application had not concerned toxoplasmosis.

Today we know of no plans in the U.S. to study roxithromycin for any AIDS-related condition. There may a toxoplasmosis study soon in France.

Roxithromycin—The Next Step

As many as 31,000 persons with AIDS may develop toxoplasmosis by 1991 (Potasman *et al.*, 1988); with conventional treatments only, most of them will die. Obviously clinical trials of promising treatments like roxithromycin are needed.

Physicians, scientists, and regulatory officials may have missed the importance of roxithromycin, thinking that it could not be a major advance because in the test tube and in animals it is no more effective than the conventional treatment for toxoplasmosis, and perhaps somewhat less effective. The implication that roxithromycin is therefore unimportant is probably erroneous, for two reasons.

First, it overlooks the strikingly high concentrations of roxithromycin in brain tissue, where the toxoplasmosis infection is located. This very good penetration into the human brain is not found in the rat, so animal experiments would not be expected to show the benefits which might be found in humans. The study (cited above) which found the high concentrations in human brain tissue was presented as a poster session at the ICAAC conference last October, and may not be widely known.

Second, the comparative efficacy against *Toxoplasma gondii* is not the important question here. Both roxithromycin and pyrimethamine/sulfadiazine (the conventional treatment) are clearly effective, though neither kills *Toxoplasma* entirely. The problem with pyrimethamine/sulfadiazine is that toxicity develops, preventing long-term use and resulting in relapse when the drugs can no longer be used. Roxithromycin has very little toxicity, so it could probably be used for a long time.

At the very least roxithromycin should be tried in cases when there is no other option.

The central problem seems to be that no one is making sure that even the most obvious and fundamental interests of persons with AIDS or at risk for AIDS are considered when drug-development decisions are made. We need leadership from the medical community, as well as from patient-advocacy groups.

Until trials can be arranged, the second best option is to obtain roxithromycin from France, or send patients there, and collect anecdotal information. The PWA Health Group recently listed roxithromycin as one of the prescription drugs it wants to make available (see "AIDS Group Organizing Imports of Drugs Not Approved by F.D.A.," *The New York Times,* March 6, 1989, page 1).

REFERENCES

Araujo, F.G. *et al.,* "Azithromycin, a Macrolide Antibiotic with Potent Activity Against Toxoplasma Gondii," *Antimicrobial Agents and Chemotherapy* 32(5) (May 1988), pp. 755-7.

Chan, J. and B.J. Luft, "Activity of Roxithromycin (RU28965), a Macrolide, Against *Toxoplasma gondii* Infection in Mice," *Antimicrobial Agents and Chemotherapy* 30(2) (August 1986), pp. 323-4.

Chang, H.R. and J.F. Pechere, "Effects of Roxithromycin on Acute Toxoplasmosis in Mice," *Antimicrobial Agents and Chemotherapy* 31(7) (July 1987), pp. 1147-9.

———, "In Vitro Effects of Four Macrolides (Roxithromycin, Spiramycin, Azithromycin (CP-62,993) and A-56268 on *Toxoplasma gondii,*" *Antimicrobial Agents and Chemotherapy* 32(4) (April 1988), pp. 524-9.

Clumeck, N. *et al.,* "The Benefit of Zidovudine on the Long-term Survival of AIDS Patients with CNS Toxoplasmosis," *Program and Abstracts of the Twenty-Eighth Interscience Conference on Antimicrobial Agents and Chemotherapy* (October 23-26, 1988), Abstract Number 1474.

Holliman, R.E., "Toxoplasmosis and the Acquired Immune Deficiency Syndrome," *Journal of Infectious Disease* 16(2) (March 1988), pp. 121-8.

Israelski, D.M. *et al.,* "AZT Antagonizes Pyrimethamine in Experimental Infection with *Toxoplasma gondii,*" *Program and Abstracts of the Twenty-Eighth Interscience Conference on Antimicrobial Agents and Chemotherapy* (October 23-26, 1988), Abstract Number 349.

Kazmierczak, A. *et al.,* "Roxithromycin Pharmacokinetic Compared with Those of Spiramycin and Trolandomycin After a Single Oral Dose," *Program and Abstracts of the Twenty-Eighth Interscience Conference on Antimicrobial Agents and Chemotherapy* (October 23-26, 1988), Abstract Number 137.

Manuel, C. *et al.,* "Penetration of Roxithromycin into Brain Tissue," *Program and Abstracts of the Twenty-Eighth Interscience Conference on Antimicrobial Agents and Chemotherapy* (October 23-26, 1988), Abstract Number 1224.

Musey, K.L. *et al.,* "Effectiveness of Roxithromycin for Treating *Isospora belli* Infection," *The Journal of Infectious Disease* 158(3) (September 1988), p. 646.

Neu, H.C., "Roxithromycin—An Overview," *The British Journal of Clinical Practice* 42(55) (1988), pp. 1-3.

Potasman, I. *et al.,* "Intrathecal Production of Antibodies Against *Toxoplasma gondii* in Patients with Toxoplasmic Encephalitis and the Acquired Immunodeficiency Syndrome (AIDS)," *Annals of Internal Medicine* 108 (1988), pp. 49-51.

HYPERICIN: NEW DOSAGE INFORMATION

The last issue of *AIDS Treatment News* (Issue Number 74) included a major report on human experience with hypericin, an experimental antiviral readily available in certain extracts of the St. John's wort plant. The following updates are based on information we received after the article was published.

Dose Calculation Error

In our February 24 article, we calculated equivalent doses for the Hyperforat tincture from Germany, and St. John's wort tablets (Yerba Prima Botanicals) which are more available and convenient, and less expensive. We calculated that the 120 drops of Hyperforat (the dose with the most human experience so far) would be equivalent to three and a half of the tablets, each of which contains 250 mg of 0.14 percent hypericin. (Both products are standardized for hypericin content, so different lots should have the same strength.)

Since the article was published, a chemist told us that our calculations were probably incorrect. According to his information, the correct dose would be about two tablets, not three and a half, to be equivalent to 120 drops of Hyperforat tincture.

Our error was that when we converted drops to milliliters, in order to calculate the amount of hypericin in 120 drops of tincture, we used a ratio of 20 drops per milliliter, a standard conversion factor in medicine. However, the chemist explained that the 20 drops applies to pure water, but that a mixture of water and alcohol, as found in herbal tinctures, has different surface characteristics resulting in smaller drops. He estimates that there would be 40 to 45 drops per milliliter.

We could not obtain the Hyperforat product by press time for a direct test, but two other hypericin tinctures we tested both fell within this range. If Hyperforat does also, then the 120-drop daily dose of that product would be equivalent to somewhat less than two of the tablets—based on the specified hypericin content of the two products.

Animal Studies Suggest Less Frequent Use

We spoke again with the team at New York University which did the laboratory and animal studies published last July in the *Proceedings of the National Academy of Sciences, USA*. In further animal studies, they have consistently found that giving hypericin less often than once a day has worked better as an antiretroviral than giving it every day.

For example, a single dose of ten micrograms was less effective than a single dose of 100 micrograms, as expected. But ten daily doses of ten micrograms each worked less well than even the *single* 10 microgram dose.

The animals were given larger doses relative to body weight than people have been using. *The scientists emphasized that this information should in no way be interpreted as recommending any specific dose at this time.*

The researchers are now preparing their animal results for publication, but the paper will not be published for several months at least. They pointed out that there is no guarantee that findings in animal studies will apply to humans—or to HIV, which in laboratory tests seems to be more sensitive to hypericin than the animal retroviruses they had been using—and that only clinical trials can determine the best dose and schedule for human use.

Editorial Comment.   At this time there is no human experience with a less frequent schedule. Everyone we have talked to who has used St. John's wort extracts has used them every day—as recommended for antidepressant use in Europe.

In the reports so far, clinical benefits have usually been found within three to four weeks of starting daily use of standardized hypericin preparations (see *AIDS Treatment News,* Issue Number 74). Therefore, within a month it might be clear whether or not the treatment is working for a patient. If not, the treatment might be discontinued; if it is working, then if the person decides to change to a less frequent dosage schedule, the benefits already seen can serve as a baseline for comparing whether or not the new schedule seems to be better.

More Good News—But Caution Needed

Before going to press, we asked Dr. Payne, four of whose patients have been using hypericin for three to four months, if there was any new information in the two weeks since we published our last issue. All four of them have continued to improve clinically. T-helper count increases have remained disappointingly slow—not surprising since these patients started with counts less than 10.

In our last issue we reported that one of the four patients had gone from P24 antigen positive to negative while using hypericin. Results are now back on two of the others. One of them has also gone from positive to negative. The other has remained positive, but the antigen level improved, from over 400 to 117. The fourth patient was P24 negative from the beginning.

Despite the continuing good results, the information so far available about hypericin is very preliminary. No one knows the best dose or dosage regimen, no one knows which patients may be most likely to benefit, and no one knows if the herbal extracts will prove effective or even safe in long-term use. It is important that some people try hypericin, so that we will find out soon whether or not it is useful; that is already happening. But it would be risky for this treatment possibility to come into widespread use before more is known.

There is no great rush to start using hypericin. The largest buyer's club, the PWA Health Group in New York, received many calls about St. John's wort extracts, but sold only a few dozen bottles in the week after our article came out. The Healing Alternatives Foundation in San Francisco has also had only moderate sales. Fortunately people are being cautious. Or perhaps a treatment which costs about 25 cents a day is unlikely to be taken very seriously.

Because there have been many dissapointments before, including some treatments which looked good at first but turned out to be harmful, we emphasize again that no one knows how hypericin will turn out, and therefore caution is important.

Note: As we went to press we heard from a physician that one patient using St. John's wort tablets and no other treatment had a liver function test result four times normal—which might or might not have been caused by the herbal extract. This case reinforces the suggestion, published in our last issue, to have one's physician monitor a blood-chemistry panel when using hypericin extracts. The research team at New York University found small, temporary changes in liver function and other blood-chemistry values in some rhesus monkeys given the chemical.

We do not know what tablets were used, or what dose, or how long.

Dr. Payne checked the records of his four patients who had used hypericin for three months or more, and found no such problem. Two had elevated liver enzymes before starting hypericin; both have improved while they have used it. A third had a slight elevation while on hypericin; however, he had done well enough to resume AZT, which could have been the cause. The fourth was normal throughout.

CHINESE HERB COMBINATION: UPDATE

Six months ago, *AIDS Treatment News* interviewed Keith Barton, M.D., a physician trained in acupuncture and Chinese herbal treatment as well as Western medicine. Dr. Barton had prepared a combination of six herbs traditionally used as anti-infection treatments in Chinese medicine, and which also had shown anti-HIV activity in laboratory tests. We reported that of the first two patients who used the combination, one had gone from P24 antigen poitive to negative in three weeks—a good early sign.

Recently Dr. Barton told us that this particular herbal combination has not proved effective. The patient whose antigen had gone to zero had started at a very low value. Later, he went off the herbs in order to begin another treatment program, and his antigen level subsequently rose.

Three other patients who took the same combination have not shown P24 antigen improvement. Some of them have a higher T-helper cell count than when they started the herbs, but the rises are not large enough to rule out laboratory error.

The six herbs used in this combination were Lonicer japonica, Lithospermum erythrorhizon, Prunella vulgaris, Viola yedoensis, Epimedium grandiflorum, and licorice root.

There are other Chinese herbal combinations which might prove effective and have not yet been evaluated. Also, Dr. Barton pointed out that only a highly effective treatment would be identified by the protocol he used.

KS: NEW TREATMENT POSSIBILITIES
by Denny Smith

In January, 1989, *AIDS Treatment News*, Issue Number 73, reported on conventional treatments for Kaposi's sarcoma which have been adapted to HIV-related KS. Those included the careful use of radiation therapy, and chemotherapy administered intravenously or intralesionally. Recently, at least three more treatments have entered the field: the Prosorba column, interferon, and laser surgery. The Prosorba column, also known as a protein A column, and the interferons alpha and beta are systemic approaches to KS (like intravenous chemotherapy). The use of lasers (like Velban injections or irradiation of specific lesion sites) is a localized treatment. Whether to consider a systemic treatment or a localized one depends on the growth and location of the lesions, as we described in the earlier article.

Lasers are currently being used to remove lesions in the mouth and esophagus, tissues which can become severely inflamed if treated with radiation. Herbert H. Dedo, M.D., of the University of California at San Francisco has used lasers for fifteen years to treat cancer and to remove warts or scar tissue. He feels that treatment of lesions in the oral cavity is warranted if they have become symptomatic—if they functionally impair swallowing or breathing. The procedure is done under general anesthesia and is usually followed by an overnight hospital stay. To gain access to the lesion, Dr. Dedo employs a retractor he designed himself, and with an operating microscope as a visual guide he aims a laser at the targeted lesion for a duration calculated in fractions of a second. The lesion is vaporized, and the surrounding blood capillaries are cauterized by the laser's action. The patient may experience some soreness at the site for a few weeks, but less than a surgical excision would cause.

The Prosorba column was first developed to treat cancer, and then was found to be useful against HIV-related ITP (idiopathic thrombocytopenic purpura). Dobri Kiprov, M.D., director of the plasmapheresis unit at Children's Hospital in San Francsico, has had over four years of experience using the Prosorba device for KS. He has seen a response rate (lesion regression or stabilization) of about 42 percent. The response in patients with ITP was higher, between 50 to 60 percent, but the KS application may still be refined to obtain a better result. The Prosorba column appears to be a simple procedure, but operates on a mechanism of action not fully understood. The object of the treatment is to remove from the bloodstream substances called circulating immune complexes (CIC), and other "blocking factors," which some researchers feel are an obstacle to a normal immune response.

According to this logic, the removal of some CIC could trigger an effective attack against the antigen responsible for KS and ITP. To accomplish this, a unit of blood is drawn from the patient and processed in a centrifuge, where cells are separated from plasma. The cells are returned unaffected to the patient, but the plasma is run through a column of silica which has been coated with "protein A." This protein binds with a type of immunoglobulin, the CIC targeted for removal. The plasma is then returned to the patient. Side effects appear to be slight but common—mostly fevers and chills. The treatment can be repeated periodically. Dr. Kiprov feels that circulating immune complexes may play a role in the development of ARC or AIDS, and that the Prosorba column, in addition to filtering out CIC, might potentiate the body's immunity by stimulating production of interleukin, and other components of the immune system.

This treatment is still under investigation and is done under a research protocol. For more information about the Prosorba column, physicians only can call in IMRE Corporation (see Appendix B).

Interferon is a protein naturally secreted by cells in response to viruses, bacteria, and other antigens. Occurring in three distinct classes, alpha, beta and gamma, interferon stimulates surrounding cells to manufacture other proteins which in turn inhibit antigen growth or replication, and which enhance an appropriate immune response. It is the body's most rapidly produced defense. In related experiments, all the interferons demonstrated *in vitro* anti-HIV activity, and interferons alpha and beta were shown to have antitumor activity. At least 12 studies presented at the IV International Conference on AIDS in Stockholm discussed the value of interferon as a treatment for KS. The results were uneven, but several reports suggested that interferon is more effective if given when T4-helper cell counts are over 200, and may work in synergy with AZT.

In November 1988 the FDA approved the use of recombinant alpha interferon for treating KS, based on a lesion-reduction response in 40 to 45 percent of patients receiving a high dose. In December 1988, *AIDS Treatment News* (Issue Number 70) spoke with Mathilde Krim, Ph.D., founding co-chair of the American Foundation for AIDS Research, who felt that the dose upon which the FDA based its approval was unnecessarily high: 20 million units or more daily. (The dose is usually lower when administered concurrently with AZT.) Trials are still in progress which will hopefully determine the optimum therapeutic index (the ratio of an effective dose to a toxic dose). In any event, the side effects of large doses almost always include persistent flu-like symptoms.

Meanwhile, other potential KS treatments are being investigated, and we will watch for any good results. They include beta interferon, tumor necrosis factor, cryotherapy, colony stimulating factor, CL246,738 and interleukin-2.

SAN FRANCISCO: CHINESE MEDICINE EXPERT TO VISIT

Dr. Wei Bei-Hai, Director and Chief Physician of the Beijing Research Institute of Traditional Chinese Medicine, will give lectures, workshops, and consultations in San Francisco, April 6–10, 1989. Dr. Wei was trained in Western medicine and has been working with the integration of Western medicine and traditional Chinese medicine (TCM) for 30 years.

Lecture topics include: Chinese medicine and the theory of immunity; treatment of chronic viral infection through combination of Western and TCM therapies; TCM treatment of diabetes; and TCM treatment of physical weakness in the elderly.

AIDS AND DISABILITY RIGHTS: YOU CAN HELP

Congress will soon consider the Americans with Disabilities Act, a landmark bill to protect all disabled persons against discrimination. Disability activists have commendably insisted on including all disabled persons equally, instead of allowing different disease constituencues to be split by political tradeoffs. The AIDS community owes a debt to the larger disability community, which has refused to abandon persons with AIDS to appease bigots. We can begin to repay the debt when the Act is introduced, by working all-out for its passage.

There are still attempts, however, to exclude persons with HIV from legislation to protect other disabled persons. To resist these attempts, the delegate from NAPWA (the National Association of People with AIDS) to the Congressional Task Force on the Rights and Empowerment of Americans with Disabilities wants to hear about cases of AIDS- or HIV-related discrimination—in medical care, employment, public accomodations, or otherwise.

If you or anyone you know has experienced such discrimination, write a short account—half a page is usually enough—and send it to David Bodenstein at the National Association of People with AIDS (see Appendix B). Please include a phone number or address where you can be contacted. Your name will be kept confidential; or you can write anonymously if you prefer.

Appendix A
Additional Information

I. PRESERVING YOUR MEDICAL AND DISABILITY BENEFITS
(from *AIDS Treatment News*, Issue Number 76, March 24, 1989)

Many persons with serious illnesses lose insurance and medical benefits to which they are entitled, because of the complex rules governing these programs. We asked benefits counselors what are the most important traps to avoid, the most important things people may need to know as "first aid" to preserve their access to benefits, even before they get to an expert adviser.

Audrey K. Doughty, executive director of AIDS Benefits Counselors, a new San Francisco organization which specializes in Social Security and employee benefits and advises other organizations as well as individual clients, suggests, "To be a friend to a person who has tested HIV positive, encourage him or her to start early on financial planning.

"Many have panicked after testing HIV positive (and especially after an AIDS or ARC diagnosis), then quit their jobs, losing benefits for which they have worked and to which they are entitled. Others lose their benefits by staying on the job longer than they are physically able and getting fired for poor performance.

"You must familiarize yourself with the provisions of your benefits package. Obtain a copy of your company's actual contract with their insurance firm. Frequently a shorter, simplified version is handed to employees, and it may not give you the precise and complete information you need."

Diana Kuderna, a benefits counselor in Alameda County, California (near San Francisco) and chair of the East Bay AIDS Response Organization, makes the same point and adds other suggestions:

"If your illness is beginning to interfere with your work, rather than leave or allow yourself to be terminated from a job that includes benefits, you and your doctor need to consider a disability leave, as benefits can be lost otherwise. In order to retain access to extended health-care benefits, and short- or long-term disability plans, you must be employed when deemed disabled."

481

Ms. Kuderna added that many people also lose benefits by going part-time without checking on requirements or negotiating retention of benefits.

A physician can declare a patient disabled entirely, or only for full-time work but still able to work part time. The employer does not need to know that disability is being considered until after the determination has been made. If you are found to be disabled only for full-time work, then if you continue to work part time, you may still receive up to 100 percent of State disability income (in California at least), in addition to your part-time earnings, providing that the total does not exceed your income before applying for disability. (For more detailed information, see the article by Ms. Kuderna described below.)

There are many more important points to know, for example:

• In most (but not all) jobs, if you leave the job for any reason, you can keep the medical insurance for up to 18 months by paying premiums yourself. However, you must make arrangements to do so within the allowed time—and pay all the premiums when due. (This right to extend a health-insurance policy by paying the premiums oneself is provided by a Federal law, known as COBRA. Unfortunately, the insurance period expires six months before the two-year disability requirement for Medicare, leaving a six-month gap in coverage. This gap needs to be fixed by legislation.)

A few employers will continue to pay premiums for about six months after an employee leaves. The employee must begin paying when the employer stops, in order to maintain the health benefits. Usually, however, the employee should apply for COBRA immediately.

Businesses of less than 20 employees are not required to offer the COBRA extension of benefits.

• If you qualify as disabled under Social Security, you may then qualify under either of two programs for disability income:

SSDI (Social Security Disability Income, sometimes called "SSA") does not require low income and assets. But you must have paid into the system for five of the last ten years (less for those age 24 and under). And no benefits will be paid until after five months of disability.

SSI (Supplemental Security Income) requires low income and assets, as well as disability. But you do not need to have paid into the system to qualify. And there is no five-month waiting period. Benefits usually take a couple months to kick in, but then they are retroactive to the initial by-phone benefits request—your "protective filing date." (SSDI is not retroactive.)

• Persons with CDC-defined AIDS are usually presumed by Social Security to be disabled. But persons with ARC are often denied disability, even if they are equally or even more disabled than many persons with AIDS. AIDS Benefits Counselors has an excellent record in appealing these denials and getting them reversed. Careful record keeping (including very detailed descriptions from physicians) is often required. (See below about getting help on benefits from AIDS service organizations.)

• There are other health-care and disability-income possibilities, including Medicaid (Medi-Cal in California), and state disability insurance. Medicaid may be valuable even for persons who have private insurance. However, the program varies greatly from state to state.

Ms. Kuderna described some advantages of Medi-Cal (California's Medicaid program) even for those who have other insurance:

"While essential for the uninsured, the program is also useful as a supplement to insurance. It will pay for care not covered in your policy—dentistry, chiropractic care, mental health services, drug detox, supplies ordered by a doctor, and nursing home care. Medi-Cal allows you to use health-care providers—those that accept Medi-Cal as partial or full payment—outside of your HMO (Health Maintenance Organization) provider list. If your policy has deductible amounts and percentages that are not payable, Medi-Cal can cover them. Some care providers and pharmacies expect you to pay now and bill insurance yourself. Medi-Cal can be used to avoid the difficult cash outlays. If your condition makes it difficult for you to take public transportation, cabs to medical appointments can be paid for by Medi-Cal. Note that there is no cash reimbursement, only 'compensatory stickers.' "

• Do not overlook miscellaneous programs available in some areas, such as private or religious AIDS emergency funds, free or low-cost food programs, greatly reduced fares on public transit for persons with disabilities, and others.

• Ms. Kuderna emphasized some practical hints which could be overlooked:

(1) in California at least, In-Home Support Services can be used to pay for anyone of your choosing, including a lover, spouse, or family member, to help with home chores—up to 283 hours of help per month at minimum wage. You must require chore service in your home (the number of hours is determined by a home visit) and be eligible for SSI, except that your income can be somewhat higher. Those paid to do the work can have any income. Other states may have similar programs.

This program may also enable you to qualify for Medi-Cal even if your income would otherwise be too high. By an arrangement with your chore helper not to bill for the first certain number of hours per month (i.e., to pay for them yourself), you can reduce your income for Medi-Cal eligibility purposes.

(2) Payment for cost of experimental treatments is often a problem. But for meeting SSI income limits, you should be able to deduct the cost of experimental treatment supervised by a physician from earned income. (We do not know about states other than California.)

(3) Ms. Kuderna encourages people to consider State disability insurance. One fact the disability office may not tell you is that you can collect disability income for more than one year maximum. If your physician releases you to go back to work for more than a 14-day period (even if you do not actually find work in that time) and then re-imposes restrictions, a new claim can begin. (Again, we do not know how eligibility varies in different states.)

Where To Get Help and Advice

• Check with your local AIDS service organization. If you do not know what is available in your locality, start by calling the National AIDS Hotline (see Appendix B). (This excellent referral service has up to 40 information specialists available 24 hours a day, so usually there is no wait to get through. It has one of the largest AIDS referral databases in the country. Unfortunately, the hotline is not well known.)

- As an example of the kinds of assistance which may be available from local AIDS service organizations, the San Francisco AIDS Foundation has weekly benefits workshops for persons with AIDS or ARC, both morning and evening sessions. The workshop includes all Federal, State, and local disability benefits, employer-sponsored benefits, and insurance. It also includes other social services available through the Foundation, and elsewhere in San Francisco. To register for the workshops, call the San Francisco AIDS Foundation (see Appendix B), and ask to speak to the on-duty social worker.

Clients can also meet individually with a social worker for a benefits review.

The Foundation also sponsors a twice-monthly benefits seminar for Federal employees with AIDS or ARC. To register, call the on-duty social worker.

- Chris Alexander, a benefits expert at the Foundation, emphasizes how much can be done early—while one is HIV-positive, before receiving an AIDS or ARC diagnosis—to preserve one's access to medical care, disability income, and insurance.

- Persons with ARC have special difficulty qualifying for Social Security disability. The San Francisco AIDS Foundation has a program for them, using a team of volunteers to explain what is required and how persons can improve their chances of qualifying. The team follows up with clients, and with the Social Security Administration. It cannot guarantee acceptance, but it can guarantee that Social Security has a complete picture of a client's background.

- On ARC disability, Diana Kuderna adds, "Documentation submitted to assist in determining the severity and probable duration of disability can include reports written by anyone closely familiar with your daily routine. Several such descriptions of limitation of function resulting from your illness can help, including what you can and cannot do as a result of fatigue, pain, mental changes, nausea, diarrhea, confusion, drug side effects, sleep interruptions, weakness, depression, rashes, anxiety or forgetfulness."

- Persons with ARC can also obtain a 95-page manual, *Guide for Social Security Disability Insurance Claims for HIV Disease, (AIDS and ARC),* by Patrick James, a founder of AIDS Benefits Counselors. In San Francisco, New York, and Los Angeles, the book is available at A Different Light bookstore; it can be ordered from AIDS Benefits Counselors (see Appendix B). This book includes forms and sample medical narratives which show the level of detail with which physicians should document ARC disabilities. It includes a checklist to be used by persons with ARC, and their friends, family, and physicians, which has been very helpful in documenting disability. It tells what sections must be changed for users in California but outside the San Francisco Bay Area, or by those outside of California. From AIDS Benefits Counselors the book costs $25 plus $5 handling for agencies, but it is free to persons with AIDS or ARC who cannot afford it.

- Diana Kuderna has prepared a ten-page writeup "AIDS/ARC Benefits Counseling in Alameda County." This article, full of detailed information about eligibility criteria and other aspects of many disability, insurance, and other benefits programs, was written primarily for training benefits counselors. Applicants may also find it useful, however; and even persons outside of Alameda County or outside of California may find valuable hints and ideas in the article, although the details will differ. You can obtain a copy by sending a self-addressed stamped envelope (with two ounces of postage) to: Diana Kuderna (see Appendix B).

• We spoke with a hospital intake worker, who urged people to have medical insurance information with them (such as the name of their insurance company or HMO, and policy numbers) in case they need to be admitted to a hospital. Many plans require pre-authorization in order to reimburse for certain procedures (or notification within a certain time afterwards, in case of emergency). Sometimes people do not know the name of their company, and while they are in the hospital there may be no one at home or at work to find out.

• Chris Alexander emphasized the importance of becoming familiar with your local AIDS service organization, and of finding out what is available in your area (including emergency funds, money to pay certain bills, and county benefits such as food stamps or general assistance which vary from county to county). Insurance and benefits problems can be overwhelming when one is dealing with everything else about an AIDS or ARC diagnosis, so be aware of how an AIDS service organization can help, for example by assistance in filing applications, or by explaining the paperwork requirements. People do not need to go it alone.

II. COMPOUND Q (GLQ223)
(from *AIDS Treatment News,* Issue Number 77, April 21, 1989)

In the last few weeks a potential AIDS treatment, so far tested only in the laboratory, has generated enormous public and scientific interest. We have followed compound Q (also called GLQ223) and do agree that it is important (we listed it as one of eight treatments to watch in 1989 in our January 13 issue). This note will refer readers to authoritative, accessible published information—and also include cautions about use of a similar drug from China, should it become available.

The reason for the interest is that laboratory studies suggest that compound Q *might* kill infected macrophages, and eliminate this major reservoir of HIV from the body. No other treatment has been found to do so.

Two good, readily-available articles summarizing information on compound Q were published in *The New York Times* (April 18, 1989, Medical Sciences section) and in *Business Week* (April 24, 1989, page 29).

For technical background, see the article by Michael S. McGrath *et al.*, "GLQ223: An Inhibitor of Human Immunodeficiency Virus Replication in Acutely and Chronically Infected Cells of Lymphocyte and Mononuclear Phagocyte Lineage," *Proceedings of the National Academy of Sciences, USA* (April 15, 1989). Also see the United States Patent, number 4,795,739, date of patent January 3, 1989.

The active ingredient in compound Q is a protein called trichosanthin, which is extracted from the root of a Chinese cucumber, *Tricosanthes kirilowii.* It must be given by injection. This protein is also used in China to induce abortions, and to treat ectopic pregnancy, hydatidiform moles, and one particular kind of cancer, choriocarcinoma. (For an overview of the Chinese medicinal use of trichosanthin, see Yu Wang *et al.*, "Scientific Evaluation of Tian Hua Fen (THF)—History, Chemistry, and Application," *Pure and Applied Chemistry* 58(5) (1986), pages 789-798. "Tian Hua Fen" is the name of the herbal preparation from which trichosanthin, the active ingredient, can be extracted.)

INJECTING IMPURE PREPARATIONS OF THE PROTEIN COULD CAUSE FATAL SIDE EFFECTS. In China, there are three different grades of trichosanthin prepared for injection: crude extract, purified extract, and crystalized, which is the highest purity. Only the crystalized form can be used safely; the others cause severe side effects. (Animal tests cited by Wang *et al.*, referenced above, showed a lethal dose to be only three times higher than the effective dose for the least pure grade, only six times for the intermediate, so-called "pure" grade, but over 75 times higher than the effective dose for the purest, crystalized grade.) Fortunately, it is fairly easy to test for impurities, using a standard chemical technique called gel chromatography, so it should be straightforward to test that a drug claimed to be the "crystalized" grade really is.

We have heard that side effects (of the Chinese "crystalized" grade) can include fever, muscle weakness, and possible electrolyte imbalance, lasting 12 to 18 hours. These problems may not start for about 12 hours. Because of the possibility of electrolyte imbalance, the patient must be monitored by a physician, so that treatment can be given if necessary. Wang *et al.*, (reference above) mention 1,042 cases of human use of the crystalized grade, by intra-amniotic or intramuscular injection, in their paper published in 1986. They said there were no significant side effects; a low fever of 37.5 C. degrees occurred in 79 percent of the cases. (Since there are no side effects of compound Q in animals unless dose is extremely high, the side effects of the Chinese crystalized version may result from some remaining impurities or from the intended killing of target cells, which presumably would not occur in animal toxicity tests.)

There may be additional precautions. For example, repeated use could conceivably cause anaphylaxis, although no such problem has been seen in animal tests. We do not know if there is any Chinese experience with repeated use.

This drug may be dangerous, and must not be used without knowledgeable professional supervision.

A story widely reported in the press claims that six people in Florida used a Chinese version of compound Q, and had to be hospitalized due to side effects. We have heard serious doubts about the truth of this rumor, and have not been able to confirm it.

COMPOUND Q WARNING, AND UPDATE
(from *AIDS Treatment News*, Issue Number 78, May 5, 1989)

Compound Q, an experimental AIDS treatment extracted from the root tuber of a Chinese cucumber, has received wide publicity in the last month. On May 5, we heard the first report of a severe adverse reaction to a bogus "compound Q," apparently homemade from the root which was obtained from a health-food store, and injected. According to Martin Delaney of Project Inform, who is now warning buyers' clubs, the person almost died as a result, and was in intensive care for three days. This case occurred in Kansas City.

We have also heard that some health-food stores are exploiting the situation and promoting a dried root or extract by suggesting that it contains compound Q. People should know (1) that the root also contains lectins, which are poisonous when injected because they cause blood cells to clump together, which can cause heart attacks or strokes, and (2) that compound Q (which is a protein called tricosanthin) is almost certainly destroyed by drying, so the dried root used as an herbal medicine for other purposes does not contain the active ingredient.

It is generally believed that a good-quality equivalent of compound Q does exist in China, and has been used there for other purposes for several years (see article above from Issue Number 77). However, this drug is tightly controlled and very difficult to obtain. We have heard from knowledgeable persons (but have not yet been able to confirm independently) that only half a million doses a year are manufactured, all by one factory in or near Shanghai, and that some of it did reach a few persons with AIDS in the U.S. While extracting the active ingredient (tricosanthin) from the Chinese cucumber root is not too difficult for a protein chemist, there are practical problems, especially the need to obtain large quantities of the fresh or frozen root, as well as the usual difficulties of setting up effective manufacturing and quality control for pharmaceuticals.

Any credible, good-quality data which may develop from use of the Chinese compound-Q equivalent would be very important in speeding the authorized clinical trials. At this time, the only clinical trial planned anywhere in the world is a "phase I" study to take place at San Francisco General Hospital. This trial may be slowed by the current budget crisis of the City and County of San Francisco, since hospitalization is required for the study but there is not enough funding to staff the nursing support for the hospital beds.

The San Francisco trial will also be slow because it is designed primarily to test for toxicity and determine the maximum tolerated dose, not to determine whether the drug can help patients. A tiny dose which no one believes could be effective will be tried first, followed by a wait to look for side effects. This process will be repeated several times, with a wait each time. This dose-escalation study could take as little as three to six months, or as long as a year. By contrast, "underground" users of the Chinese drug will test reasonable doses right away—the same which have already been used in China—so they can get results far ahead of the official trials. If such use should happen to produce credible evidence that the drug is useful in treating AIDS, then far more pressure would develop to speed the research and regulatory system and make compound Q available through authorized channels.

We have heard that a phase II trial is now being designed, and could be started before phase I is finished.

NEWS FLASH 6/28/89:
UNOFFICIAL "COMPOUND Q STUDY"
(from *AIDS Treatment News,* Issue Number 81, June 16, 1989)

A so-called "secret study" of tricosanthin, the experimental AIDS treatment also called Compound Q, became a focus of national controversy after one of the patients died. All indications so far are that the drug *did not* contribute to the cause of death. But the controversy has furthered a much-needed national discussion over the design and implementation of clinical trials during a public-health emergency.

The project, a treatment program organized by Project Inform of San Francisco, included very thorough monitoring of laboratory test results and the clinical condition of over 30 patients in four U.S. cities, treated by their physicians with tricosanthin. The drug was obtained from China, where it has been widely used for almost two decades. All patients received the lowest dose used for any purpose in China; this dose was repeated three times at weekly intervals. The patients selected were very ill and had failed all other treatments. No one was charged anything to participate; all labor and expenses were donated by the physicians, or by Project Inform or others.

While early indications are promising, Project Inform emphasizes that it is too early to tell if tricosanthin will be useful as an AIDS treatment; the organization hopes to make a full report available in one to two months. Also, the drug is similar to chemotherapy and can cause severe side effects in some patients; it must not be used without proper medical supervision. A major reason for organizing this monitoring project was that people were already using the drug as an AIDS treatment, with unknown and potentially serious risks.

We will cover the tricosanthin monitoring study (and the debate around it) in depth in future issues. Meanwhile, readers can learn the basic facts from newspapers such as the *San Francisco Chronicle, San Francisco Examiner, The New York Times,* and the *Los Angeles Times.*

Comment

This monitoring study is as thorough, professional, and careful as any trial we have seen, and it promises to be a turning point in efforts to control the AIDS epidemic. It shows that clinical trials can develop useful information very quickly when they are organized to do so, and when patients are well informed of the unavoidable risks and willing to accept them.

If tricosanthin turns out to be valuable as an AIDS treatment, then this project could save thousands of lives. Everyone involved deserves our gratitude and support.

COMPOUND Q UPDATE
(from *AIDS Treatment News,* Issue Number 82, June 30, 1989)

Our previous issue included a last-minute report on a so-called "unofficial study" of Compound Q—actually a treatment program and data monitoring project—organized by San Francisco's Project Inform and including over 30 patients and nine physicians in four U.S. cities (San Francisco, Los Angeles, New York, and Miami/Ft. Lauderdale), using a version of the drug which is in common use in China. Probably no single story in the AIDS epidemic has generated as much coverage in San Francisco's major daily newspapers, the *San Francisco Chronicle* and *San Francisco Examiner.* Some of the information released by the San Francisco press is available nowhere else. Local press coverage has been even-handed and mostly sympathetic, despite vociferous opposition from some researchers in the official Compound Q study at San Francisco General Hospital. (A spokesperson for the California Medical Association took a middle position, describing the doctors involved as "respected physicians in the community working desperately to provide effective treatment and care," but expressing serious concern about phase I— dosage or safety—studies being conducted outside of a university medical center.)

We believe that a loud debate "for" or "against" the unofficial study would be unproductive, the wrong issue for furthering the common fight against AIDS. The better question is what can we learn from this extraordinary response to an extraordinary situation. What can we learn about the drug, and also about how to improve the official system of authorized research, to get faster and better answers not only for AIDS but for other diseases as well?

Project Inform and others involved in this treatment program want to wait until it is finished, probably 30 to 60 days, to make a full report. This article is based on news already released but not widely available outside the San Francisco area.

Background

AIDS Treatment News covered Compound Q in its Issues Number 72, 77, 78, and 81 (reproduced above). The active ingredient of Compound Q is a protein called tricosanthin, extracted from the root of a Chinese cucumber. The plant extract must be highly purified before injection; otherwise it is highly toxic and could be fatal. In the test tube, tricosanthin works by selectively killing macrophages infected with HIV. Infected macrophages are believed to be the major reservoir of the virus in the body.

In China, tricosanthin is used to induce abortion, because it selectively kills "trophoblast" cells, which line the uterus during pregnancy. It is also used to treat choriocarcinoma, a cancer of these cells, and may be better for this purpose than any treatment available in the U.S.

Dr. Hin-Wing Yeung, a scientist from Hong Kong, suggested tricosanthin as an AIDS treatment, based on earlier development of the drug by researchers in Shanghai. Michael McGrath, M.D., at San Francisco General Hospital, first thought that the drug might kill every macrophage in the body—a radical but possible treatment, as macrophages are normally replaced. In laboratory tests, he unexpectedly learned that it killed only those cells infected with HIV.

The Unofficial Study

About three months ago, before Project Inform was involved with Compound Q, scattered groups of person with AIDS, especially one group in Florida, had been able to obtain supplies of the drug from China. Because this drug is more dangerous than other non-approved AIDS treatments, the effort was made to obtain some answers quickly about its safety and efficacy through a highly professional treatment and data-monitoring program, before patients were harmed by self-medication or other improper use.

At a press conference on June 28, 1989, Martin Delaney of Project Inform explained the unofficial study, and the reason it was done. We edited his comments for length:

> This treatment use (of Compound Q) is no different from things like it that have been going on for the last five years. What is different is that the media has turned this into a high-profile event.
>
> Several points guided us and made us feel compelled to organize this treatment program. One was impending community use of this drug. Like other drugs before it—like ribavirin, AL 721, dextran sulfate—patients have ways to get these drugs into the country legally. When there is hope about new drugs, patients begin

distributing and using them. Unfortunately, widespread distribution and use has often taken place before we had any sense of whether the drugs were safe, or whether they worked.

For example, in 1985 when ribavirin started coming into the U.S. from Mexico, Project Inform was formed to ask the medical community to set up prospective data monitoring on patients using that drug. Nobody did so, and three years went by of use of that drug, and the government ultimately concluded that it was not useful, and might even be harmful in some patients. That's not an intelligent way to run an epidemic.

Now Compound Q is perhaps the most hopeful drug, but also maybe a very toxic drug. Patients legitimately within their rights are preparing to use it. Once again we have the specter of hundreds if not thousands of people taking a drug that we do not know is safe or effective. Once again, it will take years to get the answer by the standard methods.

A hundred and fifty people a day are dying now because of bureaucratic delays, beccause of inability to access important drugs that are tied up in the pipeline. A good example is the drugs DDI and DDC; their promise has been known since 1986. The official researchers have now finished phase I testing on them, and now they are telling us it will be two to two and a half more years before efficacy tests are confirmed. AIDS patients don't have that long to live. That's beyond the life expectancy of most patients.

We're already two and a half years into Compound Q, as scientists learned the basic facts about it two and a half years ago, and kept the information from us while there was a good equivalent drug in China, a drug that had been used there for nearly two decades.

It is true that the ongoing official study of Compound Q might have been done in six or nine months—but it would not provide the answers we needed to guide community use. It will give limited answers about certain doses of the drug, one administration only, in certain patients. We have to answer to an entire community of people who are going to use the drug in any way they see fit, unless guidance is given.

It is not okay, it is not acceptable morally, to just turn our backs and say, 'You guys shouldn't do it,' and feel that we've done our job. We have to give guidance, if people are going to have access to these drugs—and they do have that access, whether we want it or not.

We also had experience going into this from people in Florida. We were not the first ones to use Compound Q in a clinical study. More than a dozen people in Florida had already used the (Chinese) drug for HIV, before we even began talking about doing what we are doing now. So we had considerable human experience before going in.

What did we do? First we talked to people working on importation. We asked them this time, let's not distribute the drug, let's not sell it to people. Instead, let's try to channel it into controlled clinical use, rather than the old system which was pass it out and see what happens.

We then collaborated to design a carefully controlled clinical process under which patients would be treated. This is not technically a study, it is a treatment program. People call it a study because of the extent of scientific processes being used to collect data from it. But the primary goal is treatment, not research.

For the protocol design, we called upon a researcher who had run the research on another drug similar to trichosanthin, called ricin-A, which has been used in more than a thousand patients and is in the same family as trichosanthin. We used her help in putting this protocol together, along with the experience of the physicians involved. So the data gathering, the study part of what we are doing, was based on an existing FDA-approved study of the drug ricin-A; it is not something we made up.

We also created an elaborate consent process to protect the patients and the physicians alike.

We then shared the protocol with other interested physicians, pulled together a team of four groups in four cities, looking to treat about 60 patients.

(The next section of the statement, omitted here, concerned legal implications.)

Baseline data was collected from all patients. Most of them already had more than a year of extensive laboratory work. After a complete workup, the patients were infused with a reasonable quantity of the drug—the smallest amount used for any purpose in China. It is a fraction of the dose used in China with cancer patients. It is a midpoint in the dose range proposed for the trials at San Francisco General Hospital; in another week they will have exceeded our dose. Our dose is the midpoint of expected therapeutic doses based on laboratory data—and the dose used by more than a dozen patients in Florida. It is a fifth of the dose that we've seen some patients use self-medicated.

Basic safety precautions were followed. The criteria for entrance to this study were the critera we lifted from San Francisco General's study. The same precautions were taken. Each patient was administered a test dose of the drug in a tiny quantity, to look for allergic reactions. They were followed for a 24 hour period of hospitalization, with vital signs taken constantly. They were in the physician's office nearly daily for the following week.

Elaborate data gathering is going on, just as in formal clinical study. Fourteen full physicals, 14 complete workups, blood chemistry, urinalysis, sedimentation rates, P24 antigen and antibodies, complete cellular immunity, all of what is being done in virtually every AIDS clinical study in the country.

Additional safety precautions include use of standard adverse experience reporting forms that are approved by FDA, standard side-effect ratings from FDA-approved studies, and complete tracking of concomitant medications used. There is nothing missing here in what has been done.

The outcome to date is that the vast majority of the more than 30 patients who have been treated in our treatment program have tolerated the drug very well.

We seem to have made an interesting, perhaps major discovery about the effect of the drug on patients with HIV infection of the brain. Two patients experienced mental confusion, which cleared up in one to two weeks. And as you all know, one patient entered a coma, a coma that lasted no more than 24 hours and was in the process of complete resolution when the incident occurred about a week later when the patient died.

This patient vomited in his sleep and inhaled some of the vomit, and had to be resuscitated. The evidence at the scene suggested that the resuscitation process was quite successful, his vital signs had returned to normal. However, the patient had a living will, an agreement which called for no heroic measures, which the family interpreted this as being, and the family asked that the tube be pulled. It was the opinion of physicians on site that had that not been the case, the patient could well be alive today. We cannot say at this point if the problem was related to the drug or not.

At this time we are not making statements about whether the drug is working. We have seen some interesting lab measures. But it would be irresponsible scientifically to say that therefore the drug is working. It will take time, to follow these patients for a longer period and see if these results hold up. It would give the wrong signal to our community to say we've concluded that the drug works. We need more information before people should start using this drug. The buyers' clubs and other groups that work with patients are completely cooperative with this; nobody is interested in endangering anyone.

As to the future, there are questions we set out to answer here to protect our community; we intend to get the answers to those questions. The FDA has not shut us down; we do not know whether they will try to or not. We think where we should go is cooperation; we would like collaborate, share out data with the people in San Francisco General Hospital and the Food and Drug Administration. That was the intention all along; and until the incident last week, they shared in that intention. We had discussed sharing data submissions, about the interaction of our data with theirs. It was only after this very unfortunate death that people headed for the hills.

We intend to present our data to the FDA, the National Institutes of Health, and the medical journals. If the data suggests that the drug is useful, we will fight for early access to it on behalf of AIDS patients. And whatever the outcome, we will continue to press for faster action. It is unconscionable to accept five and a half years' typical time for the development of drugs for AIDS, when patients have an average lifespan of only two years. We have fought long and hard battles in Washington to improve this process, we think progress is being made, but it isn't being made fast enough.

Neurological Side Effects: Bad News or Good?

As Delaney mentioned in the press conference above, a handful of patients with dementia or other evidence of HIV infection of the brain suffered neurological side effects—a period of mental confusion lasting one to two weeks for two patients, or a coma lasting less than 24 hours for one other.

Although no one knows for sure, it seems likely that the neurological effects may be evidence that the drug is doing its job—not a sign of toxicity.

What Delaney had heard from experts familiar with the study is that HIV does not infect neurons in the brain, but rather glial cells—supporting cells which the body can replace. The neurological effects seem to be a temporary result of killing a large number of infected cells at one time. If so, Compound Q might prove helpful for persons with HIV brain infection. It may need to be given in smaller doses at first, to control the side effects.

Further studies will be needed to answer this question. Meanwhile, because of the unknowns and risks involved, physicians are screening patients for evidence of HIV brain infection, because of the increased risk of treating them with Compound Q until more is known.

The Future

The unofficial Compound Q study will end in 30 to 60 days. Until the results are reported, we will not know whether the drug is useful for treating AIDS or HIV, or not.

Readers should realize that there are other side effects, dangers, and precautions not touched on in this article. No one should use Compound Q without expert medical supervision.

What lessons have been learned? Medically, the unofficial study has taught researchers more in the last few weeks about Compound Q as a human treatment for HIV than had ever been learned before. And according to Delaney, the official study at San Francisco General Hospital has already used this information to skip some of its low test doses, which are now unnecessary. One result of the unofficial study, therefore, is that the official trials will produce results sooner—a major purpose of the unofficial treatment program all along.

Even more importantly, the unofficial Compound Q study is demonstrating that it is possible to get useful results quickly, if a research project is organized for that purpose. How is Project Inform's program getting useful results in only four or five months, while official trials take five years or longer to do the same?

A look at specifics of the trials will show part of the answer. The official Compound Q was kept secret for at least a year and a half, between May 29, 1987 when the patent application was filed for anti-HIV use of trichosanthin, and January 3, 1989 when the patent was granted. During this time a new method for extracting the drug from the Chinese cucumber root was developed. Then after the patent was granted, it took six months to get phase I tests going; and these tests are slow because phase I tests were designed for new chemicals never given to humans before. The Chinese experience was ignored.

In contrast, the unofficial study used the drug and medical information already existing in China. It proceeded immediately with a dose well known in human use and projected, based on laboratory data, to be therapeutic for HIV. By doing so, instead of developing a new patentable technology requiring new animal tests and phase I human trials, it avoided two years or more of delay. Note that this study could have been carried out two years ago, exactly as it is being done today, if the anti-HIV use of trichosanthin had not been kept secret during that time. As far as we know, the intervening two years of official research added little or nothing to the unofficial study, which is based on pre-existing medical technology from China, not on the new technology created during the patent hiatus.

After the patent was granted on January 3 of this year (1989), there was little media interest until April 15, 1989, when an article on Compound Q (also called GLQ223) was published in the *Proceedings of the National Academy of Sciences.*

Another delay in the official research track is illustrative. After the patent was granted in January, it took some time for Genelabs, the developer of Compound Q, to get an IND (Investigational New Drug approval, meaning approval to test the drug in humans) from the FDA. We cannot know the full story of this delay, but we do know that at one point a San Francisco TV reporter called the FDA to ask why the IND had not been granted for this drug, and was told that the FDA had no application for the IND on file! Genelabs said that it had applied. Because of a misunderstanding, each party was waiting for the other. Apparently the FDA believed that what Genelabs had submitted was only a draft, not an official application—while Genelabs thought it had applied and was waiting for approval to begin the clinical trial at San Francisco General Hospital. We are all lucky that a chance call from a reporter straightened out this snafu, which had put the entire world's research program for one of the two most promising AIDS drugs on hold.

This kind of problem seems surprising only to the uninitiated. In our three years of covering AIDS treatment research, we have seen such mindless delays happen again and again. The difference is that usually there is no public interest in the details of the process, and nobody there to make the call or do what else may be needed to straighten the problem out.

For too long the public has accepted a stock answer that clinical research is going as fast as possible, that the delays are caused only by the requirements of good science. But analysis of what is actually happening shows that the system can be vastly improved.

In the field of industrial quality assurance, there are trained, professional specialists to solve just this kind of problem. If a company is taking too long to get its products developed, for example, it can hire experts to analyze what is happening and suggest solutions. Typically the problems are due to flaws in the system, not to faults of the individuals involved, as no one person alone may have the power and resources to produce results. Instead, the system must be improved, by identifying the problems and correcting them. Academic experts in quality assurance can and should be invited onto the team to examine how trials might be organized to get faster results, consistent with good science.

The unofficial study of Compound Q organized by Project Inform is now producing the most important results—practical information about whether, when, and how to use the drug—about ten times faster than the official research system has been able to do so, either for Compound Q or for other drugs.

Admittedly, there are greater risks to the patients in an accelerated study. Some patients want a role in making this decision, however, in balancing the risks of using a new treatment against the risks of doing nothing. Some may also want to contribute to the benefit of others, realizing that tens of thousands of lives are likely to be saved if an accelerated study shows unequivocally that a drug is helpful, months or years ahead of the official trials.

The take-home lesson, we believe, is *not* to blame individuals, on either side. Nor do we believe that the official system, with its safeguards and protections for research subjects, should be abandoned. Instead, we should reform the official system of clinical trials to make it faster and more efficient. If this can be done, there should be no need for bypassing the system in the future.

The right approach to reform is a win-win approach. Nobody's interest needs to be sacrificed—and certainly the quality of scientific workmanship need not be reduced. Instead, careful, professional analysis and negotiation can find intelligent ways to make the system work better.

Who can implement this approach? Ultimately the only force which can do so is a professional consensus in the medical and research communities. Without that consensus, no one else—not the AIDS community, not the FDA, the NIH, the White House, or the pharmaceutical industry—can make it happen.

What if the consensus is not there? Physicians and scientists prize their independence; no one can tell them what to do. But we can appeal to their intelligence. The AIDS community can investigate and analyze exactly what is happening, and illuminate precisely what the problems are, what their consequences are, and what should be happening instead. Usually we cannot implement the reforms by ourselves. But we can make the problems and the opportunities for improvement so obvious that they cannot be ignored.

III. PML (PROGRESSIVE MULTIFOCAL LEUKOENCEPHALOPATHY)

(from *AIDS Treatment News,* Issue Number 79, May 19, 1989)

by Denny Smith

Progressive multifocal leukoencephalopathy (PML) is an uncommon but devastating brain infection with an historically bleak outlook, and many physicians have opted not to initiate treatment, or simply rely hopefully on AZT for its antiviral and CNS access capacity. The results of intervention in the progress of PML have increased the possible options, however, enough to justify an aggressive attempt to treat.

This opportunistic infection probably results from reactivation of a latent papovirus to which most people gain immunity after childhood exposure. Some symptoms of PML, such as headaches, confusion, visual impairment in one or both eyes, aphasia (difficulty with verbal comprehension or expression) or loss of muscle coordination on one side of the body, can resemble toxoplasmosis, herpes encephalitis or meningitis. Each of those infections, as well as PML, can be imminently life-threatening and should be seem immediately by an AIDS-knowledgeable physician, who may consult a neurologist. Someone experiencing these symptoms may become too disoriented to respond quickly to the situation, so the observant help of friends or family could make a difference. The time from appearance of symptoms to diagnosis to treatment is crucial for PML or other AIDS-related neurological infections.

AIDS Treatment News recommends to interested readers a very comprehensive, well-researched report on experimental treatments for PML compiled by two concerned AIDS activists in Los Angeles, Lisa A. Muller and Peter L. Brosnan, with an introduction by Ronald Webeck, a long-term survivor of PML. The treatments discussed in this report were drawn from current medical literature and include beta interferon, vidarabine (adenine arabinoside, or ARA-A), cytarabine (cytosine arabinoside, or ARA-C), alpha-2 interferon, acyclovir, clonzepam, trimethoprim with sulfamethoxazole, and dexamethasone combined first with sulfadiazine and then with pyrimethamine. The first three in the list appeared to be more effective when administered intrathecally (injected into the spinal fluid) instead of intravenously. The others were tried only intravenously. (Clonazepam is probably useful to control convulsions which may accompany PML, but not as a primary treatment.)

Some of these drugs have side effects which people with HIV and their doctors would usually weigh carefully, but the gravity of an untreated PML infection may override these concerns, and AIDS-experienced physicians often make similar compromises in treating other opportunistic infections. None of these drugs have been proven to work repeatedly, but accumulated attempts to treat PML *have* resulted in better survival rates than nontreatment. The articles referenced from the literature are included in entirety in the report's appendix, making it self-contained and practical for outpatient clinics and AIDS-care health professionals. A copy of the report can be obtained by sending a request with a $10 donation or more to cover the cost of printing and mailing to Lisa Muller (see Appendix B for address).

Appendix B
Referral Numbers

The following listings are the names, addresses and/or telephone numbers as referred to in the body of the text.

ACT-UP/San Francisco
2300 Market Street, Suite 68
San Francisco, CA 94114
(415) 563-0724

AIDS Alternative Healing Project
513 Valencia Street
San Francisco, CA 94110

AIDS/ARC Vigil, San Francisco
(415) 771-4688

AIDS Benefits Counselors
(415) 673-3780

AIDS Fraud Task Force
Attorney General's Office
Attn: Michael R. Botwin
3580 Wilshire Boulevard
Los Angeles, CA 90010
(213) 736-2160

AIDS Information BBS
(415) 626-1246

AIDS Treatment Library
(see Healing Alternatives Foundation)

AIDS Treatment News
John S. James, Publisher
P.O. Box 411256
San Francisco, CA 94141
(415) 255-0588

AIDS Treatment News by computer access
on AIDS Information BBS,
(415) 626-1246
and also on CAIN, (213) 464-7400

Allergy Research Group/Nutricology
(415) 639-4572

Alliance 7
(619) 281-5360

American Foundation of Traditional
Chinese Medicine
2390-A Powell Street
San Francisco, CA 94133
(415) 956-3030

American Foundation for AIDS Research
(AmFAR)
1515 Broadway
New York, NY 10036-8901
(212) 719-0033

American Health Consultants
(800) 554-1032 (toll-free)

Babcock, Gary
(415) 548-5953

Badgley, Laurence E., M.D.
370 West San Bruno Avenue, Suite D
San Bruno, CA 94066
(415) 588-4495

Barton, Keith, M.D.
3099 Telegraph Avenue
Berkeley, CA 94705
(415) 845-4430

Bihari, Bernard, M.D.
Downstate Medical Center,
Brooklyn, NY
(718) 270-1094

BIOHERB, Inc., Schaumberg, IL
(312) 885-8789

BRS Colleague
(800) 468-0908 (toll-free)

CAIN (Computerized AIDS Information
Network)
(213) 464-7400

Cardiovascular Research Ltd.
1061-B Shary Circle
Concord, CA 94518
(415) 827-2636

Cascade Mushrooms, Portland, OR
(503) 644-4236

Columbia University Student Health
Services/Columbia University Gay Health
Advocacy Project
Columbia University
John Jay Hall
New York, NY 10027
(212) 854-2878

Community Research Alliance (CRA)
273 Church Street
San Francisco, CA 94114
(415) 626-2145

Community Research Initiative,
New York
(212) 481-1050

Conference Recording Service
1308 Gilman Street
Berkeley, CA 94706
(415) 527-3600

Corwin Publishers
P.O. Box 2806
San Francisco, CA 94126

DAIR (see "Documentation of AIDS
Issues and Research")

Dextran Products Limited
(416) 755-2231

DIALOG Information Services
(800) 3DIALOG (toll-free)

DNCB Information (see "Henry, Jim")

Documentation of AIDS Issues and
Research Foundation (DAIR)
150 Eureka Street, Room 107
San Francisco, CA 94114
(415) 552-1665

Dynamic Information Corp.,
Redwood City, CA
(415) 591-5900

Ethigen Corporation, Los Angeles, CA
(800) 752-5721 (toll-free)

Face to Face
P.O. Box 1599
Guerneville, CA 95446
(707) 887-1581

Family Pharmaceuticals of America
(800) 922-3444 (toll-free)

Ganciclovir Study Center
(301) 497-9888

Gay Macrobiotic Center
Attn: Tom O'Connor
(415) 821-0853

Gay Men's Health Crisis
132 W. 24th Street, Box 274
New York, NY 10011
(212) 807-6655

Golden Gate Nurses' Association
(415) 821-7400

The Healing Alternatives Foundation
(THAF) (formerly the Healing
Alternative Buyers' Club)
1748 Market Street
San Francisco, CA 94102
(415) 626-2316

Health Concerns, Alameda, CA
(800) 233-9355 (toll-free)

Henry, Jim
700 Taylor Street, Apt. 201
San Francisco, CA 94108
(415) 681-7437

Herb-Pharm
(503) 846-7178

Heritage Foundation
214 Massachusetts Avenue, N.E.
Washington, DC 20002
(202) 546-4400

Human Energy Press
370 West San Bruno Avenue, Suite D
San Bruno, CA 94066
(415) 588-4495

Huntington Plaza Pharmacy
(818) 397-3072

IMRE Corporation
(206) 448-1000 (physicians only)

InfoMedix
(800) 992-9286 (toll-free within
California)
(800) 367-9286 (toll-free nationwide)

Information Network Against War and
Fascism
Attn: Paul Bernardino
747 Ellis Street, #4
San Francisco, CA 94102
(415) 673-4609

Information on Demand
(800) 999-4463 (toll-free)

Institute for Traditional Medicine
and Preventive Health Care
2442 S.E. Sherman
Portland, OR 97214
(503) 233-4907

Intrend
(408) 429-1596

Jarrow Formulas
(213) 204-6936

Kalvert Personnel Services
(516) 567-2444

Kotler, Donald, M.D.
(212) 870-6154

KPIX Channel 5
Public Relations Department
855 Battery Street
San Francisco, CA 94111
(415) 765-8874

Kuderna, Diana
871½ 52nd Street
Oakland, CA 94608

Levin, Alan S., M.D.
(415) 788-4535

LyphoMed Hotline
(800) 727-7003 (toll-free)

Medicorp
(212) 674-4680

MegaHealth Society
Attn: Stephen Fowkes
P.O. Box 60637
Palo Alto, CA 94301
(415) 949-0919

Mobilization Against AIDS (MAA)
1540 Market Street, Suite 60
San Francisco, CA 94102
(415) 863-4676

Muller, Lisa
3031 Angus Street
Los Angeles, CA 90039
(213) 666-0751

National Academy of Sciences
(202) 334-2000

National Association of People with AIDS
(NAPWA)
2025 "I" Street, N.W., Suite 415
Washington, DC 20006

National AIDS Hotline
(800) 342-AIDS (toll-free)
(800) 344-SIDA (toll-free,
Spanish-speaking)

National Gay Rights Advocates
540 Castro Street
San Francisco, CA 94114
(415) 863-3624

National Institute of Allergy and
Infectious Diseases (NIAID)
Trimetrexate Information line
(800) 537-9978 (physicians only)

National Institutes of Health (NIH)
Clinical Trials of Experimental AIDS
Treatments Hotline
(800) TRIALS-A (toll-free)

New York Native
P.O. Box 1475
Church Street Station
New York, NY 10008

Nutricology, San Leandro, CA
(800) 545-9960 (toll-free)

Nutritional Products Buyers' Club
(213) 855-0533

Options+
(301) 229-0882

Oriental Healing Arts Institute
1945 Palo Verde Avenue, Suite 208
Long Beach, CA 90815
(213) 431-3544

Passive Immunotherapy Project
(415) 626-8455

Pathology Institute
(800) 438-8674 (toll-free)
(415) 540-1638

People Taking Action Against AIDS
(PTAAA)
P.O. Box 378
Belport, NY 11713
(516) 286-2374

Pfizer Central Research
(203) 441-4112

Preferred Rx
5755 Granger Road, Suite 305
Independence, OH 44131
(800) 445-4519 (toll-free within
New York state)
(800) 227-1195 (toll-free nationwide)

Project Inform
347 Dolores Street, Suite 301
San Francisco, CA 94110
(415) 558-9051 (local/international)
(415) 558-0684 (FAX)
(800) 334-7422 (toll-free within Calif.)
(800) 822-7422 (toll-free nationwide)

People With AIDS Coalition (PWA
Coalition)
31 West 26th Street, 5th Floor
New York, NY 10010
(212) 532-0290

PWA Health Group
(212) 532-0280

Quan Yin Acupuncture and Herb Center
1748 Market Street
San Francisco, CA 94103
(415) 861-1101

San Francisco AIDS Foundation
P.O. Box 6182
San Francisco, CA 94101
(415) 863-AIDS (local/international)
(800) FOR-AIDS (toll-free nationwide)

San Francisco City Clinic
(415) 864-8100

Significant Other Records
P.O. Box 1545
Canal Street Station
New York, NY 10013

Source Naturals
(800) 776-7701 (toll-free)

Specialty Laboratories, Inc.
(213) 828-6543 (local)
(800) 882-1345 (toll-free within
California)
(800) 421-7110 (toll-free nationwide)

Task Force on Nutrition Support in AIDS
Wang Associates, Inc.
19 West 21st Street
New York, NY 10010

Vitamin Trader
(800) 334-9300 (toll-free within
California)
(800) 334-9310 (toll-free nationwide)

Yerba Prima Botanicals
(415) 632-7477 (local)
(800) 421-9972 (toll-free)

Appendix C
PWA Coalitions, ACT-UP Affiliates, and Buyers' Clubs

A Resource List Compiled by Debra Kelly and Denny Smith

We continue to focus on three kinds of organization which are important in the HIV treatment movement, and which seldom find their way into established resource manuals.

Entries on the list which are followed by an "A" are local chapters of ACT NOW, a national organization advocating nonviolent direct action in the interests of PWAs (people with AIDS, ARC, or HIV). "B" on the list indicates buyers' clubs, a network of outlets which provides access to alternative treatments, often at cost plus overhead. And "C" denotes PWA coalitions, although some of these phone numbers are for umbrella organizations which agreed to extend their resources until the local coalition had a number of its own.

Please let us know of any changes or additions.

ALABAMA
Birmingham, Living with AIDS Coalition of Alabama (205) 934-3262 C

ALASKA
Anchorage, PWA Coalition (907) 338-0835 C

ARIZONA
Phoenix, Buyers' Club (602) 264-7033 B
Phoenix, PWA Coalition (602) 224-5486 C
Tucson, PWA Coalition (602) 322-9808 C

CALIFORNIA
Los Angeles, ACT UP (213) 668-2357 A
Los Angeles, Nutritional Products (213) 855-0533 B

San Diego, ACT UP (619) 233-9337 A
San Diego, Alliance 7 (619) 281-5360 B
San Francisco, ACT UP (415) 563-0724 A
San Francisco, Healing Alternatives (415) 626-2316 B
San Francisco, PWA Coalition (415) 553-2560 C
West Hollywood, Being Alive (213) 667-3262 C

COLORADO
Denver, ACT UP (303) 830-0730 A
Denver, Health Action Project (303) 894-8650 B
Denver, PWA Coalition (303) 837-8214 C

CONNECTICUT
New Milford, PWA Coalition (203) 624-0947 C

DELAWARE
Wilmington, PWA Coalition (302) 652-6776 C

DISTRICT OF COLUMBIA
Carl Vogel Foundation (202) 547-5651 B
Lifelink (202) 833-3070 C
NAPWA (National Association of PWAs) (202) 429-2856 C

FLORIDA
Broward Country, PWA Coalition (305) 763-5311 C
Coconut Grove, Cure AIDS Now (305) 856-8378 A
Dade County, PWA Coalition (305) 576-1111 C
Jacksonville, PWA Coalition (904) 396-2562 C
Key West, PWA Coalition (305) 296-5701 C
Orlando, Action Now (407) 351-6930 A & B
Palm Beach, PWA Coalition (407) 845-0800 C

GEORGIA
Atlanta, PWA Coalition (404) 874-7926 C

ILLINOIS
Chicago, ACT UP (312) 509-6802 A
Chicago, Kapuna Wellness Network (312) 536-3000 C
Chicago, Test Positive Aware (312) 728-1943 B

INDIANA
Indianapolis, PWA Coalition, Rick Buell (317) 637-2720 C
Lafayette, PWA Coalition (317) 742-2305 C

LOUISIANA
New Orleans, PWA Coalition (504) 944-1959 C

MAINE
Portland, PWA Coalition (207) 774-6877 C

MARYLAND
Baltimore, PWA Coalition (301) 625-1677 or 625-1688 C
Hyattsville, PWA Coalition (301) 464-6964 C

MASSACHUSETTS
Boston, ACT UP (617) 492-2887 A
Boston, PWA Coalition (617) 437-6200 C
Westfield, PWA Coalition (413) 562-8465 C

MICHIGAN
Ann Arbor, Friends Huron Valley (313) 747-9068 C
Detroit, Friends PWA Alliance (313) 543-8310 C

MINNESOTA
Minneapolis, The Aliveness Project (612) 822-7946 B & C

MISSISSIPPI
Jackson, PWA Coalition (601) 353-7611 C

MISSOURI
Kansas City, Heartland AIDS Resource Council (816) 753-3215 C

NEW JERSEY
Bergenfield, PWA Coalition (201) 387-1805 C
Orange, ACT UP (201) 836-8645 A

NEW YORK
Buffalo, Niagara Frontier AIDS Alliance (716) 852-6778 C
Long Island, PWA Coalition (516) 324-2076 C
New York City, ACT UP (212) 533-8888 A
New York City, PWA Health Group (212) 532-0280 B
New York City, PWA Coalition (212) 532-0290 C

OHIO
Dayton, PWA Coalition (513) 223-2437 C

OKLAHOMA
Oklahoma City, PWA Coalition (405) 525-9887 C

OREGON
Portland, ACT UP (503) 224-8809 A
Portland, Genesis (503) 234-5611 C

PENNSYLVANIA
Allentown, PWA Coalition (215) 433-5444 C
Philadelphia, We The People (215) 545-6868 B & C

RHODE ISLAND
Providence, Project AIDS (401) 277-6545 C

SOUTH CAROLINA
Columbia, Healing Circle Support Group (803) 771-7300 C

TENNESSEE
Nashville, People Living With AIDS (615) 385-1510 C

TEXAS
Austin, PWA Coalition (512) 472-3792 C
Dallas, Buyers' Club (214) 526-5068 B
Dallas, PWA Coalition (214) 941-0523 C
Fort Worth, PWA Coalition (817) 332-7966 C
Houston, PWA Coalition (713) 522-5428 C
Port Arthur, PWA Coalition (409) 724-2437 C
San Antonio, PWA Coalition (512) 821-6218 C

UTAH
Salt Lake City, PWA Coalition of Utah (801) 359-5555 C

VIRGINIA
Richmond, Awakening (804) 746-2178 C

WASHINGTON
Seattle, ACT UP (206) 623-5061 A
Seattle, People Living With AIDS (206) 329-3382 C

CANADA
Toronto, AIDS Action Now (416) 591-8489 A
Vancouver, PWA Coalition (604) 683-3381 C

UNITED KINGDOM
London, Vanmount, LTD 299-1409

WEST GERMANY
Berlin, Deutsche AIDS-Hilfe 030-8969-060

Appendix D
Recommended AIDS Newsletters
and Directories

The AIDS/HIV Experimental Treatment Directory is compiled and published quarterly by the American Foundation for AIDS Research, and includes a comprehensive list of antivirals and immune modulators for which clinical trials are currently ongoing or are planned. Treatments for opportunistic infections are described more briefly. The directory also includes information about the current status of clinical trials, such as the purpose and duration of the trial, the criteria for being included or excluded, and the names of the manufacturers and investigators. It often has information not otherwise published or available, obtained from interviews with researchers. A single copy is $10—free for persons with HIV who cannot afford it. Annual subscription is $30. To order the directory by phone, call (212) 719-0033; by mail, send a check to: AmFAR, 1515 Broadway, Suite 3601, New York, New York 10036. (*Note:* the February 1989 issue is a special edition titled *A Practical Guide to Clinical Research.* It is a handbook for people considering volunteering for clinical trials.)

AIDS Medical Report, published monthly by American Health Consultants is a journal of in-depth articles on the treatment of HIV-related disorders. Articles are written for physicians but are usually quite readable by patients. To subscribe, write *AIDS Medical Report,* 67 Peachtree Park Drive, N.E., Atlanta, Georgia 30309; subscriptions are $109 per year. *Note:* We do *not* recommend the "special reports" also sold by the publisher. The ones we have seen seem overpriced, and not as useful as the newsletter itself.

AIDS Targeted Information Newsletter (ATIN) is a monthly collection of abstracts selected from recent medical literature. Many are highly technical, written for scientists and physicians. They are grouped into eight areas: molecular, virological, immunological, epidemiological and clinical research, treatment and assay methods, and ethical/legal concerns. To order *ATIN*, call (800) 638-6423. In Maryland call 528-4105 collect. Subscription price is $125 per year individual; $275 for institutions.

Bulletin of Experimental Treatments for AIDS (BETA) is published by the San Francisco AIDS Foundation. Issues have appeared that focused on AZT, experimental antivirals, with an update on AZT, and provide a very good overview of promising options for HIV intervention. *BETA* is free to residents of San Francisco. To subscribe, call (415) 861-3397.

The Directory of Antiviral and Immunomodulatory Therapies for AIDS (DAITA) is published by *CDC AIDS Weekly* (a privately published AIDS newsletter not connected with the Centers for Disease Control). This directory aims to be complete, to review "current published research on every drug or therapy that has been presented as a potential treatment for AIDS"— but as the name implies, it does not include treatments for opportunistic infections. *DAITA* differs from the AmFAR directory (see review above) in several ways. It includes all antivirals or immune modulators (AmFAR often omits those which appear unpromising), usually reviews published information only (AmFAR also includes original reporting), and does not have the detailed information about clinical trials which AmFAR's directory does. We find *DAITA* a handy reference for basic information when we hear about proposed treatments with which we are not familiar. *DAITA* costs $26 for the current issue. For ordering information, call *CDC AIDS Weekly* at (205) 991-6920.

P.I. Perspectives is a quarterly journal from Project Inform. It often covers public policy issues (drug access, FDA regulations), as well as treatment information. Project Inform has long endorsed early intervention for HIV infection, and has developed a "treatment strategy" to help people who are HIV-positive make choices about monitoring and treatment to stay healthy. To receive the treatment strategy information, *P.I. Perspectives,* and in-depth writeups of several popular treatments, people outside of California can call (800) 822-7422; from California outside of San Francisco call (800) 334-7422; from San Francisco (and from outside the United States) call (415) 558-9051. There is no charge, but a donation is requested.

Treatment Issues is published ten times a year by the Gay Men's Health Crisis. A wide range of excellent articles has covered new anti-HIV drugs, immunomodulators and treatments for all the major opportunistic infections. Articles are useful for both patients and physicians. To subscribe, write to GMHC, Dept. of Medical Information, 129 W. 20th Street, New York, New York 10011. A $20 donation is requested from those who can afford it.

Index

To order additional copies of this book:

INDIVIDUALS may order copies of this book by sending $18.00 for each copy ordered (includes first class postage and any applicable sales tax) to: ATN Publications, P.O. Box 411256, San Francisco, CA 94141. Outside North America, add $6 for airmail postage *per book*.

BOOKSTORES, DISTRIBUTORS, AND OTHER RETAILERS may order directly from the publisher, Celestial Arts, P.O. Box 7327, Berkeley, CA 94707; phone (415) 524-1801. The toll-free number—for orders only—is (800) 841-2665.

GROUPS, ORGANIZATIONS, AND INSTITUTIONS: Special bulk rates are available from the publisher, Celestial Arts. Please write or call our special sales department at: Celestial Arts, P.O. Box 7327, Berkeley, CA 94707; phone (415) 524-1801.

How to subscribe to *AIDS Treatment News:*

Write or call for current subscription rates and information: ATN Publications, P.O. Box 411256, San Francisco, CA 94141; (415) 255-0588.

To protect your privacy, we mail first class without mentioning AIDS on the envelope, and we keep our subscriber list confidential.